AMBULATORY COLORECTAL SURGERY

AMBULATORY COLORECTAL SURGERY

EDITED BY

LAURENCE R. SANDS

University of Miami Medical Center
Miami, Florida, USA

DANA R. SANDS

Cleveland Clinic Florida
Weston, Florida, USA

CRC Press
Taylor & Francis Group
Boca Raton London New York

CRC Press is an imprint of the
Taylor & Francis Group, an **informa** business

First published 2009 by Informa Healthcare USA, Inc.

Published 2019 by CRC Press
Taylor & Francis Group
6000 Broken Sound Parkway NW, Suite 300
Boca Raton, FL 33487-2742

First issued in paperback 2019

ISBN 13: 978-0-367-45249-0 (pbk)
ISBN 13: 978-0-8247-2792-5 (hbk)

Visit the Taylor & Francis Web site at
http://www.taylorandfrancis.com

and the CRC Press Web site at
http://www.crcpress.com

Library of Congress Cataloging-in-Publication Data

Ambulatory colorectal surgery / edited by Laurence R. Sands, Dana R. Sands.
p. ; cm.
Includes bibliographical references and index.
ISBN-13: 978-0-8247-2792-5 (hardcover : alk. paper)
ISBN-10: 0-8247-2792-4 (hardcover : alk. paper)
1. Colon (Anatomy)–Surgery. 2. Rectum–Surgery. 3. Ambulatory surgery. I. Sands, Laurence R. II. Sands, Dana R.
[DNLM: 1. Colon–surgery. 2. Ambulatory Surgical Procedures–methods. 3. Digestive System Surgical Procedures–methods. 4. Rectum–surgery. WI 520 A497 2008]

RD544.A533 2008
617.5'547–dc22

2008039614

Foreword

The Editors are to be congratulated on their collaborative effort to provide colon and rectal surgeons and their trainees with an excellent resource for the management of anorectal and outpatient problems in colon and rectal diseases. The table of contents is comprehensive and contemporary. The chapters have been authored by young colon and rectal surgeons with experienced senior surgeons as coauthors in certain circumstances. The approach to each topic is well organized with adequate historical comment to provide background to modern therapy. This is a rapidly changing field and the authors have provided evidence for the use of each physiologic test, imagining technique, and therapeutic maneuver (medical or surgical). This is a concise, detailed, and practical treatise, which will be easily used as a reference in the clinic, physiology lab, and outpatient operating room.

James W. Fleshman, M.D.
Washington University School of Medicine,
St. Louis, Missouri, U.S.A.

Preface

The face of medicine has changed significantly in the 21st century. Emphasis is placed on minimally invasive techniques and shorter hospitalization. This medical climate has challenged physicians to provide excellent care of increasingly complex problems often in the outpatient setting and frequently using multidisciplinary approaches.

As such, we have been motivated to write a new colon and rectal surgery textbook capitalizing on the shifting practices of medicine in the 21st century. This book represents a compilation of office-based diagnoses, conditions, and treatments that are commonly encountered in general and colon and rectal surgical practices. Attention is paid to all facets of outpatient colorectal surgery including the evaluation and treatment of complex pelvic floor pathology.

Many office-based outpatient conditions and anorectal diseases in general are often poorly understood. This disease spectrum is frequently glossed over in surgical training programs. Most surgical trainees today have limited access to the outpatient office setting, especially within the confines of the restricted working hours of residents. Conditions such as the ones reviewed in this book make up the core of many surgical practices. Therefore, we believe that this book will be useful to all practicing colon and rectal surgeons, general surgeons with an interest in anorectal disease, and particularly those young surgeons just completing their surgical training and starting in practice.

The chapters are listed by condition and include a comprehensive review of the disease entity followed by the available diagnostic modalities and treatment options. The perioperative care is also included in order to provide the reader with a guide to the complete management of these patients. A review of the literature, both classic and new, will help the reader to gain a thorough understanding of each disease process. Prominent authors who have expertise in these areas have been brought together in this effort to bring some simplicity to the treatment of a group of common conditions, which are often ineffectively managed by physicians.

Our hope is that this book will give surgeons the ability to manage the spectrum of diseases encountered in the outpatient setting and make a strong contribution to the welfare of all patients.

The editors are especially thankful to the contributors who have taken time from their busy clinical practices to help in this endeavor and to Elektra McDermott, without whom, this project would not have been possible. We also wish to acknowledge and dedicate this book to our dear children, Ryan and Cory, from whom we have taken much time in the preparation of this project.

Laurence R. Sands
Dana R. Sands

Contents

Foreword James W. Fleshman .... *iii*
Preface .... *v*
Contributors .... *ix*

Section I: Evaluation Tools

1. **Patient Evaluation** *1*
Sanjay Jobanputra, T. Cristina Sardinha, and Marc E. Sher

2. **Anatomy of the Rectum and Anus** *7*
José Marcio Neves Jorge and Newton Luiz T. Gasparetti, Jr.

3. **Anorectal Physiology** *21*
Sherief Shawki and Dana R. Sands

4. **Anorectal Ultrasound** *45*
Tracy Hull and Massarat Zutshi

5. **Biofeedback Treatment for Functional Anorectal Disorders** *55*
Dawn Vickers

Section II: Functional Disorders

6. **Hemorrhoids: Office-Based Management** *79*
Dean C. Koh and Martin A. Luchtefeld

7. **Hemorrhoids: Surgical Treatment** *87*
David J. Maron and Steven D. Wexner

8. **Anal Fissure** *103*
Miguel del Mazo and Laurence R. Sands

9. **Fecal Incontinence: Evaluation** *109*
Jaime L. Bohl and Roberta L. Muldoon

10. **Fecal Incontinence: Office-Based Management** *121*
Tisha Lunsford and Jonathan Efron

11. **Fecal Incontinence: Surgical Management** *135*
Juan J. Nogueras and Anne Y. Lin

12. **Constipation: Evaluation and Management** *141*
Badma Bashankaev, Marat Khaikin, and Eric G. Weiss

13. Urogynecologic Pelvic Floor Dysfunction *163*
Vivian C. Aguilar and G. Willy Davila

14. Anorectal Pain *181*
Jill C. Genua and David A. Vivas

Section III: Septic Disorders

15. Anorectal Abscess *187*
Orit Kaidar-Person and Benjamin Person

16. Fistula-in-Ano *203*
Rodrigo Ambar Pinto, Cesar Omar Reategui Sanchez, and Mari A. Madsen

17. Pilonidal Disease *217*
Jorge A. Lagares-Garcia and Matthew Vrees

18. Perianal Crohn's Disease *225*
Marat Khaikin and Oded Zmora

19. Pruritis Ani *239*
Eliad Karin and Shmuel Avital

Section IV: Infectious Diseases

20. Viral Sexually Transmitted Diseases *245*
Peter M. Kaye and Mitchell Bernstein

21. Bacterial Sexually Transmitted Diseases *251*
David E. Beck and Johnny B. Green

22. Anal Intraepithelial Neoplasia *259*
Patrick Colquhoun

Section V: Perioperative Care

Postoperative Care

23. Wound Management *267*
Hao Wang, Badma Bashankaev, and Helen Marquez

24. Ostomy Management *283*
Mary Lou Boyer

25. Perioperative Pain Management *305*
Lawrence Frank

26. Perioperative Counseling *321*
Norma Daniel and Arlene Segura

Index 327

Contributors

Vivian C. Aguilar Section of Urogynecology, Department of Gynecology, Cleveland Clinic Florida, Weston, Florida, U.S.A.

Shmuel Avital Department of Surgery A, Sourasky Medical Center, Tel Aviv, Israel

Badma Bashankaev Department of Colorectal Surgery, Cleveland Clinic Florida, Weston, Florida, U.S.A.

David E. Beck Department of Colon and Rectal Surgery, Ochsner Clinic Foundation, New Orleans, Louisiana, U.S.A.

Mitchell Bernstein Columbia University College of Physicians and Surgeons, and St. Luke's/Roosevelt Hospital Center, New York, New York, U.S.A.

Jaime L. Bohl Department of Surgery, Colon and Rectal Surgery Program, Vanderbilt University, Nashville, Tennessee, U.S.A.

Mary Lou Boyer Department of Colorectal Surgery, Cleveland Clinic Florida, Weston, Florida, U.S.A.

Patrick Colquhoun Department of Surgery, University of Western Ontario, London, Ontario, Canada

Norma Daniel Department of Colorectal Surgery, Cleveland Clinic Florida, Weston, Florida, U.S.A.

G. Willy Davila Section of Urogynecology, Department of Gynecology, Cleveland Clinic Florida, Weston, Florida, U.S.A.

Miguel del Mazo University of Miami Medical Center, Miami, Florida, U.S.A.

Jonathan Efron Division of Colorectal Surgery, Mayo Clinic Arizona, Scottsdale, Arizona, U.S.A.

Lawrence Frank Division of Anesthesiology, Cleveland Clinic Florida, Weston, Florida, U.S.A.

Newton Luiz T. Gasparetti, Jr. Department of Gastroenterology, Colorectal Unit, Hospital das Clínicas, University of Sao Paulo, Sao Paulo, Brazil

Jill C. Genua Colon and Rectal Surgeons of Connecticut, Stamford, Connecticut, U.S.A.

Johnny B. Green Kitsap Colorectal Surgery, Bremerton, Washington, U.S.A.

Tracy Hull Cleveland Clinic Foundation, Cleveland, Ohio, U.S.A.

Sanjay Jobanputra North Shore-Long Island Jewish Medical System, New Hyde Park, New York, U.S.A.

José Marcio Neves Jorge Department of Gastroenterology, Colorectal Unit, Hospital das Clínicas, University of Sao Paulo, Sao Paulo, Brazil

Orit Kaidar-Person Department of General Surgery B, Rambam Healthcare Campus, Haifa, Israel

Eliad Karin Department of Surgery A, Sourasky Medical Center, Tel Aviv, Israel

Peter M. Kaye Department of Surgery, St. Luke's/Roosevelt Hospital Center, New York, New York, U.S.A.

Marat Khaikin Department of Surgery and Transplantation, Sheba Medical Center, Sackler School of Medicine, Tel Aviv, Israel

Dean C. Koh The Ferguson Clinic, MMPC, Grand Rapids, Michigan, U.S.A. and Colorectal Unit, Department of Surgery, Tan Tock Seng Hospital, Singapore

Jorge A. Lagares-Garcia R.I. Colorectal Clinic, LLC, Pawtucket, Rhode Island, U.S.A.

Anne Y. Lin Department of Surgery, Division of Colorectal Surgery, Washington University, St. Louis, Missouri, U.S.A.

Martin A. Luchtefeld The Ferguson Clinic, MMPC, Grand Rapids, Michigan, U.S.A.

Tisha Lunsford Division of Gastroenterology and Hepatology, Mayo Clinic Arizona, Scottsdale, Arizona, U.S.A.

Mari A. Madsen Department of Colon and Rectal Surgery, Cedars Sinai Medical Center, Los Angeles, California, U.S.A.

David J. Maron Department of Colon and Rectal Surgery, University of Pennsylvania School of Medicine, Philadelphia, Pennsylvania, U.S.A.

Helen Marquez Department of Colorectal Surgery, Cleveland Clinic Florida, Weston, Florida, U.S.A.

Roberta L. Muldoon Department of Surgery, Colon and Rectal Surgery Program, Vanderbilt University, Nashville, Tennessee, U.S.A.

Juan J. Nogueras Department of Colorectal Surgery, Cleveland Clinic Florida, Weston, Florida, U.S.A.

Benjamin Person Department of General Surgery B, Rambam Healthcare Campus, Haifa, Israel

Rodrigo Ambar Pinto Department of Colorectal Surgery, Cleveland Clinic Florida, Weston, Florida, U.S.A.

Arlene Segura Surgical Services, Cleveland Clinic Florida, Weston, Florida, U.S.A.

Cesar Omar Reategui Sanchez Department of Colorectal Surgery, Cleveland Clinic Florida, Weston, Florida, U.S.A.

Dana R. Sands Department of Colorectal Surgery, Cleveland Clinic Florida, Weston, Florida, U.S.A.

Laurence R. Sands University of Miami Medical Center, Miami, Florida, U.S.A.

T. Cristina Sardinha North Shore-Long Island Jewish Medical System, New Hyde Park, New York, U.S.A.

Sherief Shawki Department of Colorectal Surgery, Cleveland Clinic Florida, Weston, Florida, U.S.A.

Marc E. Sher North Shore-Long Island Jewish Medical System, New Hyde Park, and Albert Einstein College of Medicine, Bronx, New York, U.S.A.

Dawn Vickers GI-GU Functional Diagnostics, Fort Lauderdale, Florida, U.S.A.

David A. Vivas Cleveland Clinic Florida, Weston, Florida, U.S.A.

Matthew Vrees R.I. Colorectal Clinic, LLC, Pawtucket, Rhode Island, U.S.A.

Hao Wang Department of Colorectal Surgery, Cleveland Clinic Florida, Weston, Florida, U.S.A.

Eric G. Weiss Department of Colorectal Surgery, Cleveland Clinic Florida, Weston, Florida, U.S.A.

Steven D. Wexner Department of Colorectal Surgery, Cleveland Clinic Florida, Weston, Florida; Ohio State University Health Sciences Center, Columbus, Ohio; University of South Florida College of Medicine, Tampa, Florida, U.S.A.

Oded Zmora Department of Surgery and Transplantation, Sheba Medical Center, Sackler School of Medicine, Tel Aviv, Israel

Massarat Zutshi Cleveland Clinic Foundation, Cleveland, Ohio, U.S.A.

1 Patient Evaluation

Sanjay Jobanputra and T. Cristina Sardinha
North Shore-Long Island Jewish Medical System, New Hyde Park, New York, U.S.A.

Marc E. Sher
North Shore-Long Island Jewish Medical System, New Hyde Park,
Albert Einstein College of Medicine, Bronx, New York, U.S.A.

INTRODUCTION

Over the past few decades, there have been vast changes in the practice of surgery. Sutures and sewing have been ever increasingly replaced by stapling devices. Generous incisions are being replaced by small port sites. These advances have also been accompanied by cost-reducing measures. Elective inguinal hernia repair is no longer a three day hospital stay, but rather a three hour experience. During this time period, the concept of ambulatory surgery, surgery not requiring in-patient hospitalization, has become a reality. This includes patients who undergo surgery where they are admitted a few hours prior to surgery and discharged a few hours after surgery, or patients who are admitted for a 23-hour stay. The field of colorectal surgery, especially anorectal surgery, has accepted and welcomed this change.

Ambulatory colorectal surgery has proven to be both safe and cost-effective (1). However, careful preoperative patient assessment and optimization, along with proper surgical planning, are required to ensure a safe outcome.

In addition to a thorough history and physical examination, appropriate laboratory, radiologic, and endoscopic tests are part of the preoperative armamentarium. Moreover, anesthetic and surgical technique must be individualized for every patient and explained to the patient during the office consultation. During this evaluation, a risk-assessment system is also used to better predict the outcome of the procedure to be performed. Furthermore, adequate preoperative education to be provided by the colorectal surgeon or by a member of the surgical team familiar with the procedure will provide comfort and minimize the patient's anxiety.

CHOICE OF PROCEDURE

Despite a growing number of procedures being safely performed at ambulatory centers, there are still limitations. Therefore, the choice of the procedure must be carefully made by the colorectal surgeon prior to determining the setting of the surgery.

In the realm of colorectal surgical procedures, ambulatory surgery is limited predominantly to anal and rectal surgery. Although not comprehensive, a list of acceptable ambulatory procedures is outlined in Table 1. Intra-abdominal colorectal surgery, whether by conventional laparotomy or laparoscopic approach, has not yet made its way to the ambulatory setting. Postoperative issues such as prolonged ileus, intravenous fluid requirements, and postoperative pain management continue to require inpatient care after intra-abdominal colorectal surgery. Table 2 lists some of the relative contraindications to ambulatory surgery.

PATIENT EVALUATION

Patient evaluation for ambulatory surgery begins with a thorough history and physical examination. The history should first focus on the nature of the disease process to assist in making the correct diagnosis. The history should also elicit information that would be important for planning different treatment options. From the history, the physician should be able to assess

Table 1 Acceptable Ambulatory Procedures

Examination under anesthesia
Incision and drainage of peri-rectal abscess
Treatment of anal fistula
Treatment of anal fissure
Treatment of pilonidal sinus
Treatment of anal condyloma
Treatment of hemorrhoidal disease
Transanal excision of rectal lesions
Endoscopy

what type of surgery the patient will require, and also based on the patient's condition and proposed procedure, the appropriate setting for the planned procedure. For example, a 25-year-old healthy female undergoing an elective hemorrhoidectomy will differ greatly from a 65-year-old male with a history of congestive heart failure, recent myocardial infarction, and defibrillator on antiplatelet therapy.

After obtaining a history, a complete physical examination should be performed. The examination should not be limited to the area of pathology so as to not miss associated conditions which may affect the ultimate treatment plan. As surgeons, we are eager to correct our patients' problems quickly and efficiently, but this should not interfere with thoroughness. For example, the treatment plan for a patient with hemorrhoidal disease would be very different if the patient was noted on physical examation to have abdominal distention secondary to ascites. Therefore, all major organ systems should be evaluated, even though the patient's chief complaint only involves an anorectal problem.

Based on the history and physical, and often some diagnostic tests to be discussed later, a variety of risk-assessment scores have been developed (Table 3). The most commonly used is the American Society of Anesthesiologists Classification (ASA) (Table 4) (2). The advantage of the ASA is its ease of use, its lack of other testing needed for use, and its correlation with perioperative morbidity and mortality (2). The disadvantage of the ASA is that it is a subjective and very generalized score. The ASA should not be used as the sole criteria for determining the appropriateness of an ambulatory setting for surgery; however, patients over an ASA of II should strongly be considered for nonambulatory surgery.

Organ-specific risk-assessment indexes are also available. The most widely used is the Goldman cardiac risk index (3). This index assigns point values for different clinical variables and then patients are divided into different classes based on the total score (Table 5). With increasing class, there is an increase in life-threatening complications and cardiac death risk. There are no official guidelines on what class of patient based on the Goldman risk index should not be considered a candidate for ambulatory surgery. However, patients who fall in Class III and IV should definitely be evaluated by the surgeon, cardiologist, and anesthesiologist prior to scheduling a procedure at an ambulatory center.

Table 2 Relative Contraindications to Ambulatory Surgery

Expected ileus
Expected fluid shifts
Expected intravenous fluid requirements
Intravenous analgesics
Expected electrolyte abnormalities

Table 3 Risk-Assessment Scores

American Society of Anesthesiologists Classification
Goldman Cardiac Risk Index
Prognostic Nutritional Index
Pulmonary Complication Risk

Table 4 ASA Classification

I.	Normal healthy patient
II.	Mild systemic disease
III.	Severe, noncapacitating systemic disease
IV.	Incapacitating systemic disease, threatening life
V.	Moribund, not expected to survive 24 hr
VI.	Emergency

Source: From Ref. 2

Scores such as the Prognostic Nutritional Index, although potentially useful for major colon and rectal procedures, do not play a significant role in cases that would be considered for an ambulatory setting. Other physiologic scores including the Acute Physiology and Chronic Health Evaluation (APACHE), APACHE II, and the Physiological and Operative Severity Score for enUmeration of Mortality (POSSUM) do not play a significant role in the evaluation of patients for ambulatory surgery.

SPECIAL PATIENT CONSIDERATIONS

As the decision to proceed with surgery is underway and the decision between ambulatory surgery and hospital admission is being considered, there are certain patient characteristics that require special attention.

There is no official age limit that would be considered safe to undergo ambulatory surgery; however, the literature has shown an increased rate of readmission, morbidity, and mortality for patients undergoing ambulatory surgery over the age of 85 (4). Nonetheless, age alone should not prevent ambulatory surgery, but it should be evaluated in conjunction with associated comorbidities which may lead toward an in-patient setting.

Obesity is another growing problem in the United States and throughout the western world. There is no recommended maximum body mass index or weight that should be considered a contraindication for ambulatory colorectal surgery; however, obese patients should be considered higher risk for surgery from many perspectives, especially from an airway protection standpoint. When obese patients are being evaluated for surgery, the surgeon should be familiar with the capabilities of the operative facility in terms of dealing with obese patients including equipment matters and adequate resources to safely care for this patient population. When surgery is planned for the prone position, as is often the case in anorectal procedures, special consideration should be given to general anesthesia in obese patients for airway protection.

Obstructive sleep apnea (OSA) is another concern when scheduling surgery, whether ambulatory or in-patient. OSA is often associated with obesity; however, normal weight patients may also suffer from OSA. All patients should be questioned about potential symptoms including apneic events during sleep, heavy snoring, or the feeling of fatigue after a full night's sleep.

Table 5 Goldman Cardiac Risk

	# Points
Myocardial infarction within 6 mo	10
Age greater than 70	5
S3 gallop or jugular venous distension	11
Aortic stenosis	3
Nonsinus rhythm or atrial premature contractions	7
Greater than 5 premature ventricular contractions	7
Poor general medical condition	3
Intraperitoneal, thoracic, aortic operation	3
Emergency operation	4
Class I	0–5
Class II	6–12
Class III	13–25
Class IV	≥26

Source: From Ref. 3

The use of a Continuous Positive Airway Pressure (CPAP) device is also an obvious indicator of sleep apnea. OSA is not an absolute contraindication to outpatient procedures; however, the surgeon should ensure that the ambulatory surgery center has adequate monitoring capabilities for a longer than normal recovery and monitoring period. The possibility of in-patient admission should also be considered and arrangements made prior to surgery, especially if the patient is likely to require narcotics for analgesia.

The presence of a pacemaker and/or of a defibrillator is not a contraindication for ambulatory surgery; however, adequate cardiology back-up must be available to handle any issues which may arise, including reprogramming the device both pre- and postoperatively. In our institution, the presence of a defibrillator prohibits surgery at the Ambulatory Surgery Center; however, the patient may have surgery at the main hospital operating room and still be discharged home the same day of surgery.

Malignant hyperthermia is a rare complication of anesthesia. A known history or known family history of malignant hyperthermia should be considered a relative contraindication to ambulatory surgery. If the patient will only have intravenous sedation and local anesthesia, this would be less of a concern; however, this should be discussed with the anesthesia and nursing team prior to surgery.

PREOPERATIVE WORK-UP

Once the decision to proceed with surgery has been made and the appropriate location and setting for surgery has been selected, the patient must undergo a preoperative work-up.

All patients must have a complete history and physical examination prior to surgery. As discussed earlier, all organ systems should be evaluated with a thorough review of systems. Physical examination should also include all organ systems.

The use of "routine" preoperative laboratory tests is becoming a subject of historical interest. Patients undergoing ambulatory colon and rectal surgery, as with all ambulatory surgical patients, should have preoperative laboratory tests, only as needed, specific to the patient, diagnosis, and proposed surgery. Each institution has specific guidelines and requirements for ambulatory and major surgery. The following are guidelines at our institution. These guidelines apply to adult patients undergoing ambulatory colorectal surgery who have no specific comorbidities.

All patients at our institution have a preoperative complete blood count (CBC) within seven days of surgery. The basic metabolic panel (BMP) is officially reserved for all patients over the age of 65; however, many patients over the age of 50 will also undergo a BMP prior to surgery if comorbid conditions are present. Patients who undergo mechanical bowel preparation will also benefit from electrolyte evaluation, especially potassium levels. This is often performed in the morning of surgery. If the potassium is low, it is replaced prior to or intraoperatively. Diabetic patients should undergo fingerstick blood glucose levels on the day of surgery. Routine coagulation studies including prothrombin time (PT) and partial thromboplastin time (PTT) are not necessary unless the patient has a personal or family history of bleeding disorders or the patient is taking anticoagulants such as warfarin. Bleeding time is rarely assessed prior to surgery unless there is a significant concern over the patient's platelet function. Other hematology or chemistry studies are usually not necessary. Despite the clear lack of need for "routine" preoperative laboratory values for all patients, both surgeons and primary care physicians continue to order and anesthesiologists demand these tests with a significant cost to the health-care system. Better education is required for all members of the health-care team to help reduce the number of unnecessary tests and thus reduce costs.

For female patients of child bearing age, a urine or serum pregnancy test should be performed on the day of surgery or within a few days prior to surgery. Exceptions to this testing exist (Table 6); however, many institutions have adopted a policy of mandatory testing, except for the postmenopausal women and women who have had a hysterectomy.

The use of an electrocardiogram (ECG) is based on age and gender. All males over the age of 40 are required to have an ECG as are all females over the age of 50. Any patient with a cardiac history or pulmonary history should also undergo an ECG prior to surgery. Patients with many other comorbidities including obesity and diabetes mellitus should also undergo ECG.

Table 6 Exceptions to Pregnancy Testing

Absolute
Total hysterectomy
Bilateral oopherectomy
Menopause
Relative
Consistent oral contraceptive use and normal menses
Consistent intrauterine device or levonorgestrel implants
Bilateral tubal ligation

Radiologic studies for ambulatory surgery are usually unnecessary except to aid in confirming the diagnosis for the proposed surgery. Preoperative chest X-ray for ambulatory surgery patients should only be performed in patients over the age of 75. Patients with significant cardiac and/or pulmonary disease should also undergo a preoperative chest X-ray.

There is no specific age at which patients should have a medical work-up prior to surgery; however, patients over the age of 40 are usually referred to a primary care physician for evaluation prior to elective surgery. The surgeon should be aware of the proper preoperative work-up of patients.

Cardiac evaluation prior to surgery is determined based on the patient's history. A simplified protocol follows (5). Patients who had a recent cardiac evaluation with either invasive or noninvasive testing which was normal or unchanged compared with prior evaluation should require no further work-up prior to elective ambulatory surgery. Patients who have excellent functional status and report no cardiac or pulmonary symptoms should also require no further work-up other than a normal ECG. Patients with poor functional status and a normal/stable ECG undergoing a low-risk ambulatory procedure should require no further work-up unless deemed necessary by the cardiologist. Patients with cardiac symptoms including congestive heart failure, prior myocardial infarction, valvular disease, or significant arrhythmias should have a full cardiac work-up prior to an elective ambulatory procedure. This work-up should include evaluation by a cardiologist, ECG, noninvasive studies, and cardiac catheterization, if indicated. These guidelines are simplified and should be tailored to each patient individually. High-risk patients would also benefit from the anesthesiologist's evaluation prior to surgery.

All patient medications should be taken into account during the preoperative evaluation. Anticoagulants should ideally be stopped five days prior to surgery, unless contraindicated. Aspirin and other antiplatelet agents should be stopped at least 7 to 10 days prior to the proposed surgery. A history of cardiac drug-eluting stents often requires that the patient remain on the antiplatelet agents, especially for the first 9 to 12 months. If this is the case, surgery should be postponed, if possible. Otherwise, a discussion should be undertaken with the cardiologist regarding the discontinuation of these agents prior to surgery. Based on the risks/benefits of the surgery compared with the risks/benefits of discontinuing these agents, a decision should be made. The use of herbal supplements should also be elicited from the patient as many of these agents can cause increased bleeding tendencies. Thus, depending on the agent, they often must be discontinued prior to surgery.

A very important aspect of the patient evaluation is preoperative counseling relative to postoperative expectations. This is important for all types of surgery; however, even more important in ambulatory surgery as the patient will be discharged home postoperatively. Patients should be given realistic expectations of the level of pain to expect; for example, patients should be told that significant pain should be expected for at least one week after hemorrhoidectomy. Discussion with the patient should include all aspects of postoperative recuperation including wound care, bowel regimes, analgesics, and postoperative follow-up. A detailed discussion with the patient prior to ambulatory surgery will lead to a better postoperative experience and faster recovery. Ideally, the nursing and anesthesia staff should also discuss the expected postoperative course from their perspectives.

In addition to the overall medical evaluation, a dedicated preoperative anorectal assessment is required. This starts with careful inspection of the anus and perianal area followed by a detailed digital examination. Most anorectal pathologies treated as outpatient procedures are diagnosed based on the physical examination, including but not limited to hemorrhoids, pilonidal cyst, condyloma, and chronic anal fissure.

The majority of anorectal abscesses are also diagnosed based on the physical examination. However, supralevator or deep postanal space abscesses may require endorectal ultrasonography or computerized tomography scan for complete evaluation, especially in patients with Crohn's disease or immunosuppressive disorders.

Patients with anorectal fistula should also undergo preoperative and/or intraoprative evaluation to determine the fistulous tract in order to guide the optimum surgical approach and prevent iatrogenic tract creation. This includes anorectal ultrasonography with hydrogen peroxide injection through the external opening, magnetic resonance imaging with or without anorectal probe, and fistulogram. Intraoperatively, injection of hydrogen peroxide, normal saline, or methylene blue via the external opening will aid in the identification of the internal opening allowing the safe introduction of a fistulous probe through the tract and further direct management of the fistula.

CONCLUSION

The cost-effectiveness of ambulatory colorectal surgery has been well established. Nonetheless, these procedures can only be safely performed after adequate preoperative evaluation and cautious patient selection.

REFERENCES

1. Place R, Hyman N, Simmang C, et al. Practice parameters for ambulatory anorectal surgery. Dis Colon Rectum 2003; 46(5):573–576.
2. Menke H, Klein A, John KD, et al. Predictive value of ASA classification for the assessment of perioperative risk. Int Surg 1993; 78:266–270.
3. Goldman L, Caldera DL, Nussbaum SR, et al. Multifactorial index of cardiac risk in noncardiac surgical procedures. New Engl J Med 1977; 297:845–850.
4. Fleisher LA, Pasternak LR, Herbert R, et al. Inpatient hospital admission and death after outpatient surgery in elderly patients: Importance of patients and system characteristics and location of care. Arch Surg 2004; 139:67–72.
5. Eagle KA, Berger PB, Calkins H, et al. ACC/AHA guideline update for perioperative cardiovascular evaluation for noncardiac surgery-executive summary. A report of the American College of Cardiology/American Heart Association Task Force on Practice Guidelines (Committee to Update the 1996 Guidelines on Perioperative Cardiovascular Evaluation for Noncardiac Surgery). Anesth Analg 2002; 94(5):1052–1064.

2 Anatomy of the Rectum and Anus

José Marcio Neves Jorge and Newton Luiz T. Gasparetti, Jr.
Department of Gastroenterology, Colorectal Unit, Hospital das Clínicas, University of Sao Paulo, Sao Paulo, Brazil

INTRODUCTION

Concepts concerning the anatomy of the anorectum are constantly changing in light of new scientific methodology. In addition, the anatomy of this region is so intrinsically related to its physiology that many aspects are appreciated only in the living. Therefore, it is a region in which the colorectal surgeon has, as advantages over the anatomist, the experience on "in vivo" dissection, and on both physiological and endoscopic examinations. Recent advances in anorectal physiology, along with the advance of surgical techniques, have renewed the interest in more detailed studies of anatomy (1–8). Conversely, studies matching 3-D reconstructions of specific muscle groups of the anorectum and pelvic floor, with level oriented resting and squeeze pressure profiles, have provided more data to reevaluate concepts of the high-pressure zone or functional anal canal length (9,10).

RECTUM

The rectum is a 12 to 15 cm long segment of large bowel involved in the entire process of defecation—its sensibility initiates the process and its capacity makes the patient able to control it, among several other mechanisms involved. It occupies the sacral concavity and ends 2 to 3 cm anteroinferiorly to the tip of the coccyx, where it angulates backward to pass through the levators to become the anal canal (Figs. 1 and 2). The proximal limit of the rectum, the rectosigmoid junction, has been considered as an externally indistinct segment which to most surgeons comprises the last 5 to 8 cm of sigmoid and the uppermost 5 cm of the rectum. However, it is well defined endoscopically as a narrow and sharply angulated segment and, in fact, is the narrowest portion of the large intestine. In a more clear definition, the rectosigmoid junction is the "point" where the tenia libera and the tenia omentalis fuse to form a single anterior tenia and where both haustra and mesocolon terminate, usually situated at 6 to 7 cm below the sacral promontory (Fig. 3) (4). Likewise, the distal limit of the rectum is debatable, regarded as the muscular anorectal ring by surgeons and as the dentate line by anatomists.

Anatomical characteristics of the rectum include a wide and easily distensible lumen and the absence of teniae, epiploic appendices, and haustra. The rectal mucosa is smooth, pink, and transparent which allows visualization of submucosal vessels. This typical "vascular pattern" disappears in inflammatory diseases and melanosis coli. The rectum is characterized by three lateral curves: the upper and lower curves are convex to the right and the middle is convex to the left. These curves correspond on the intraluminal aspect to the folds or valves of Houston. There are usually three folds: two on the left side (at 7–8 cm and at 12–13 cm) and one at 9 to 11 cm on the right side. The middle valve is the most consistent (Kohlrausch's plica) and corresponds to the level of the anterior peritoneal reflection. The valves of Houston must be negotiated during rectosigmoidoscopy, and they disappear after straightening of the rectum, which is attributed to the 5-cm length gained during rectal mobilization; they do not contain all the rectal wall layers and do not have a specific function; however, from a clinical point of view, they are an excellent location for rectal biopsy (11).

Anatomical Relationships of the Rectum

The upper third of the rectum is invested by peritoneum on both its anterior and lateral aspects. The middle rectum is only anteriorly covered by peritoneum, as the posterior peritoneal reflection is usually 12 to 15 cm from the anal verge. Finally, the lower third of the rectum is entirely extraperitoneal, as the anterior peritoneal reflection occurs at 9 to 7 cm from the anal verge, in men, and a little lower at 7.5 to 5 cm from the anal verge in women. The rectum is, therefore,

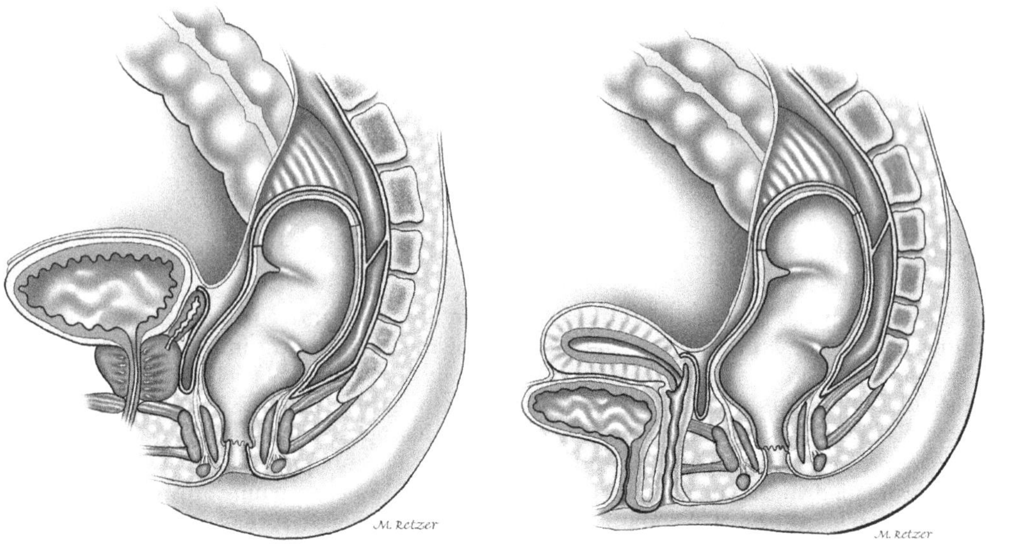

(A) (B)

Figure 1 Sagittal diagram of the (**A**) male and (**B**) female pelvis.

entirely extraperitoneal on its posterior aspect. According to anatomists, the rectum is characterized by the absence of a mesorectum. However, the areolar tissue on the posterior aspect of the rectum, containing terminal branches of the inferior mesenteric artery and enclosed by the fascia propria, is often referred to by surgeons as the mesorectum (Fig. 4). A more distinct mesorectum, however, may be noted in patients with complete rectal prolapse. In addition, the mesorectum may be a metastatic site from a rectal cancer and it can be removed without clinical sequelae, as no functionally significant nerves pass through it (12).

Anteriorly, the rectum is related to the cervix uteri and the posterior vaginal wall in women; in men, the rectum lies behind the bladder, vas deferens, seminal vesicles, and prostate. Posteriorly, the rectum is related to the concavity of the sacrum and coccyx, the median sacral vessels, and the roots of the sacral nerve plexus.

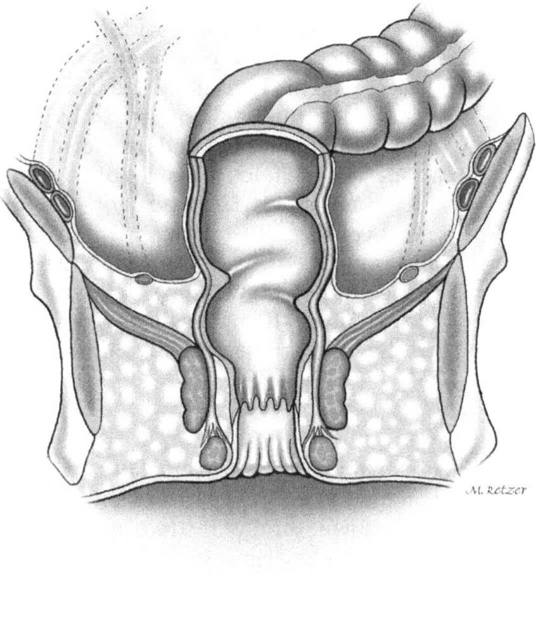

Figure 2 Frontal diagram of the rectum.

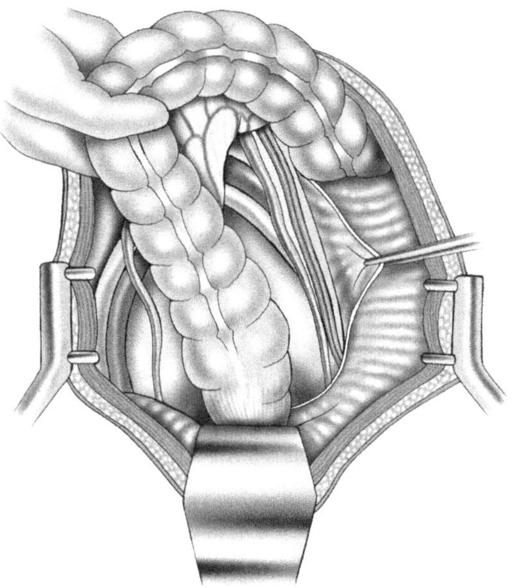

Figure 3 The rectosigmoid junction and its anatomical relationship, after division of the mesosigmoid and medial retraction of the sigmoid colon.

Fascial Attachments of the Rectum

The walls and the floor of the pelvis are lined by the parietal endopelvic fascia, which continues on the pelvic organs as a visceral fascia and attaches them to the pelvic walls. Because the parietal fascia is intimately attached to the pelvic viscera, it is also referred to as the viscero–fascial layer. The fascia propria of the rectum is then an extension of the pelvic fascia that encloses the rectum and fat, nerves and blood, and lymphatic vessels, present mainly in the lateral and posterior extraperitoneal portion of the rectum [Figs. 5(A) and (B)].

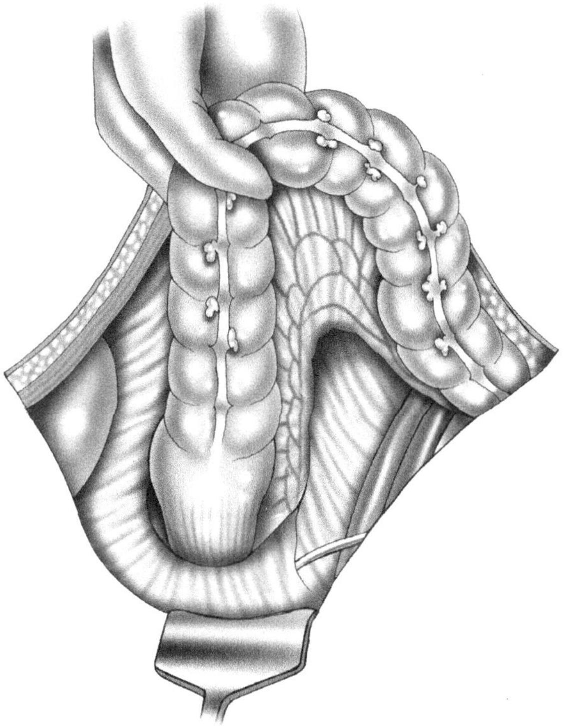

Figure 4 The mesorectum.

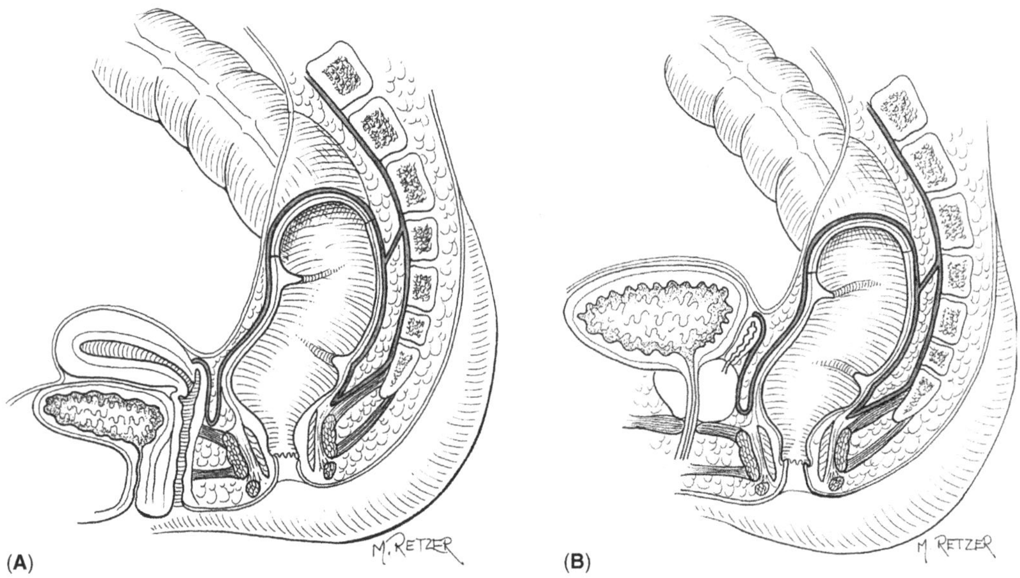

Figure 5 Fascial attachments of the rectum in the (**A**) female and (**B**) male pelvis.

The rectum is attached to the lateral pelvic wall by distal condensations of the fascia propria of the rectum, known as lateral ligaments or lateral stalks of the rectum (Fig. 6). These ligaments comprise essentially connective tissue and nerves; the middle rectal artery does not traverse the lateral stalks of the rectum but sends minor branches through them, uni- or bilaterally, in approximately 25% of cases (13). Consequently, division of the lateral stalks during rectal mobilization carries out a 1:4 chance of bleeding. However, from a practical point of view the stalks rarely require ligation; electrocautery is sufficient in the vast majority of cases.

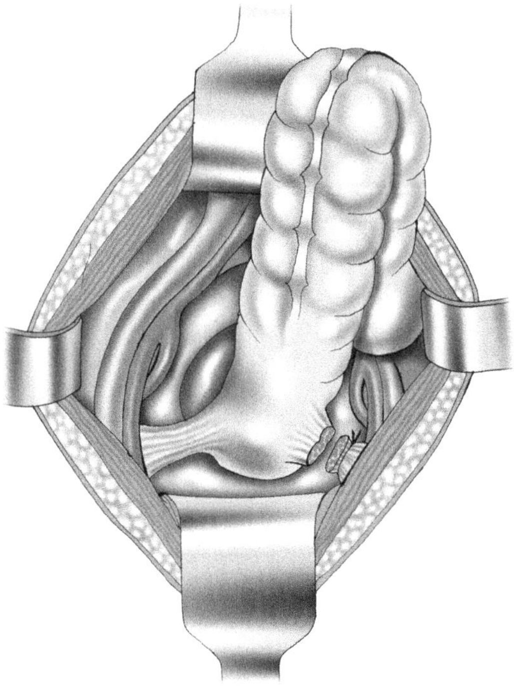

Figure 6 Lateral stalks of the rectum.

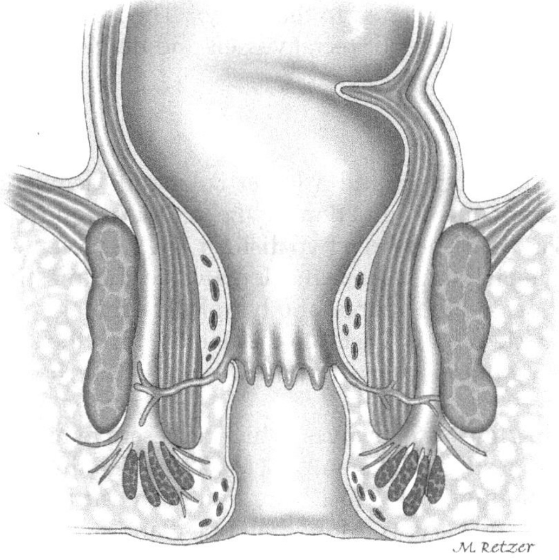

Figure 7 The anal canal.

Furthermore, ligation of the stalks implies leaving behind lateral mesorectal tissue, which may preclude obtaining oncologically adequate lateral or mesorectal margins.

The presacral fascia is a thickened part of the parietal endopelvic fascia that covers the concavity of the sacrum and coccyx, nerves, the middle sacral artery, and presacral veins. Intraoperative rupture of the presacral fascia may cause troublesome hemorrhage, related to the underlying presacral veins, in 4.6% to 7% of cases after surgery for rectal neoplasms (14,15). These veins are avalvular and communicate, via basivertebral veins, with the internal vertebral venous system. This system can attain hydrostatic pressures of 17 to 23 cm H_2O, about two to three times the normal pressure of the inferior vena cava, in the lithotomy position (14). In addition, the adventitia of the basivertebral veins adheres firmly, by structures "in anchor," to the sacral periosteum at the level of the ostia of the sacral foramina found mainly at the level of S3–S4 (14). Consequently, despite its venous nature, presacral hemorrhage can be life-threatening due to the high hydrostatic pressure and difficult to control due to retraction of the vascular stump into the sacral foramen.

The rectosacral fascia is an anteroinferior-directed thick fascial reflection from the presacral fascia at the S4 level, on the upper surface of the anococcygeal ligament to the fascia propria of the rectum, just above the anorectal ring. Although William Waldeyer had described the entire pelvic fascia without specifically emphasizing the rectosacral fascia, this fascia became classically known as fascia of Waldeyer (1). Anteriorly, close to the urogenital diaphragm, the rectum is separated from the prostate and seminal vesicle or the vagina by a condensation of visceral pelvic fascia, known as the fascia of Denonvilliers. Both Waldeyer's and Denonvilliers' fascia are important anatomical landmarks during rectal mobilization [Figs. 5(A) and (B)].

ANAL CANAL

The anal canal has a peculiar anatomy and a complex physiology, which accounts for its vital role in continence and its susceptibility to a variety of diseases. It is distinctly defined by anatomists and surgeons as the "anatomical" or "embryological" anal canal, which is shorter (2.0 cm), extends from the anal verge to the dentate line which corresponds to the procotodaeal membrane, and the "surgical" or "functional" anal canal, which is longer (4.0 cm) and extends from the anal verge to the anorectal ring (Fig 7). The anorectal ring, or the upper end of the sphincter, is more precisely the puborectalis (PR) and the upper border of the internal anal sphincter (IAS) and is an easily recognized boundary of the anal canal on physical examination. Despite lacking embryological significance, the anorectal ring is of clinical relevance since division of this structure, as during surgery for abscesses and fistula, will inevitably result in fecal incontinence. The anterior-directed contraction of the sling of PR can also be easily palpated around the anorectal junction during rectal examination. Anteriorly, the anal canal is related to the urethra in the male and to the perineal body and to the lowest part of the posterior vaginal wall in the female. Posteriorly, the anal canal is related to the coccyx. The ischiorectal fossa is situated on either side and contains fat and the inferior rectal vessels and nerves which traverse it to enter the wall of the anal canal.

Lining of the Anal Canal

The lining of the anal canal consists of an upper mucosal and a lower cutaneous segment. The dentate (pectinate) line represents the "sawtoothed" junction of the ectoderm and the endoderm and, thus, represents an important landmark between two distinct origins of venous and lymphatic drainage, nerve supply, and epithelial lining. Above the dentate line, the intestine has sympathetic and parasympathetic innervation and the venous and lymphatic drainage and the arterial supply are to and from the hypogastric vessels. Distal to the dentate line, the anal canal has somatic nerve supply and its vascularization is related to the inferior hemorrhoidal system.

The pectinate or dentate line corresponds to a line of anal valves, which represent remnants of the proctodeal membrane. Above each valve is situated a small pocket known as the anal sinus or crypt. A variable number of glands, ranging from 4 to 12, are more concentrated in the posterior quadrants and are connected to the anal crypts. More than one gland may open into the same crypt, while half the crypts have no communication. The anal gland ducts, in an outward and downward route, enter the submucosa; two-thirds enter the IAS; and half of these terminate into the intersphincteric plane (16). Obstruction of these ducts, presumably by accumulation of foreign material in the crypts, may cause perianal abscesses and fistulas (17). Above the dentate line, 8 to 14 longitudinal folds, known as the rectal columns (columns of Morgagni), have their bases connected in pairs to each valve at the dentate line. At the lower end of the columns are the anal papillae. The mucosa in the area of the columns consists of several layers of cuboidal cells and acquires a deep purple color due to the underlying internal hemorrhoidal plexus. This 0.5 to 1 cm strip of mucosa above the dentate line is known as the anal transition or cloacogenic zone, and it is the source of some anal tumors. Above this area, the epithelium becomes a single layer of cuboidal columnar cells and macroscopically acquires the characteristic pink color of the rectal mucosa.

Anus and Anal Verge

The anus or anal orifice is an anteroposterior cutaneous slit which, at rest, as well as the anal canal, is kept virtually closed due to both tonic circumferential contraction of the sphincters and the anal cushions. The cutaneous part of the anal canal consists of a modified squamous epithelium, which is thin, smooth, pale, and stretched and devoid of hair and glands. The terms "pectin" and "pecten band" have been used to define this segment (18). However, the round band of fibrous tissue called "pecten band," divided in cases of anal fissure (pectenectomy), represents probably the spastic IAS. The anal verge (linea Alban, anocutaneous line of Hilton) marks the lowermost edge of the anal canal, usually the level of reference for measurements taken during colonoscopy. Others prefer to evert the anus and consider the dentate line as a landmark because it is more precise; the difference between the two is nearly 1 cm. Distal to the anal verge, the lining becomes thicker, pigmented, and arranged in radiating folds around the anus; it then acquires hair folicules, glands including large apocrinal glands, and other features of normal skin. For this reason, perianal hidradenitis suppurative—inflammation of the apocrinal glands—may be excised with preservation of the anal canal.

Muscles of the Anorectal Region

Based on phylogenetical studies, two muscle groups derive from the cloaca—the "sphincter" and "lateral compressor" groups (19). The sphincteric group is present in almost all animals; in higher mammals this group is divided into ventral (urogenital) and dorsal (anal) groups; in primates, the latter forms the external anal sphincter (EAS). The lateral compressor or pelvicaudal group connects the rudimentary pelvis to the caudal end of the vertebral column. This group is more differentiated and subdivided in lateral and medial compartments, but only in reptiles and mammals. The homologue of the lateral compartment is apparently the ischiococcygeus, and the pubo and ileococcygeus in the medial pelvicaudal compartment. In addition, most primates possess a variable-sized group of muscle fibers close to the inner border of the medial

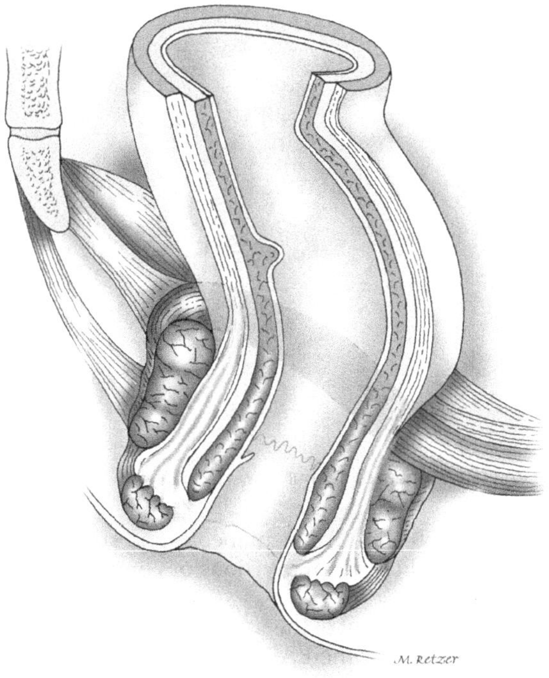

Figure 8 Muscles of the anal canal.

pelvicaudal muscle, which attach the rectum to the pubis; these fibers are more distinct and known in man as the PR muscle.

Internal Anal Sphincter

The IAS represents the distal 2.5 to 4 cm long condensation of the inner circular muscle layer of the rectum (Fig. 8). The lower rounded edge of the IAS can be felt on physical examination, about 1.2 cm distal to the dentate line; the groove between it and the EAS, the intersphincteric sulcus, can be visualized or easily palpated. The different echogenic patterns of the anal sphincters facilitate their visualization during endosonography. The IAS is a 2 to 3 mm thick circular band and shows a uniform hypoechogenicity. The PR and the EAS, despite their mixed linear echogenicity, are both predominantly hyperechogenic, and the distinction is made by position of their shape and topography.

Conjoined Longitudinal Muscle

Whereas the inner circular layer of the rectum gives rise to the IAS, the outer longitudinal layer, at the level of the anorectal ring, mixes with some fibers of the levator ani muscle to form the conjoined longitudinal muscle (CLM) (Fig. 8). This muscle descends between the IAS and EAS and ultimately some of its fibers, referred to as the corrugator cutis ani muscle, traverse the lowermost part of the EAS to insert into the perianal skin. There is still controversy regarding the anatomy of the CLM: other sources for the striated component include the PR and deep EAS, the pubococcygeus, and top loop of the EAS and lower fibers of the PR (20–22). On its descending course, the CLM may give rise to medial extensions that cross the IAS to contribute the smooth muscle of submucosa (musculus canalis ani, sustentator tunicae mucosae, Treitz muscle, and musculus submucosae ani) (23). Others have described outward filamentous extensions of the CLM crossing the entire length of the EAS to enter the fat of the ischiorectal fossa (24).

External Anal Sphincter

The EAS is the elliptical cylinder of striated muscle that envelops the entire length of the inner tube of smooth muscle, but ends slightly more distal to the terminus of the IAS. It is a continuous sheet of muscle which forms, along with the PR and levator ani, one funnel-shaped sheet of skeletal muscle; the deepest part of the EAS is intimately related to the PR, which is actually considered a component of both the levator ani and EAS muscle complexes (25). The EAS is also

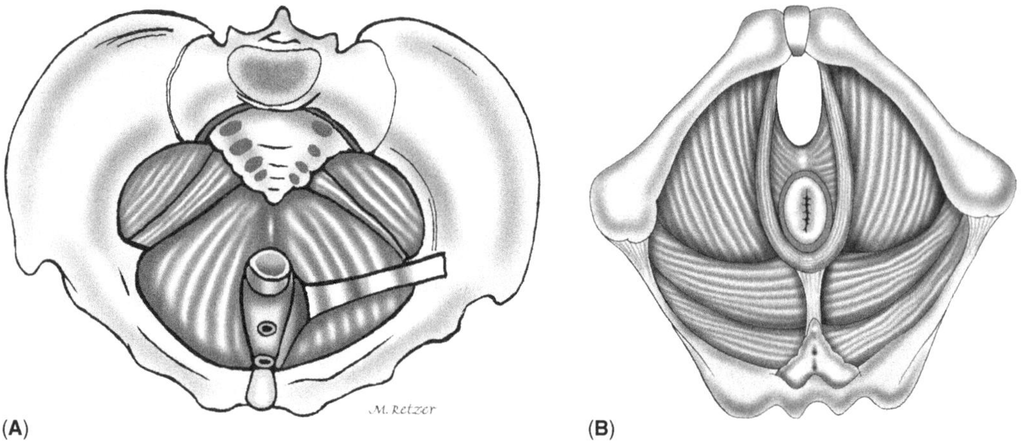

(A) (B)

Figure 9 The pelvic floor: (**A**) pelvic or superior view and (**B**) perineal or inferior view.

described as composed of two [(1) deep sphincter and PR and (2) subcutaneous and superficial sphincter] or three [(1) subcutaneous, (2) superficial, and (3) deep] divisions or compartments (Fig. 8) (2,26).

Oh and Kark (26) also noted differences in the arrangement of the EAS according to gender and site around the anal canal. In the male, the upper half of the EAS is enveloped anteriorly by the CLM, while the lower half is crossed by it. In the female, the entire EAS is grossly encapsulated by a mixture of fibers derived from both longitudinal and IAS muscles. Based on an embryological study, the EAS also seems to be subdivided into two parts, superficial and deep, without any connection to the PR (5). Shafik (2) proposed the three U-shaped loop system concept, in which each loop is a separate sphincter with distinct attachments, muscle bundle directions, and innervations and each loop complements the others to help maintain continence. However, clinical experience has not supported Shafik's three part scheme; the EAS is more likely a one muscle unit, not divided into layers or laminae, attached by the anococcygeal ligament posteriorly to the coccyx and anteriorly to the perineal body.

Levator Ani

The levator ani muscle or pelvic diaphragm is a pair of broad symmetrical sheets composed of three striated muscles: iliococcygeus, pubococcygeus, and PR (Figs. 9 and 10). A variable fourth component, the ischiococcygeus or coccygeus, is, in humans, rudimentary and is represented by a few muscle fibers on the surface of the sacrospinous ligament (27). The coccyx, the sacrospinous ligament, and the ischial tuberosities, when palpated during rectal examination, are landmarks for procedures involving the pudendal nerve such as anesthetic block and evaluation of the pudendal nerve terminal motor latencies. The pelvic floor is "defective" in the midline where

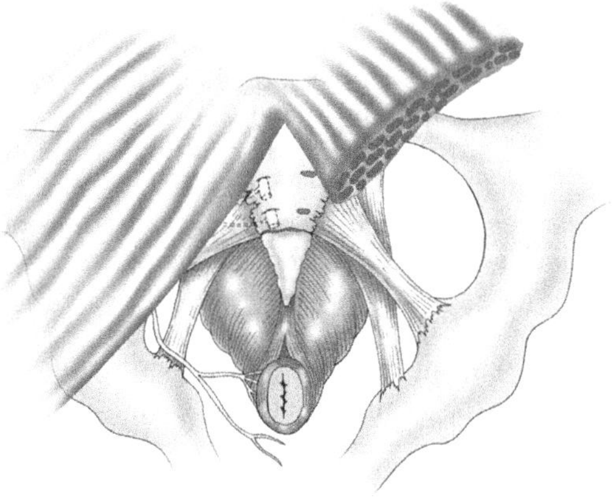

Figure 10 Posterior view of the pelvic floor and sphincteric muscles.

the lower rectum, urethra, and either the dorsal vein of the penis in men or the vagina in women pass through it. This defect is called levator hiatus and consists of an elliptical space situated between the two pubococcygeus muscles (11). The hiatal ligament, originating from the pelvic fascia, maintains the intrahiatal viscera together and prevents their constriction during levator ani contraction.

The ileococcygeus arises from the ischial spine and posterior part of the obturator fascia, and courses inferiorly and medially to insert into the lateral aspects of S 3 and S 4, the coccyx, and the anococcygeal raphe. The pubococcygeus fibers arise from the posterior aspect of the pubis and the anterior part of the obturator fascia, run dorsally alongside the anorectal junction, to decussate with fibers of the opposite side at the anococcygeal raphe and insert into the anterior surface of the fourth sacral and first coccygeal segments. The PR muscle is a U-shaped strong loop of striated muscle which slings the anorectum junction to the back of the pubis. The anorectal angle, the result of the anatomic configuration of the U-shaped sling of PR muscle around the anorectal junction, is thought to maintain gross fecal continence. The PR is the most medial portion of the levator muscle and is situated immediately cephalad to the deep component of the EAS. Since the junction between the two muscles is indistinct and they have similar innervation (pudendal nerve), the PR has been regarded by some authors as a part of the EAS rather than the levator ani complex (26). Anatomical and phylogenetic studies suggest that the PR is either a part of the levator ani (28) or of the EAS (19). Based on microscopic examinations in human embryos, Levi et al. (5) observed that the PR muscle has a common primordium with the ileo and pubococcygeus muscles; the PR is, in various stages of development, never connected with the EAS. Additionally, neurophysiologic studies have implied that the innervation of these muscles may not be the same because stimulation of sacral nerves resulted in electromyographic activity in the ipsilateral PR muscle, but not in the EAS (29). This is, therefore, a controversial issue, and as a consequence of all this evidence, the PR has been considered to belong to both the EAS and levator ani muscular groups (30).

PARANAL AND PARARECTAL SPACES

Potential spaces of clinical significance in the anorectal region include ischiorectal, perianal, intersphincteric, submucous, superficial postanal, deep postanal, supralevator, and retrorectal spaces [Figs. 5(A) and (B)]. The ischiorectal fossa is subdivided by a thin horizontal fascia into two spaces: the ischiorectal and perianal. The ischiorectal space comprises the upper two-thirds of the ischiorectal fossa. It is a pyramid-shaped space situated, on both sides, between the anal canal and lower part of the rectum medially, and the side wall of the pelvis laterally. The apex is at the origin of the levator ani muscles from the obturator fascia, and the base is represented by the perianal space. Anteriorly, the fossa is bounded by the urogenital diaphragm and transverse perinei muscles. Posterior to the ischiorectal fossa is the sacrotuberous ligament and the inferior border of the gluteus maximus. On the superolateral wall, the pudendal nerve and the internal pudendal vessels run in the pudendal canal (Alcock's canal). The ischiorectal fossa contains fat and the inferior rectal vessels and nerves.

The perianal space is the area corresponding to the anal verge that surrounds the lower part of the anal canal. It is continuous with the subcutaneous fat of the buttocks laterally and extends into the intersphincteric space medially. The external hemorrhoidal plexus lies in the perianal space and communicates with the internal hemorrhoidal plexus at the dentate line. This space is a typical site of anal hematomas, perianal abscesses, and anal fistula tracts. The perianal space also encloses the subcutaneous part of the EAS, the lowest part of the IAS and fibers of the longitudinal muscle. These fibers function as septa, dividing the space into a compact arrangement, which may account for the severe pain caused by a perianal hematoma or abscess (11).

The intersphincteric space is a potential space between the IAS and the EAS, where most anal glands end. Therefore, its importance lies in the genesis of perianal abscesses.

The submucous space is situated between the IAS and the mucocutaneous lining of the anal canal. This space contains the internal hemorrhoidal plexus and the muscularis submucosae ani. Cephalad is continuous with the submucous layer of the rectum and, inferiorly, it ends at the level of the dentate line.

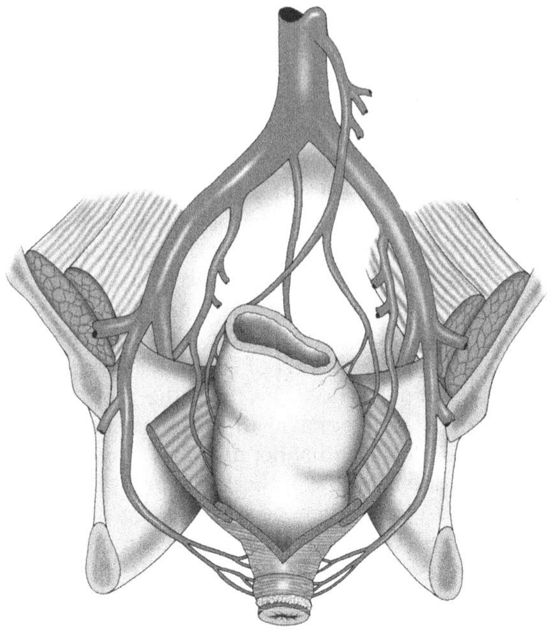

Figure 11 The arterial supply of the anorectum.

The superficial postanal space is interposed between the anococcygeal ligament and the skin. The deep postanal space, also known as the retro-sphincteric space of Courtney, is situated between the anococcygeal ligament and the anococcygeal raphe. Both postanal spaces communicate posteriorly with the ischiorectal fossa, and are potential sites of horseshoes abscesses.

The supralevator spaces are situated between the peritoneum superiorly and the levator ani inferiorly. Medially, these bilateral spaces are related to the rectum and, laterally, to the obturator fascia. Supralevator abscesses may occur as a result of upward extension of a cryptoglandular source or from a pelvic origin.

The retrorectal space is located between the fascia propria of the upper two-thirds of the rectum anteriorly and the presacral fascia posteriorly. Laterally are the lateral rectal ligaments, inferiorly is the rectosacral ligament and, above, it is continuous with the retroperitonium. The retrorectal space is a site for embryological remnants and the rare presacral tumors.

ARTERIAL SUPPLY

The superior and inferior rectal (or hemorrhoidal) arteries represent the major blood supply to the anorectum (Fig. 11). The contribution of the middle rectal artery (middle hemorrhoidal artery) varies inversely with the magnitude of the superior rectal artery, which may explain its variable and controversial anatomy. Some authors report absence of the middle rectal artery in 40% to 88% (31,32), whereas others have identified it in 94% to 100% of specimens (33). It originates more commonly from the anterior division of the internal iliac or the pudendal arteries and reaches the rectum. The middle rectal artery reaches the lower third of the rectum anterolaterally, close to the level of the pelvic floor and deep to the levator fascia; therefore it does not run in the lateral ligaments, which are inclined posterolaterally. The middle rectal artery is more prone to be injured during low anterior resection, when anterolateral dissection of the rectum, close to the pelvic floor, is performed from the prostate and seminal vesicles or from the upper part of the vagina. Although scarce in extramural anastomoses, the anorectum has a profuse intramural anastomotic network, which probably accounts for the fact that division of both superior rectal and middle rectal artery does not result in necrosis of the rectum.

The paired inferior rectal artery (IRA) or inferior hemorrhoidal artery is a branch of the internal pudendal artery, which is a branch of the internal iliac artery. The IRA arises within the pudendal canal and is, on its course, entirely extrapelvic; it traverses the obturator fascia, the ischiorectal fossa, and the EAS to reach the submucosa of the anal canal and ultimately ascend in this plane. The IRA needs to be ligated during the perineal stage of the abdominoperineal resection. Kloesterhalfen et al. (3), based on postmortem angiographic, manual, and histologic preparations, found two topographic variants of the IRA. In the so-called type I, which is the most common (85%), the posterior commissure is less perfused than the other sections of the anal canal. In addition, the blood supply may be jeopardized by contusion of the vessels passing vertically through the muscle fibers of the IAS during increased sphincter tone. These authors postulated that, in a pathogenetic model of the primary anal fissure, the resulting decrease in blood supply would lead to a relevant ischemia at the posterior commissure.

VENOUS DRAINAGE

Blood from the rectum along with the left colon, via the inferior mesenteric vein, reaches the intrahepatic capillary bed through the portal vein. The anorectum also drains, via middle and inferior rectal veins, to the internal iliac vein and then to the inferior vena cava. Although it is still a controversial subject, the presence of anastomoses among these three venous systems may explain the lack of correlation between hemorrhoids and portal hypertension (34).

The paired inferior and middle rectal veins and the single superior rectal vein originate from three anorectal arteriovenous plexuses. The external rectal plexus, situated subcutaneously around the anal canal below the dentate line, constitutes the external hemorrhoids when dilated. The internal rectal plexus is situated submucosally around the upper anal canal, above the dentate line. The internal hemorrhoids originate from this plexus. The perirectal or perimuscular rectal plexus drains to the middle and inferior rectal veins.

LYMPHATIC DRAINAGE

The lymphatic drainage of the large intestine, similar to the venous drainage, basically follows its arterial supply. The lymph nodes in the rectum, however, are particularly more numerous as compared to the other parts of the large bowel. The nodes situated between the peritoneum and the bowel wall, equivalent to the epicolic group in the colon, are known as "nodules of Gerota." Lymph from the upper 2/3 of the rectum drains exclusively upward, via superior rectal vessels, to the inferior mesenteric nodes and then to the paraortic nodes. Lymphatic drainage from the lower third of the rectum occurs not only cephalad, along the superior rectal and inferior mesentery arteries, but also laterally along the middle rectal vessels to the internal iliac nodes. Studies using lymphoscintigraphy failed to demonstrate communication between inferior mesenteric and internal iliac lymphatics (35). In the anal canal, the dentate line is a landmark for two different systems of lymphatic drainage: above, to the inferior mesenteric and internal iliac nodes and, below, along the inferior rectal lymphatics to the superficial inguinal nodes, or, less frequently, along the IRA. Block and Enquist (36) have demonstrated that, in the female, after injection of dye 5 cm above the anal verge, lymphatic drainage may also spread to the posterior vaginal wall, uterus, cervix, broad ligament, fallopian tubes, ovaries, and cul-de-sac. After injection of dye at 10 cm above the anal verge, spread occurred only to the broad ligament and cul-de-sac, and at the 15 cm level, no spread to the genitals was seen.

INNERVATION

Rectum

The sympathetic and parasympathetic components of the autonomic innervation of the large intestine closely follow the blood supply (Fig. 12). The sympathetic supply arises from L1, L2, and L3. Preganglionic fibers, via lumbar sympathetic nerves, synapse in the preaortic plexus, and the postganglionic fibers follow the branches of the inferior mesenteric artery and superior rectal artery to the upper rectum and left colon. The lower rectum is innervated by the presacral nerves, which are formed by fusion of the aortic plexus and lumbar splanchnic nerves. Just below the sacral promontory, the presacral nerves form the hypogastric plexus (or superior hypogastric plexus). Two main hypogastric nerves, on either side of the rectum, carry sympathetic innervation from the hypogastric plexus to the pelvic plexus. The pelvic plexus lies on the lateral side of the pelvis at the level of the lower third of the rectum, adjacent to the lateral

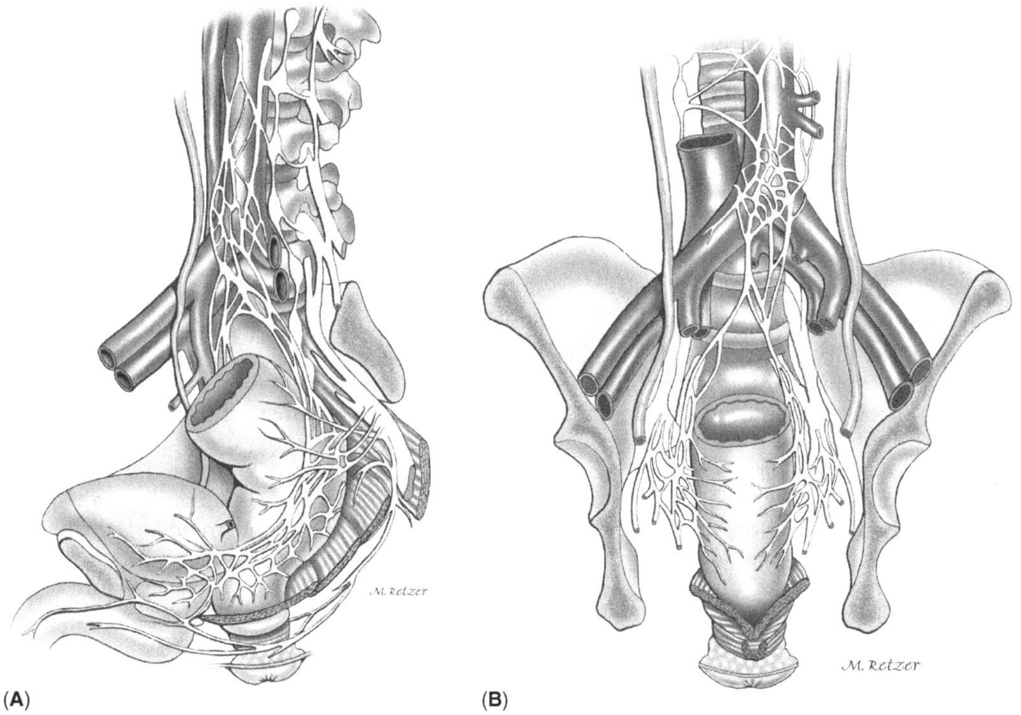

(A) (B)

Figure 12 The parasympathetic and sympathetic nerve supply to the rectum: (**A**) sagittal and (**B**) coronal diagrams.

stalks. The term inferior hypogastric plexus has been used to mean the hypogastric nerves or the pelvic plexus; therefore it is inaccurate.

The parasympathetic supply derives from S2, S3, and S4. These fibers emerge through the sacral foramen and are called the nervi erigenti. They pass laterally, forwards, and upwards to join the sympathetic hypogastric nerves at the pelvic plexus. From the pelvic plexus, combined postganglionic parasympathetic and sympathetic fibers are distributed to the upper rectum and left colon, via inferior mesenteric plexus, and to the lower rectum and upper anal canal. The periprostatic plexus, a subdivision of the pelvic plexus situated on the Denonvilliers'fascia, supplies the prostate, seminal vesicles, corpora cavernosa, vas deferens, urethra, ejaculatory ducts, and bulbourethral glands.

Sexual function is regulated by cerebrospinal, sympathetic, and parasympathetic components; locally the latter plays the main role. Erection of the penis is mediated by both parasympathetic (arteriolar vasodilatation) and sympathetic (inhibition of vasoconstriction) inflow. Sympathetic activity is responsible for emission and parasympathetic activity for ejaculation. Urinary and sexual dysfunction is commonly seen after a variety of pelvic surgical procedures, including low anterior resection and abdominoperineal resection. Permanent bladder paresis occurs in 7% to 59% of patients after abdominoperineal of the rectum (37). The incidence of impotence is approximately 15% and 45% and that of other ejaculatory dysfunction is 32% and 42% after low anterior resection and abdominoperineal resection, respectively (38). The overall incidence of sexual dysfunction after proctectomy may reach up to 100% for malignant disease (39,40); however, these rates are much lower (0–6%) for benign conditions, such as inflammatory bowel disease (40–43). This occurs because dissection performed for benign disease is closer to the bowel wall and avoids nerve injury (44).

All pelvic nerves lie in the plane between the peritoneum and the endopelvic fascia and are endangered during rectal dissection. Injury to the autonomic nerves may occur at several points: during flush ligation of the IMA, close to the aorta, the sympathetic preaortic nerves may be injured. Lesion of both the superior hypogastic plexus and hypogastric nerves may occur during dissection at the sacral promontory or in the presacral region; in this case, sympathetic denervation with intact nervi erigentes results in retrograde ejaculation and bladder dysfunction. The nervi erigentes are located in the posterolateral aspect of the pelvis and, at the point of fusion with the sympathetic nerves, they are closely related to the middle hemorrhoidal artery. An isolated injury of these nerves may completely abolish erectile function. The pelvic plexus may be damaged either by excessive traction on the rectum, particularly laterally, or during division of the lateral stalks, when it is performed closer to the pelvic lateral wall. Finally, dissection near the seminal vesicles and prostate may damage the periprostatic plexus (mixed parasympathetic and sympathetic injury) resulting in erectile impotence and flaccid neurogenic bladder; sexual function may preserved by dissection below the Denonvilliers'fascia. Sexual complications after rectal surgery predominate in men, but are probably underdiagnosed in women (45). Some discomfort during intercourse is reported in 30% (46) and dyspareunia in 10% (47), after proctocolectomy and ileostomy.

Anal Canal

The IAS is supplied by sympathetic (L5) and parasympathetic (S2, S3, S4) nerves following the same route as the nerves to the rectum. The levator ani is supplied by sacral roots (S2, S3, and S4) on its pelvic surface and by the perineal branch of the pudendal nerve on its inferior surface. The PR receives additional innervation from the inferior rectal nerves. The EAS is innervated on each side by the inferior rectal branch (S2, S3) of the pudendal nerve and the perineal branch of S4. Despite the fact that the PR and EAS have somewhat different innervations, these muscles seem to act as an indivisible unit. After unilateral transection of a pudendal nerve, the EAS function is still preserved due to the crossover of the fibers at the spinal cord level.

Sensory Innervation

The upper anal canal contains a rich profusion of both free and organized sensory nerve–endings, especially in the vicinity of the anal valves. Organized nerve-endings include Meissner's corpuscles (touch), Krause's bulbs (cold), Golgi–Mazzoni bodies (pressure), and genital corpuscles (friction). Anal sensation is carried in the inferior rectal branch of the pudendal nerve and is thought to play a role in anal continence (27).

REFERENCES

1. Church JM, Raudkivi PJ, Hill GL. The surgical anatomy of the rectum—a review with particular relevance to the hazards of rectal mobilisation. Int J Colorect Dis 1987; 2:158–166.
2. Shafik A. A concept of the anatomy of the anal sphincter mechanism and the physiology of defecation. Dis Colon Rectum 1987; 30:970-–982.
3. Klosterhalfen B, Vogel P, Rixen H, et al. Topography of the inferior rectal artery. A possible cause of chronic, primary anal fissure. Dis Colon Rectum 1989; 32:43–52.
4. Stoss F. Investigations of the muscular architecture of the rectosigmoid junction in humans. Dis Colon Rectum 1990; 33:378–383.
5. Levi AC, Borghi F, Garavoglia M. Development of the anal canal muscles. Dis Colon Rectum 1991; 34:262–266.
6. Lunniss PJ, Phillips RKS. Anatomy and function of the anal longitudinal muscle. Br J Surg 1992; 79:882–884.
7. Tjandra JJ, Milsom Jw, Stolfi VM, et al. Endoluminal ultrasound defines anatomy of the anal canal and pelvic floor. Dis Colon Rectum 1992; 35:465–470.
8. Garavoglia M, Borghi F, Levi AC. Arrangement of the anal striated musculature. Dis Colon Rectum 1993; 36:10–15.
9. Williams AB, Cheetham MJ, Bartram CI, et al. Gender differences in the longitudinal pressure profile of the anal cnal related to anatomica estructure as demonstrated by three-dimensional anal endosonography. Br J Surg 2000; 87:1674–1679.
10. Zbar AP. Anorectal anatomy: The contributuion of new technology. In: Wexner SD, Zbar AP, Pescatori M, eds. Complex Anorectal Disorders: Investigation and Management. Springer-Verlag, London, 2005:3–16.
11. Nivatvongs S, Gordon PH. Surgical anatomy. In: Gordon PH, Nivatvongs S, eds. Principle and Practice of Surgery for the Colon, Rectum and Anus. St Louis: Quality Medical Publishing Inc., 1992:3–37.
12. Heald RJ, Husband EM, Ryall RD. The mesorectum in rectal cancer surgery—the clue to pelvic recurrence? Br J Surg 1982; 69:613–616.
13. Boxall TA, Smart PJG, Griffiths JD. The blood–supply of the distal segment of the rectum in anterior resection. Br J Surg 1963; 50:399–404.
14. Quinyao W, Weijin S, Youren Z, et al. New concepts in severe presacral hemorrhage during proctectomy. Arch Surg 1985; 120:1013–1020.

15. Jorge, JMN, Habr-Gama A, Souza AS Jr., et al. Rectal surgery complicated by massive presacral hemorrhage. Arq Bras Cir Dig 1990; 5:92–95.
16. Lilius HG. Investigation of human fetal anal ducts and intramuscular glands and a clinical study of 150 patients. Acta Chir Scand (Suppl) 1968; 383:1–88.
17. Parks AG. Pathogenesis and treatment of fistula-in-ano. Br Med J 1961; 1:463–469.
18. Abel AL. The pecten: The pecten band: Pectenosis and pectenectomy. Lancet 1932; 1:714–718.
19. Wendell-Smith CP. Studies on the Morphology of the Pelvic Floor. Ph.D. Thesis. University of London, 1967.
20. Milligan ETC, Morgan CN. Surgical anatomy of the anal canal: With special reference to anorectal fistulae. Lancet 1934; 2:1150–1156.
21. Shafik A. A new concept of the anatomy of the anal sphincter mechanism and the physiology of defecation III. The longitudinal anal muscle: Anatomy and role in sphincter mechanism. Invest Urol 1976; 13:271–277.
22. Lawson JON. Pelvic anatomy II. Anal canal and associated sphincters. Ann R Coll Surg Engl 1974; 54:288–300.
23. Roux C. Contribution to the knowledge of the anal muscles in man. Arch MikrAnat 1881; 19:721–723.
24. Courtney H. Anatomy of the pelvic diaphragm and anorectal musculature as related to sphincter preservation in anorectal surgery. Am J Surg 1950; 79:155–173.
25. Goligher JC, Leacock AG, Brossy JJ. The surgical anatomy of the anal canal. Br J Surg 1955; 43:51–61.
26. Oh C, Kark AE. Anatomy of the external anal sphincter. Br J Surg 1972; 59:717–723.
27. Miller R, Bartolo DCC, Cervero F, et al. Anorectal sampling: A comparison of normal and incontinent patients. Br J Surg 1988; 75:44–47.
28. Paramore RH. The Hunterian lectures on the evolution of the pelvic floor in non-mammalian vertebrates and pronograde mammals. Lancet 1910; 1:1393–1399, 1459–1467.
29. Percy JP, Swash M, Neill ME, et al. Electrophysiological study of motor nerve supply of pelvic floor. Lancet 1981; 1:16–17.
30. Russell KP. Anatomy of the pelvic floor, rectum and anal canal. In: Smith LE. Practical guide to anorectal testing. New York: Ygaku-Shoin Medical Publishers, Inc., 1991:744–747.
31. Ayoub SF. Arterial supply of the human rectum. Acta Anat 1978; 100:317–327.
32. Didio LJA, Diaz-Franco C, Schemainda R, et al. Morphology of the middle rectal arteries: A study of 30 cadaveric dissections. Surg Radiol Anat 1986; 8:229–236.
33. Michels NA, Siddharth P, Kornblith PL, et al. The variant blood supply to the small and large intestines: Its importance in regional resections. A new anatomic study based on four hundred dissections with a complete review of the literature. J Int Col Surg 1963; 39:127–170.
34. Bernstein WC. What are hemorrhoids and what is their relationship to the portal venous system? Dis Colon Rectum 1983; 26:829–834.
35. Miscusi G, Masoni L, Dell'Anna A, et al. Normal lymphatic drainage of the rectum and the canal anal revealed by lymphoscintigraphy. Coloproctology 1987; 9:171–174.
36. Block IR, Enquist IF. Studies pertaining to local spread of carcinoma of the rectum in females. Surg Gynecol Obstet 1961; 112:41–46.
37. Gerstenberg TC, Nielsen ML, Clausen S, et al. Bladder function after abdominoperineal resection of the rectum for anorectal cancer. Am J Surg 1980; 91:81–86.
38. Orkin BA. Rectal carcinoma: Treatment. In: Beck DE, Wexner SD, eds. Fundamentals of Anorectal Surgery. New York: McGraw-Hill, Inc., chapter 18, 1992:260–369.
39. Weinstein M, Roberts M. Sexual potency following surgery for rectal carcinoma. A followup of 44 patients. Ann Surg 1977; 185:295–300.
40. Danzi M, Ferulano GP, Abate S, et al. Male sexual function after abdominoperineal resection for rectal cancer. Dis Colon Rectum 1983; 26:665–668.
41. Balslev I, Harling H. Sexual dysfunction following operation for carcinoma of the rectum. Dis Colon Rectum 1983; 26:785–795.
42. Bauer JJ, Gerlent IM, Salky B, et al. Sexual dysfunction following proctectomy for benign disease of the colon and rectum. Ann Surg 1983; 197:363–367.
43. Walsh PC, Schlegel PN. Radical pelvic surgery with preservation of sexual function. Ann Surg 1988; 208:391–400.
44. Lee ECG, Dowling BL. Perimuscular excision of the rectum for Crohn's disease and ulcerative colitis. A conservative technique. Br J Surg 1972; 59:29–32.
45. Metcalf AM, Dozois RR, Kelly KA. Sexual function in women after proctocolectomy. Ann Surg 1986; 204:624–627.
46. Burnham WR, Lennard-Jones JE, Brooke BN. Sexual problems among married ileostomists. Gut 1977; 18:673–677.
47. Petter O, Gruner N, Reidar N, et al. Marital status and sexual adjustment after colectomy. Scand J Gastrol 1977; 12:193–197.

3 Anorectal Physiology

Sherief Shawki and Dana R. Sands
Department of Colorectal Surgery, Cleveland Clinic Florida, Weston, Florida, U.S.A.

INTRODUCTION

Anorectal physiology is complex and relies on a delicate interplay of the neuromuscular function and structural integrity of the pelvic floor. Alterations in pelvic floor physiology result in an increasing number of visits to colorectal surgeons from patients complaining of functional disorders. It has been estimated that more than four million people complain of constipation every year, representing a prevalence rate of 2% of the total population. This is associated with more than 3 million prescriptions, and over 200 million spent, for cathartics and over-the-counter laxatives (1). Conversely, fecal incontinence is estimated to occur in more than 6.5 million Americans with a prevalence of up to 11% (2).

While the spectrum of disease is often not life-threatening, pelvic floor pathology has a significant impact on quality of life. The physician with a comprehensive understanding of anorectal physiology and the available diagnostic modalities will be able to offer relief to many patients with an accurate diagnosis and appropriate therapeutic recommendations.

Determination of the etiology of constipation, fecal incontinence, rectal prolapse, and anorectal pain can be facilitated in the anorectal physiology laboratory. Often, the cause of functional disorders is multifactorial. Physiologic testing after a careful history and physical examination can provide the physician with the needed insight to offer the most effective treatment regimen.

This chapter will present the most widely used diagnostic modalities with emphasis on their underlying principle, technique, interpretation, and clinical application.

ANORECTAL MANOMETRY

Background and Basic Concepts

Since the classic experiments of Denny-Brown and Robertson (3) in 1935, explaining the mechanisms underlying human defecation based on a manometric study, anorectal manometry (ARM) has become widely used for studying anorectal functional disorders (3). Measurements are obtained by inserting a pressure-sensitive device into the anal canal, which is connected via a nondistended tubing system to a transducer. The transducer transforms the pressure signals into electronic ones that are transformed and processed through an amplifier and subsequently presented as measurements (4).

Instrumentation

There are three basic systems used to perform ARM: Fluid or air-filled balloon systems, Water perfused systems, and Microtransducers.

Fluid or Air-Filled Balloon Systems

In 1965, Schuster et al. (5) described a method for measuring anal sphincter pressures. The air-filled balloon device consisted of a latex balloon was tied around a hollow cylinder, through which another balloon could be passed, thus creating two compartments. Both of the balloons are connected to pressure transducers (5). After placing the probe in the anal canal, one balloon is in the region of the internal anal sphincter (IAS) while the other is encircled by the superficial portion of the external sphincter (EAS).

Although, theoretically, both regions of the anal sphincter could be separately assessed, the considerable overlap of both IAS and EAS does not allow this method to accurately differentiate the two sphincters. Therefore, the pressure readings obtained represent the sum of all forces acting upon the balloon (4).

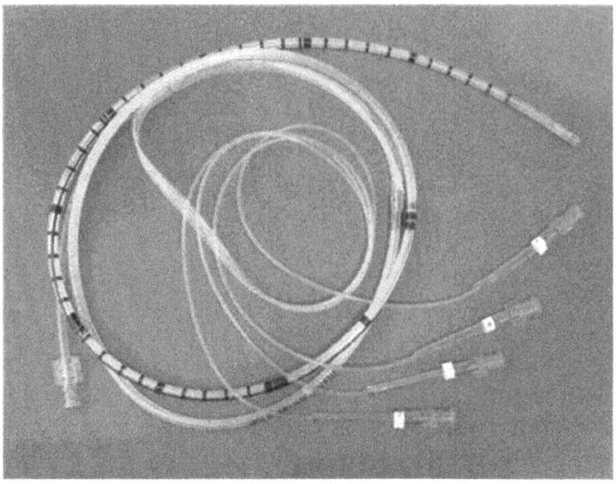

Figure 1 Four-channel water-perfused manometry catheter.

Since the size of the catheter introduced into the anal canal can alter the sphincter tone, which in turn results in artifactual distortion of the resting pressure, the smaller the size of the catheter the more accurate the results (6). However, smaller catheters allow a relatively smaller area of the anal canal to be measured (7). The pressure distribution inside the anal canal is asymmetric along its longitudinal as well as radial axes. As the pressure increases gradually from proximal to distal, there are unequal forces acting from each sidewall. The balloon system does not take into account the radial asymmetry of the anal canal sphincter and recording regions are restricted to two regions—the upper and lower anal canal.

Air or water can be used to distend the balloon, but since air is distensible, using water provides lower variation in pressure measurements. This requires complete evacuation of air bubbles to avoid damping of the recorded pressures, which can be a challenging task (3).

Water-Perfused Systems

Water-perfused systems are the most commonly used in North America and are considered reliable methods for performing ARM (Fig. 1) (8). Originally, developed by Arndorfer et al. (9) in the late 1970s for esophageal manometry, the principle of this method depends on continuous water flow in a constant rate through the catheter. By means of measuring the resistance to this water outflow exerted by the surrounding anal sphincters, pressures can be eventually recorded (Fig. 2) (10).

While the catheter is properly situated inside the rectum, there is a potential space between the catheter and the anal canal wall. Once this space is filled by perfusate, the water flows cephalad toward the rectum or outside the anal canal. The pressure required to overcome the initial resistance after the space has been filled is termed the "yield pressure" (4,11,12).

A constant flow rate, usually 0.3 mL/channel/min is required to enable the sensors to measure the outflow resistance or pressure (13). The greater the sphincter strength, the more resistance impeding the water flow, the higher the pressure recorded. Low flow rates may interfere with accuracy of detecting pressure changes, whereas high rates are associated with more fluid accumulation in the rectum, which can then affect the reproducibility of the procedure (8,14).

Microtransducers

Microtransducers have a fixed location on the anorectal probe, from which measurements are provided with respect to radial pressures. The use of microtransducers is convenient as they

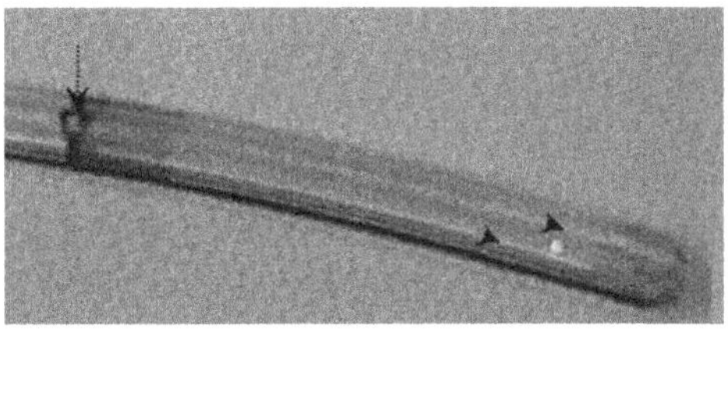

Figure 2 Tip of the catheter showing one of the four openings for the water outflow (*arrow*) and two of the channels (*arrow heads*).

are easy to set up and calibrate. They require the use of relatively small-size catheters, thus minimizing the amount of artifactual stimulation, and there is no water leak. Since there is no hydraulic transmission, pressures measured are thought to be more accurate than those from perfused catheters. (3,4) Furthermore, microtransducers eliminate concerns regarding positioning, thereby allowing ambulatory measurements and recordings to be taken in the sitting position, creating a more physiologic evaluation. Drawbacks associated with these transducers, however, are that they are expensive and very fragile, and require handling with great amount of care (15–17).

Manometry Catheters

Sleeve catheters consist of a thin silastic membrane adhered to a catheter formed of a silastic tube with a second tube formed on one side. Water flows between the two silastic interfaces along the sphincter, thus any resistance to the water flow would be recorded in terms of pressure (4,18). As with the balloons system, sleeves provide an assessment of the global pressures of the anal canal but cannot provide information regarding pressures at a specific location within the sphincter complex.

Water-perfused catheters are the most commonly used. The outer diameter of the catheter ranges from 4 to 8 mm, which helps reduce the artifactual distortion from larger catheters when inserted into the anal canal. While rigid catheters are easy to insert and orient in the anal canal, the more flexible catheters cause less distortion (8).

The commonly used catheters have multiple channels, ranging from 2 to 8 mm with the channel ports opening on the side of the catheter. These openings can be displayed in a radial or a stepwise pattern.

Catheters are irrigated with sterile water and are connected to a transducer via a low compliance, nondistensible capillary tubing system. This feature is important for transmitting any small pressure changes occurring inside the anal canal. Unlike microtransducers, water-perfused catheters cannot be used in an ambulatory setting as any movements of the patient will result in considerable pressure artifacts (4).

Measurements

Resting Pressure

Resting pressure represents the sphincter tone during the resting state, which is produced mainly by the IAS. This is a smooth muscle, which is in a state of continuous involuntary contraction as a result of both intrinsic myogenic and extrinsic autonomic supply, and it provides a natural barrier to the involuntary loss of stool (19).

The IAS is responsible of 50% to 85% of the resting tone, while the EAS accounts for 25% to 30%. This extra pressure is essential to minimize voluntary attention to the anal sphincters. Finally, anal cushion expansion makes up the remaining 5% to 15%, which seems to be essential for perfect anal control (19–22). As pressure increases gradually in anal canal from proximal to distal, the highest resting pressure is recorded generally 1 to 2 cm proximal to the anal verge. This corresponds anatomically to the condensation of distal fibers of the IAS.

The mean anal canal resting pressure in healthy volunteers is generally in the range of 50 to 70 mmHg. This is lower in women as well as in the elderly (Fig. 3) (8,23,24).

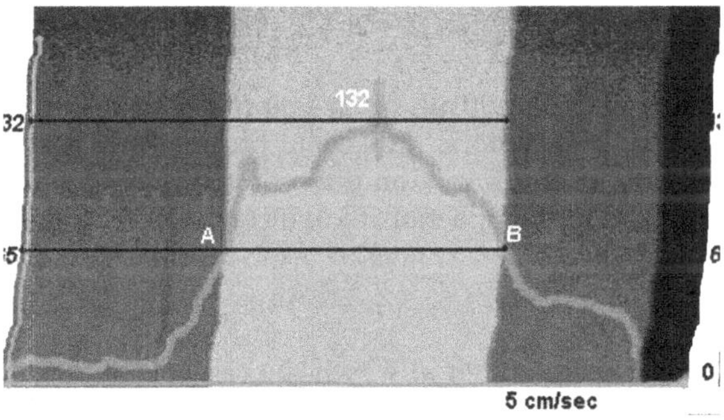

Figure 3 Schematic representation of a "resting" pressure. Points A and B represent the 50% of maximum pressure. Distance A–B represents "high pressure zone."

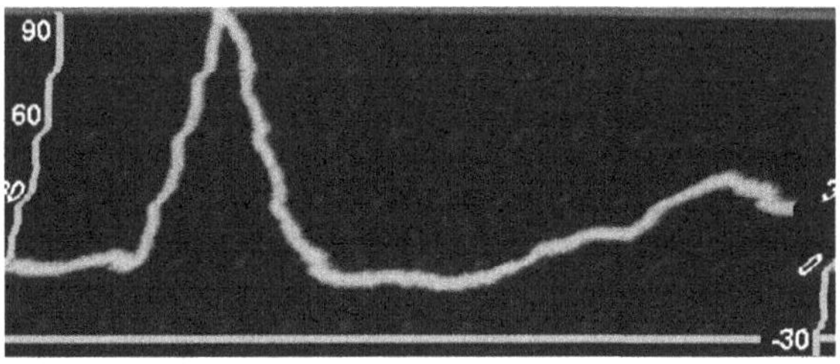

Figure 4 Typical rectoanal inhibitory reflex (RAIR). *Note*: Ascending curve represents the EAS contraction followed by pronounced relaxation of the internal anal sphincter.

Squeeze Pressure

Squeeze pressure is the result of voluntary contraction of the EAS and puborectalis muscles. During maximal squeeze contractions, intra-anal pressures usually reach two to three times their baseline values (100–180 mm Hg), which can be maintained for about 40 to 60 seconds because of the muscle fatigue that occurs afterward. However, the EAS undergoes reflex contraction in response to rectal distension, increased intra-abdominal pressure, and posture alteration. This mechanism prevents leakage during such activities as coughing (25–27).

High Pressure Zone

The high pressure zone (HPZ) is defined as the length of the IAS in which the pressures are greater than half of the maximum pressure at rest. (28) Using this definition, the HPZ will always be at least 1 cm, which could be inaccurate in patients with a patulous anus (29). Alternatively, the HPZ can be defined as that zone which is bounded caudally by a rise in pressure of 20 mm Hg and cephalad by a decrease in pressure of 20 mm Hg in at least 50% of the circumference of the anal canal (Fig. 3). This latter definition may present a more accurate picture of the sphincters in incontinent patients, as pressures are so low that there is no true HPZ. The length of the HPZ is generally about 2 to 3 cm in women and 2.5 to 3.5 cm in men (8,29,30).

Rectoanal Inhibitory Reflex

The Rectoanal Inhibitory Reflex (RAIR) is defined as a transient contraction of the EAS followed by pronounced reflex relaxation of the IAS in response to rectal distension. The RAIR is normally evoked with as little as 10 to 30 mL distension of the rectum, and the response is usually maximal at 40 to 60 mL. (8) This reflex, which was initially described by Gowers in 1877 (17) and subsequently by Denny-Brown and Robertson in 1935, is believed to enable rectal contents to reach the highly sensitive area of the anal mucosa. This "sampling" mechanism provides accurate distinction between fluid, flatus, and feces and has an important role in the fine adjustment of anal continence (Fig. 4) (3,29).

Impaired anal sensation is correlated with childbirth, perineal descent syndrome, and prior transanal mucosectomy. Patients with Hirschsprung's disease, Chagas' disease, dermatomyositis, and scleroderma all have abnormal RAIR (31,32). Failure to induce a reflex at any volume is strong evidence for Hirschsprung's disease (33,34).

Chagas' disease is an endemic protozoan infection in certain rural areas in South America. It is caused by the parasite Trypanosoma cruzi, which destructs the nerve cells of the autonomic enteric nervous plexus. In patients with Chagas' disease, the IAS relaxation is absent and, instead, a contraction is occasionally observed. (35,36)

Patients with dermatomyositis have normal IAS relaxation but no EAS contraction; conversely, patients with scleroderma have no IAS relaxation but normal EAS contraction (8).

Sensory Threshold

Rectal sensation is usually achieved when between 10 and 20 mL of air is introduced into the intrarectal balloon. The rectum itself does not have receptors; rather, the proprioceptors are probably located in the levators, puborectalis, and IAS and EAS. Conditions in which conscious sensation of rectal fullness is reduced might result in fecal impaction, fecal incontinence, or both (8,37).

Rectal Capacity

Rectal capacity is the maximum volume that can be tolerated at which the call of defecation cannot be further delayed. Normal capacity usually ranges from 100 to 300 mL. Rectal capacity tends to be higher in younger and constipated patients, and is generally lower in the elderly and in patients with fecal incontinence (8).

Rectal Compliance

When defecation must be delayed, the rectal contents have to be accommodated. This deferral of stool is achieved through the mechanism of rectal compliance, which enables the rectum, by means of its viscous and elastic properties, to maintain a low pressure while being filled, thus continence is not threatened. The compliance of the normal rectum ranges from 2 to 6 mL H_2O per mmHg (8). However, great variation in rectal capacity and compliance can occur. This can be attributed to the method used, balloon compliance, and rate of balloon inflation.

Normal rectal compliance appears to depend on the intrinsic nervous system and viable muscles. Therefore, rectal compliance is impaired in diseases such as ulcerative colitis, Hirschsprung's disease, and radiation proctitis (38,39). Measuring rectal compliance is not a diagnostic test. Instead, it supplements other investigations while evaluating the pathophysiology of anorectal disease. For example, in a patient with radiation proctitis and fecal incontinence, it is important to distinguish whether the incontinence is due to loss of reservoir function of the rectum or due to diminished anal tones; similarly, the presence of abnormally high compliance in a patient with constipation can reflect a sensory element in the outlet obstruction (8).

Other Measured Variables During Manometry

Cough Reflex Test

This test evaluates the change in anal canal pressure in response to any sudden change in intra-abdominal pressure. Anal pressure should raise secondary to any increase in intra-abdominal pressure in order to preserve continence.

Pressures During Attempted Defecation

Normally during defecation there is an increase in intrarectal pressure associated with a decrease in intra-anal pressure. However, with the presence of paradoxical contraction of the puborectalis or absent/incomplete relaxation of the anal sphincters, this physiological decrease in anal canal pressures may not occur. (3)

Technique of Manometric Evaluation

There are two main methods of performing ARM: stationary pull-through and continuous pull-through.

While the patient is in the left lateral decubitus position, the catheter is inserted to 6 cm inside the rectum. After insertion of the catheter, it is important to wait for approximately 20 to 30 seconds before starting the test. This gives the IAS a chance to recover from the initial stimulus, thus avoiding artifactual measurements as well as allowing the potential space between the anal canal and catheter to fill with water and reach the yield pressure (3).

Subsequently, various wave patterns may be observed on the monitor. This demonstrates some intrinsic activity that is attributable primarily to the IAS. These patterns are described in Table 1.

Table 1 Manometric Wave Patterns

Wave pattern	Finding	Frequency	Amplitude	Description
Slow waves	Most frequently observed	10 to 20 cycles/min	Small amplitude	Identified in the region between cephalic end of the sphincter and the area of max resting pressure (40,41)
Ultraslow wave	Second most common	0.5 to 1.5 cycles/min	Large amplitude	Seen in region of max average resting pressure Usually found in patients with high resting tones (42,43)
Intermediate wave	Least frequent	4 to 8 cycles/min	Moderate amplitude	Noted in neurogenic FI, after IPAA (42,43)

Stationary Pull-Through Method

In the stationary pull-through method, the patient is asked to actively perform a maximum squeeze effort followed by a period of rest. This is repeated at 5 further points, at 1 cm increments and directed caudally toward the anal verge. In this way, rest and squeeze pressures are obtained over the entire length of the anal sphincter. From these measurements mean resting and squeeze pressures, and the HPZ can be calculated (29).

The catheter is then positioned at 2 cm from the anal verge and the balloon is inflated with 30 mL of air over two to three seconds in order to elicit the RAIR. In some cases, especially those patients with megarectum and decreased anal sensation, higher volumes are required to induce the reflex. The air is then removed and, with the balloon in the same position, re-insufflated with 40 mL, 50 mL, or higher, until a reflex is obtained. If the reflex is still undetectable, the test can be repeated with the catheter positioned 3 cm from anal verge.

In our laboratory, we record only the presence or absence of the reflex. Other parameters are sometimes calculated including duration of the reflex, percentage of excitation, and latency of excitation (8). The catheter is subsequently reinserted to 6 cm (positioning the balloon in the rectal ampulla) and the balloon is filled with core temperature water at a rate of 1 mL/sec.

The first sensation the patient perceives is recorded as the first sensation (minimal sensory volume) and the mean intraballoon pressure is noted at this volume. The balloon is continuously filled until the maximum tolerable volume is reached. This volume is recorded again with the intraballoon pressure. Using theses variables, the rectal compliance can be calculated as ($\Delta V / \Delta P$) (29).

Continuous Pull-Through Method

In the continuous pull-through method, the equipment includes a motor that results in automated continuous withdrawal of the catheter rather than manually pulling it out. The addition of computerized software helps calculate all the measurements and presents the data in a predesigned form.

Measuring Cough Reflex

In this maneuver, the patient is asked to cough or to blow up a balloon while the pressures in the rectal ampulla and in the anal canal are measured. This is done by calculating the difference between the baseline and the highest intraluminal pressure in both the rectum and anal canal. Normally, these pressures should show considerable increment compared to the resting state (3).

Measuring Pressure During Attempted Defecation

While the catheter is situated inside the anal canal, the patient is asked to bear down in an attempt to defecate and the changes in pressures are observed. Normally there should be a drop in these pressures; however, in cases of dyssynergia, pressures may stay the same or even increase, indicating paradoxical puborectalis contraction.

Potential Pitfalls

Considerable water accumulation in the rectum may occur in the lengthy water-perfused method, which is associated with false observations. This can be avoided by controlling the perfusion rate (usually 0.3 mL/channel/min) (8) or in the case of an extended examination, the patient is asked to evacuate the accumulated rectal contents. (4) Air in the water-perfused channel system may result in a considerable change in pressure interception by the transducers. Adequate perfusion of the system before examination will help avoid this problem.

If close apposition between the catheter and the anal canal is not present, which is important for establishing a continuous column of fluid, then no resistance to the flow of water will be detected with subsequent lowered pressures. This is clinically important during the assessment of patients with rectal prolapse and patulous anus or in patients who have had surgery for imperforate anus. A larger catheter may help to avoid this problem.

Technical errors may result in the false absence of RAIR. Presence of stool in the rectum may interfere with proper placement of the balloon as well as inflation of the balloon. In a patient with a megarectum, more volume is required to inflate the balloon in order to cause rectal distension and induce a reflex. A leaking balloon may not distend the rectum enough to elicit a reflex.

Patients with fecal incontinence often use accessory muscles to accommodate for poor sphincter function, thus falsely elevated squeeze pressures can arise from gluteal muscle contraction (3).

Clinical Application

There is no doubt that physical examination is an important step in the evaluation of anorectal functional disorders; however, manometry seems to provide more accurate and essential information which promotes objective therapeutic decisions (40,41). It has been demonstrated that digital examination does not always correlate well with objective measurements of sphincter function (42). In addition, it has been shown that the specificity, sensitivity, and predictive values of digital examination with respect to the estimation of normal resting and squeeze pressures are less than optimal (43).

ARM is widely implemented in the assessment of common anorectal functional conditions such as chronic constipation and fecal incontinence. It can provide a baseline for comparison with functional results after surgical treatment as well as objective evidence of improvement in continence (41). It has been shown that improvement in HPZ of 57%, squeeze pressure of 71%, and resting tone of 79% is correlated with good functional results (42). Although ARM is not accepted as routine prior to all colon and anorectal procedures, it should be considered prior to procedures which may jeopardize anal sphincter function and threaten continence, such as low colorectal, coloanal, and ileoanal procedures.

ELECTROMYOGRAPHY

Background and Basic Concepts

The first recorded human electrical activity was obtained from a human forearm muscle by Piper in 1908. At that time, a string galvanometer was used to detect the electrical activity. In 1929, Adrian and Bronck devised the concentric needle electrode, which was followed by successful recording of anal sphincter electromyography (EMG) by Beck in 1930. Since that time, anal EMG was further developed and widely used to assess the functional activity of the pelvic floor (44).

Anal EMG entails observing and recording the electrical activity from the striated muscle fibers constituting the EAS and puborectalis muscles at rest and during voluntary contraction, simulated defecation, and various reflexes. In general, electrical activity can be measured from individual fibers, or more commonly, from a group of muscle fibers as part of a motor unit which is composed of the anterior horn cell, its axon and terminal branches, and the muscle fibers supplied by it.

In order to detect an electrical activity, an action potential must occur. As nerve impulses move down the axon reaching the neuromuscular end plate, this results in depolarization of the muscle fibers (i.e., an electrical activity which can be recorded during EMG). This electrical activity is known as motor unit potential (MUP). Anal EMG can be used for mapping the electrical activity of the EAS muscle fibers providing information about its integrity in incontinent patients or about its functionality when evaluating pelvic floor function in patients suffering from constipation.

With the exception of the cricopharyngeal muscle and the paraspinous muscle, the EAS and the levator complex are the only striated muscles in tonic contraction. Histological studies have shown that these muscles have a predominance of type I fibers which are characteristic of skeletal muscles of tonic contractile activity (8,19).

The EAS tone is mediated by a low sacral reflex arc at the level of the cauda equine during waking hours; however, during sleep it is significantly reduced although still present (45). This tone is increased in response to distension of the rectum or urinary bladder, change in body position, cough or physical activity, and finally to anal scratch and bulbocavernosus stimulation (44). EMG activity should normally cease during defecation as both the puborectalis and EAS relax allowing evacuation of the rectal contents. MUPs recorded during EMG are usually biphasic or triphasic; however, polyphasic potentials with four or more phases may be observed in normal sphincters in between 7% and 25% of individuals (46,47).

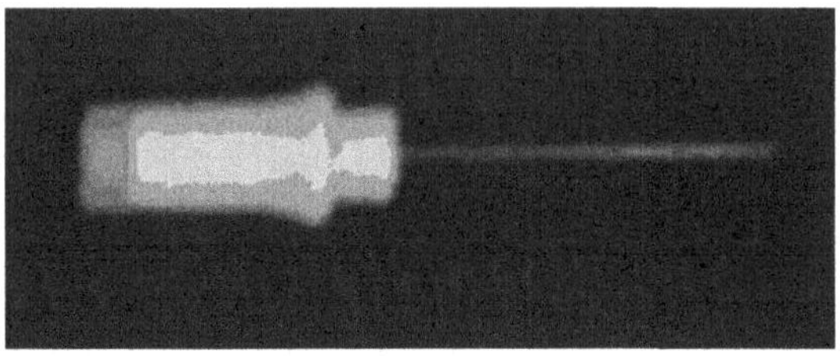

Figure 5 Disposable concentric needle.

Instrumentation and Technique

The instrumentation required for EMG evaluation includes recording electrodes, preamplifier, amplifier, oscilloscope for display of the electrical activity, and a loudspeaker to provide an audible signal that correlates with the level of EMG activity. Modern EMG equipment is associated with computer software that allows analysis and provides more detailed information regarding amplitude and time-based duration of a wave. There are four different techniques used to record pelvic floor electrical activity.

Single-Fiber EMG

A single-fiber EMG electrode consists of a needle that is slightly less than 0.1 mm in diameter, filled with resin, and allows an electrode of 25 um to project through it. A separate surface electrode is required for grounding (8). Single-fiber EMG can detect electrical activity and record single MUPs, thus allowing calculation of fiber density and neuromuscular jitter. By obtaining 20 different measurements in each half of the sphincter, fiber density is calculated as the mean number of single muscle fiber action potentials in each position. The mean normal fiber density is 1.5 ± 0.6. The neuromuscular jitter is the time interval between two consecutive action potentials in a single motor unit detected in the uptake area of a single-fiber EMG (44,48,49). Although this parameter is a reflection of the variability of impulse transmission across the neuromuscular end plate, its clinical relevance is unclear.

Concentric Needle EMG

The concentric needle was first designed by Adrian and Bronck in 1929 and consisted of 0.1 mm steel wire surrounded by resin insulation from the outer thin-pointed cannula (Fig. 5). The concentric needle EMG can detect electrical activity in a small area that includes several motor units; therefore, it cannot identify individual muscle fiber action potential. While concentric needle can provide objective data on sphincter integrity, reinnervation, and is useful in sphincter mapping, it is a painful procedure for patients and is often difficult to undergo follow-up evaluation using the same technique (8,29,44,49).

Surface Anal Plug EMG

As a result of the pain and discomfort associated with needle electrodes, in 1988, O'Donnell and his colleagues (50) used surface electrodes during studying the electrical activity of the EAS. The relatively inaccurate recordings as a result of electrical interference from the other adjacent muscles as well as the difficulty in assessment of surface electrodes prompted the development of disposable anal plug electrodes (Fig. 6) (50).

These are plastic or sponge plugs that consist of two longitudinal or circular electrodes mounted on their surfaces. The former is considered superior since longitudinal electrodes correlate better with fine-wire electrodes (44,51). Although surface plugs can be easily inserted inside the anal canal and hence are much more tolerable by the patients, they provide only generalized information about the sphincter.

It has been shown that surface electrodes have good correlation with concentric needle electrodes in the diagnosis of paradoxical anal sphincter contractions. As a consequence, they are useful in evaluating patients with constipation, especially those with muscle discoordination. Surface plugs, however, cannot provide adequate data when sphincter mapping is essential for assessment of patients with fecal incontinence (52).

Monopolar Wire Electrode EMG

In 1973, Basmajian introduced a thin Teflon-coated silver wire monopolar electrode with a hook at its tip to help secure the electrode in place. As the Teflon is removed 4 mm from the tip,

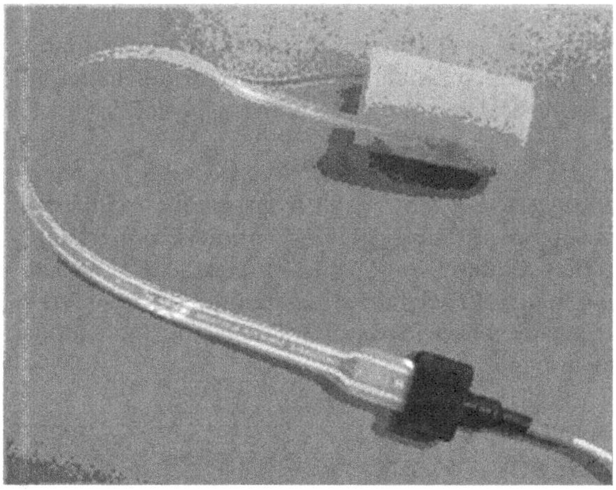

Figure 6 Anal plug for surface EMG.

the electrode is inserted under the guidance of a lumbar puncture needle. An electrocardiogram electrode, used as a ground electrode, is applied to the patient's back (44). Monopolar wire electrodes have been shown to be of especially beneficial in the diagnosis of paradoxical puborectalis contraction (53,54).

Findings and Interpretation

Since the EAS has a continuous simultaneous tone, a constant baseline EMG activity should be observed while recording at rest (Fig. 7) (46).

During maximum contraction and induced reflexes such as cough, more electrical activity appears in the form of higher wave frequencies and amplitudes; however, this activity disappears or is significantly reduced during feigned defecation. Wave amplitude varies depending on the number of discharging fibers in the motor unit and the distance from the electrode; therefore, amplitude values are not reliable for comparative purposes (47).

In patients with paradoxical contraction or nonrelaxing puborectalis, the EMG will remain unchanged or even increase during attempted defecation (55–58). Damage of the anal sphincter muscle results in scarring that is characterized histologically by the presence of scattered hypertrophied muscle fibers surrounded by fibrous and adipose tissue. This results in decreased motor units and a marked decrease in MUPs at rest, during squeeze, and at reflex elicitation (59,60).

In case of severe injury to the nerve supply of a muscle, some or all of the fibers become atrophic due to denervation, which is observed as absent electrical activity and a silent audible signal. Incomplete injury initiates reinnervation through regeneration of the damaged axons or through sprouting of nearby unaffected axons. This latter process results in redistribution of the muscle fibers within the motor unit with clustering of fibers supplied by a single motor neuron; this process is known as fiber-type grouping (44). These immature nerve fibers are slow conductors of nerve impulses and in addition to the subsequent new distribution of injured muscle fibers among motor units, results in motor potentials of increased amplitude and prolonged duration associated with increased polyphasic potentials (46,59–61).

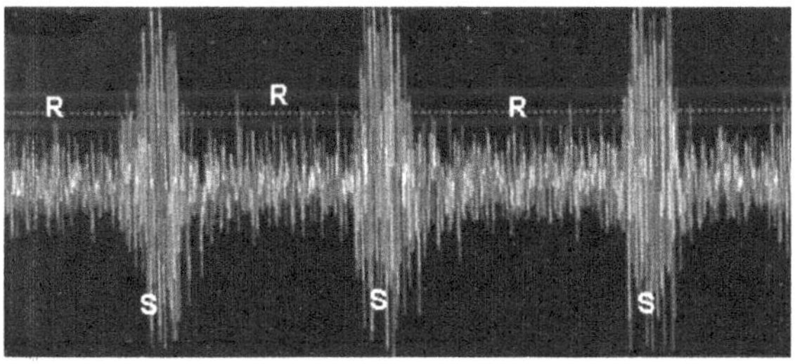

Figure 7 An electromyographic tracing taken by concentric needle during squeeze. *Note*: the pre- and postsqueeze electrical activity.

Clinical Application and Indications

Clinically, EMG can provide both quantitative as well as objective information in the evaluation of functional anorectal disorders. It has been proven that EMG has an important role in sphincter mapping in the assessment of patients with fecal incontinence with suspected sphincter damage (62).

Constipation may be caused by functional pelvic outlet obstruction secondary to nonrelaxing or paradoxical contraction of the puborectalis, or may result from colonic inertia. It is important to distinguish between both causes before any surgical intervention is contemplated (40,63,64). EMG can objectively identify and detect nonrelaxation and/or paradoxical contractions of the puborectalis as either no change or increased MUPs during attempted feigned defecation, respectively (55,56). Anal EMG is also considered as an important tool in the biofeedback retraining of paradoxical puborectalis contraction (44).

PUDENDAL NERVE TERMINAL MOTOR LATENCY

Background and Basic Concepts

The EAS is supplied by the pudendal nerve (S2, S3, and S4) and its assessment is considered to be an important component in the evaluation of patients with fecal incontinence. Based on Brendley's technique for electro-ejaculation (65), in 1984 Kiff and Swash (66) introduced a device that combined stimulating and recording electrodes. This was followed by the development of a simple disposable model by Rogers and associates (67). Assessment includes evaluating the time taken from stimulation of the nerve to the onset of muscle depolarization; alternatively, it can be described as the time consumed for transmitting an impulse via the pudendal nerve to the beginning of the action potential of the motor units. The combination of neurophysiological tests, EMG and PNTML, provides objective evidence relative to the neuromuscular integrity of the EAS.

Instrumentation and Technique

Electrode

The St Mark's electrode (Figs. 8 and 9), used universally, is a disposable thin elastic strip of plastic with adhesive surface to be placed on the volar aspect of the gloved index finger of the examiner's hand. It has two stimulating electrodes, representing an anode and a cathode, at the tip and another two recording electrodes about 4 cm apart at the base. This design allows the electrodes to sit on the tip and on the base of the examiner's finger, respectively.

Electromyographic Equipment

The EMG unit provides the electrical source for delivering a 50-volt square-wave stimulus of 0.1 milliseconds in duration. An amplifier is also needed to record the obtained electrical activity.

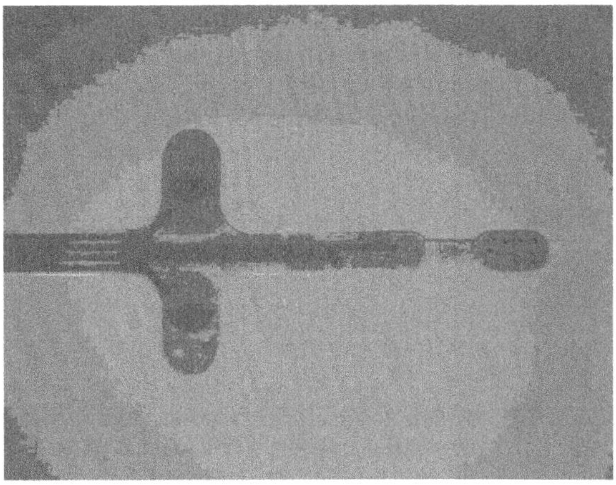

Figure 8 St Mark's electrode.

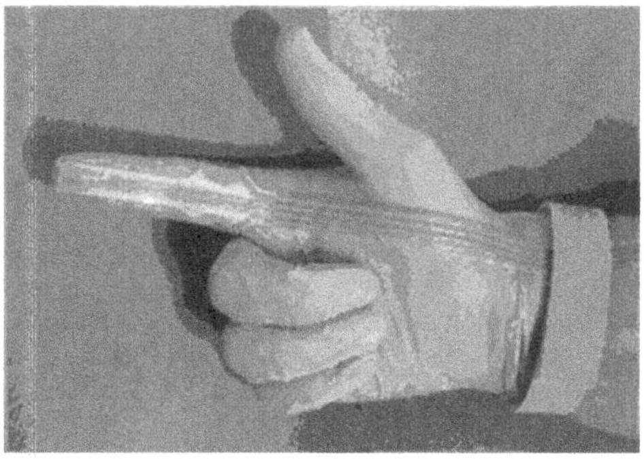

Figure 9 St Mark's electrode mounted to the examiner's index finger.

A foot switch enables controlling the timing of delivering the electrical stimulus in coordination with the examiner's finger position intrarectally.

Technique

While the patient is grounded and placed in the left lateral position, a gentle rectal examination with a St Mark's electrode mounted to the examiner's gloved hand and localization of the pudendal nerve is performed. This is achieved by aiming the tip of the index finger to the end of coccyx, then turning toward the ischial tuberosity where the nerve is in close proximity to the stimulating electrode. An electrical stimulus starting at 22 to 35 mA to a maximum of 50 mA is delivered while the examiner's fingertip is moved across the pelvic sidewall in order to determine the most appropriate site to assess the nerve latency. This is recognized by observing the MUP amplitude, which can be associated with a coincident EAS contraction felt around the examiner's finger (29).

The time interval from stimulation of the nerve to the beginning of the muscle depolarization is considered to be the nerve terminal motor latency. A normal value is considered to be 2.0 $\pm$ 0.2 milliseconds. Three recordings are taken for each nerve on each side. Prolonged PNTML indicates pudendal neuropathy (Figs. 10 and 11) (68,69).

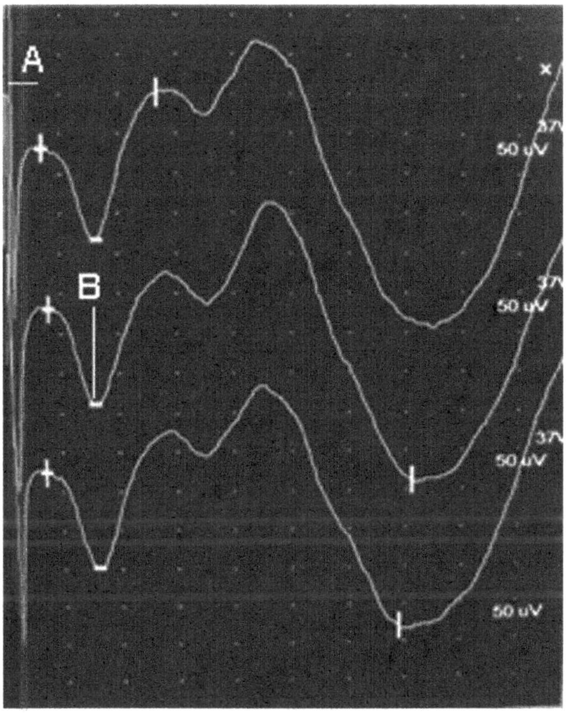

Figure 10 Normal left pudendal nerve terminal motor latency. *Note*: Distance "A" represents the nerve latency time, "+" represents the beginning of muscle depolarization, and distance "B" represents the amplitude of the action potential.

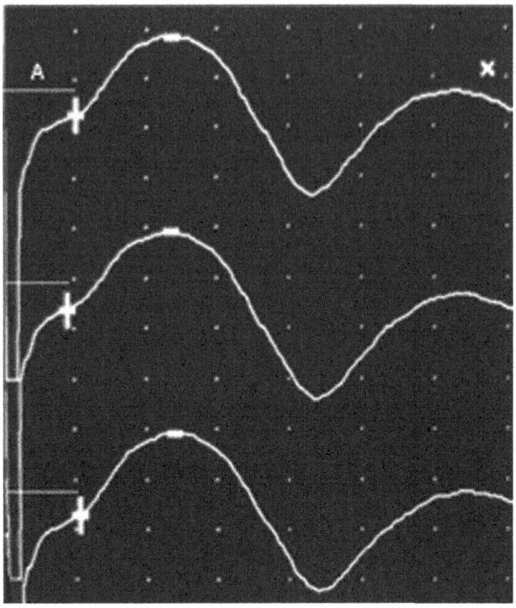

Figure 11 Abnormal right pudendal nerve terminal motor latency. *Note*: The longer distance for the nerve latency and the different direction of the wave.

Clinical Application and Technique

The quantitative assessment of the efficacy of impulse transmission along the pudendal nerve has been shown to provide useful information in patients with fecal incontinence (62,70). Pudendal nerve neuropathy assessment occupies an integral part in the preoperative evaluation for overlapping sphincter repair in patients with fecal incontinence. It has been considered as a predictive factor for the success of overlapping sphincteroplasty.

Furthermore, bilateral functionally normal pudendal nerves have been found to be associated with "good" or "excellent" functional outcome compared to those patients with only unilaterally normal PNTML (71,72). This provides a useful tool in preoperative counseling prior to sphincteroplasty. Abnormal PNTML is usually associated with other pelvic floor disorders such as descending perineal syndrome, rectal prolapse, rectal ulcer, and chronic constipation (73,74).

DEFECOGRAPHY (EVACUATION PROCTOGRAPHY)

Background and Basic Concepts

The fluoroscopic examination of the process of rectal evacuation was first described by Walldén in 1954 (75). Since then, it has been shown that defecography is important in the evaluation of the anatomic causes involved in pelvic floor functional disorders. Defecography helps to provide a better understanding of the different facets involved in disordered defecation (76). The procedure is undertaken in a fluoroscopic suit and the fluoroscopic device should be equipped with an examining table that can be positioned horizontally and vertically, as needed. A videocassette recorder connected to the fluoroscopic output unit is imperative for evaluation of the dynamic process of defecation. Radiation exposure during defecography is considered to be significantly low when compared to barium enema studies (77,78). During a standard examination, a dose of 0.02 to 0.66 cGy and 0.036 to 0.053 cGy will be delivered to the skin of the right hip and to the ovaries, respectively (79). Exposure to radiation can be minimized by reducing the duration of the study and using radiation only when needed (80).

Instrumentation and Technique

Commode

A chair or a commode is needed in order to perform the study in the seated position. It should be radiolucent so that there is no interference with the X-ray beam to the pelvis.

Contrast Media

Approximately 50 mL of barium suspension is required to coat the rectal mucosa and enhance the contrast imagery. Another 250 cc of thick barium sulfate, or less if the patient experiences rectal fullness earlier, is instilled to simulate the presence of stool in the rectum. Other examiners use "home" recipes that help with a thickening effect on the barium sulfate paste (81–83). The vagina is then opacified in order to provide valuable information about the presence of an enterocele.

Technique

In the fluoroscopic unit, while the patient is in the left lateral decubitus position on the examining table with both hips and knees are flexed, the amount of liquid barium is injected into the rectum followed by the paste (29). Some investigators perform additional maneuvers in order to visualize the entire pelvic floor. These include water-soluble contrast or a barium-soaked tampon placed in the vagina, outlining the bladder by introducing a water-soluble contrast via a urinary catheter, or an oral contrast ingested about two hours prior to the study to help delineate an enterocele during the study (84–86).

The patient is then seated on the commode after the fluoroscopic table has been repositioned in the upright position, thus a lateral view of the filled and centered rectum is obtained. The patient is asked to evacuate the rectum completely. Static films are taken at rest, and during squeeze and maximum evacuation. A simultaneous video recording is taken to allow for interpretation of the dynamic process of defecation.

Findings and Interpretations

Measurements

Certain measurements are obtained from the static imaging including the anorectal angle, perineal descent, and puborectalis length. They are measured at rest, squeeze, and push. Calculating the difference between rest and push in each parameter provides a global idea about the dynamics of the pelvic floor during evacuation. Each of these values has a wide range of normal values which rendered comparison among patients and other control groups difficult (29,80).

Anorectal Angle

The anorectal angle (ARA) is defined as the angle between the axis of the rectum and the anal canal. The former is drawn as a line corresponding to the distal half of the distal posterior rectal wall, and the later as a line passing through the anal canal (Figs. 12 and 13) (80,82,87,88).

Others draw the rectal axis through the middle of the rectal ampulla (81,89,90).

The normal range of the resting ARA is between 70 and 140 degrees (82,91,92). However, during evacuation it becomes more obtuse, ranging from 110 to 180 degrees. The ARA becomes more acute during squeeze and ranges from 75 to 90 degrees (81,93,94). It is believed that the

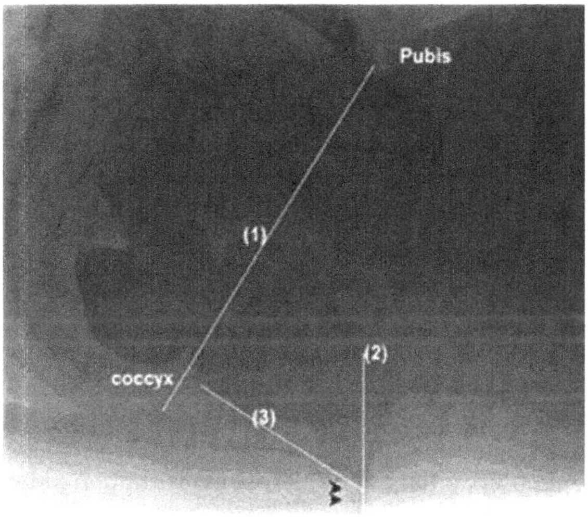

Figure 12 Landmarks used in obtaining measurements from static pictures taken during defecography.
1. Pubococcygeal line
2. Anal Axis
3. Rectal Axis

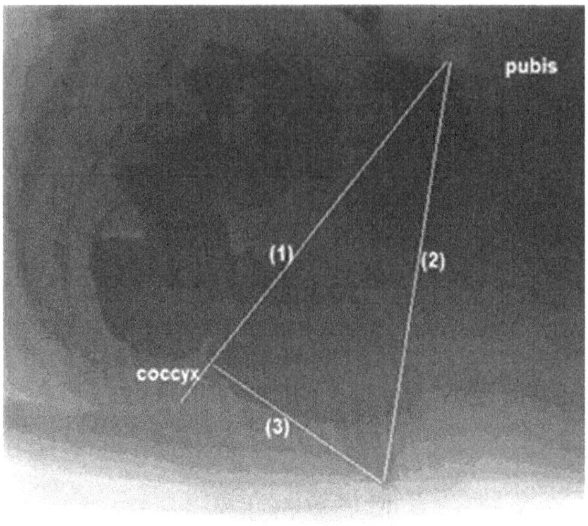

Figure 13 Measurements of:
1. Pubococcygeal line
2. Puborectalis length
3. Perineal descent
4. Arrow head: anorectal angle

ARA is not affected by gender (89,92). These variations in range can be attributed partly to discrepancies in technique and to patient position during the examination. Values are higher in the seated position than in the left lateral decubitus position. However, it is the difference in the ARA observed during rest and push that is more important than the absolute measurement itself (95).

Perineal Descent

Perineal descent (PD) is identified by measuring a line drawn from the anorectal junction perpendicular on the pubococcygeal line. The latter is more representative of the levator ani to the pelvic floor (Fig. 13) (29,80). As such, the normal pelvic floor position is about 1.8 cm below the pubococcygeal line at rest and does not exceed 3 cm during maximal push (82,88,94). Increased PD is considered dynamic when the difference between descent during maximum evacuation and at rest is more than 3 cm. Increased PD is defined as fixed when perineal descent is more than 4 cm at rest (80,94).

Puborectalis Length

Puborectalis length (PRL) is measured as the distance between the pubic symphysis and the anorectal junction (80). The normal resting PRL ranges from 14 to 16 cm, while during squeeze it ranges from 12 to 15 cm, and on maximum push, ranges from 15 to 18 cm (Fig. 13) (28). It has been shown that the disappearance of a prominent puborectalis impression during evacuation and the absence of increased PD at defecography are predictors of good outcome after biofeedback retraining (96,97).

Structural and Anatomic Findings

Normal defecography should demonstrate relaxation, lengthening of the puborectalis, and blunting of its impression. These findings should occur in accordance with symmetrical opening of the anal canal with widening of the ARA. This process takes about four to five seconds and allows the rectal contents to be subsequently evacuated through the anus (98,99). When thickened contrast medium is used, complete evacuation takes about 10 to 12 seconds, and takes less time (8–9 seconds) with softer paste (29,100).

Nonrelaxing Puborectalis

Nonrelaxing puborectalis syndrome was first described by Wassermann in 1964 (101).

Although many theories have been proposed to explain the cause of this problem, the exact etiology remains unknown (80). Proposed theories include muscular dystonia with or without generalized pelvic floor disorder, voluntary suppression of the normal inhibitory reflex, sympathetic nerve abnormalities, and psychological factors (97,102–104). It seems that the behavior theory based upon lack of coordinated relaxation upon the call for defecation is supported by the noticeable improvement after biofeedback retraining (105–107).

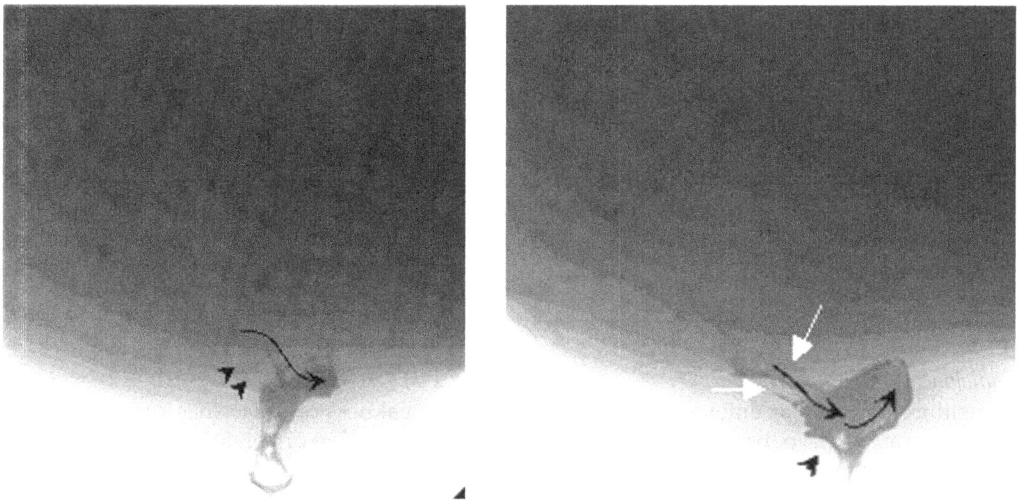

(A) (B)

Figure 14 (**A**) Nonrelaxing puborectalis at the beginning of pushing (*arrow heads*) with "re-direction" of forces to the anterior rectal wall instead of the physiological exit, anal canal. (**B**) Redirection of forces by the nonrelaxing puborectalis results in development of rectocele. *Note*: The association of the rectoanal intussusception (*white arrows*).

Criteria on defecography include persistence of puborectalis impression and failure of opening and widening of the ARA, which may be associated with poor rectal emptying [Fig. 14 (A)] (108).

Parks et al. (97) showed that nonrelaxing syndrome can be considered as of two types, based on defecographic findings. Type A, without persistent puborectalis indentation and with widening of the ARA but with anal canal hypertonia, and Type B in which puborectalis is persistent and ARA does not increase. Whereas biofeedback was successful in treating only 25% of Type A, 86% of Type B showed improvement in response to this mode of therapy (80). A nonrelaxing puborectalis has been observed in normal individuals with normal evacuation; therefore, some tend to treat only those patients whose complaint is outlet obstruction confirmed by other physiologic tests such as EMG and/or defecography (70,105).

Rectocele

Rectocele is a bulging or herniation of the rectal wall into the surrounding structures. It is more common anteriorly than posteriorly and more prevalent in females than in males. This is attributed to female-related factors such as multiparity and difficult vaginal delivery, which can result in weakness of the pelvic floor as well as the rectovaginal septum.

Rectoceles are present in about 70% of normal females. Consequently, an anterior rectocele of 2 cm in size that empties on evacuation is considered normal (29,80,100). However, a rectocele with a maximum diameter of $\geq$4 cm that is not emptying is considered significant if the appropriate symptoms are present (Fig. 15) (94). The fact that a rectocele can occur with other structural findings, such as increased PD, intussusception, colonic inertia, and nonrelaxing puborectalis syndrome, makes it imperative to correlate clinical findings with other concomitant functional disorders prior to establishing rectocele as diagnosis.

Intussusception

Folding of the posterior rectal wall mucosa can be observed in anatomically normal individuals and is considered to be a normal finding during evacuation (109). However, when these infoldings are circumferential, forming a ring pocket of more than 3 mm thickness by invagination of the rectal wall, then a true intussusception exists. Internal rectoanal intussusception is feared as the early phase of rectal prolapse or procidentia. Intussusception may be a significant cause of evacuatory dysfunctions (Fig. 15). As with rectocele, intussusception is usually found in association with a constellation of other structural abnormalities, thus this finding should be interpreted based upon the clinical history [Fig. 14(B)] (80).

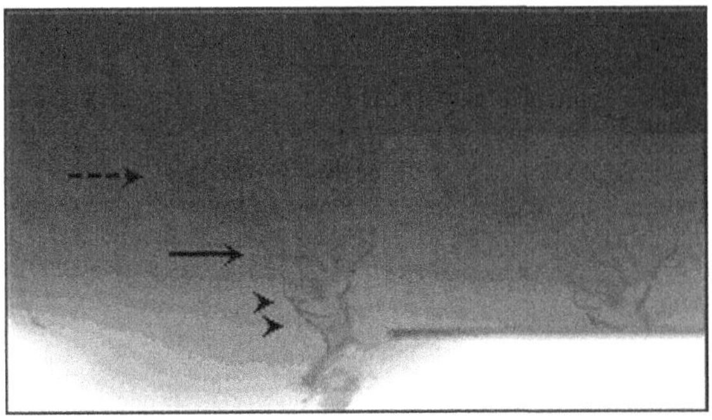

Figure 15 "Significant intussusception." *Note*: Solid arrow shows the intussusception filling the rectal lumen causing outflow obstruction. Arrow heads show normally relaxing puborectalis. Dashed arrow shows residual rectal contents "incomplete evacuation."

Sigmoidocele

Sigmoidocele as well as enterocele is characterized by weakness of the tissues supporting the pelvic floor as well as pelvic organs, also known as pelvic relaxation or pelvic laxity. Based on the extent of descent of the sigmoid loop during maximum straining into the pelvis, sigmoidoceles are graded as first, second, and third degree sigmoidocele (see chap. 12 for full definition) (Fig. 16) (85).

CLINICAL APPLICATIONS AND INDICATIONS

Since defecography is performed in the seated position, which is more closely resembles the correct physiological position for defecation, it offers an accurate assessment of evacuation. It has been proven that defecography is important in evaluating pelvic floor functional disorders, as it enables the assessment of anatomical and structural abnormalities associated with this problem. Paradoxical puborectalis syndrome, sigmoidocele, rectocele, and rectoanal intussusception can all be easily demonstrated on defecography.

As such, it is of particular value in assessing patients with chronic constipation in order to exclude causes of obstructed defecation prior to establishing other diagnoses. This is imperative in patients with colonic inertia. Defecography may be also indicated in patients with suspected solitary rectal ulcer syndrome (92,110,111).

The role of defecography is of less value for assessing fecal incontinence. However, in incontinent patients who have a concomitant history of chronic straining, defecography is helpful to rule out chronic obstruction with overflow incontinence (29,82,89,93,112).

Finally, the incidental finding of a structural abnormality does not necessarily constitute the etiology of the patient's symptoms. Furthermore, some anatomic findings such as a small rectocele and intussusception are considered as variants of normal, and failure of recognizing this fact could result in unnecessary interventions.

TRANSIT STUDIES

Colonic Transit

Constipation is a complex constellation of symptoms including infrequent bowel movements and difficult or incomplete evacuation. When there is no obvious dietary cause, it can be generally stratified to either outlet obstruction or delay in delivery time (colonic transit time). In order to distinguish the exact cause of constipation, colonic transit time should be evaluated.

Historically, transit time was assessed by the ingestion of nonabsorbable materials such as glass or plastic beads, which were collected after defecation or using chemically detectable materials; all these methods were unpleasant for both the patient and the physician and are no longer in use (113–115).

Hinton and Lennard (116) proposed a simple method for assessment. A 5.6 mm diameter radio-opaque tube is cut into 20, 2-mm thick, rings that are then placed in a gelatin capsules to be ingested by the patient. This method required daily X-rays to follow the markers. This was followed by further modifications that also required daily X-ray studies in order to assess segmental colonic transit times, which, in turn, exposed the patient to more radiation than necessary.

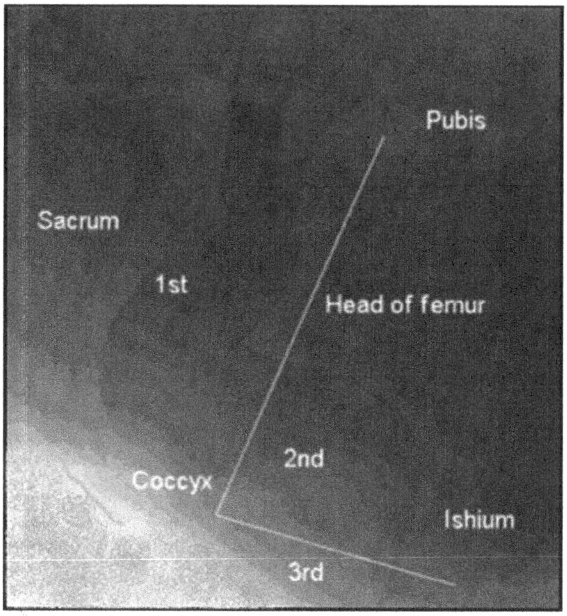

Figure 16 Degrees of sigmoidocele in correlation to the pelvic landmarks.

In normal adults, markers enter the right colon in about 8 hours after ingestion, where they remain for up to 38 and 37 hours in the right and left colon, respectively, and finally in the rectosigmoid region for about 34 hours (116).

Technique

Most patients who are asked to undergo this test are laxative dependent and rely on cathartics, enemas, and/or suppositories. It is important to instruct the patients to avoid using any of these methods to purge themselves for the duration of the study.

Patients are asked to take a commercially available single capsule containing 24 radio-opaque rings (Sitzmark^{TM}; Konsyl Pharmaceuticals, Lafayette, Texas). This is followed by abdominal X-rays on days 3 and 5. Patients are instructed to take psyllium supplements and to eat a high-fiber diet as well as drink plenty of water during the duration of the study (113).

Interpretation

Basically, three results to this single capsule test can be obtained. If less than 20% of the markers are retained, this should be considered normal. If more than 20% are retained in the rectosigmoid region, an outlet functional problem is thought to be the cause of the constipation. Conversely, when retained markers are scattered throughout the colon, this is an indication of colonic inertia (Fig. 17).

Clinical Application

This test is important in evaluating patients suffering from constipation, especially those with infrequent bowel movements. The combination with another anatomical study such as defecography to assess pelvic floor function during defecation is often useful for proper judgment and decision-making. Since the results of this study may shift the management to subtotal colectomy for a constipated patient, instructions must be strictly followed. If any doubt exists about validity of the study or patients cooperation, the study should be repeated (115).

SMALL BOWEL TRANSIT

Background and Basic Concepts

Colonic inertia is sometimes the reflection of a generalized motility disturbance of the gastrointestinal tract, as many patients may have a generalized gastrointestinal motility disorder.

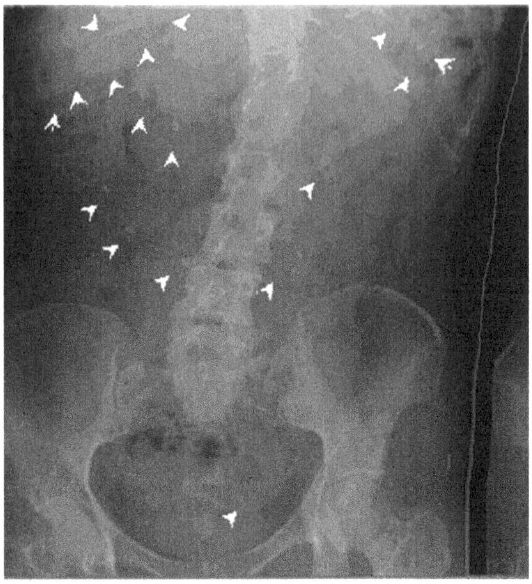

Figure 17 Colonic transit study in a patient with colonic inertia.

It is important to distinguish the cause of the problem (29). Many laboratories use the breath hydrogen analysis test to investigate small bowel transit time.

The patient ingests a nonabsorbable carbohydrate such as lactulose or baked beans as an indicator of liquid or solid transit, respectively (117). Once these substrates reach the cecum, colonic bacteria start to act upon them, resulting in production of hydrogen. Since it is a highly diffusible gas and relatively insoluble in water, hydrogen is rapidly absorbed in the blood and reaches the lungs where it gets exhaled and subsequently measured during the test, using gas chromatography (117). However, there are some factors that may render interpretation difficult: 5% to 20% of the population does not produce hydrogen (the so-called "non-fermenters") (118,119); some of the substrate may be metabolized by oral bacteria, in which case mouthwash before ingesting the test material is helpful (120); small intestinal bacterial overgrowth will result in shorter time as a consequence of rapid metabolism; antibiotic administration may be associated with bacterial depletion and thereby prolong the transit time, therefore it is advisable to prevent patients from taking antibiotics within 10 days prior to the study; and smoking has been shown to influence the concentration of hydrogen in the exhaled breath (29).

There are different criteria upon which different centers estimate transit time. Some consider that a rise of 20 parts per million (ppm) is indicative of transit time, (121,122) while others use a rise of 2 ppm (123), 3 ppm (124), or 5 ppm (125) as indicators of transit time. In our laboratory, a two- to threefold rise of the baseline is considered positive.

Instrumentation and Technique

Source of Lactulose

Ten gram of lactulose with 100 mL of water produces accurate values of orocecal transit, as larger amounts may result in shorter transits due to osmotic effects (126).

Gas Chromatography Device

This device is required to analyze the concentration of hydrogen in the patients' breath.

An air/hydrogen mixture is used for calibration. Calibration is important prior to every test and it may also be required for some devices during the test.

Collection Bags

Samples are collected in specific collection bags (Fig. 18).

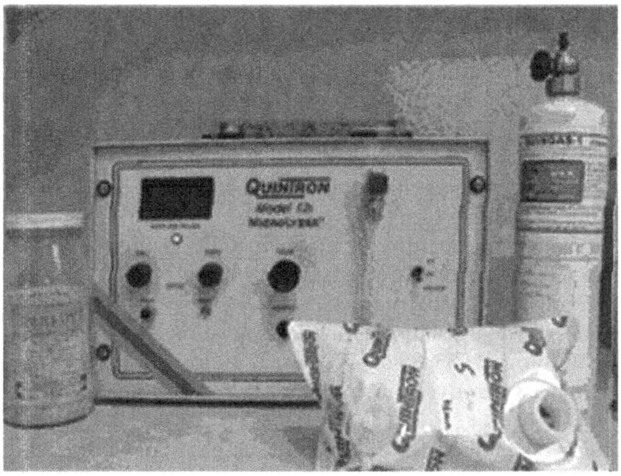

Figure 18 Microanalyzer with the accessories for hydrogen breath test.

Technique

Care is taken to instruct the patient to fast (including refraining from smoking) and refrain from taking antibiotics and bowel cleansing preparations within a period of seven days prior to the test. On the morning of the test, the device is calibrated and set ready to use.

The patient is instructed to ingest 10 g lactulose with approximately 100 mL of water. A baseline measurement of breath hydrogen is taken. Samples are collected by instructing the patient to slowly exhale into the collecting bag. This is continued for up to three hours, or until the hydrogen levels reach a plateau (29).

Clinical Application and Indications

Small bowel transit study is used as an adjunct to colonic transit study to enable in identifying patients with isolated colonic inertia from those with generalized hypomotility. The breath hydrogen test is simple and is a noninvasive test. In evaluating small bowel transit, the breath hydrogen test has been found to be reliable, reproducible, and well tolerated by patients (124).

CONCLUSION

Colorectal surgeons see patients with a wide range of functional complaints. The ability to arrive at an accurate diagnosis relies, in part, on the tools available in the Anorectal Physiology Laboratory. The use of ARM, neurophysiologic evaluation, defecography, anal ultrasound, and transit studies provide valuable information to the physician treating this complex group of patients.

REFERENCES

1. Johnson JF. Geographic distribution of constipation in the United States. Am J Gastroenterol 1998; 93:188–191.
2. Nyam DCNK. Fecal incontinence: Hope for an under diagnosed condition. Singapore Med J 2000; 41:188–192.
3. Meunier PD, Gallavardin D. Anorectal manometry: The state of the art. Dig Dis 1993; 11:252–264.
4. Stein BL, Roberts PL. Manometry and the rectoanal inhibitory reflex. In: Steven D. Wexner, David C. Bartolo C, eds. Constipation: Etiology, Evaluation and Management. Oxford: Butterworth-Heinemann, 1995:63–76.
5. Schuster MM, Hookman P, Hendrix TR, et al. Simultaneous manometric recording of the internal and external anal sphincter reflexes. Bull Johns Hopkins Hosp 1965; 116:79–88.
6. Duthie HL, Watts JM. Contribution of the external anal sphincter to the pressure zone in the anal canal. Gut 1965; 6:64–68.
7. Hill JR, Kelly ML Jr, Schlegel JF, et al. Pressure profile of the rectum and anus of healthy persons. Dis Colon Rectum 1960; 3:203–209.
8. Jorge JMN, Wexner SD. Anorectal manometry: Techniques and clinical applications. South Med J 1993; 86:924–931.

9. Arndorfer RC, Steff JJ, Dodds WF, et al. Improved infusion system for intraluminal esophageal manometry. Gastroenterology 1977; 73:23–27.
10. Karulf RE, Coller JA, Bartolo DCC, et al. Anorectal physiologic testing: A survey of availability and use. Dis Colon Rectum 1991; 34:464–468.
11. Harris LD, Winans CS, Pope CE II. Determination of yield pressures: A method of measuring anal sphincter competence. Gastroenterology 1966; 50:754–760.
12. Katz LA, Kaufman HJ, Spiro HM. Anal sphincter pressure characteristics. Gastroenterology 1967; 52:513–518.
13. Pemberton JH. Anatomy and physiology of the anus and rectum. In: Zuidema GD, ed. Shackelford's Surgery of the Alimentary Tract. 3rd ed. Philadelphia, PA: WB Saunders Co, 1991:242–274.
14. Coller JA. Clinical application of anorectal manometry. Gastroenterol Clion North Am 1987; 16:17–33.
15. Bartolo DC, Read NW, Jarratt JA, et al. Differences in anal sphincter function and clinical presentation in patients with pelvic floor descent. Gastroenterology 1983; 85:68–75.
16. Roberts JP, Womack NR, Hallan RI, et al. Evidence from dynamic integrated proctography to refine anismus. Br J Surg 1992; 73:310–312.
17. Womack NR, Williams NS, Holmfield JH, et al. New method for the dynamic assessment of anorectal function in constipation. Br J Surg 1985; 72:994–998.
18. Dent JA. A new technique for continuous sphincter pressure measurement. Gastroenterology 1976; 71:263–267.
19. Jorge JMN, Wexner SD. Anatomy and physiology of the rectum and anus. Eur J Surg 1997; 163:723–731.
20. Gibbons CP, Bannister JJ, Trowbridge EA, et al. An analysis of anal cushions in maintaining continence. Lancet 1986; 1:886–887.
21. Frenckner B, Euler CHRV. Influence of pudendal block on the function of the anal sphincters. Gut 1975; 16:482–489.
22. Lestar B, Penninckx F, Kerremans R. The composition of anal basal pressure. An in vivo and in vitro study in man. Int J Colorect Dis 1989; 4:118–122.
23. Bannister JJ, Abouzekry L, Read NW. Effect of aging on anorectal function. Gut 1987; 28:353–357.
24. Laurberg S, Swash M. Effects of aging on the anorectal sphincters and their innervation. Dis Colon Rectum 1989; 32:737–742.
25. Parks AG, Porter NH, Melzak J. Experimental study of the reflex mechanism controlling the muscles of the pelvic floor. Dis Colon Rectum 1962; 5:407–414.
26. Philips SF, Edwards DAW. Some aspects of anal continence and defecation. Gut 1965; 6:394–406.
27. Duthie HL, Watts JM. Contribution of the external anal sphincter to the pressure zone in the anal canal. Gut 1963; 4:179–182.
28. Jorge JMN, Wexner SD. A practical guide to basic anorectal physiology investigations. Contemp Surg 1993; 43:214–224.
29. Wexner SD, Sardinha TC, Gilliland R. Setting up a colorectal physiology laboratory. In: Corman ML, ed. Colon and Rectal Surgery. Philadelphia, PA: Lippincott Williams & Wilkins, 2004:129–167.
30. Wexner SD, James K, Jagelman DG. The double-stapled ileal reservoir and ileoanal anastomosis: A prospective review of sphincter function and clinical outcomes. Dis Colon Rectum 1991; 34:487–494.
31. Duthie HL, Watts JM. The relation of sensation in the anal to the function sphincter length: A possible factor in anal incontinence. Gut 1963; 4:179–182.
32. Miller R, Bartolo DCC, Cervero F, et al. Anorectal sampling: A comparison of normal and incontinent patients. Br J Surg 1988; 75:44–47.
33. Aaronson I, Nixon HH. A clinical evaluation of anorectal pressure studies in the diagnosis of Hirschsprung's disease. Gut 1972; 13:138–146.
34. Meunier P, Marechal J-M, Mollard P. Accuracy of the manometric diagnosis of Hirschsprung's disease. J Pediatr Surg 1978; 12:411–415.
35. Habr-gama A, Raia A, Correa Netro A. Motility of the sigmoid colon and rectum. Contribution to the physiopathology of megacolon in Chagas disease. Dis Colon Rectum 1971; 14 291–304.
36. Habr-gama A, Raia A, Correa Netro A. Chagas disease of the bowel. In: Allan RN, Keighly MRB, Alexander-Williams J, et al., eds. Inflammatory Bowel Disease. Edinburgh: Churchill-Livingstone, 190:609–616.
37. Buser WD, Miner PB Jr. Delayed rectal sensation with fecal incontinence. Successful treatment using anorectal manometry. Gastroenterology 1986; 91:1186–1191.
38. Denis PH, Colin R, Galmiche JP, et al. Elastic properties of the rectal wall in normal adults and in patients with ulcerative colitis. Gastroenterology 1982; 83:970–980.
39. Devroede G, Vobecky S, Masse S, et al. Ischemic fecal incontinence and rectal angina. Gastroenterology 1982; 83:970–980.
40. Wexner SD, Daniel N, Jagelman DG. Colectomy for constipation: A physiologic investigation is the key to success. Dis Colon Rectum 1991; 34:851–856.

41. Wexner SD, Marchetti F, Jagelman DG. The role of sphincteroplasty for fecal incontinence re-evaluated: A physiologic and functional review. Dis Colon Rectum 1991; 34:22–30.
42. Fleshman JW, Dreznik Z, Fry RD, et al. Anal sphincter repair for obstetric injury: Manometric evaluation of functional results. Dis Colon Rectum 1990; 33:479–486.
43. Felt-Bersma RJF, Klinkerberg-Knol LB, Meuwissen SGM. Investigation of anorectal function. Br J Surg 1988; 75:53–55.
44. Ger GC, Wexner SD. Electromyography and pudendal nerve terminal motor latency. In: Steven D. Wexner, David C, Bartolo C, eds. Constipation: Etiology, Evaluation and Management. Oxford: Butterworth-Heinemann, 1995:91–102.
45. Floyd WF, Walls EW. Electromyography of the sphincter ani externus in man. J Physiol 1953; 122:599–609.
46. Adrian ED, Bronck DW. The discharge of impulses in motor nerve fibers. J Physiol 1929; 67:119–151.
47. Farouk R. Electromyographic techniques. In: Smith LD, ed. Practical Guide to Anorectal Testing. 2nd ed. New York: Igaku-shoin, 1995:195–206.
48. Ekstedt J. Human single fiber action potentials. Acta Physiol Scand 1964; 61:1–98.
49. Neill ME, Swash M. Increased motor unit fiber density in the external anal sphincter muscle in anorectal incontinence: A single fiber EMG study. J Neurol Neurosurg Psychiatry 1980; 43:343–347.
50. O'Donnell P, Beck C, Doyle R, et al. Surface electrodes in perineal electromyography. Urology 1988;34:375–379.
51. Binnie NR, Kawimbe M, Papachrysostomou M, et al. The importance of the orientation of the electrodes plates in recording the external anal sphincter EMG by non-invasive anal plug electrodes. Int J Colorectal Dis 1990; 6:5–8.
52. Lopez A, Nilsson BY, Mellgren A, et al. Electromyography of the external anal sphincter: Comparison between needle and surface electrodes. Dis Colon Rectum 1999; 42:482–485.
53. Johansson C, Nilson BY, Holstrom B, et al. Is paradoxical sphincter reaction provoked by needle electrode electromyography? Dis Colon Rectum 1991; 34:1109–1112.
54. Keighley MRB, Henry MM, Bartolo DCC, et al. Anorectal physiology measurement: Report of a working party. Br J Surg 1989; 76:356:357.
55. Rutter KR. Electromyographic changes in certain pelvic floor abnormalities. Proc R Soc Med 1974; 78:690–692.
56. Preston DM, Lennard-Jones JE. Anismus in chronic constipation. Dig Dis Sci 1985; 30:413–418.
57. Dahl J, Lindquist BL, Tysk C, et al. Behavioural medicine treatment in chronic constipation with paradoxical anal sphincter contraction. Dis Colon Rectum 1991; 34:769–776.
58. Fleshman JW, Dreznik Z, Meyer K, et al. outpatient protocol for biofeedback of pelvic floor outlet obstruction. Dis Colon Rectum 1992; 35:1–7.
59. Enck P, Von Giensen HJ, Schafer A, et al. Comparison of anal sonography with conventional needle electromyography in the evaluation of anal sphincter defects. Am J Surg 1996; 91:2534–2539.
60. Ferrara A, Lujan JH, Cebrian J, et al. Clinical manometric and EMG characteristics of patients with fecal incontinence. Tech Coloproctol 2001; 5:13–18.
61. Snooks SJ, Barnes PR, Swash M, et al. Damage to the innervation of the pelvic floor musculature in chronic constipation. Gastroenterology 1985; 89:977–981.
62. Neill ME, Parks AG, Swash M. Physiological studies of the anal sphincter musculature in fecal incontinence and rectal prolapse. Br J Surg 1981; 68:531–536.
63. Wexner SD, Jagelman DG. Chronic constipation. Postgrad Adv Colorectal Surg 1989; 1:1–22.
64. Wasserman IF. Puborectalis syndrome (rectal stenosis due to anorectal spasm). Dis Colon Rectum 1964; 7:87–98.
65. Brindley GA. Electroejaculation: Its technique, neurological implications and uses. J Neurol Neurosurg Psych 1981; 44:9–18.
66. Kiff ES, Swash M. Slowed conduction in the pudendal nerves in idiopathic (neurogenic) fecal incontinence. Br J Surg 1984; 74:614–616.
67. Rogers J, Henry MM, Misiewiscz JJ. Disposable pudendal nerve stimulator: Evaluation of standard instrument and new device. Gut 1988; 29:1133–1137.
68. Snooks SJ, Swash M. Nerve stimulation techniques. In: Henry MM, Swash M, eds. Coloproctology and the Pelvic Floor: Pathophysiology and Management. London: Butter-Worth, 1985:112–128.
69. Wexner SD, Marchetti F, Salanga VD, et al. Neurophysiologic assessment of the anal sphincter. Dis Colon Rectum 1991; 34:616–612.
70. Jones PN, Lubowski DZ, Swash M, et al. Is paradoxical contraction of the puborectalis muscle of functional importance? Dis Colon Rectum 1987; 30:667–670.
71. Cheong DM, Vaccaro CA, Salanga VD, et al. Electrodiagnostic of fecal incontinence. Muscle Nerve 1995;18:612–619.
72. Gilliland R, Heymen S, Altomare DF, et al. Outcome and predictors of success of biofeedback for constipation. Br J Surg 1997; 84:1123–1127.

73. Kiff ES, Barnes PRM, Swash M. Evidence of pudendal neuropathy in patients with perineal descent and chronic straining at stool. Gut 1984; 11:1279–1284.
74. Lubowski DH, Swash M, Henry MM. Neural mechanisms in disorders of defecation. Clin Gastroenerol 1988; 2:201–223.
75. Wallden L. Defecation block in cases of deep rectogenital pouch. A surgical, roentgenological and embryological study with special reference to morphological conditions. Acta Scand 1952; 165:1–22.
76. Krulf RE, Coller JA, Bartolo DCC,et al. Anorectal physiology testing: A survey of availability and use. Dis Colon Rectum 1991; 34:464–468.
77. Rannikko S, Servomaa A, Ermakoff I, et al. Calculation of the estimated collective effective dose equivalent (SE) due to x-ray diagnostic examinations: Estimate of the SE I Finland. Health Phys 1987; 53:31–36.
78. Goei R, Kemerink G. Radiation dose in defecography. Radiology 1990; 176:137–139.
79. Rafert JA, Lappas JC, Wilkins W. Defecography: Techniques for improved imaging quality. Radiol Technol 1990; 61:368–373.
80. Jorge JMN, Habr-Gama A, Wexner SD. Clinical application and techniques of Cinedefecography. Am J Surg 2001; 182:93–101.
81. Lesaffer LPA. Digital subtraction defecography. In: Smith LE, ed. Practical Guide to Anorectal Testing. 2nd ed. New York: Igako-shoin, 1995:161–184.
82. Mahieu P, Pringot J, Bodart P. Defecography: I. Description of a new procedure and results in normal patients. Gastrointest Radiol 1984; 9:247–251.
83. Sentovich SM, Rivela LJ, Thorson AG, et al. Simultaneous dynamic proctography and peritoneography for pelvic floor disorders. Dis Colon Rectum 1995; 38:912–915.
84. Bremmer S, Ahlback S-O, Uden R, et al. Simultaneous defecography and peritoneography in defecation disorders. Dis Colon Rectum 1995; 38:969–973.
85. Glassman LM. Defecography. In: Smith LE, ed. Practical Guide to Anorectal Testing. 2nd ed. New York: Igaku-shoin, 1995:143–160.
86. Hock D, Lombard R, Jehaes C, et al. Colopocystodefecography. Dic Colon Rectum 1993;36:1015–1021.
87. Bartram CI, Mahieu PHG. Evacuation proctography and anal endosonography. In: Henry MM, Swash M, eds. Coloproctology and the Pelvic Floor. London: Butterworth, 1991:146–172.
88. Jorge JMN, Wexner SD, Marchetti F, et al. How reliable are currently available methods of measuring the anorectal angle? Dis Colon Rectu 1992; 35:332–338.
89. Felt-Bersma RJF, Luth WJ, Janssen JJWM, et al. Defecography in patients with anorectal disorders: Which findings are clinically relevant? Dis Colon Rectum 1990; 33:227–284.
90. Penninckx F, Debruyne C, Lestar B, et al. Observer variation in the radiologic measurement of the anorectal angle. Int J Colorect Dis 1990; 5:94–97.
91. Turnbull GK, Bartram CI, Lennard-Jones JE. Radiologic studies of rectal evacuation in adults with idiopathic constipation. Dis Colon Rectum 1988; 31:190–197.
92. Goei R, Van Engelshoven J, Schouten H, et al. Anorectal function: Defecographic measurement in asymptomatic subjects. Radiology 1989;173:137–141.
93. Ferrante Sl, Perry RE, Schreiman JS, et al. The reproducibility of measuring the anorectal angle in defecography. Dis Colon Rectum 1991; 34:51–55.
94. Finaly IG, Bartolo DCC, Bartram CI, et al. Symposium: Proctography. Int J Colorect Dis 1988; 3:67–89.
95. Jorge JMN, Ger GC, Gonzalez L, et al. Patient position during cinedefecography. Influence on perineal descent and other measurements. Dis Colon Rectum 1994; 37:927–931.
96. Karlbom U, Hallden M, Eeg-Olofsson KE, et al. Results of biofeedback in constipated patients: A prospective study. Dis Colon Rectum 1997; 40:1149–1155.
97. Parks UC, Choi SK, Piccirillo MF, et al. Patterns of anismus and relation to biofeedback therapy. Dis Colon Rectum 1996; 39:768–773.
98. MacDonald A, Paterson PJ, Baxter JN, et al. Relationship between intra-abdominal and intrarectal pressure in the proctometrogram. Br J Surg 1993; 80:1070–1071.
99. Shafik A, El-Sibai O. Study of the levator ani muscle in the multipara: Role of levator dysfunction I defecation disorders. J Obstet Gynecol 2002; 22:187–192.
100. Kuijpers HC. Defecography. In: Wexner SD, Bartolo DCC, eds. Constipation: Etiology, Evaluation and Management. Oxford: Butterworth-Heinmann, 1995:77–85.
101. Wasserman IF. Puborectalis syndrome (rectal stenosis due to anorectal spasm). Dis Colon Rectum 1964; 7:87–98.
102. Mathers SE, Kempster PA, Swash M, et al. Constipation ad paradoxical puborectalis contraction in anismus and Parkinson's disease: A dynamic phenomenon? J Neurosurg Psychiatry 1988; 51:1503–1507.
103. Kuijpers HC, Bleijenberg G, Morree H. The spastic pelvic floor syndrome. Large bowel outlet obstruction caused by pelvic floor dysfunction: Radiological study. Int J Colorect Dis 1986; 1:44–48
104. MacDonald A, Shearer M, Paterson PJ, Finlay IG. Relationship between outlet obstruction constipation and obstructed urinary flow. Br J Surg 1991; 78:693–695.

105. Wexner SD, Cheape JD, Jorge JMN, et al. Prospective assessment of biofeedback for the treatment of paradoxical puborectalis syndrome. Dis Colon Rectum 1992; 35:145–150
106. Lestar B, Penninckx F, Kerremans R. Biofeedback defecation training for anismus. Int Colorectal Dis 1991; 6:202–207.
107. Fleshman JW, Dreznik Z, Meyer K, et al. Outpatient protocol for biofeedback therapy of pelvic floor outlet obstruction. Dis Colon Rectum 1992; 35:1–7.
108. Jorge JMN, Wexner SD, Jagelman DG. Cinedefecography and EMG in the diagnosis of nonrelaxing puborectalis syndrome. Dis Colon Rectum 1993; 36:6668–676.
109. Shorvon PJ, McHugh S, Diamant NE, et al. Defecography in normal volunteers: Results and implications. Gut 1989; 30:1737–1749.
110. Mahieu P. Barium enema and defecography in the diagnosis and evaluation of the solitary rectal ulcer syndrome. Int J Colorectal Dis 1986; 1:85–90.
111. Kuijpers HC, Schreve RH, Hoedemakers HTC. Diagnosis of functional disorders of defecation causing the solitary rectal ulcer syndrome. Dis Colon Rectum 1986; 29:126–129.
112. Goei R. Anorectal dysfunction in patients with defecation disorders and asymptomatic subjects: Evaluation with defecography. Radiology 1990; 174:121–123.
113. Arhan P, Devroede G, Jehannin B, et al. segmental colonic transit time. Dis Colon Rectum 1981; 24:625–629.
114. Dick M. Use of Cuprous thiocyanate as a short-term continuous marker for faeces. Gut 1969; 10:408–412.
115. Maousos ON, Truelove SC, Lumsden K. Transit times of food in patients with diverticulosis or irritable colon syndrome and normal subjects. Br J Surg 1967; 3:760–762.
116. Pfeifer J, Agachan F, Wexner SD. Surgery for Constipation: A review. Dis Colon Rectum 1996; 39:444–460.
117. Levitt MD. Production and excretion of hydrogen gas in man. N Engl J Med 1969; 281:122–127.
118. Bjorneklett A, Jenssen E. Relationships between hydrogen (H2) and methane (CH4) production in man. Scand J Gastroenterol 1982; 17:985–992.
119. Bleijenberg G, Kuijpers HC. Treatment of the spastic pelvic floor syndrome with biofeedback. Dis Colon Rectum 1987; 30:108–111.
120. Thompson DG, Binfield p, De Belder A, et al. Extra intestinal influences on exhaled breath hydrogen measurements during the investigation of gastrointestinal disease. Gut 1985; 26:1349–1352.
121. Read NW, Miles CA, Fisher D, et al. transit of a meal through the stomach, small intestine, and colon in normal subjects ad its role in the pathogenesis of diarrhea. Gastroenterology 1980; 79:1276–1282.
122. Caride VJ, Prokop EK, Troncale FJ, et al. Scintigraphic determination of small intestinal transit time: Comparison with the hydrogen breath technique. Gastroenterology 1984; 86:714–720.
123. Basilisco G, Bozzani A, Camboni G, et al. Effect of loperamide and naloxone on mouth-to-cecum transit time evaluated by lactulose hydrogen breath test. Gut 1985; 26:700–703.
124. Jorge JMN, Wexner SD, Ehrenpreis ED. The lactulose hydrogen breath test as a measure of orocaecal transit time. Eur J Surg 1994; 160:409–416.
125. Rubinoff MJ, Piccionne PR, Holt PR. Clonidine prolongs human small intestinal transit time: Use of the lactulose-breath hydrogen test. Am J Gastroenterol 1989; 84:372–374.
126. Bond JH, Levitt MD, Prentiss R. Investigation of small bowel transit time in man utilizing pulmonary hydrogen (H2) measurements. J Lab Clin Med 1975; 85:546–555.

4 Anorectal Ultrasound

Tracy Hull and Massarat Zutshi
Cleveland Clinic Foundation, Cleveland, Ohio, U.S.A.

INTRODUCTION

In the armamentarium of a colorectal surgeon, a good history and physical examination are the first steps toward treatment. A popular tool to augment the physical examination is endorectal ultrasound (AUS). This is due to its ease of availability in the office, easily mastered technique, comparative less expense, and a high degree of accuracy.

The problems that can be evaluated by AUS range from benign conditions such as abscesses and anal fistulae to rectal tumors, both benign and malignant, extent of spread of rectal cancers, node positivity in rectal tumors, and presacral tumors. Other modalities of diagnosis for these problems include magnetic resonance imaging (MRI) with or without a body coil, and three-dimensional ultrasound (3-DUS). The latter is still an office procedure, while MRI is performed in a radiology setting. Both procedures are more expensive than an AUS and are not available at all centers. Although the accuracy of all three is comparable (1–7), AUS may be more operator dependent (6,8).

EQUIPMENT

Most AUS machines currently in use utilize a two-dimensional (2-D) view. The 2-D AUS utilizes an ultrasound transducer crystal of 7.0 or 10 mHz. The focal range of the 7.0 m mHz transducer is between 2 and 5 cm. This provides optimal visualization of the mesorectum while searching for abnormal lymph nodes. Theoretically, the 10 mHz transducer with its shorter focal length provides superior resolution of the wall structures, and is used to visualize the anal sphincters. However, some studies have shown that accuracy is greater for T1 tumors with the 10 mHz transducer, which is reportedly superior in assessing the mucosa and submucosa (9).The difference between an adenoma and a T1 lesion may also be more accurately staged with the 10 mHz transducer. However, visualization of the mesorectum is better using the 7 mHz transducer, thus there may be a trade-off when selecting which transducer to employ.

PROCEDURE

For rectal tumors, the probe is covered by a balloon that has the capacity to instill approximately 90 cc of degassed water. If the water is poured into a container and then quickly drawn into the syringe, it creates bubbles, in the balloon, which distort the image. Allowing the bubbles to disperse and then slowly instilling the fluid down the shaft result in less gas in the water and, hence, less distortion. The water is needed for the coupling necessary for the sound waves from the probe to be emitted and then the reflected waves detected. Air is the enemy—thus it is imperative to ensure that there is no air between the wall and the transducer.

The probe is introduced either directly through the anus or more commonly through the lumen of a proctoscope, especially when the tumor is exophytic. The proctoscope is inserted under direct vision and the probe is then advanced down the shaft after the maximum proximal distance is achieved. This level is preferably proximal to the tumor. It is of note that tumors higher than 12 cm are not well visualized and in our practice are staged and managed similar to sigmoid cancers (vs. rectal cancer). The transducer rotates 360° and the plane of visualization is 90° to the shaft of the probe. Images are viewed in real time and can be printed and/or saved electronically.

An enema is administered prior to the procedure to eliminate stool in the rectum, which can alter the image by creating an impermeable shadow. The patient is placed in the left lateral position with hips and knees flexed. A digital examination is performed to judge the location of the tumor. The proctoscope is advanced beyond the tumor and the probe is then inserted through the proctoscope. The balloon is inflated with approximately 40 cc of degassed water. The right hand is used to guide the probe into the rectum which is at the end of the shaft. It centralizes the probe by moving the end, which in turn will shift the position of the transducer in the rectum. The goal is to keep the probe in the middle of the rectum. The right hand is used to grasp the proctoscope and keep the apparatus aligned 90°. The probe is moved proximally to distally, scrutinizing tumor location, depth of tumor penetration, and nodal involvement. It is difficult to move proximally with the balloon inflated, thus any proximal movement requires the proctoscope be removed along with the transducer, then repositioned and then placed again. The probe may be passed a few times through the proctoscope to fully view the tumor and examine the mesorectum. If the tumor is large and the lumen is obstructed, it may be impossible to pass the proctoscope proximal to the tumor. Simply placing the probe against the lumen may yield information regarding depth of penetration without actually advancing proximal to the lesion.

In order to view the anal sphincters, the 10 mHz crystal is usually covered with a plastic cone, although some centers use the same type of balloon used for rectal lesions. The same method is used to insert the probe and transducer, although it needs to be passed above the anorectal ring into the distal rectum, thus the proctoscope is not required. Visualization is initiated from the upper anal canal where the puborectalis is identified. The probe is gradually withdrawn through the anal canal to end at the anal verge. The procedure is performed with the patient in the left lateral or supine position and occasionally, in women, a finger may have to be placed in the vagina to help determine the position of the probe.

Traditionally images are obtained in the upper anal canal where the puborectalis is seen, the mid anal canal where both the internal and external muscles should be seen, and in the lower anal canal where the external muscle may be the only portion of the sphincters visualized. Additional views between these three areas may also be observed to fully evaluate the sphincters.

IMAGING FOR A RECTAL TUMOR

Normal Image

AUS displays five layers (Fig. 1) as described by Hildebrand and Fifel (10–12). The layers appear alternatively as bright (hyperechoic) and dark (hypoechoic) layers. The first layer is bright and is located in the interphase of the balloon with the rectal wall. The next dark layer is the mucosal layer (mucosa and muscularis mucosa). The next bright layer is the submucosa. Adjacent to this is a dark layer, which is of great significance and is the muscularis propria. The last bright layer

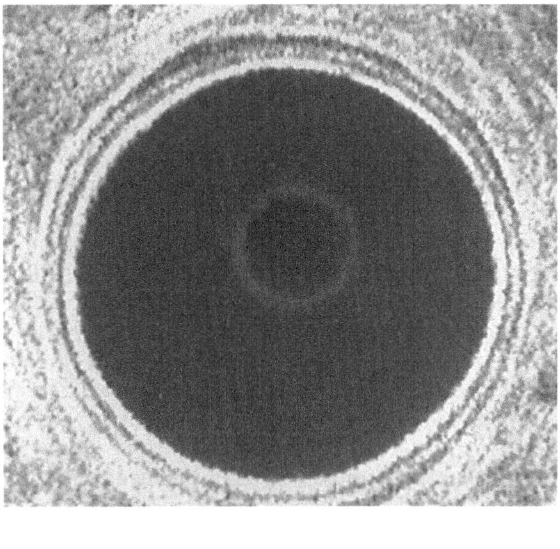

Figure 1 Normal ultrasound image of a rectal wall using the 7 mHz crystal. *Source*: Photo courtesy of The Cleveland Clinic, Cleveland, Ohio, U.S.A.

Table 1 Ultrasound Staging and Its Image Characteristics

Staging by ultrasound	Image description (Based on a description by Hildebrandt and Feifel)
uT0	Tumor lying within the mucosa—first dark (hypoechoic) layer
uT1	Tumor lying within the submucosa—second bright (hyperechoic) layer
uT2	Tumor breaching the submucosa—second bright (hyperechoic) layer
uT3	Tumor infiltrating the submucosa—second bright (hyperechoic) layer into the perirectal fat—last bright (hyperechoic) layer
uT4	Tumor infiltrating the perirectal fat—last bright (hyperechoic) layer into the adjacent organs, like prostate, seminal vesicles, and vagina
uN0	No nodes identified as dark structures in the perirectal fat
uN1	One or more nodes identified as dark structures in the perirectal fat at or just above the level of the tumor

is the perirectal fat layer. Anatomical location of the tumor is defined by identifying anteriorly the prostate and seminal vesicles in males and the vagina in females.

IMAGING A RECTAL MASS

A tumor appears dark on the AUS, as do any accompanying infiltrated nodes, which have the same echogenicity. It is important during an examination to start identifying the layers of the rectum at the point where they are normal and then trace the layers toward the tumor (Table 1). uT1 tumors are located in the submucosa and are hence within the first dark line (Fig. 2). Any breach of this dark line identifies the tumor at the T2 level (Fig. 3). A deep uT2 tumor and an early uT3 tumor can be difficult to differentiate. The dark circle that represents the muscularis propria can become thickened and appear wavy when uT2 tumor is deep, before the tumor penetrates through the layer to become uT3 (Fig. 4). uT4 tumors invade the surrounding organs, which include the prostate and seminal vesicles in males and the vagina in females (Fig. 5).

Nodes appear dark and are staged based on size and location. Blood vessels also appear dark. However, as the probe is moved up and down in the rectum, blood vessels appear as longitudinal structures, are constant in shape, and appear over a larger distance than lymph nodes. Nodes that are hyperechoic are usually benign. Pathological lymph nodes typically are those that are in close proximity to the tumor, more than 5 mm[12] in size and appear hypoechoic (Fig. 6). Inflammatory nodes have a hypoechoic center due to germinal center hyperactivity. Lymph nodes with small tumor deposits and those beyond the depth of the transducer resolution will not be detected (11,12).

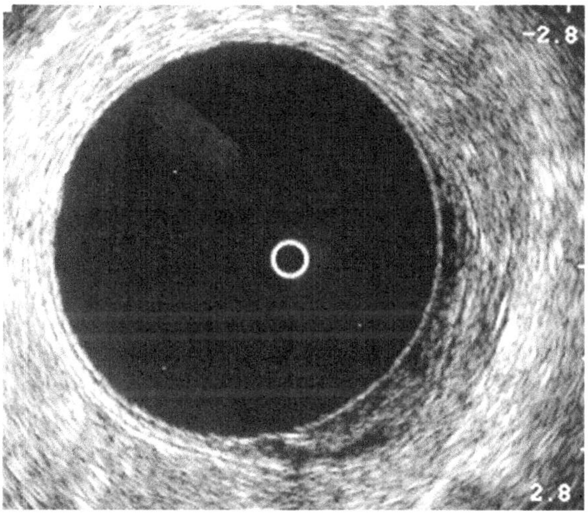

Figure 2 uT1 lesion: Tumor in the mucosa; muscular propria intact. *Source*: Photo courtesy of The Cleveland Clinic, Cleveland, Ohio, U.S.A.

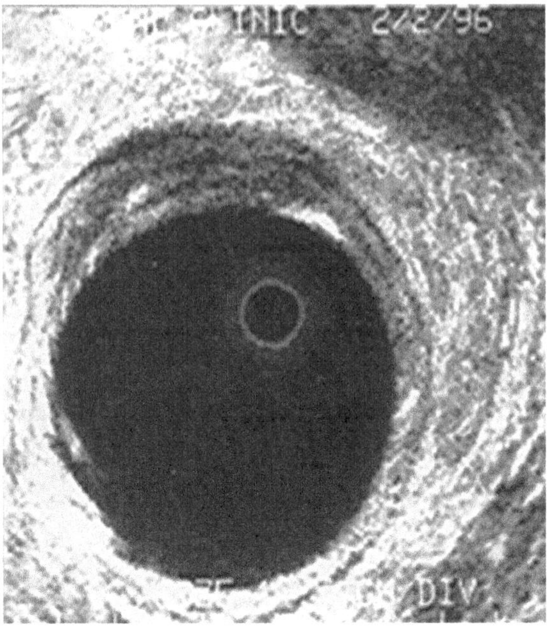

Figure 3 uT2 lesion: Tumor in the submucosa; muscularis propria intact. *Source*: Photo courtesy of The Cleveland Clinic, Cleveland, Ohio, U.S.A.

ACCURACY OF IMAGING RECTAL TUMORS

Accuracy in predicting the tumor stage is between 69% and 97% (a median of 84%). There have been published reports related to the accuracy in the 90% range (13); however, a study from the University of Minnesota (2) found a less optimistic accuracy of 68%.

Viewing the stages more closely, the accuracy (14) for uT1 tumors is approximately 47% and approximately 68% for uT2 tumors (7). uT2 tumors are the most often overstaged, in approximately 18% to 19% (9), while understaging in these tumors is approximately 12%. Overstaging may be due to peritumoral inflammation, which also appears dense, making differentiation between tumor and inflammation difficult (14). Understaging is due to the inability to visualize microscopic invasion due to the limits of the resolution of the transducer. The accuracy decreases for tumors that are low in the rectum (15). Some studies have shown higher accuracy of uT prediction when tumors are less than 6 cm from the anal verge (16), while others (2)

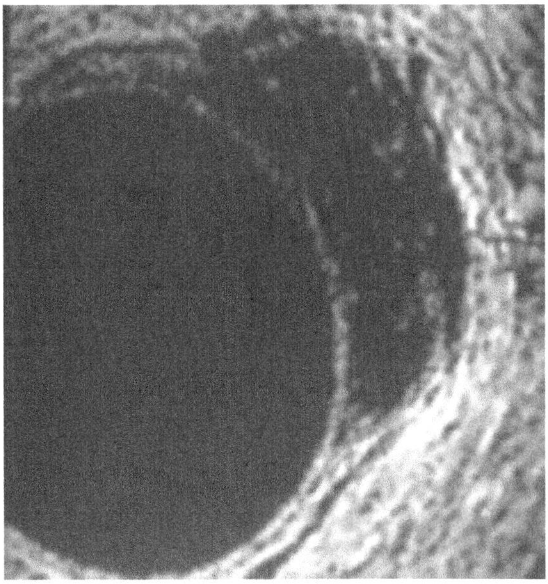

Figure 4 uT3 lesion: Tumor infilltrating the perirectal fat; muscular propria breached. *Source*: Photo courtesy of The Cleveland Clinic, Cleveland, Ohio, U.S.A.

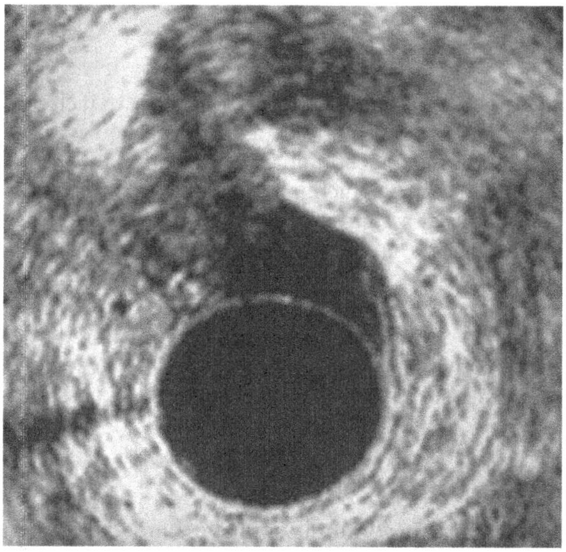

Figure 5 uT4 lesion: Tumor infiltrating the prostate. *Source*: Photo courtesy of The Cleveland Clinic, Cleveland, Ohio, U.S.A.

have shown that the distance of the tumor from the anorectal ring does not influence accuracy. Staging accuracy is improved when there is a uniform contact between the balloon and the rectal wall. Suboptimal delineation of the rectal wall may occur just above the anorectal ring where the rectum dips posteriorly toward the sacrum. Another factor that may hinder accurate staging is a large tumor with exophytic components. These lesions may produce artifacts due to portions of the tumor folding back over on itself.

According to Detry and Kartheuser (17) the positive predictive value for staging T1 and T2 tumors is 93% and that of T2 and T3 tumors is 100%. The penetration of the rectal wall can be accurately predicted in 94%, with a sensitivity of 82%, specificity of 81%, positive predictive value of 70%, and negative predictive value of 90%.

Lymph nodes add more complexity to the staging process with AUS. Kwok et al. (13) estimated accuracy of lymph node staging to be approximately 74% with a range between 44 to 87%. The accuracy for defining lymph nodes is higher if they are greater than 5 mm in size (12). The accuracy decreases to approximately 30% when nodes are less than 5 mm in size. Herzog et al. (15) have shown the accuracy to be approximately 79% for nodes 0 to 5 mm, 92% for nodes between 6 and 10 mm, and 100% for those greater than 10 mm. However, others have found the shape, size, and outer borders were not predictive of metastasis (18).

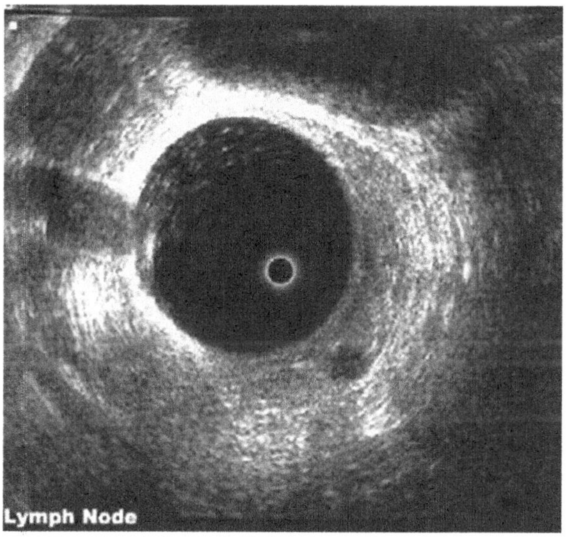

Figure 6 uN1 lesion: Lymph node in perirectal fat. *Source*: Photo courtesy of The Cleveland Clinic, Cleveland, Ohio, U.S A.

IMAGING FOR SPHINCTER DEFECTS

Normal Sphincter

The puborectalis is visualized in the upper anal canal as a sling or U shaped structure that circles the rectum posteriorly, and is hyperechoic (appearing more white) due to its striated nature. As the probe is retracted down the anal canal, the external anal sphincter (EAS) comes into view in the upper and mid anal canal as another white structure which is a full circle and normally has a uniform thickness if the probe is held correctly at a right angle to the muscle. The EAS runs oblique to the probe and, as it is not enclosed in a fascia, its margins appear indistinct (19). As the probe is withdrawn, the internal anal sphincter (IAS) comes into view in the mid low anal canal as a hypoechoic (dark) band due to the smooth muscles that is made up of water. As with the balloon and cone, the sound waves pass through water without being altered and give the dark appearance to the IAS. As the probe is further withdrawn, the IAS disappears and only the EAS is seen normally at the anal verge. Measurements of the sphincter thickness and any defect in the anal sphincter can be made.

Sphincter Abnormalities

Abnormal sphincters demonstrate a defect or disruption in continuity, or have marked thinning of the IAS and EAS, but may have no defect. The most common causes of injury are obstetrical trauma, post surgical trauma, or trauma from rectal prolapse. Thinning can also occur for no apparent reason.

Between the "arms" of a disrupted muscle, scarring can be detected, which is of differing density. A defect in the EAS is demonstrated in Figure 7 while a defect in the IAS is shown in Figure 8. Attenuation or thinning of the IAS is seen in Figure 9. After a sphincter repair, the overlap of the "arms" performed during surgery can be detected. In addition, if the overlap has become disrupted or is incomplete, these changes can also be visualized.

ACCURACY OF IMAGING SPHINCTER DEFECTS

A sphincter defect is clearly demonstrated on AUS. However, not all sphincter defects are pathognomonic of incontinence nor do they correlate to the degree of incontinence. EAS defects have been demonstrated in postpartum women without any symptoms of incontinence (20). However, the demonstration of a sphincter defect in a woman with incontinence is an indication for operative reconstruction of the anal sphincters.

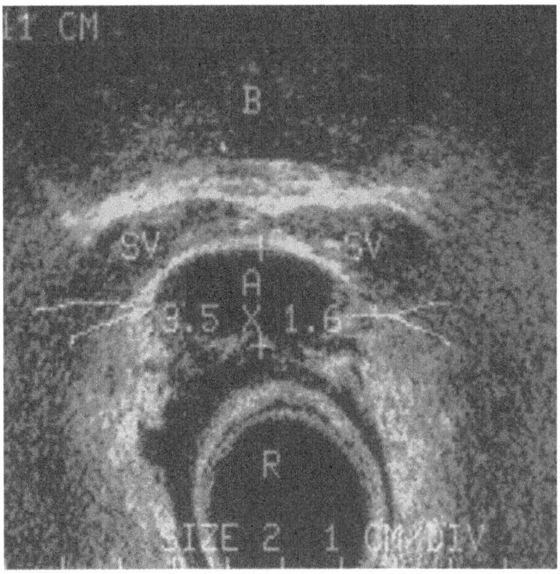

Figure 7 Abscess cavity (*marked "A" and white arrows*) between seminal vesicle (SV) and internal anal sphincter (IAS). R, rectum; B, bladder. *Source*: Photo courtesy of The Cleveland Clinic, Cleveland, Ohio, U.S.A.

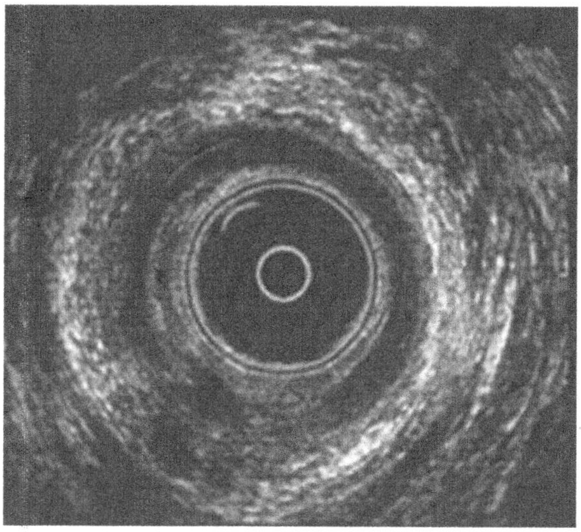

Figure 8 Internal anal sphincter defect (*arrows depict the two ends*). *Source*: Photo courtesy of The Cleveland Clinic, Cleveland, Ohio, U.S.A.

Thinning of the anal sphincters may be indicative of denervation of the muscle, and this can be further demonstrated by electromyography (EMG) and pudendal nerve terminal motor latency (PTNML) studies, both of which have been described in other chapters.

AUS IN ABSCESSES

Most perianal abscesses are easily seen and diagnosed clinically. The use of the AUS is reserved for those patients who have severe anal pain without a clearly demonstrated pathology. An abscess appears as a dark (hypoechoic) area. The procedure can be performed in the office setting, but if the patient is too uncomfortable, examination with AUS in the operating room under anesthesia may be required. Supralevator and ischiorectal abscesses, which are situated out of the focal length of the probe, may be most difficult to visualize. MRI is more accurate in these cases (21). However, AUS may be most advantageous in demonstrating an intersphincteric abscess that may be difficult to appreciate on physical examination (Fig. 9).

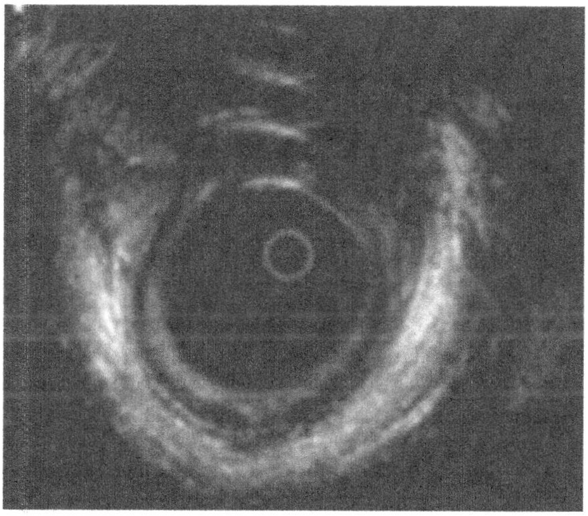

Figure 9 Internal anal sphincter defect (*white arrow*), external anal sphincter defect (*thick arrow*). *Source*: Photo courtesy of The Cleveland Clinic, Cleveland, Ohio, U.S.A.

FISTULA IN ANO

Simple fistulae are easily demonstrable by probing in the office setting. More complex fistulous tracts are difficult to delineate. The internal opening may be difficult to locate in the office setting or in the operating room. AUS may demonstrate both the internal and external openings. MRI is felt to have a higher accuracy (22) than AUS; however, this is not an office-based procedure. The description of the tract and the openings on AUS have been defined by Seow–Choen et al. (23). The internal opening is a hypoechoic defect in the subepithelial layer of the anorectum, a defect in the circular muscles of the internal sphincter, and a hypoechoic lesion of the normally echoic longitudinal muscle abutting on the normally echoic circular smooth muscle. The internal opening was further defined by Cho (24) as having one of the three criteria:

1. An appearance of a root-like budding formed by the intersphincteric tract, which contacts the internal sphincter;
2. An appearance of a root-like budding with an internal sphincter defect;
3. A subepithelial breach connecting to the intersphincteric tract through an intersphincteric defect.

The accuracy of detecting fistulous tracts with AUS is 60% to 70% (23,25,26). Delineation of a tract can be further enhanced using hydrogen peroxide, after which the accuracy improves to 96% (26). Hydrogen peroxide is injected through the external opening and the external opening is blocked to avoid the liquid from pouring out. The oxidation reaction produces a gas that fizzes, causing the tract to become highlighted and more hypoechoic. Instillation of hydrogen peroxide may be of particular value in evaluating horse-shoe fistulae (26). The downside of its use is that a secondary tract may not fill if all the fluid escapes through the internal opening. Identification of high fistulae with this technique may be instrumental in changing the treatment strategy to a sphincter saving procedure (i.e., endoanal flap), or planning surgery in two steps if a secondary tract is delineated (27).

AUS IN RECTOVAGINAL FISTULA

Rectovaginal fistulae are best demonstrated clinically. AUS is of value when a fistula is suspected, but cannot be demonstrated. In one study, Baig et al. (28) reported a fistulous connection in four patients who did not have a demonstrable connection. They reported an accuracy of 73% for identifying rectovaginal fistulae using AUS (28). In addition, AUS can delineate the location of the fistulous tract in relation to the anal sphincters along with the presence of an occult sphincter defect. MRI is equally comparable to AUS with a positive predictive value of 100% versus 92% with AUS (26).

AUS IN EXTRARECTAL MASSES

Although not common, tumors occurring outside the rectum such as presacral cysts and chordomas and their relationship to the rectal wall can be demonstrated with AUS. Although MRI is perhaps the preferred imaging modality, AUS is a relatively quick procedure, which can initiate the treatment plan and may augment information gained with an MRI.

SUMMARY

AUS is inexpensive and conveniently performed in the office setting. The degree of accuracy is operator dependant. Sphincter defects associated with fecal incontinence or rectovaginal fistulae may be best demonstrated by AUS, although clinical correlation is required. Complex fistulae, deep abscesses, and suspected rectovaginal fistulae may be demonstrated by AUS. Suspected intersphincteric abscesses may be best demonstrated with AUS. The drawbacks of AUS are associated with the inability to visualize beyond the focal length of the probe and its limitation with rectal tumors in relation to (1) detect distant metastases; (2) pass the probe beyond near obstructing lesions in approximately 17% of stenotic lesions (29); (3) detect subtle differences in wall penetration; and (4) detect positive lymph nodes with a great deal of accuracy.

CONCLUSION

AUS is a valuable imaging modality for several anorectal conditions and is available conveniently in the office. The simplicity involved in performing the procedure and the high degree of accuracy make it a user-friendly and valuable tool for the colorectal surgeon.

REFERENCES

1. Drew PJ, Farouk R, Turnbull LW, et al. Preoperative magnetic resonance staging of rectal cancer with an endorectal coil and dynamic gadolinium enhancement. Br J Surg 1999; 86(2):250–254.
2. Garcia-Aguilar J, Pollack J, Lee SH, et al. Accuracy of endorectal ultrasonography in preoperative staging of rectal tumors. Dis Colon Rectum 2002;45:10–15.
3. Huch Boni RA, Meyenberger C, Pok LJ, et al. Value of endorectal coil versus body coil MRI for diagnosis of recurrent pelvic malignancies. Abdom Imaging 1996;21(4):345–352.
4. Kim JC, Cho YK, Kim SK, et al. Comparative study of three-dimensional and conventional endorectal ultrasonography in rectal cancer staging. Surg Endosc 2002;16:1280–1285.
5. Rifkin MD, Ehrlich SM, Marks G. Staging of rectal carcinoma: prospective comparison of endorectal US and CT. Radiology 1989; 170: 319–322.
6. Solomon MJ, McLeod RS. Endoluminal transrectal ultrasonography: accuracy, reliability, and validity. Dis Colon Rectum 1993; 36:200–205.
7. Waizer A, Powsner E, Russo I, et al. Prospective comparative study of magnetic resonance imaging versus transrectal ultrasound for preoperative staging and follow-up of rectal cancer. Preliminary report. Dis Colon Rectum 1991; 37:1189–1193.
8. Orrom WJ, Wong WD, Rothenberger DA, et al. Endorectal ultrasound in the preoperative staging of rectal tumors: a learning experience. Dis Colon Rectum 1990: 33:654–659.
9. Kauer WKH, Prantl L, Dittler HJ, Jr. S. The value of endographic rectal carcinoma staging in routine diagnostics. Surg Endosc 2004; 18:1075–1078.
10. Hildebrandt U, Feifel G. Preoperative staging of rectal cancer by intrarectal ultrasound. Dis Colon Rectum 1985; 28; 42–46.
11. Beynon J, Mortensen NJ, Foy DM, et al. Pre-operative assessment of local invasion in rectal cancer: digital examination, endoluminal sonography or computer tomography? Br J Surg 1986; 73(12):1015–1017.
12. Dworak O. Number and size of lymph node metastases in rectal carcinomas. Surg Endosc 1989; 3:96–99.
13. Kwok H, Bissett I, Hill GL. Preoperative staging of rectal cancer. Int J Colorectal Dis 2000; 15:9–20.
14. Starck M, Bohe M, Simanaitis M, et al. Rectal ultrasonography can distinguish benign rectal lesions from invasive early rectal cancers. Colorectal Dis 2002; 5:246–250.
15. Herzog U, von Flue M, Tondelli P, et al. How accurate is endorectal ultrasound in the preoperative staging of rectal cancer? Dis Colon Rectum 1993; 36:127–134.
16. Sentovich SM, Blatchford GJ, Falk PM, et al. Transrectal ultrasound of rectal tumors. Am J Surg 1993; 166(16): 638–641.
17. Detry R, Kartheuser A. Endorectal ultrasonography in staging small rectal tumors. Br J Surg 1992; 79(suppl): 30.
18. Hildebrandt U, Feifel G. Endosonography in the diagnosis of lymph nodes. Endoscopy 1993;25: 243–245.
19. Law PJ, CI B. Anal ultrasonography: technique and normal anatomy. Gastrointest Radiol 1989; 14:349–353.
20. Varma A, Gunn J, Gardiner A, et al. Obstetrical anal sphincter injury: prospective evaluation of incidence. Dis Colon Rectum 1998; 42:423–427.
21. Maruyama R, Noguchi T, Takano M, et al. Usefulness of magnetic resonance imaging for diagnosing deep anorectal abscesses. Dis Colon Rectum 2000; 43:S2–5.
22. Bartram CI, G B. Imaging anal fistula. Radiol Clin North Am 2003; 41(2):443–457.
23. Choen S, Burnett S, Bartram CI, et al. Comparison between anal ultrasonography and digital examination in theevaluation of anal fistulae. Br J Surg 1991; 78(26):69–80.
24. Cho DY. Endosonographic criteria for an internal opening of fistula in ano. Dis Colon Rectum 1999; 42:515–518.

25. Cheong DM, Nogueras JJ, Wexner SD, et al. Anal ultrasonography for recurrent anal fistulas:image enhancement with hydrogen peroxide. Dis Colon Rectum 1993; 36:1158–1160.
26. Stroker J, Rociu E, Wiersma TG, et al. Imaging of anorectal disorders. Br J Surg 2000; 87:10–27.
27. Navarro-Luna A, Garcia-Domingo M, Rius-Macias J, et al. Ultrasound study of anal fistulas with hydrogen peroxide enhancement. Dis Colon Rectum 2004; 47(1):108–114.
28. Baig MK, Zhao RH, Yuen CH, et al. Simple rectovaginal fistulas. Int J Colorectal Dis 2000; (15):323–327.
29. Hawes RH. New staging techniques. Endoscopic ultrasound. Cancer 1993; 71(suppl 12):4207–4213.

5 Biofeedback Treatment for Functional Anorectal Disorders

Dawn Vickers
GI-GU Functional Diagnostics, Fort Lauderdale, Florida, U.S.A.

INTRODUCTION

Over the past 20 years, biofeedback has been used for the treatment of functional anorectal disorders. In the current Rome ll diagnostic system, which provides the most widely recognized criteria for diagnosing and classifying functional gastrointestinal disorders, three anorectal disorders are recognized: functional fecal incontinence (FI), functional anorectal pain, and pelvic floor dyssynergia (PFD) (1).

PELVIC FLOOR DYSSYNERGIA

Constipation and its associated symptoms are the most common chronic gastrointestinal complaint, accounting for 2.5 (2) million physician visits per year with a prevalence of 2% in the U.S. population (3). Rome II diagnostic criteria for a diagnosis of constipation are specified in Table 1 (4). After identification and exclusion of extracolonic or anatomic causes, many patients respond favorably to medical and dietary management. However, patients unresponsive to simple treatment may require further physiologic investigation to evaluate the pathophysiologic process underlying the symptoms. Physiologic investigation generally includes colonic transit time study, cinedefecography, anorectal manometry, and electromyography (EMG) (5), which allows for definitive diagnosis of treatable conditions including colonic inertia, rectocele, sigmoidocele, and anismus (6). Functional constipation is commonly classified as slow colonic transit or outlet delay; however, some patients may fulfill criteria for both. Functional defecation disorders are characterized by inadequate propulsive forces during attempted defecation or PFD, a paradoxical contraction or inadequate relaxation of the puborectalis muscle during attempted defecation (7). PFD—also termed, anismus, spastic pelvic floor syndrome, paradoxical puborectalis contraction, and nonrelaxing puborectalis syndrome—accounts for an estimated 50% of patients with symptoms of chronic constipation (8). Rome II diagnostic criteria for a diagnosis of PFD is specified in Table 2 (4). Invasive surgical therapies or injection of botulinum neurotoxin (9) are associated with an unacceptable incidence of incontinence. In 1993, Enck's critical review summarized that biofeedback has become widely accepted as the treatment of choice for PFD (10).

FUNCTIONAL FECAL INCONTINENCE

Fecal incontinence (FI) is defined as the uncontrolled passage of fecal material recurring for ≥3 months (7). Fecal incontinence can have a devastating psychological and social impact on otherwise functional individuals, causing fear, anxiety, and perceived shame and often leading to progressive isolation and depression. It is estimated that 7.15% of the general population experiences fecal soiling and 0.7% experiences gross incontinence (11). Because of the perceived shame, FI is not often spontaneously reported by patients.

Fecal incontinence is a complex and challenging dilemma of multifactorial etiology. A careful history, physical examination, and selected objective test of the continence mechanisms are recommended so that appropriate therapy can be instituted. Continence depends on the presence of a series of anatomic barriers to the movement of feces through the anus. These barriers include the puborectalis muscle of the pelvic floor as well as the internal and external anal sphincters. Continence requires normal sensation of rectal distention, intact innervation of

Table 1 Rome II Criteria for Diagnosis of Constipation

Straining >25% of defecations
Lumpy or hard stools >25% of defecations
Sensation of incomplete evacuation >25% of defecations
Sensation of anorectal obstruction/blockage >25% of defecations.
Manual maneuvers to facilitate >25% of defecations (i.e., digital evacuation, support of the pelvic floor) and/or <3 defecations per week.
Loose stools are not present, and there are insufficient criteria for irritable bowel syndrome

the muscles, and adequate reservoir capacity of the rectum. Although the pelvic floor muscles (PFMs) and external anal sphincter are tonically active, entry of stool into the rectum or upper anal canal calls for heightened contraction of these muscles to preserve continence (11). Anal sphincter weakness has long been associated with fecal incontinence. Although attention is usually focused on external sphincter weakness, dysfunction of the internal anal sphincter also contributes to incontinence (11). Enck's critical review concluded that rehabilitation of the PFMs utilizing biofeedback applications for the treatment of FI has shown to improve anorectal function in the majority of patients (12).

FUNCTIONAL ANORECTAL PAIN

Two forms of functional anorectal pain have been described: levator ani syndrome and proctalgia fugax. Their diagnosis is based on symptoms alone. Levator ani symptoms are usually described as a vague, dull ache, or pressure sensation high in the rectum, often worse with sitting or lying down, lasting hours or days. Proctalga fugax symptoms are usually sudden, severe pain in the anal area lasting several seconds or minutes, then spontaneously disappearing completely (1). Results with biofeedback therapy for this condition are still scarce in the literature, with an overall success rate ranging from 34% to 91% (13).

EFFICACY OF BIOFEEDBACK THERAPY: LITERATURE REVIEW

When interpreting the clinical outcome of the studies listed for FI and constipation, one should keep in mind that there are no established guidelines regarding the number of sessions, teaching methods, clinician qualifications, type of equipment used, and patient inclusion criteria (Tables 3 and 4). In addition, there are no subjective or objective data used to establish success of the therapy. All of these factors vary considerably. Hyman's critical review reports that, perhaps most importantly, there is no identified standard for training biofeedback clinicians to treat pelvic floor disorders. As with any therapy, the competence of the clinician is likely to have a significant impact on the outcome of treatment (14). Norton reports that many patients lack the motivation or are unconvinced about the possible value of what they perceive to be simple exercises; therefore, results of treatment are largely patient dependent, unlike drug or surgical therapy (15). Gilliland et al. (24) reported that patient motivation and willingness to comply with treatment protocols were the most important predictor of success.

It has been suggested that when researchers understand the essential components of biofeedback training, research studies are often successful. These components are: (1) The biofeedback instrument which is no more and no less than a mirror. Like a mirror, it feeds back information, but has no inherent power to create change in the user; (2) To maximize results, biofeedback training, like any type of complex skill training, involves clear goals, rewards for

Table 2 Rome II Criteria for Pelvic Floor Dyssynergia

The patient must satisfy diagnostic criteria for functional constipation in Diagnostic Criteria listed in Table 1
There must be manometric, electromyographic, or radiological evidence for inappropriate contraction or failure to relax the pelvic floor muscles during repeated attempts to defecate
There must be evidence of adequate propulsive forces during attempts to defecate, and
There must be evidence of incomplete evacuation

Table 3 Biofeedback Studies in Constipation

Author/year	*n*	Pre-evaluation	Diagnosis	Mean age (yrs)	Feedback method	No. of sessions	Follow up	Evaluation assessment	% Improved	Defined success
Emmanuel 2001 (14)	49	BE, EMG, CTT, CRAFT, Rectal Laser Doppler Flowmetry	IC	39	EMG + BD	4–7	28 mo	Diary, Rectal Laser Doppler, BE, CTT Cardio respiratory autonomic function testing	59	Pre vs. Post BF: <3 BM/wk (27v9) Need to strain (26v9) Laxative or suppository (34v9) Slow transit (22v9) Rectal mucosal blood flow: (improved vs. not improved) (29% vs. 7%)
Dailianas 2000 (15)	11	CTT, MN, DF, EMG	PPC	43	MN	2	6 mo	Diary	54.5	Symptom improvement
Lau 2000 (16)	173	DF	PPC	67	EMG	4–7	4–7	Diary	55	Improved bowel function
Mollen 1999 (17)	7	CTT, DF, BE, MN	PPC	30	NR	10	NR	MN	NR	Effects rectocolonic inhibitory reflex
McKee 1999 (18)	30	DF, CTT, BEN, Colo, EMG, MN	PPC	35	MN	3–4	12 mo	Diary, BE	30	Symptom improvement
Chiotakakou 1998 (19)	100	CTT, MN, EMG	PPC + IC	40	EMG	4–5	23 mo	Phone Interview	57	Symptom improvement
Rieger 1997 (20)	19	MN, DF, CTT, EMG, BE	IC	63	EMG + BD	6	6 mo	Interview	12.5	>50% symptom reduction @ 6 mo
Glia 1997 (21)	26	MN, DF, CTT, EMG, BE	PPC	55	EMG, MN	1–2/wk< 10wk	6 mo	Diary	58 (75% completed therapy)	Symptom improvement
Ko 1997 (22)	32	EMG, DF, CTT, BE	PPC	50	EMG	4 (2–9)	7 M	Diary	80	Symptom improvement
Patankar 1997 (23)	116	EMG, DF MN, CTT, DF, AUS,	IC	73	EMG	8 (2–14)		Diary	73	Satisfaction rate
Gilliland 1997 (24)	194	EMG, DF, MN	PPC	71	EMG	11 (5–30)	72 M	Return to normal (>3unassisted BM per wk)	35 (63% completed therapy)	Normal bowel habits
Karlbom 1997 (25)	17	EMG,DF, MN, CTT	PPC	46	EMG, BE	8	14 M	Questionnaire	43	Improved rectal emptying
Rao 1997 (26)	25	MN, DF, CTT, BE		50	MN, BE	2–10	<2 M	Diary MN, BE	92	>% Anal relaxation >Intrarectal pressure >Defecation index <BE time <Laxative use <Straining
Patankar 1997 (27)	30			65.3	EMG	5–11	No	Diary EMG	84	>Frequency of spontaneous BM> 2/wk >EMG endurance and net strength of external anal sphincter

(continued)

Table 3 Biofeedback Studies in Constipation (*Continued*)

Author/year	*n*	Pre-evaluation	Diagnosis	Mean age (yrs)	Feedback method	No. of sessions	Follow up	Evaluation assessment	% Improved	Defined success
Park 1996 (28)	68	MN, DF, CTT, EMG	PPC	65.9	EMG	11	NO	Diary & Questionnaire	25/85	Improved or unimproved
Ho 1996 (29)	62	MN, DF, CTT, EMG	PPC	48	MN, BE	4	14.9	Diary	90.3	>Frequency of spontaneous BM <Laxative and enema use >Symptom improvement
Leroi 1996 (30)	15	MN, EMG,	PPC	41.2	Psychotherapy, MN, EMG	16	6–10 M	Not reported (NR)	66.7	Complete recovery of symptoms
Siproudhis 1995 (31)	27	MN, DF, BE	PPC	46	MN, BE	1–10	1–36 M	NR	51.8	Complete recovery of symptoms
Koutsomanis 1995 (32)	60	CTT, EMG, BE	PPC	40.5		1–7	2–3 M	Diary	50	<EMG activity with Valsalva >Anismus index
Koutsomanis 1994 (33)	20	MN, DF, CTT, BE,	IC	34		2–6	6–12 M	Diary	50	>BM frequency <Staining >Symptom improvement
Bleijenberg 1994 (34)	21	MN, EMG, DF, BE	PPC	37	EMG vs Balloon	8–11	NO	Diary constipation score	EMG: 73 BE: 22	Symptom improvement
Papachrysostmou 1994 (35)	22	MN, DF, CTT, EMG, BE	PPC	42	EMG	>3	NO	MN, DF, EMG Clinical improvement	89 vs 86	<EMG activity >Improved DF >Rectal sensation
Keck 1994 (36)	12	MN, DF, CTT, EMG, BE	IC	62	EMG	3	1–8 M	Tel interview	58	Symptom improvement
Trunbull 1992 (37)	7	MN, DF, CTT, EMG	PPC	35.7	MN, Relax	4–5	2–4 yr	Diary	85.7	Stool frequency <Symptoms of bloating and pain
Fleshman 1992 (38)	9	MN, DF, CTT, ENG, BE	PPC	49.4	EMG, BE, Relax	2 × 6	>6 M	BE, EMG	100	<EMG activity during strain BE 60cc Eliminate psyllium slurry
Wexner 1992 (39)	18	MN, DF, CTT, EMG	PPC	67.7	EMG	9	1–17	Diary	88.9	Spontaneous BM frequency <Laxative use
Dahl 1991 (40)	9	MN, DF, CTT, EMG, BE	IC	41	EMG	5	6	Diary	77.8	BM frequency <Laxative use
Kawimbe 1991 (41)	15	MN, BE	PPC	45	EMG	2/D	6.2	DF, diary	86.7	<Anismus index >Anorectal angel straining BM frequency
Lestar 1991 (42)	16	MN, DF, BE, CTT, EMG	PPC	42.5	Defae-cometer	1	0	Defaecometer	68.7	Ability to expel balloon
Webber 1987 (43)	22	MN	IC		MN	2–4	0	NR	18.2	Daily spontaneous BM
Bleijenberg 1987 (44)	10	DF, CTT, EMG	PPC	32	EMG, BE	Daily	7	NR	70	Spontaneous BM

Abbreviations: MN, manometry; CTT, colon transit time; colo, colonoscopy; IC, idiopathic constipation; BE, balloon expulsion; DF, cinedefecography; BE, barium enema; PPC, paradoxical puborectalis contraction; BF, biofeedback; EMG, electromyography; BM, bowel movement.

Table 4 Biofeedback for Fecal Incontinence: Published Series

Author/year	*n*	Mean age (yrs)	Pre-evaluation	Post evaluation	Feedback method	Treatment method	No. of Sessions	Defined success	% Improved
Engel 1974 (45)	7	40.7 (6–54)	MN	MN	MN	Coordination	1–4	Subjective	57
Cerulli 1979 (46)	50	46 (5–97)	No	MN	MN	Coordination sensitivity	1	>90%	72
Goldenberg 1980 (47)	12	12	MN	No	MN	Sensitivity	>1	Subjective	83
Wald 1981 (48)	17	47 (10–79)	MN	No	MN	Coordination sensitivity PME	1–2	>75%	71
Whitehead 1985 (49)	18	73 (65–92)	MN	MN	MN	PME	8	>75%	77
Buser 1986 (50)	13	53.6	MN	MN	MN	Sensitivity PME	1–3	Subjective	92
McLeod 1987 (51)	113	56 (25–88)	No	EMG	EMG	PME	3.3	>90%	63
Enck 1988 (52)	19	47 (10–80)	MN	MN	MN	Coordination	5–10	Subjective	63
Riboli 1988 (53)	21	61 (14–84)	MN	MN	MN	Coordination sensitivity PME	12	>90%	86
Miner 1990 (54)	25	54 (17–76)	MN	MN	MN	Coordination sensitivity PME	3	Subjective	76
Loening-Baucke 1990 (55)	8	63 (35–78)	MN	MN	MN	Coordination sensitivity PME	3	>75%	50
Keck 1994 (56)	15	39 (29–65)	MN	MN	EMG	Sensitivity PME	1–7	Subjective	53
Guillemot 1995 (57)	24	(39–78)	MN	MN	MN	PME	4	Incontinence score (IS)	Improved IS 19
Sangwan 1995 (58)	28	52 (30–74)	MN	MN	MN	Sensitivity PME	1–7	Complete continence to solid stool	46 Excellent 29 Good 25 Bad
Ho 1996 (59)	13	62.1	MN	MN	MN	PME	11	>90%[a]	76.9
Rao 1996 (60)	19	50 (17–78)	MN EMG	MN EMG	MN	Coordination sensitivity PME	4–13	>67%	53
Jensen 1997 (61) 1997 (*86*)	28	34 (23–57)	MN		EMG	PME	3–4	>80% + Incontinence score	89
Reiger 1997 (62)	30	68 (29–85)	MN	MN	EMG	PME	6	Incontinence score	67 Incontinence score
Ko 1997 (63)	25	63 31–82)	MN EMG	EMG	EMG	PME	2–13	Subjective	92
Pantankar 1997 (64)	25	34 (23–57)	EMG	EMG	EMG	PME	5–11	>75%	83
Glia 1998 (65)	26	61 (32–82)	MN	MN	MN	Sensitivity PME	4–10	>50% Decrease in soiling episodes	23 Excellent 41 Good 36 No Improvement
Leroi 1998 (66)	27	53 (29–74)	MN, PNTML USG	MN	MN	Coordination sensitivity PME	4–14	Subjective	29.6

[a]Decrease in frequency of incontinent episodes.

Abbreviations: MN, manometry; EMG, electromyography; PNTML, pudendal nerve terminal motor latency; PME, pelvic muscle exercises.

approximating the goals, ample time and practice for achieving mastery, proper instruction, a variety of systematic training techniques, and feedback of information; (3) The individual using the feedback must have a cognitive understanding of the process and goals, positive expectations and positive interaction with the trainer, and must be motivated to learn (67). Therefore, establishing a double blind, placebo controlled research protocol for biofeedback therapy, based on the principals used for medication trials, becomes inherently difficult. Studies based on understanding the essentials of biofeedback training are often successful (67). In 1991, Dahl defined his teaching methods of sensory awareness by teaching patients the correct sphincter responses, using home practice, physiological quieting methods, generalization, and weaning of equipment. There was a reported symptom improvement success rate of 78% for patients with anismus (68). Rao's study is another example of defined teaching methods employing the essentials of biofeedback training and reporting 100% success, which is defined as >50% symptomatic improvement. They concluded that biofeedback therapy effectively improves objective and subjective parameters of anorectal function in patients with FI. In addition, they noted that customizing the number of sessions and providing periodic reinforcement may improve success (69).

Constipation

The many variants in these clinical trials may account for the wide range of success rates from 30% to 100% (Table 3). The number of treatment sessions varies significantly from one session of outpatient training to two weeks of daily inpatient training, followed by additional subsequent home training. Rao's review noted that the end-point for successful treatment has not been clearly defined and the duration of follow up has also been quite variable (8). Enck points out that comparing clinical symptoms prior to and after treatment usually assesses treatment efficacy; however, other studies have reported evaluation of sphincter performance during physiological testing. Outcome was sometimes assessed by diary cards; however, reviews, telephone interviews, and questionnaires were more often used. These evaluation techniques are unreliable when the recorded event, such as defecation, is infrequent in nature (12). Furthermore, diagnostic data from physiologic testing beyond confirmation of spastic pelvic floor syndrome are often not reported. The patient's concomitant conditions disclose a significant variance in inclusion criteria (e. g., presence of rectoceles, rectal sensory thresholds, previous surgery), which presumably contribute to the success of treatment (12). Park described two varieties of anismus, anal canal hypertonia and nonrelaxation of the puborectalis muscle, that appear to correlate with the success of biofeedback; specifically, anal canal hypertonia may be responsible for failure of biofeedback therapy (28). McKee concluded that biofeedback for outlet obstruction constipation is more likely to be successful in patients without evidence of severe pelvic floor damage (18). The study by Emmanuel in 2001 (14) reported on 49 patients with idiopathic constipation pre and post biofeedback using objective measurements as well as patient symptom diaries; symptomatic improvement occurred in 59% of patients. Twenty-two patients had slow transit before treatment, of which 14 felt symptomatic improvement and 13 developed normal colonic transit. There was a significant increase in rectal mucosal blood flow in patients who subjectively improved. These authors concluded that successful response to biofeedback for constipation is associated with specifically improved autonomic innervation to the large bowel and improved transit time. In 1998, Chiotakokowi's study (19) of 100 patients treated with biofeedback therapy reported that 65% had slow transit and 59% had paradoxical puborectalis contraction on straining. Long-term follow up at 23 months revealed that 57% of patients felt their constipation had improved (19). More recent studies have been published with more sophisticated designs, methodologies, and often more adequate sample sizes compared to earlier studies. In 2007 Roa et al. (70) reported a randomized controlled trial of biofeedback, sham feedback, and standard therapy for dyssynergic defecation. They showed symptomatic improvement in physiologic characteristics of colorectal function. During attempted defecation, the dyssynergic pattern was corrected in 79% of patients who received biofeedback, but was unchanged in the other two therapies. More recently, Heyman et al. (71) showed biofeedback to be superior to alternative treatments for patients with PFD. Biofeedback is a conservative treatment option for patients with idiopathic constipation, although some studies have shown to have less favorable results. Reiger (20) evaluated the results of biofeedback to treat 19 patients with intractable constipation of no specific etiology and concluded that biofeedback had little therapeutic effect. In these cases, Wexner et al. (72) reported patients remain symptomatic requiring the inconvenience and expense associated with the use of cathartics. Engel and Kamm (73) showed that excessive straining has both acute and chronic effects on pudendal nerve latencies. Long-term symptom duration with intense straining would thus induce nerve damage. It has also been reported that the chronic use of laxatives induces changes in the myenteric nerve plexa (74). Wexner et al. (72) suggested that an alternate course of action would be to explain to patients that, although success of only 40% to 60% can be anticipated, the success rate is determined by their willingness to complete the course of therapy. Patients should be counseled that biofeedback therapy is the only recourse other than the continued use of laxatives and cathartics. Chiarioni's more recent study (75) compared biofeedback to polyethylene glycol for the treatment of PFD. Results at six months showed significant improvement reported by 80% of the biofeedback patients versus 22% of the laxative-treated patients.

Fecal Incontinence

In 2007, Byrne et al. (76) published the largest retrospective review of 385 patients who completed the biofeedback treatment program and reported that more than 75% of the patients had clinically and statistically significant improvement in outcome, including incontinence scores, quality of life, and physiologic measure of sphincter function. Heymen's critical review (77) of 35 studies published in 2001 compared the results of coordination training (coordinating PFM contraction with the sensation of rectal filling) with a mean success rate of 67% to strength training (PFM contraction) with a mean success rate of 70%. Enck's critical review (10) summarized a total of 13 clinical studies published between 1974 and 1990 using biofeedback therapy for the treatment of fecal incontinence. He reported that weighting the number of patients included into each study yields an overall success rate of 80%. Despite the wide variety in almost all criteria used to compare these studies, the therapy outcome is homogenous, ranging between 50 to 90%. In a review of 14 biofeedback studies performed between 1988 and 1997, Rao et al. (26) reported that 40% to 100% of patients were improved. The mechanism by which training effects are achieved is controversial (78). Some have argued that the most important ingredient is sensory discrimination training in which patients are taught to recognize and respond to increased intrarectal pressure (79). Others believe it is important to squeeze more quickly in response to rectal distention (54). Still others believe that biofeedback works primarily by strengthening the external anal sphincter muscles (in conjunction with Kegel exercises) (49). On one hand, sensations consistently improve with biofeedback. As this improvement occurs rapidly, it is likely associated with relearning neurophysiological patterns that are essentially intact but not used because of faulty sensation. Conversely, it is unlikely that short-term sensory discrimination training and coordination training will alter muscle tone or strength sufficiently to modify a condition where weakness is the primary contributor to the incontinence. Thus, when the muscles are weak but sensation is intact, symptom reduction would depend on changing muscle strength through extended and well-designed exercise protocols (10). This approach was clearly shown by Chiarioni (78) and Rao (69) who both outlined specific goals to improve the strength of the anal sphincter, improve rectoanal coordination, and improve rectal sensory thresholds. Visual and verbal feedback techniques were used to reinforce their appropriate responses as they were being performed. Fernandez-Fraga's study demonstrated the significance of the pelvic floor by showing that the levator ani contraction is the independent variable with the strongest relation to the severity of incontinence, as well as the strongest predictive factor of the response to treatment. Furthermore, in contrast to other physiologic parameters, marked and significant levator ani strengthening was associated with clinical improvement in response to biofeedback therapy (51). In general, most experts believe that all components are useful and that the treatment program should be customized for a given patient depending on the underlying dysfunction (69). The degree to which biofeedback will be successful often depends upon the complexity of the underlying pathophysiology (80).

BIOFEEDBACK DEFINED

Schwartz (10) defines the biofeedback process as "a group of therapeutic procedures that utilizes electronic instruments to accurately measure, process, and feed back to persons and their therapists, meaningful physiological information with educational and reinforcing properties about their neuromuscular and autonomic activity, both normal and abnormal, in the form of analog, binary, auditory, and/or visual feedback signals." This process helps patients develop a greater awareness of, confidence in, and an increase in voluntary control over physiological processes. This is best achieved with a competent biofeedback professional. Employing biofeedback instruments without proper cognitive preparation, instruction, and guidance is not appropriate biofeedback therapy. As with all forms of therapy, the therapist's skill, personality, and attention to the patient, all affect the outcome (80).

COMPONENTS OF BIOFEEDBACK THERAPY FOR THE COLON AND RECTAL PRACTICE

Practical aspects of biofeedback therapy for the colon and rectal practice for the treatment of PFM dysfunction including symptoms of PFD, FI, and functional anorectal pain, include technical, therapeutic, behavioral, and pelvic muscle rehabilitation (PMR) components.

Technical Component

The technical component involves the instrumentation used to provide meaningful information or feedback to the user. There are several technical systems available and the advantages of any one device have not been scientifically tested. Devices include surface EMG (sEMG), water-perfused manometry systems, and the solid-state manometry systems with a latex balloon. Although each system has inherent advantages and disadvantages, most systems provide reproducible and useful measurements. The choice of any one system depends on many factors, including cost and the goals of training. A solid-state system is preferable to a water-perfused system because there is no distraction or embarrassment from leakage of fluid and the patient can be moved to a sitting position without adversely affecting calibration. Although this instrumentation is of proven effectiveness, this method is relatively cumbersome, complicated, and expensive (51). sEMG instrumentation is widely used and proven effective for biofeedback training. Although not suitable for coordination training or sensory conditioning for FI (52). sEMG is more cost effective and suitable for office use (51). Patients are able to remain fully clothed during the session, and position changes are easily accomplished to assist with functional maneuvers.

sEMG Instrumentation

There is no standardization for sEMG recordings among manufacturers of biofeedback instrumentation; therefore, it is important for clinicians to understand basic technical aspects such as signal detection, signal processing, data acquisition, and display.

Signal Detection

Surface electrodes summate the electrical action potentials from the contracting muscle and establish electrical pathways from skin contact of the monitored muscle site (Fig. 1) (80). The sEMG instrument receives and processes this electrical correlate of a muscle activity measured in microvolts (μV) (Fig. 2). Muscle contraction involves the pulling together of the two anchor points; therefore, active electrodes should be placed between the anchor points along the long axis of the muscle (80). The interelectrode distance determines the volume of muscle monitored. Various types of electrodes are used with sEMG devices for PMR. The most direct measure of the sEMG activity from the pelvic musculature occurs when using internal sensors. Binni et al. (81) compared fine-wire electrodes to sensors with longitudinal electrodes and circumferential electrodes during rest, squeeze, and push. Internal sensors with longitudinal electrodes correlated better with fine-wire electrodes in all three categories (Fig. 3). Current internal sensors may detect one or two channels of sEMG activity. The two-channel multiple electrode probe anal EMG sensor (MEP) (Fig. 4) allows discrimination between proximal and distal external anal sphincter (EAS) activity, thereby, allowing the clinician to target specific areas of EAS inactivity in the rehabilitation process.

Signal Processing

The majority of the sEMG signal from the pelvic floor musculature is less than 100 Hz. The instrumentation should have the ability to filter noise interference allowing for a clear signal to be displayed. In order to detect the majority of the pelvic musculature signal the instrumentation

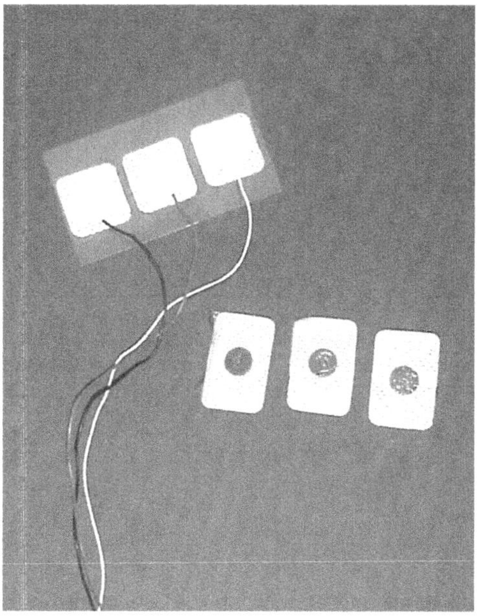

Figure 1 Disposable surface electromyography electrodes.

should have a wide bandwidth filter of 30–500 Hz. As muscle encounters fatigue, a shift to the lower frequencies (Hz) occurs; therefore, a wide bandwidth allows signal detection of low amplitude contractions (80). A 60 Hz "notch" filter rejects power-line interference. As all electronic instrumentation have internally generated noise, it is important for the clinician to know the internal noise level in order to distinguish noise from the sEMG signal.

Data Acquisition and Feedback Display

The sEMG instrument is designed to separate the electrical correlate of muscle activity from other extraneous noise and to convert this signal into forms of information or feedback meaningful to the user (10). Adjusting the sensitivity settings of the feedback display permits the clinician to tailor the shaping process according to the patient's ability to perform an isolated pelvic muscle contraction. If the sensitivity setting of the feedback display is 0 to 20 μV, expanding the display to a scale of 0 to 10 μV provides reinforcement for submaximal contractions of weak muscles.

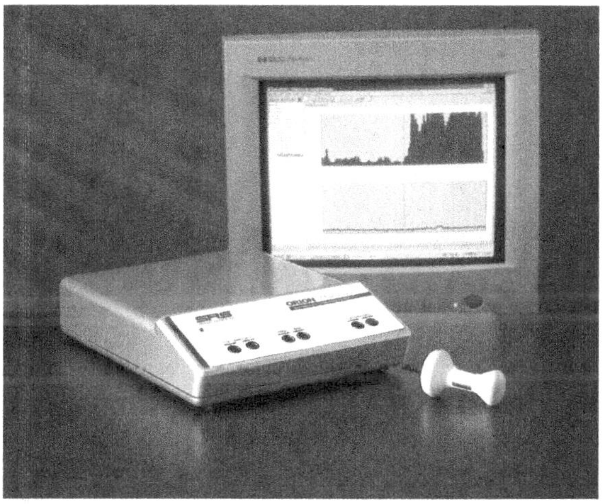

Figure 2 The Orion Platinum multimodality biofeedback system show a typical display during a PFM contraction. *Source*: Courtesy of SRS Medical, Redmond, Washington, U.S.A.

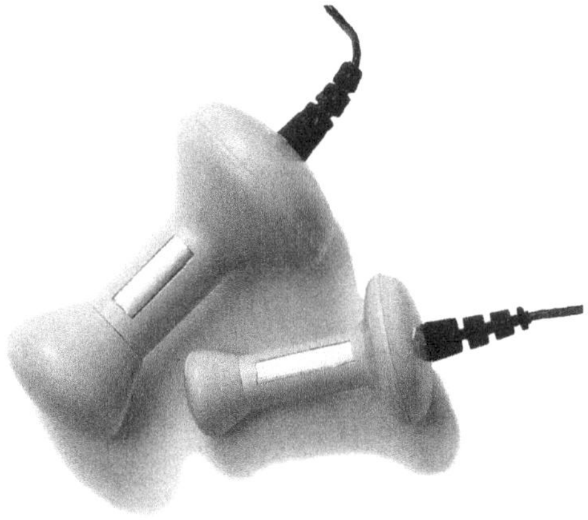

Figure 3 The SenseRx internal vaginal and anal sensors with longitudinal electrodes that maintain proper orientation to muscle fiber for accurate EMG monitoring. *Source*: Courtesy of SRS Medical, Redmond, Washington, U.S.A.

Pelvic Floor Musculature sEMG Evaluation

Abdominal and Pelvic Floor

The two channels of sEMG muscle activity, abdominal and pelvic floor, should be monitored simultaneously during the sEMG evaluation and the sEMG biofeedback-assisted pelvic muscle exercise training. Interpretative problems arise when monitoring only PFMs without controlling changes in the intra-abdominal pressure. The transmission of abdominal artifact to perennial measurements invalidates changes in the PFM measurements and can inadvertently reinforce maladaptive abdominal contractions (80). The recommended surface electrode placement for monitoring abdominal muscle activity is along the long axis on the lower right quadrant of the abdominal oblique muscles. Perianal placement of surface electrodes may be used to monitor the PFMs when internal sensors are inappropriate as in young pediatric patients. Placing the active electrodes in the 10 and 4 o'clock position around the anal opening and placing the reference electrode on the gluteus maximus or coccyx reduces artifact (Fig. 5). In order to obtain an evaluation, patients are instructed to simply relax, then to perform an isolated pelvic muscle contraction over a 10 second period. This sequence is repeated two to four times for accuracy (Table 5). During contraction, the abdominal muscle activity should remain relatively low and stable indicating the patient's ability to isolate PFM contraction from abdominal contraction (Fig. 6). This is followed by a Valsalva maneuver in which patients are instructed to push or bear down as if attempting to evacuate. During the Valsalva maneuver, PFM muscle activity should drop below the resting baseline to ($<2\ \mu V$), while the abdominal sEMG activity increases with elevated intra-abdominal pressure (Fig. 7). These objective measurements are documented and reviewed with the patient. This also provides the clinician with initial objective measurements to gauge training and recommend home practice according to meet individual capabilities.

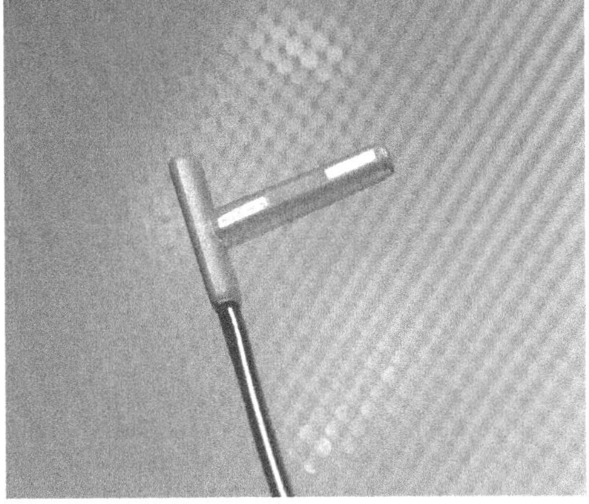

Figure 4 The Multiple electrode Probe (MEP) internal sensor. *Source*: Courtesy of SRS Medical, Redmond, Washington, U.S.A.

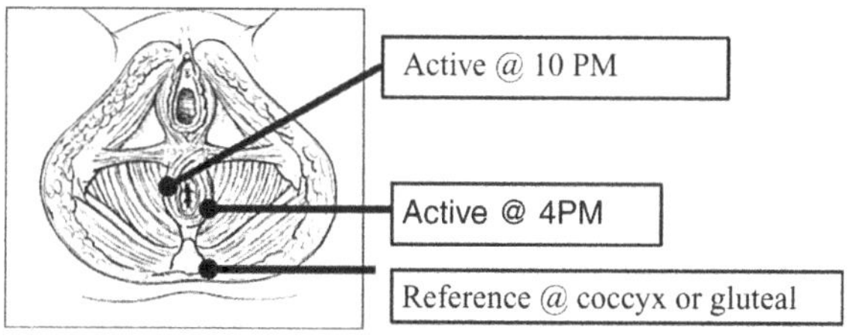

Figure 5 sEMG Perianal placement.

Therapeutic Component

The therapeutic component involves the clinician taking an active role by establishing a rapport with the patient, listening to concerns, reviewing the patient's medical history including current medications as well as over-the-counter and herbal preparations, reviewing bowel and bladder habits, educating the patient, and interpreting data. Clinicians must have a complete understanding of bowel and bladder function considering the coexistence of multifactorial concomitant PFM dysfunction. A patient with symptoms of constipation and dysfunctional defecation can also have a dysfunctional voiding pattern and associated symptoms of urinary urgency, frequency, and incontinence. Chronic straining with stool is another source of PFM denervation that contributes to PFM weakness and, ultimately, FI (19). Patients with FI may complain of multiple daily bowel movements and a feeling of incomplete evacuation resulting in postdefecation see page (80). Many patients who present with FI frequently have concomitant symptoms of urinary incontinence. For these reasons, it is difficult to offer a specific standard biofeedback therapy protocol that is beneficial for all patients. Therefore, the clinician must address all bowel and bladder symptoms and develop an individualized program for each patient with progressive realistic goals. After identifying functional problems and sEMG abnormalities, the clinician should prepare a treatment plan with specific short- as well as long-term goals. Short-term goals describe the training components by which the patient may achieve functional changes, whereas long-term goals refer to the expected functional outcomes (Table 6) (80).

Behavioral Component

The behavioral component is aimed toward systematic changes in the patient's behavior to influence bowel and bladder function. Operant-conditioning utilizing trial and error as an essential part of learning is merely one aspect of the learning process. Treatment is aimed at shaping the patient's responses toward a normal model by gradually modifying the patient's responses through positive reinforcement of successive approximations to the ideal response (80). As a behavioral program, the patient's active participation is paramount in achieving subjective treatment goals which include symptom improvement, quality of life improvement, and patient satisfaction.

Behavioral Strategies

Patient Education and Behavior Modification

Many misconceptions can be dispelled as patients gain a better understanding of their disorder. This begins with reviewing the anatomy of the PFM along with a review of normal bowel and bladder function with the use of visual aids. This is followed by reassurance that irregular

Table 5 Pelvic Floor Muscle sEMG Evaluation

sEMG resting baseline
sEMG peak amplitude the contraction
sEMG mean amplitude of the contraction during a 10-sec period
Duration of the contraction: 0 if <5 sec, 1 if 5 sec, 2 if >5 sec, 3 if >10 sec
sEMG muscle recruitment scale 0 = slow, 10 = fast
Pelvic muscle isolation during contraction: 0 = none, 10 = good
Valsalva maneuver
Progress this week: 0 = worse to 10 = excellent

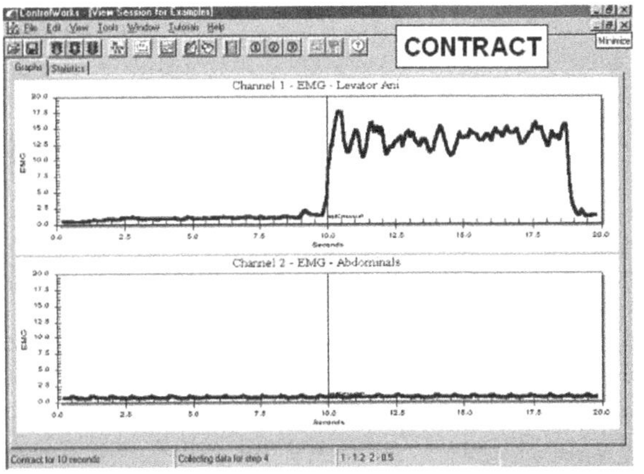

Figure 6 *Channel* 1: sEMG tracing of the PFM during contraction. Note the quick recruitment of appropriate PFM, ability to maintain the contraction, and ability to return to a normal resting tone. *Channel* 2: Abdominal sEMG tracing. Note the stability of the abdominal muscle activity.

bowel habits and other defecatory symptoms are common in the healthy general population. Patients may exhibit a variety of behavioral patterns, thus requiring tailored education specific to the underlying functional disorder. Some patients feel they need to have daily bowel movements and resort to laxative and enema misuse. Some patients may make several daily attempts straining to evacuate, while others may postpone the urge or make hurried attempts for convenience. Another frequently observed behavioral pattern, common among elderly women with symptoms of urinary incontinence, is the restriction of fluid intake to avoid leakage. This may, in fact, worsen symptoms of constipation as well as symptoms of urinary incontinence. Patients who have difficulty evacuating often do not tolerate the symptoms of gas and bloating associated with fiber intake. Once emptying improves, these patients are encouraged to slowly begin weaning their laxative use and instead slowly add fiber to their diet.

Habit Training

Habit training is recommended for patients with symptoms of incomplete, difficult, or infrequent evacuation. Patients are encouraged to set aside 10 to 15 minutes approximately the same time each day for unhurried attempts to evacuate. The patient should not be overly concerned with any failure as another attempt later in the day is acceptable. This is best initiated after a meal, which stimulates the gastrocolic reflex (82).

Most commodes are approximately 35 to 40 cm in height; if a patient's feet or legs hang free or dangle above the floor while sitting, simulation of the squatting position will not be accomplished. Flexion of the hips and pelvis provides the optimal body posture. Full flexion of the hips stretches the anal canal in an anteroposterior direction and tends to open the anorectal angle, which facilitates rectal emptying. This may be achieved by use of a footstool to elevate the legs and flex the hips (82).

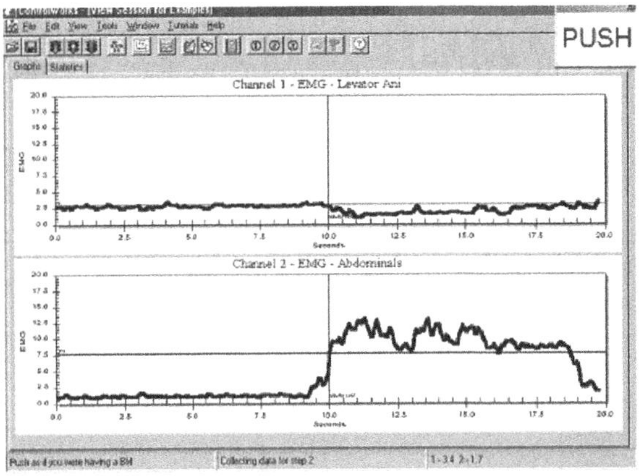

Figure 7 *Channel* 1: sEMG tracing of the PFM during a Valsalva maneuver. Note the decreased muscle activity. *Channel* 2: Abdominal sEMG tracing.

Table 6 sEMG PRM Treatment Goals

Short–term goals
Reinforce pelvic floor muscle contractions isolated from abdominal and gluteal contraction
Reinforce pelvic floor muscle contractions toward greater amplitude and duration to improve strength and tone
Improve the coordination of pelvic floor muscle by shaping pelvic floor muscle contractions with short repose latency and immediate recovery to baseline after voluntary contraction ceases
Reduce chronically elevated pelvic floor muscle activity if implicate in perineal muscle pain, voiding dysfunction, or associated bowel disorders
Reduce straining pattern by reinforcing pelvic floor relaxation during defecation or micturation
Generalize skills learned in the office to the home situation
Long–term goals
Decrease laxative, enema or suppository uses
Increase number of spontaneous bowel movements
Decrease frequency of incontinent episodes
Improved symptoms of incomplete evacuation
Decreased straining

Dietary Modification

Dietary information is reviewed with all patients to assist in improving bowel function. Patients are provided written informational handouts regarding foods that are high in fiber or foods that stimulate or slow transit. Offering creative fiber alternatives may be more appealing for the individual to easily incorporate into their daily diet regime also facilitates patient compliance. Such alternatives include unrefined wheat bran that can be easily mixed with a variety of foods such as cereals and muffins as well as over-the-counter bulking agents. Adequate fluid intake and limiting caffeine intake is essential for normal bowel and bladder function. Therefore, patients are encouraged to increase their fluid intake to 64 ounces per day, unless otherwise prescribed by their physician. Patients who are incontinent of liquid stools may benefit from an antidiarrheal medication. However, these medications typically slow colonic transit time. Therefore, this is contraindicated in patients with overflow incontinence from impaction or postdefecation seepage due to incomplete evacuation (80).

Urge Suppression Strategies for Incontinence

Burgio's urge suppression strategies assist with maintaining bowel and bladder control by educating patients to respond adaptively to the sensation of urgency. Rather than rushing to the toilet, which increases intra-abdominal pressure and exposes patients to visual cues that can trigger incontinence, patients were encouraged to pause, sit down if possible, relax the entire body, and contract PFMs repeatedly to diminish urgency, inhibit detrusor contraction, and prevent urine loss. When urgency subsides, patients are instructed to proceed to the toilet at a normal pace. Patients with mixed urinary incontinence are also taught stress strategies, which consists of contracting PFMs just prior to and during any physical activities such as coughing or sneezing that may trigger stress incontinence (83). These strategies, although intended for urinary incontinence, are quite helpful in maintaining control for patients with fecal incontinence. Hulme recommends the use of physiological quieting techniques three to five times per day for 30 to 60 seconds each time as a preventative measure for overwhelming urgency rather than waiting for it to occur. This technique affects detrusor tone through autonomic nervous system balancing (84). Whitehead et al. (49) showed that relaxation was more effective than conventional medical treatment for reducing diarrhea, and the number of medical consultations over 3.25 years. Norton and Kamm (85) reported that enhanced ability to contract the anal sphincter is likely to diminish large bowel peristalsis, may even induce retrograde peristalsis, or may simply allow continence to be preserved until the urge (bowel contractions) ceases. This appears to relate to the ability of biofeedback treatment to modify urgency.

PMR COMPONENT

The PMR component involves designing an exercise program suitable for each patient to achieve the ultimate goal of efficient PFM function (Table 3).

Pelvic Muscle Exercise Training Principles

Training principles that are important in any exercise program include the overload principle, the specificity principle, and the maintenance principle. The overload principle states that for pelvic muscles to strengthen, they must be pushed to the limit and just a little beyond. If muscles are under-exercised, they are not challenged enough to increase in strength, endurance, or speed; therefore, length and resting tone remain constant. The specificity principle states that the pelvic muscles are composed of fast and slow twitch fibers in roughly a ratio of 35% to 65%; some fibers have a combination of fast and slow twitch components. Fast twitch fibers improve in speed and strength with quick contractions, while slow twitch fibers strengthen and gain optimal resting length and tone with longer "hold" contractions. Fast twitch fibers fatigue quickly, while slow twitch fibers are designed for endurance and postural tone; therefore, repetitions are low for fast twitch fibers and higher for slow twitch fibers. The maintenance principle describes exercising for continence as a lifelong endeavor. The pelvic muscle strength is maintained by one daily 7 to 10 minute session. The reversibility principle states that if, after exercising and symptomatic improvement, discontinuing exercises will result in symptom reoccurrence over time (Table 6) (80,84).

Pelvic Muscle Exercise: Kegel Exercises

In the late 1940s Arnold Kegel developed a vaginal balloon perineometer to teach pelvic muscle exercises for poor tone and function of the genital muscles. He was instrumental in developing a standardized program for treating urinary stress incontinence. Kegel's program included evaluation and training utilizing visual feedback for patients to receive positive reinforcement as they monitored improvements in the pressure readings. Kegel also recommended structured home practice with the perineometer along with symptom diaries. His clinical use of these techniques showed that muscle reeducation and resistive exercises guided by sight sense to be a simple and practical means of restoring tone and function of the pelvic musculature. This perineometer was developed before the term "biofeedback" was coined in the late 1960s (84).

Unfortunately, clinicians taught Kegel exercises without the use of instrumentation. Bump et al. (86) showed that verbal or written instructions alone are not adequate, concluding that 50% of patients performed Kegel exercises incorrectly. There are disadvantages to teaching Kegel exercises without specific feedback from muscle contractions. There is a strong tendency to substitute abdominal and gluteal contractions for weak PFMs. This incorrect manner of performing Kegel exercises is reinforced by sensory proprioceptive sensations, giving faulty feedback for the desired contraction and, in effect, rendering the Kegel exercise useless (80). For patients with fecal or urinary incontinence, abdominal contractions raise intra-abdominal pressure, thus increasing the probability of an accident. For patients to begin performing isolated pelvic muscle contractions, patients are instructed to contract their PFM without contracting abdominal, gluteal, or leg muscles, and to hold this contraction to the best of their ability. This is done while using the instrumentation display of the simultaneous sEMG activity of the abdominal and PFM for feedback. The patient must tighten the pelvic diaphragm (levator ani) in a manner similar to stopping the passage of gas or to stop the flow of urine. Patients should be advised that the initial aim of treatment is not to produce a contraction of maximum amplitude, but to contract the PFM in isolation from other muscles without undue effort. In order to build muscle endurance, training proceeds with gradual increases in the duration of each contraction, along with gradual increases in the number of repetitions. Rhythmic breathing patterns during contractions should be encouraged.

Recommended home practice is tailored according to the patient's ability and the degree of muscle fatigue observed during the session. At each stage of treatment, patients are encouraged to practice these exercises daily without instrumentation feedback. While Kegel asked patients to perform approximately 300 contractions daily during treatment and 100 during maintenance, there is no known optimal specific number of exercise sets. The goal of Kegel exercises is to facilitate rehabilitation of the PFM to achieve efficient muscle function. This includes normal resting tone, quick recruitment of the PFM, sustained isolated pelvic muscle contraction, quick release to a normalized resting tone, and appropriate relaxation during defecation or micturation.

Pelvic Muscle Exercise: Beyond Kegels

The Beyond Kegels, a complete rehabilitation program for pelvic muscle dysfunction developed by Hulme, is based on the principal that the support system for the pelvic organs includes more

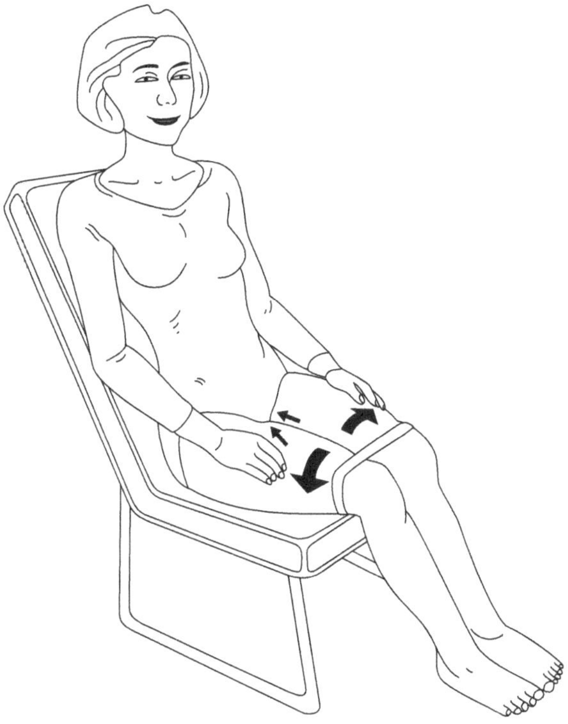

Figure 8 Beyond Kegel's obturator assist resistive exercise.

than just the PFMs. This support system, referred to as the pelvic rotator cuff (PRC), includes the obturator internus, the pelvic diaphragm (levator ani), the urogenital diaphragm, and adductor muscles. In summary, these muscles function as an interdigitated and interrelated synergistic unit, rather than separate entities, to support abdominal organs, stabilize the lumbopelvic and sacroiliac region, and reflexively act for continence. Thus, as the obturator internus muscle contracts, it acts as a pulley, lifting the pelvic diaphragm and facilitating closure of the urogenital diaphragm. As the adductor contracts, it lifts the pelvic diaphragm through overflow (proprioceptive neuromuscular facilitation) principles via the close approximation of their attachments on the symphysis pubis. The balance and work/rest cycle of the obturator and adductor muscles function as an integral part of the urogenital continence system to maintain bladder and bowel continence and to facilitate effective and efficient elimination.

One portion of the PRC protocol includes resistive exercises including the: (1) obturator assist and (2) adductor assist (Figs. 8 and 9).

This simple and effective exercise is often the one with which to begin. As the pelvic muscles become more efficient, patients can progress to performing the Kegel exercises. The PRC protocols provide a detailed progressive PMR exercise program that has shown to significantly improve and expedite the PMR process to achieve efficient muscle function (84). A study comparing traditional Kegel exercises with PRC exercises indicated that treatment length decreased an average of 46% when PRC exercises were added to an incontinence home training program and 48% of individuals were totally dry on discharge (87).

Anorectal Coordination Maneuver

Patients with symptoms of difficult, infrequent, or incomplete evacuation or those with increased muscle activity while performing the Valsalva maneuver during the initial evaluation are taught the anorectal coordination maneuver.

The goal is to produce a coordinated movement that consists of increasing intra-abdominal (intrarectal) pressure while simultaneously relaxing the pelvic muscles. During the initial sEMG evaluation of the Valsava maneuver, patients are asked to bear down or strain as if attempting to evacuate, which may elicit an immediate pelvic muscle contraction and closure of the anorectal outlet (Fig. 10). This correlates with symptoms of constipation including excessive straining and incomplete evacuation. The results of the sEMG activity observed on the screen display must first be explained and understood by the patient before awareness and change can occur. Change

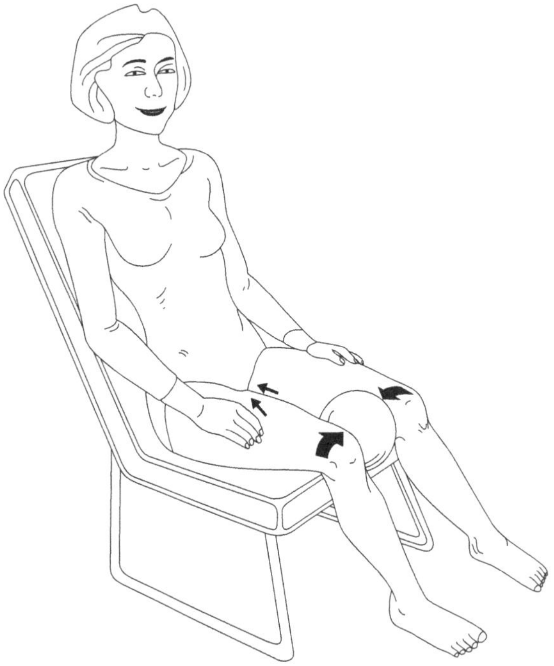

Figure 9 Beyond Kegel's adductor assist resistive exercise.

begins with educating the patient on diaphragmatic breathing, proper positioning, and habit training. Relaxation and quieting the muscle activity while observing the screen are reviewed. Initially, patients are instructed to practice these behavioral strategies; however, some patients may continue to feel the need to "push" or strain to assist with expulsion. While observing the sEMG muscle activity on the screen, they are instructed to slowly inhale deeply while protruding the abdominal muscles to increase the intraabdominal pressure. They are then asked to exhale slowly through pursed lips. The degree of the abdominal and anal effort is titrated to achieve a coordinated relaxation of the PFMs. Patients are encouraged to reproduce this maneuver during defecation attempts.

Quick Contract and Relax Exercises

This exercise improves the strength and function of the fast twitch muscle fibers primarily of the urogenital diaphragm and external sphincter muscles. These fast twitch muscle fibers are important for preventing accidents caused by increased intra-abdominal pressure exerted during lifting, pulling, coughing, or sneezing. Once the patient has learned to perform isolated pelvic muscle exercises, they are instructed to perform quick contract and release repetitions 5 to 10 times at the beginning and end of each exercise session they practice at home (84).

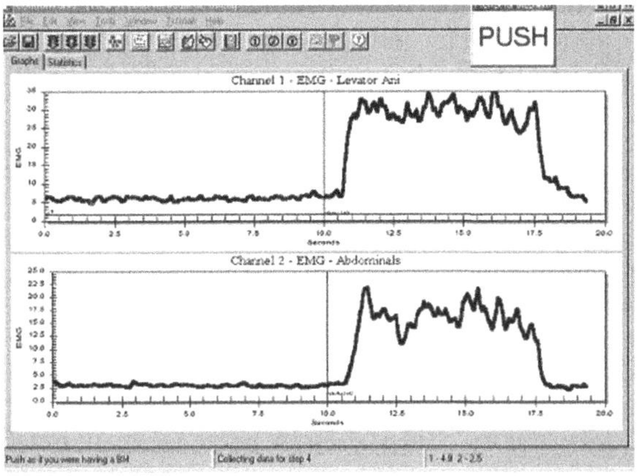

Figure 10 *Channel* 1: sEMG tracing of the PFM during a valsalva maneuver. Note the increase muscle activity indicative of a paradoxical contraction. *Channel* 2: Abdominal sEMG tracing.

Physiological Quieting

Physiological quieting is designed to balance the autonomic nervous system, so it mediates activity in the bowel and bladder most effectively and efficiently. Diaphragmatic breathing and hand warming are two techniques to directly affect the autonomic nervous system balance. The breathing diaphragm is the largest striated (voluntary) muscle in the body and is directed to act 12 to 14 times a minute by the autonomic nervous system. Cognitively training breathing patterns directly alters sympathetic input to the bladder and bowel since the sympathetic system is a global one. Hand warmth is determined to a large extent by sympathetic nervous system input to the blood vessel wall causing it to dilate or constrict. Cognitively training hand temperature directly alters sympathetic input to the bowel and bladder (84).

Diaphragmatic Breathing

The breathing cycle is intimately connected to both sympathetic and parasympathetic action of the autonomic nervous system (88). Bowel and bladder function is also mediated by the autonomic nervous system (80). Conscious, deep diaphragmatic breathing is one of the optimal methods of quieting the autonomic nervous system. This effectively initiates a cascade of visceral relaxation responses. The aim of this exercise is to make the shift from thoracic breathing to abdominal breathing (88). Patients are instructed to slowly inhale through the nose while protruding the abdomen outward as if the abdomen is a balloon being inflated, or allowing the abdomen to rise. This is followed by slow exhalation through the mouth as the abdominal balloon deflates or as the abdomen falls. Patients are encouraged to practice this in a slow rhythmical fashion.

Hand Warming

The basic strategy for stress management is to be able to achieve, and eventually maintain warm hands. This is accomplished by lowering sympathetic nervous system tone, promoting quiet emotions and relaxed muscles, and ultimately promoting a quiet body (62). Visualization and progressive relaxation techniques in conjunction with diaphragmatic breathing may be used to achieve hand warming.

BIOFEEDBACK SESSIONS

The initial session begins with a history intake. The learning process begins with a description of the anatomy and physiology of the bowel and pelvic muscle function using anatomical diagrams and visual aids. Verbal and written instructions are simplified for easy comprehension using laymen terminology. This is followed by a description of the biofeedback process, instrumentation, and PMR exercises. Patients should be aware that physicians cannot make muscles stronger nor can they change muscle behavior. However, patients can learn to improve symptoms and quality of life by active participation and commitment to making changes. Results are not immediate; as with any exercise program, muscle improvement requires time and effort. Patients are given instructions on proper insertion of the internal sensor and remain fully clothed during the session. They are placed in a comfortable semirecumbent position for training; however, internal sensors work in a variety of positions for functional maneuvers such as standing while reviewing urge suppression or sitting while performing the Valsalva. Surface electrodes are then placed on the right abdominal quadrant along the long axis of the oblique muscles, below the umbilicus used to monitor abdominal accessory muscle use.

The cables are attached to the SRS Orion PC/12 (SRS Medical Systems, Inc., Redmond, Washington, U.S.A.) multimodality instrumentation that provides the ability to simultaneously monitor up to four muscle sites (Fig. 2). EMG specifications include a bandwidth of 20 to 500 Hz and a 50/60 Hz notch filter. A sEMG evaluation is performed and reviewed with the patient. Beginning goals of isolated pelvic muscle contractions are established and an example of a sEMG tracing showing efficient muscle function is reviewed.

Training for dyssnergia, incontinence, or pain begins with the systematic shaping of PRC or isolated pelvic muscle contractions. Observation of other accessory muscle use such as the gluteal or thigh during the session is discussed with the patient. Excessive pelvic muscle activity with an elevated resting tone $>2\ \mu V$ may be associated with dyssnergia, voiding dysfunction, and pelvic pain. Jacobson's progressive muscle relaxation strategy implicated that after a muscle

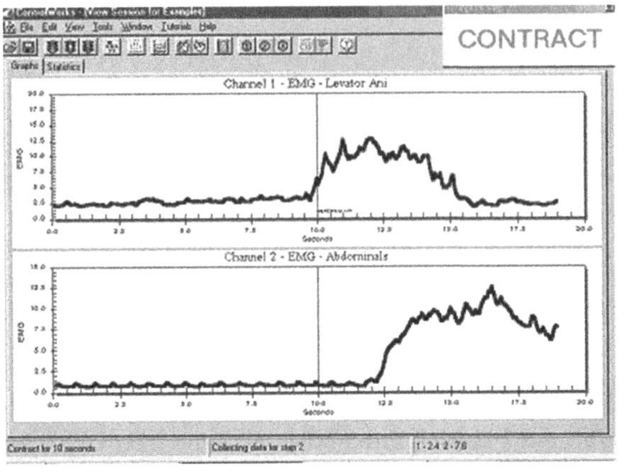

Figure 11 *Channel* 1: PFM sEMG tracing indicative of poor muscle function as seen with the slow recruitment. *Channel* 2: Inablilty to maintain the contraction along with the recruitment of abdominal muscles.

tenses, it automatically relaxes more deeply when released (23). This strategy is used to assist with hypertonia, placing emphasis on awareness of decreased muscle activity viewed on the screen as the PFM becomes more relaxed. This repetitive contract—relax sequence of PRC or isolated pelvic muscle contractions also facilitates discrimination between muscle tension and muscle relaxation. Some patients, usually women, have a greater PFM descent with straining during defecation associated with difficulty in rectal expulsion. Pelvic floor weakness may result in intrarectal mucosal intussusception or rectal prolapse, which contributes to symptoms of constipation. Furthermore, the PFM may not have the ability to provide the resistance necessary for extrusion of solid stool through the anal canal. Multifactorial concomitant PFM dysfunction accounts for the rationale to initiate all patients with PRC or isolated pelvic muscle rehabilitative exercises. Home practice recommendations for Kegel exercises depend on the observed decay in the duration of the contraction accompanied by the abdominal muscle recruitment (Fig. 11). The number of contractions the patient is able to perform before notable muscle fatigue occurs gauges the number of repetitions recommended at one time. Fatigue can be observed in as few as three to four contractions as seen in patients with weak PFMs. An example of home practice would occur with the patient performing an isolated PFM contraction, holding for a five-second duration, relaxing for 10 seconds, and repeating 3 to 10 times (one set). One set is performed three to five times daily, at designated intervals, allowing for extended rest periods between sets. The lower the number of repetitions, the more frequent interval sets should be performed daily. Excessive repetitions may overly fatigue the muscle and exacerbate symptoms. If patients are unable to perform an isolated contraction on the initial evaluation, they are given instructions for the PRC exercises. The goal for patients is to be able to perform isolated pelvic muscle contractions alternating with the PRC exercises, to ultimately achieve efficient PFM function. All patients are requested to keep a daily diary of bowel habits, laxative, enema or suppository use, fluid intake, number of home exercises completed, fiber intake, and any associated symptoms of constipation or incontinence.

Subsequent sessions begin with a diary review and establishing further goals aimed toward individualized symptom improvement. This is followed by a sEMG evaluation which may include the addition of quick contract and release repetitions, Valsalva maneuver, or PRC exercises, depending on the patient's progress. These objective measurements gage improvements in muscle activity that should be noted at each visit and occur prior to symptomatic improvement; this provides positive reinforcement for the patient to continue treatment. To assist with compliance, additional tasks should be limited to no more than three at any given time. These tasks, tailored to the individual needs, may include increasing the duration and number of PFM exercises, alternating PRC exercises, habit training, physiological quieting, anorectal coordination maneuvers, increasing fiber and fluid intake, increasing activity, and/or modifying laxative use or other methods of evacuatory assistance. Although the ideal goal may be to abolish all symptoms, this may not always be accomplished due to underlying conditions. However, patients' individual goals are significantly important. Some patients may be satisfied simply with the ability to leave home without fear of a significant relative fecal accident. Improved quality of life and patient satisfaction should be considered a treatment success.

At the onset of biofeedback therapy, it may be difficult to ascertain how many sessions are required for successful training. The number of biofeedback training sessions should be customized for each patient depending on the complexity of their functional disorder as well as the patient's ability to learn and master a new skill. Sessions are commonly scheduled as 1 to 1.5 hourly visits, once or twice weekly. Additionally, periodic reinforcement is recommended to improve long-term outcome (69).

ADJUNCTIVE TREATMENT METHODS

Various adjunctive biofeedback treatment methods have been employed throughout the years. Balloon expulsion has been used as an objective diagnostic tool and reportedly enhances sensory awareness in patients with pelvic outlet obstruction. It remains unclear which of the three components, sphincter training, sensory conditioning, or rectoanal coordination, is most useful in the treatment for FI (8). However, most agree that additional treatment methods may be helpful with symptomatic improvement depending on the underlying condition.

Balloon Expulsion for Constipation

This training technique involves inserting a balloon into the rectum and inflating with 50 ml of air so that the patient has the sensation of the need to defecate. Adherent perianal placement of surface electrodes allows the patient to see the resultant sEMG pattern made by voluntary sphincter contraction. The patient is then asked to expel the balloon and if there is an increased, rather than decreased sphincter activity, the patient is instructed on straining without increasing sphincter activity (14).

Sensory Discrimination Training for Fecal Incontinence

The sensory discrimination training technique involves a series of brief balloon inflations, noting the volume that induces a sensation of the urge to defecate, thereby establishing a current sensory threshold. The volume is subsequently reduced by 25% and a series of insufflations are repeated until the patient is able to promptly recognize the new stimuli (20). Once patients learn to associate the rise in intrarectal pressure with balloon inflation, they are encouraged to recognize sequentially smaller volumes of distention. Thus, after each session, new sensory thresholds are established (69). The mechanisms by which biofeedback training improves rectal perception are unclear. It has been suggested that biofeedback training may recruit sensory neurons adjacent to damaged afferent pathways. However, the speed with which sensory thresholds improve during biofeedback suggests that patients use existing afferent pathways, but learn to focus more on weak sensations and to recognize their significance (discrimination training) (78).

Coordination Training for Fecal Incontinence

The aim of coordination training is to achieve a maximum voluntary squeeze in less than one to two seconds after inflation of the rectal balloon and to control the reflex anal relaxation by consciously contracting the sphincter muscles. This maneuver mimics the arrival of stool in the rectum and prepares the patient to react appropriately by using the appropriate muscle group. With each balloon insufflation, the patient is asked to signal when they have perceived rectal distention and react to this distention by promptly contracting the PFM and maintaining this contraction without increasing intraabdominal pressure; this maneuver is performed while the patient observes changes on the visual display. The key element is to condition the external anal sphincter responses to improve the squeeze profile and the ability to respond to small volumes of rectal distention (8).

SUMMARY

Despite the many variants in the clinical trials for biofeedback, most experts agree that biofeedback is an attractive outpatient, conservative treatment option that is cost effective, relatively noninvasive, easy to tolerate, and morbidity free. It also does not interfere with any future treatment options that may be recommended by the physician. It is gratifying to note that this simple technique can ameliorate symptoms and improve the quality of life in many patients with functional bowel and bladder symptoms attributed to pelvic muscle dysfunction.

REFERENCES

1. Whitehead WE, Wald A, Diamant, NE, et al. Functional disorders of the anus and rectum. In: Drossman DA, Corazziari W, Talley NJ, Thompson GW, Whitehead WE, eds. Rome II: The Functional Gastrointestinal Disorders. 2nd ed. McLean, VA: Degnon Associates, 2000:483–532.
2. Sonnenberg A, Koch TR. Physician visits in the United States for constipation. Dig Dis Sci 1989; 34: 606.
3. Sonnenberg A, Koch TR. Epidemiology of constipation in the United States. Dis Colon Rectum 1989; 32:1–8.
4. Thompson WG, Longstreth GF, Drossman DA, et al. Functional bowel disorders and functional abdominal pain. Gut 1999; 45:1143–1154.
5. Jorge JMN, Wexner SD. Physiologic evaluation. In: Wexner SD, Vernava AM, eds. Clinical Decision Making in Colorectal Surgery. New York: Igaku-Shoin, 1995:11–22.
6. Wexner SD, Jorge JMN. Colorectal physiological tests: Use or abuse of technology? Eur J Surg 1994; 160:167–174.
7. Bharucha A, Wald A, Enck P, et al. Functional anorectal disorders. Gastroenterology 2006; 130:1510–1518.
8. Rao SSC, Welcher KDP, Leistikow JS. Obstructive defecation: A failure of rectoanal coordination. Am J Gastroenterol 1998; 93:1042–1050.
9. Hallan RI, Williams NS, Melling J, et al. Treatment of anismus in intractable constipation with botulinum toxin. Lancet 1988; 2:714–717.
10. Enck P. Biofeedback training in disordered defecation: a critical review. Dig Dis Sci 1993; 38:1953–1959.
11. Schiller LR. Fecal incontinence. In: Feldman M, Friedman L, Sleisenger MH, Slesinger, eds. Fordtan's Gastrointestinal and Liver Disease: Pathophysiology/Diagnosis/Management. 7th ed. Philadelphia: W. B. Saunders, 2002:164–180.
12. Enck P, Musial F. Biofeedback in pelvic floor disorders. In: Pemberton JH, Swash M, Henry MM, eds. The Pelvic Floor: Its Function and Disorders. London: W.B. Saunders, 2002:393–404.
13. Jorge JM, Habr-Gama A, Wexner SD. Biofeedback therapy in the colon and rectal practice. Appl Psychophysiol Biofeedback 2003; 28:47–61.
14. Emmanuel AV, Kamm MA. Response to a behavioral treatment, biofeedback in constipated patients is associated with improved gut transit and autonomic innervation. Gut 2001; 49:214–219.
15. Dailianas A, Skandalis N, Rimikis MN, et al. Pelvic floor study in patients with obstructive defecation. J Clin Gastroenterol 2000; 30:176–180.
16. Lau C, Heymen S, Albaz O, et al. Prognostic significance of rectocele, intussusception, and abnormal perineal descent in biofeedback treatment for constipated patients with paradoxical puborectalis contraction. Dis Colon Rectum 2000; 43:478–482.
17. Mollen RMHG, Salvioli B, Camilleri M, et al. The effects of biofeedback on rectal sensation and distal colonic motility in patients with disorders of rectal evacuation: evidence of an inhibitory rectocolonic reflex in humans. Am J Gastroenterol 1999; 94:751–756.
18. McKee RF, McEnroe L, Anderson JH, et al. Identificatioin of patients likely to benefit from biofeedback for outlet obstruction constipation. Br J Surg 1999; 86:355–359.
19. Chiotakakou-Faliakou E, Kamm MA, Roy AJ, et al. Biofeedback provides long term benefit for patients with intractable slow and normal transit constipation. Gut 1998; 6:517–521.
20. Rieger NA, Wattchow DA, Sarre RG, et al. Prospective study of biofeedback for treatment of constipation. Dis colon Rectum 1997; 40:1143–148.
21. Glia A, Gylin M, Gullberg K, et al. Biofeedback retraining in patients with functional constipation and paradoxical puborectalis contraction. Dis colon Rectum 1997; 40:889–895.
22. Ko CY, Tong J, Lehman RE, et al. Biofeedback is effective therapy for fecal incontinence and constipation. Arch Surg 1997; 132:829–834.
23. Patankar SK, Ferrara A, Larach WS, et al. Electromyographic assessment of biofeedback training for fecal incontinence and chronic constipation. Dis Colon Rectum 1997; 40:907–911.
24. Gilliland R, Heymen S, Altomare DF, et al. Outcome and predictors of success of biofeedback for constipation. Br J Surg 1997; 84:1123–1126.
25. Karlbohm U, Hallden M, Eeg-Olofssson KE, et al. Result of biofeedback in constipated patients. A prospective study. Dis colon Rectum 1997; 40:1149–1155.
26. Rao SSC, Welcher KD, Pelsan RE. Effects of biofeedback therapy on anorectal function in obstructive defecation. Dig Dis Sci 1997; 42:2197–2205.

27. Patankar SK, Ferrera A, Levy JR, et al. Biofeedback in colorectal practice. A multicenter, statewide, three-year experience. Dis Colon Rectum 1997; 40:827–831.
28. Park UC, Choi SK, Piccirillo MF, et al. Patterns of anismus and the relation to biofeedback therapy. Dis Colon Rectum 1996; 39:768–773.
29. Ho YH, Tan M, Goh HS. Clinical and physiologic effects of biofeedback in outlet obstruction defecation. Dis Colon Rectum 1996; 39:520–524.
30. Leroi AM, Duval V, Roussignol C, et al. Biofeedback for anismus in 15 sexually abused women. Int J Colorect Dis 1996; 11:187–190.
31. Siproudhis L, Dautreme S, Ropert A, et al. Anismus and biofeedback: who benefits? Eur J Gastroenterol Hepatol 1995; 7:547–552.
32. Koutsomanis D, Lennard-Jones JE, Roy AJ, et al. Controlled randomized trial of visual biofeedback versus muscle training without a visual display for intractable constipation. Gut 1995; 37:95–99.
33. Koutsomanis D, Lennard-Jones JE, Kamm MA. Prospective study of biofeedback treatment for patients with slow and normal transit constipation. Eur J Gastroenterol Hepatol 1994; 6:131–137.
34. Bleijenberg G, Kuijpers HC. Biofeedback treatment of constipation: Comparison of two methods. Am J Gastroenterol 1995; 89:1021–1026.
35. Papachrysostomou M, Smith AN. Effects of biofeedback on obstructed defecation —reconditioning of the defecation reflex. Gut 1994; 35:252–256.
36. Keck JO, Staniunas RJ, Coller YES, et al. Biofeedback training is useful in fecal incontinence but disappointing in constipation. Dis colon Rectum 1995; 37:1271–1276.
37. Turnbull GK, Ritivo PG. Anal sphincter biofeedback relaxation treatment for women with intractable cconstipaion symptoms. Dis Colon Rectum 1992; 35:530–536.
38. Fleshman JW, Dreznik Z, Meyer K, et al. Outpatient protocol for biofeedback therapy of pelvic floor outlet obstruction. Dis Colon Rectum 1992; 35:1–7.
39. Wexner SD, Cheape JD, Jorge JMN, et al. Prospective assessment of biofeedback for the treatment of paradoxical puborectalis contraction. Dis Colon Rectum 1992; 35:145–150.
40. Dahl J, Lindquist BL, Tysk C, et al. Behavioral medicine treatment in chronic constipation with paradoxical anal sphincter contraction. Dis Colon Rectum 1991; 34:769–776.
41. Kawimbe BM, Papachrysostomou M, Clare N, et al. Outlet obstruction constipation (anismus) managed by biofeedback. Gut 1991; 32:1175–1179.
42. Lestar B, Penninckx F, Kerremans R. Biofeedback defecation training for anismus. Int J Colorect Dis 1991; 6:202–207.
43. Weber J, Ducrotte P, Touchais JY, et al. biofeedback training for constipation in adults and children. Dis Colon Rectum 1987; 30:844–846.
44. Bleijenberg G, Kuijpers HC. Treatment of the spastic pelvic floor syndrome with biofeedback. Dis Colon Rectum 1987; 30:108–111.
45. Engel BT, Nikoomanesh P, Schuster MM. Operant conditioning of rectosphincteric responses in the treatment of fecal incontinence. N Egnl J Med 1974; 290:646–649.
46. Cerullli M, Nikoomanesh P, Schuster MM. Progress in biofeedback conditioning for fecal incontinence. Gastroenterology 1979; 76:742–746.
47. Goldenberg DA, Hodges K, Hersh T, et al. Biofeedback therapy for fecal incontinence. Am J Gastroenterol 1980; 74:342–345.
48. Wald A. Biofeedback therapy for fecal incontinence. Ann Int Med 1981; 95:146–149.
49. Whitehead WE, Burgio KL, Engel BT. Biofeedback treatment of fecal incontinence in geriatric patients. J Am Geriatr Soc 1985; 33:230–324.
50. Buser WE, Miner PB. Delayed rectal sensation with fecal incontinence. Gastroenterology 1986; 91:1186–1191.
51. MacLeod JH. Management of anal incontinence by biofeedback. Gastroenterology 1987; 93:291–294.
52. Enck P, Kranzle U, Schwiese J, et al. Biofeedback training in fecal incontinence. Deutsch Med Wochenschirift 1988; 113:1789–1794.
53. Riboli EB, Frascio MD, Pitto G, et al. Biofeedback conditioning for fecal incontinence. Arch Phys Med Rehabil 1988; 69:29–31.
54. Miner PB, Donnelly TC, Read NW. Investigation of mode of action of biofeedback in treatment of fecal incontinence. Dig Dis Sci 1990; 35:1291–1298.
55. Loening-Baucke V, Desch L, Wolraich M. Biofeedback training for patients with myelomeningocele and fecal incontinence. Dev Med Child Neurol 1988; 30:781–790.
56. Keck JO, Staniunas RJ, Coller JA, et al. Biofeedback is useful in fecal incontinence but disappointing in constipation. Dis Colon Rectum 1994; 37:1271–1276.
57. Guillemot F, Bouche B, Gower-Rosseau C, et al. biofeedback for the treatment of fecal incontinence: long-term clinical results. Dis Colon Rectum 1995; 38:393–397.

58. Sangwan YP, Coller JA, Barrett RC, et al. Can manometric parameters predict response to biofeedback therapy in fecal incontinence? Dis Colon Rectum 1995; 38:1021–1025.
59. Ho YH, Tan M. Biofeedback therapy for bowel dysfunction following low anterior resection. Ann Acad Med Singapore 1997; 26:299–302.
60. Rao SS, Welcher KD, Happel J. Can biofeedback therapy improve anorectal function in fecal incontinence? Am J Gastroenterol 1996; 91:2360–2366.
61. Jensen LL, Lowry AC. Biofeedback improves functional outcome after sphincteroplasty. Dis Colon Rectum 1997; 40:197–200.
62. Rieger NA, Wattchow DA, Sarre RG, et al. Prospective trial of pelvic floor retraining in patients with fecal incontinence. Dis Colon Rectum 1997; 40:821–826.
63. Ko CY, Tong J, Lehman RE, et al. Biofeedback is effective therapy for fecal incontinence and constipation. Arch Surg 1997; 132:829–834.
64. Patankar SK, Ferrara A, Larach SW, et al. Electromyographic assessment of biofeedback training for fecal incontinence and chronic constipation. Dis Colon Rectum 1997; 40:907–911.
65. Glia A, Gylin M, Akerlund JE, et al. Biofeedback training in patients with fecal incontinence. Dis Colon Rectum 1998; 41:359–364.
66. Leroi AM, Dorival MP, Lecouturier MF, et al. Pudendal neuropathy and severity of incontinence but not presence of anal sphincter defect may determine the response to biofeedback therapy in fecal incontinence. Dis Colon Rectum 1999; 42:762–769.
67. Shellenberger R, Green JA. From the Ghost in the Box to Successful Biofeedback Training. Greeley, CO: Health Psychology Publication, 1986.
68. Dahl J, Lindquist BL, Leissner P, et al. Behavioral medicine treatment in chronic constipation with paradoxical anal sphincter contraction. Dis Colon Rectum 1991; 34:769–776.
69. Rao SSC, Welcher KD, Happel J. Can biofeedback therapy improve anorectal function in fecal incontinence? Am J of Gastroenterol 1996; 91:2360–2365.
70. Roa S, Seaton K, Miller M, et al. Randomized controlled trial of biofeedback, sham feedback, and standard therapy for dyssynergic defecation. Clin Gastroenterol Hepatol 2007; 5:311–338.
71. Heyman S, Scarlett Y, Jones K, et al. Randomized controlled trial shows biofeedback to be superior to alternative treatments for patients with pelvic floor dyssynergia-type constipation. Dis Colon Rectum 2007; 50:428–441.
72. Wexner SD. Biofeeback for constipation. Dis Colon Rectum 1998,41:670–671.
73. Engel AF, Kamm MA. The acute effect of straining on pelvic floor neurological function. Int J Colorectal Dis 1994; 9:8–12.
74. Smith B. Effect of irritant purgatives on the myenteric plexus in man and the mouse. Gut 1968; 9:139–143.
75. Chiarioni G, Heyman S, Whitehead W. Biofeedback therapy for dyssynergic defecation. World J Gastroenterol 2006; 12:7069–7074.
76. Byrne C, Solomon M, Young J, et al. Biofeedback for fecal incontinence: short-term outcomes of 513 consecutive patients and predictors of successful treatment. Dis Colon Rectum 2007; 50:417–427.
77. Hyman S, Jones KR, Ringel Y, et al. Biofeedback treatment of fecal incontinence. Dis Colon Rectum 2001; 44:728–736.
78. Chiarioni G, Bassotti G, Stegagnini S, et al. Sensory retraining is key to biofeedback therapy for formed stool fecal incontinence. Am J Gastroenterol 2002; 97:109–117.
79. Latimer PR, Campbell D, Dasperski J. A component analysis of biofeedback in the treatment of fecal incontinence. Biofeedback Self Regul 1984; 9:311–324.
80. Schwartz MS. Biofeedback: A practitioner's guide. 2nd ed. New York: The Guilford Press, 1995.
81. Binnie NR, Kawimbe BM, Papachrysotomou M, et al. The importance of the orientation of the electrode plates in recording the external anal sphincter EMG by non-invasive anal plug electrodes. Int J Colorectal Dis 1991; 6:8–11.
82. Lennard-Jones JE. Constipation. In: Feldman M, Friedman L, Sleisenger MH, Sleisinger J, eds. Fordtan's Gastrointestinal and Liver Disease: Pathophysiology/Diagnosis/Management. 7th ed. Philadelphia: W.B.. Saunders, 2002:181–209.
83. Burgio KL, Goode PS, Locher JL, et al. Behavioral training with and without biofeedback in the treatment of urge incontinence in older women. J Am Med Assoc 2002; 288:2293–2299.
84. Kegel A. The physiologic treatment of poor tone and function of the genital muscles and of urinary stress incontinence. West J Surg Obstet Gynecol 1949; 57:527–535.
85. Norton C, Kamm MA. Outcome of biofeedback for faecal incontinence. Br J Surg 1999; 86:1159–1163.
86. Bump RC, Hurt WG, Fantl JA, et al. Assessment of Kegel pelvic muscle exercise performance after brief verbal instruction. Am J Obstet Gynecol 1991; 165:322–329.
87. Hulme J, Nevin G. Comparison of traditional Kegel exercises with obturator internus exercise protocol for treating incontinence. Presented at American Physical Therapy Association Combined Sections, Seattle, WA, 1999.

88. Basmajian JV. Biofeedback: Principles and Practice for Clinicians. Williams & Wilkins: Baltimore, 1989.
89. Rao SSC. The technical aspects of biofeedback therapy for defecation disorders. Gastroenterologist 1998; 6:96–103.
90. Charlesworth EA, Nathan RG. Stress Management: A Comprehensive Guide to Wellness. Ballantine Books: New York, 1985.

6 Hemorrhoids: Office-Based Management

Dean C. Koh
The Ferguson Clinic, MMPC, Grand Rapids, Michigan, U.S.A. and Colorectal Unit, Department of Surgery, Tan Tock Seng Hospital, Singapore

Martin A. Luchtefeld
The Ferguson Clinic, MMPC, Grand Rapids, Michigan, U.S.A.

INTRODUCTION

Hemorrhoidal disease is a common problem encountered in any colorectal practice, affecting as many as 10 million Americans. However, there has been a decline in the number of hemorrhoidectomies performed (1). This has been attributed to the popularity of newer nonsurgical treatment methods available today. This chapter describes the common modalities of treatment that can be employed in the office setting.

ETIOLOGY

Hemorrhoids are connective tissue cushions surrounding arteriovenous communications connecting the superior rectal arteries to superior, inferior, and middle rectal veins. Subepithelial smooth muscles arising from the longitudinal muscle layer insert into the subepithelial vascular space, providing suspension and contributing to the bulk of the cushion. There are commonly three cushions that act to ensure complete closure of the anal canal. This has an essential role in the maintenance of continence.

The loss of support to these cushions results in stagnation and stasis of the blood in the vascular plexus (2). Clinical symptoms result when internal hemorrhoids enlarge and stretch the suspensory muscles. This causes the submucosal arteriovenous plexus to dilate, and prolapse of the tissues through the anal canal. Trauma to these engorged tissues results in the typical bright red bleeding seen in many patients. Symptoms of itch and discomfort are due to mucus deposition on the perianal skin (3).

The predisposing factors causing the enlargement and/or prolapse of hemorrhoidal tissues have not been proven conclusively although numerous theories exist. What has been proven, however, is that the elevated anal resting pressure seen in patients with symptomatic hemorrhoids normalizes after hemorrhoidectomy (4).

EVALUATION

Initial symptom assessment should include a history of the frequency and quantity of bleeding and the timing and reducibility of prolapse. The latter is an unusual presentation in the absence of any thrombosis or concomitant fissures. Fissures have been observed in up to 20% of patients presenting with hemorrhoids (5).

The physical examination should not only evaluate the presence and extent of the hemorrhoids, but aim to exclude any presence of abscesses or fistulae. The minimum evaluation modalities for symptoms of rectal bleeding should include anoscopy and a flexible sigmoidoscopy (6). The patient is placed in a left lateral decubitus position on an examination table or couch; adequate lighting and appropriate instruments are essential. Initial inspection of the perineum by gently parting the buttocks allows for easy visualization of the anoderm. This is followed by a gentle digital examination, followed by an anoscopic evaluation. We recommend a side viewing anoscope (Fig. 1) which allows the hemorrhoidal cushion to fill the beveled end and be properly evaluated. The patient is asked to perform a Valsalva maneuver to create the

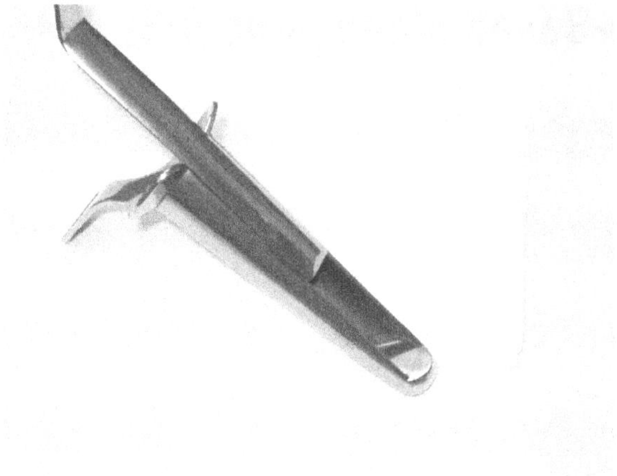

Figure 1 Side viewing anoscope.

prolapse. More sinister and proximal causes of the symptom of bleeding are excluded with a flexible sigmoidoscopy and, if necessary, a full colonoscopy.

Internal and external hemorrhoids are classified in relation to their location relative to the dentate line. The grading of hemorrhoids classically follows that described by Banov et al. (table 1) (7).

MEDICAL TREATMENT

Hemorrhoidal symptoms tend to be cyclical. Simple advice to avoid straining during defecation and defecation errors such as postponing the urge to defecate and prolonged sitting on the toilet bowl may help to reduce minor symptoms.

Diet Counselling

Avoidance of certain food and drinks such as nuts, coffee, spicy foods, and alcohol is often recommended. A high-fiber diet is associated with improvement in bowel habits and a reduction in symptoms of constipation. Recommendations include at least 20 to 30 g of fiber per day such as bran or bran products, fresh fruits, and vegetables. This should be accompanied by an adequate fluid supplementation. Bulking agents, most of which contain ispaghula husk, sterculia, or methylcellulose, help to minimize the trauma to the anal canal epithelium and decrease the incidence of ulceration and bleeding (8).

Symptom Relief

Warm soaks and Sitz baths are often advocated to help relieve symptomatic hemorrhoids. Fifteen minute durations, three to four times per day is the most commonly advocated regimen. Local skin care by cleansing the anorectal area with mild unscented soap and water after defecation may be a useful habit to acquire. The use of ice packs to decrease edema often provides some relief.

Topicals

Common commercial topical preparations used and prescribed include astringents, protectants, vasoconstrictors, keratolytics, antipruritics, local anesthetics, and steroids. These have been used

Table 1 Hemorrhoid Classification (by Degree)

First degree	Bleeding, no prolapse
Second degree	Prolapsed but reduces spontaneously
Third degree	Prolapsed, requiring manual reduction
Fourth degree	Prolapsed, irreducible manually

Table 2 Common Topical Preparations

Agent	Common dosage
Pramoxine HCl 1%	Topical ointment application up to 5 times/day
Phenylephrine HCl 0.25%	Topicals/suppositories
(Preparation H)	Up to 4 times a day
Hydrocortisone acetate 1%	Topical application up to 4 times/day
Hydrocortisone acetate 1%	Suppositories up to twice/day
Hydrocortisone 2.5%	Topical application 2 to 3 times/day
Tetracaine 2%	Application prior to bowel movement, before suppository insertion

to improve symptoms, especially that of itching and pain. The more popular preparations are shown in Table 2. The efficacy of these products has not been conclusively proven in significant studies, but there is anecdotal evidence to suggest that symptom relief is achieved to a certain extent with the use of these topical agents. Whether or not this is related to the natural cyclical variation in symptoms remains speculative. The important point is that it is unlikely that these preparations will ultimately completely ameliorate symptoms or cure the patient.

Micronized Purified Flavonoid Fraction

These are semisynthetic micronized preparations of the γ-benzopyrone family. The contents are 90% diosmine and 10% flavonoids expressed as hesperidine. Common trade names include Arvenum 500®, Alvenor®, Ardium®, Capiven®, Daflon® 500 mg, Detralex®, Elatec®, Flebotropin®, Variton®, and Venitol®. Increased absorption of the active components from the human gastrointestinal tract is achieved by the technique of micronization (9).

The achieved effect of micronized purified flavonoid fractions (MPFFs) is a reduction in capillary hyperpermeability, resulting in the inhibition of the inflammatory process and reduced edema. Studies have shown that venous tone is improved (10), capillary resistance is reinforced (11), lymphatic drainage is increased (12), and the microcirculation is protected from inflammatory mediators (13).

As an adjunct to other treatment modalities, MPFF–fiber combinations have resulted in a more rapid relief of bleeding when compared to fiber alone or fiber–rubber band ligation combinations (14). More recently, La Torre et al. (15) demonstrated in a randomized controlled trial that MPFF combined with ketorolac and antibiotics (metronidazole) significantly reduced the extent and duration of typical postoperative symptoms including pain, tenesmus, pruritus, and bleeding following hemorrhoidectomy.

An added benefit of MPFFs has been its safety profile and efficacy in symptom alleviation in pregnant women (16). This product, however, is not FDA approved for use in the United States and remains a widely prescribed treatment mainly in Europe and Asia.

RUBBER BAND LIGATION

The rubber band ligator for hemorrhoids was first described by Barron in 1963 (17) and has since evolved into an easy office-based procedure, in any colorectal surgeon's practice. No anesthetic is required since somatic sensory nerve afferents are only present distal to the anal transition zone. In addition, this procedure can be performed without an assistant.

The more modern equipment utilizes a suction device to draw redundant tissue into the applicator (Fig. 2). Once the rubber band has been placed in the proper position, fibrosis and scarring fix the connective tissue to the rectal wall, thereby reducing the prolapse. Rubber band ligation is commonly advocated for use in managing first to third degree hemorrhoids. One must bear in mind that this method addresses only the internal component of hemorrhoids and not external hemorrhoids.

The patient is typically placed in the left lateral decubitus position. Again, adequate lighting and the appropriate equipment are essential for the procedure to be performed properly (Fig. 3). We advocate placement of the band on the redundant mucosa above the hemorrhoid, as described by Nivatvongs and Goldberg (18). This provides the advantages of preserving the

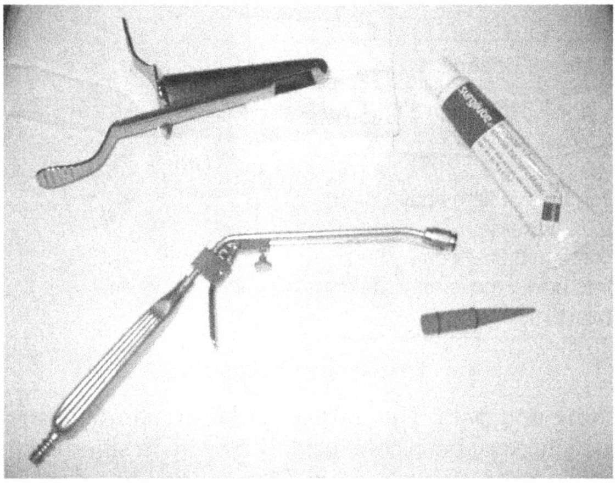

Figure 2 Standard hemorrhoid ligation equipments.

anal cushions and ensuring that the ligations are well above the dentate line, minimizing the risk of postligation pain (Fig. 4).

Typically, one to two columns are ligated each time, although ligation of up to three columns at one sitting has been described (19–21). Three-column ligation has been proven effective but is associated with a 37% incidence of prolonged postligation pain (22). Therefore, most surgeons will advise against placement of more than two bands per session to avoid the unfortunate experience of excessive discomfort and pain for the patient. Some surgeons have even recommended banding for fourth degree hemorrhoids presenting in an emergent setting (23).

Good success rates have been universally described. Patient satisfaction has been reported to be in the 80% to 90% range (24). Sixty percent to 70% of patients are cured in one treatment session, and the procedure is generally associated with a low complication rate (<2%) (24). Pain is by far the predominant complaint following ligation and has been described in 5% to 60% of patients (25). This is usually relieved with warm Sitz baths and oral analgesics. Abscess formation and urine retention can also occur. Thrombosis of adjacent hemorrhoids occurs in 2% to 11% of patients (26). Postligation bleeding is rare with a described incidence of 0.5% (27). Even less common is the occurrence of pelvic sepsis, although it has been described after single hemorrhoid banding in young and healthy patients (28,29). The triad of severe pain, fever, and urine retention must be looked out for in patients suspected with this unusual complication.

Due to limited maneuverability and a narrower field of vision with the anoscope, flexible videoendoscopic elastic band ligation (VE-EBL) has recently been described by surgeons recently (30). This technique was analyzed as a comparison to the standard anoscopic technique, and the results showed comparable long-term efficacy and safety; significantly fewer sessions were required (1.8 vs. 2.4).

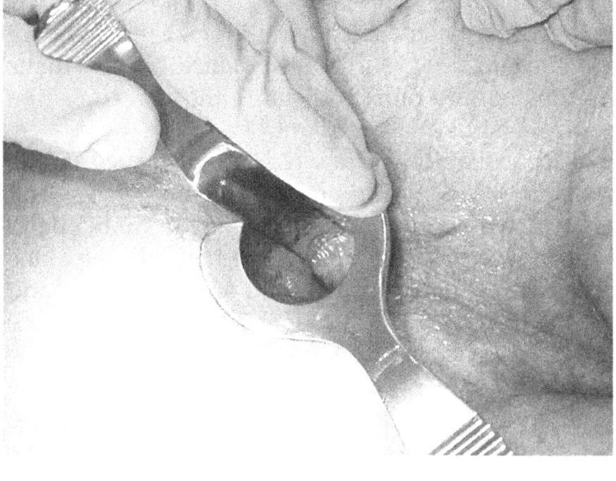

Figure 3 Visualization of hemorrhoidal cushion with anoscope.

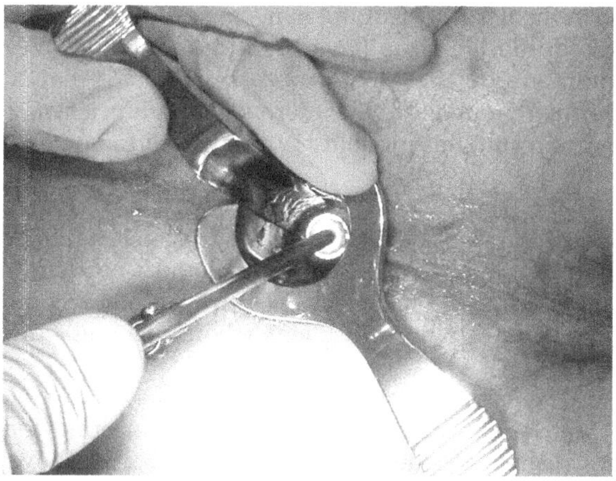

Figure 4 Placement of rubber band just proximal to hemorrhoidal cushion.

Injection Sclerotherapy

This modality of treating hemorrhoidal disease was first described in 1869 with the use of iron persulphate (31). Since then, several other sclerosants have been used, including phenol (5%) in vegetable oil, quinine, urea hydrochloride, sodium morrhuate, and sodium tetradecyl sulfate. The ultimate aim is to cause fibrosis of the vascular cushions, thereby obliterating them. Injection sclerotherapy is usually recommended for treating first- and second-degree hemorrhoids. It is contraindicated in the management of thrombosed external hemorrhoids or ulcerated internal hemorrhoids.

The patient can be placed in either the left lateral decubitus or prone jackknife position. Similar to rubber band ligation, no anesthetic is required. Anoscopy is performed in the standard fashion. Using a small gauge needle, a submucosal injection of the sclerosant is performed. This should be aimed at the base of the hemorrhoidal complex located 1 cm or more above the dentate line in order to cause thrombosis of the underlying vessels and sclerosis of the connective tissues, resulting in shrinkage and fixation of overlying mucosa. It is recommended that 1–3 mL of sclerosant be injected per hemorrhoid.

Symptom improvement has been described in up to 90% of patients with first- and second-degree hemorrhoids (32). Some trials, however, have shown no difference in bleeding rates when compared to bulk laxatives alone. There are potential complications despite the simplicity of the technique. Pain can occur in 12% to 70% of patients. Impotence, urinary retention, and abscess formation have also been described (25). Recurrence rates after initial success have been described in up to 30% of patients after four years (33).

Cryotherapy

Cryotherapy was initially introduced as a painless and effective method of treating both internal and external hemorrhoids. The concept is to use a probe of liquid nitrogen or nitrous oxide to

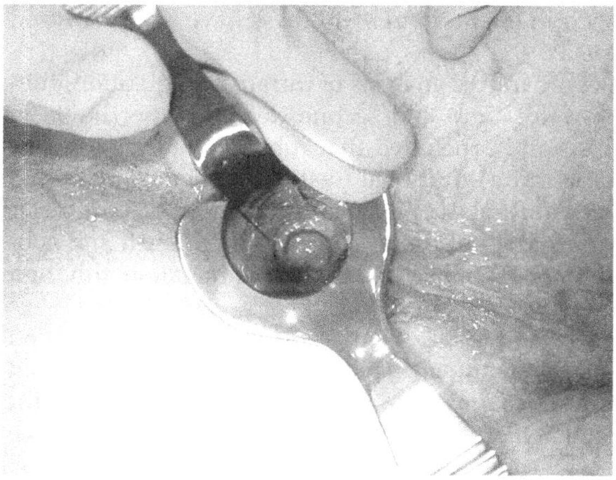

Figure 5 Post-rubber band ligation.

cause rapid freezing and cellular destruction in the tissues, resulting in necrosis of the vascular cushions (34). However, the results reported in the literature have been disappointing (36). Prolonged drainage from the wound is a common side effect (35). Another problem is that of prolonged wound pain (36). If used inappropriately, damage to the internal anal sphincter may result in anal stenosis or fecal incontinence. As a result, this modality is rarely used today.

Infrared Coagulation

Described by Neiger in 1979 (37), the technique of infrared coagulation uses a tungsten–halogen lamp with a polymer probe tip that emits infrared light. This is converted to heat in tissues, resulting in their destruction; temperatures up to 100°C are achieved. The manufacturer recommendation of three to five pulses of 0.5 to 2 second durations per hemorrhoid maintains the depth of tissue injury at 2.5 to 3 mm.

Randomized controlled trials have shown successful control of bleeding in 67% to 79% of patients (33,38). With the patient in the left lateral position, an anoscopy is inserted for exposure. Direct application of the tip of the instrument to the mucosal surface, 1 to 2 cm above the dentate line, is then performed. Appropriate application is evidenced by a visible small white dot appearing on the mucosa. This area will then ulcerate and scar down. Symptoms of discharge and edema may be noted after the procedure.

Infrared coagulation has been proven to be equally efficacious compared to sclerotherapy and rubber band ligation, and is typically recommended for smaller hemorrhoids presenting with symptoms of bleeding that are not amenable to rubber band ligation.

THROMBOSED EXTERNAL HEMORRHOIDS

This condition represents one of a few instances when hemorrhoidal disease manifests with symptoms of pain. Predisposing factors involve the increased pelvic floor pressure seen in diarrhea, constipation, straining at defecation, pregnancy, childbirth, and lifting heavy weights.

Simple excision under local anesthesia is the recommended treatment and is associated with a low incidence of complications (39). Postprocedural bleeding is seen in only 0.3% to 4% of patients while abscess or fistula formation occurs in approximately 2%. Two-thirds of patients will have no further complaints and will remain symptom-free at follow-up. Recurrence rates of up to 22% following excision have been reported.

Patients who present after more than 48 to 72 hours with improved symptoms should be given a trial of conservative management. This includes the use of warm Sitz baths, stools softeners, and local analgesics. Resolution of the thrombosis usually results after 8 to 10 days. We do not recommend simple incision and clot extraction because of the higher recurrence and the risk of infection involved.

COMPARISON STUDIES

With the numerous modalities available, making the best choice for the patient is often difficult. Many comparison studies have been published in the literature and these have been analyzed in two recent meta-analyses (40–42).

Johanson and Rimm (40) performed a comparative analysis of infrared coagulation, rubber band ligation, and injection sclerotherapy for first- and second-degree hemorrhoids in 1992. They included five trials in their analysis and concluded that rubber band ligation was associated with significantly fewer patients requiring additional treatment when compared to injection sclerotherapy and infrared coagulation. Rubber band ligation demonstrated greater long-term efficacy, possibly related to the better depth of tissue destruction achieved and subsequent submucosa fixation. Overall symptomatic response was better with ligation although a significantly higher incidence of post-treatment pain was noted.

MacRae and McLeod (41,42) analyzed 16 and subsequently 23 randomized controlled trials comparing two or more various methods of treatment. They found rubber band ligation to be superior to both sclerotherapy and infrared coagulation, with significantly less need for further therapy. In fact, it was recommended as the therapy of choice for first- and second-degree hemorrhoids. Although it was less effective when compared to hemorrhoidectomy, it was also recommended for third degree hemorrhoids because it was associated with significantly less pain and fewer complications.

CONCLUSION

Hemorrhoidal disease presenting in an office setting should first be given a trial of medical therapy. Patients who fail to respond to this conservative management should then be offered rubber band ligation. Injection sclerotherapy and infrared coagulation are reserved for the treatment of small symptomatic hemorrhoids which are not amenable to rubber band ligation.

REFERENCES

1. Johanson JF, Sonnenberg A. Temporal changes in the occurrence of hemorrhoids in the United States and England. Dis Colon Rectum 1991; 34:585–593.
2. Thomson WH. The Nature of Hemorrhoids. Br J Surg 1975; 62:542–552.
3. Loder PB, Kamm MA, Nicholls RJ, et al. Hemorrhoids: Pathology, pathophysiology and aetiology. Br J Surg 1994; 81:946–954.
4. Read MG, Read NW, Haynes WG, et al. A prospective study of effect of hemorrhoidectomy on sphincter function and fecal incontinence. Br J Surg 1982; 69: 396–398.
5. Bleday R, Pena JP, Rothenberger DA, et al. Symptomatic hemorrhoids: Current incidence and complications of operative therapy. Dis Colon Rectum 1992; 35:477–481.
6. American Society for Gastrointestinal Endoscopy. The role of endoscopy in the patient with lower gastrointestinal bleeding. Guidelines for clinical application. Gastrointestinal Endoscopy 1988; 34:235–255.
7. Banov L Jr, Knoepp LF Jr, Erdman LH, et al. Management of hemorrhoidal disease. JSC Med Assoc 1985; 81:398–401.
8. Moesgaard F, Nielsen ML, Hansen JB et al. High-fiber diet reduces bleeding and pain in patients with hemorrhoids. Dis Colon Rectum 1982; 25:454.
9. Garner RC, Leong D, Gregory S, et al. Comparison of the absorption of micronized (Daflon 500 mg) and non micronized diosmin tablets after oral administration to healthy volunteers analyzed by Accelerator Mass Spectrometry. J Pharm Sci 2001; 91:32–40.
10. Ibegbuna V, Nicolaides AN, Sowade O et al. Venous elasticity after treatment with MPFF. Angiology 1997; 48:45–49.
11. Bouskela E, Donyo KA, Verbeuren TJ. Effects of Daflon 500 mg on increased microvascular permeability in normal hamsters. Int J Microcirc 1995; 15:22–26.
12. McHale NG, Hollywood MA. Control of lymphatic pumping: interest of Daflon 500 mg. Phlebology 1994; 9:23–25.
13. Shoab SS, Porter JB, Scurr JH, et al. Endothelial activation response to oral micronized flavonoid therapy in patients with chronic venous disease—a prospective study. Eur J Vasc Endovasc Surg 1999; 17:313–318.
14. Ho YH, Tan M, Seow-Choen F. Micronized purified flavonoid fraction compared favorably with rubber band ligation and fiber alon in the management of bleeding hemorrhoids: Randomized control trial. Dis Colon Rectum 2000; 43:66–69.
15. La Torre F, Nicolai AP. Clinical use of micronized purified flavonoid fraction for treatment of symptoms after hemorrhoidectomy. Results of a randomized clinical trial. Dis Colon Rectum 2004; 47:704–710.
16. Buckshee K, Takkar D, Aggarwal N. Micronized flavonoid therapy in internal hemorrhoids of pregnancy. Int J Gynaecol Obstet 1997; 57(2):145–151.
17. Barron J. Office ligation treatment of hemorrhoids. Dis Colon Rectum 1963; 6:109–113.
18. Nivatvongs S, Goldberg SM. An improved technique of rubber band ligation of hemorrhoids. Am J Surg 1982; 144(3):378–380.
19. Lee HH, Spencer RJ, Beart RW Jr. Multiple hemorrhoidal bandings in single session. Dis Colon Rectum 1994; 37:37–41.
20. Lau WY, Chow HP, Poon GP, et al. Rubber band ligation of 3 first degree hemorrhoids in a single session. A safe and effective procedure. Dis Colon Rectum 1982; 25:336–339.
21. Khubchaudani IT. A randomized comparison of single and multiple rubber band ligations. Dis Colon Rectum 1983; 26:705–708.
22. Law WI, Chu KW. Triple rubber band ligation for hemorrhoids: Prospective randomized trial of use of local anesthetic injection. Dis Colon Rectum 1999; 42: 363–366.
23. Rasmussen OO. Larsen KGL, Naver L,et al. Emergency haemorrhoidectomy compared with incision and banding for the treatment of acute strangulated haemorrhoids. Eur J Surg 1991; 157:613–614.

24. Sardinha TC. Corman ML. Hemorrhoids. Surg Clin N Am 2002; 82:1153–1167.
25. American Gastroenterological Association Clinical Practice Committee. American Gastroenterological Association Technical Review on the Diagnosis and Treatment of Hemorrhoids. Gastroenterology 2004; 126(5):1463–1473.
26. Beck DE. Hemorrhoidal disease. In: Beck DE, Wexner SD, ed. Fundamentals of Anorectal Surgery, 2nd ed. London: W.B. Saunders, 1998:237–253.
27. Rotheberg R, Rubin RJ, Eisenstat T, et al. Rubber band ligation hemorrhoidectomy: Long term results. Am Surg 1983; 49:167.
28. O'Hara VS. Fatal Clostridial infection following hemorrhoidal banding. Dis Colon Rectum 1980; 23:570–571.
29. Russell TR, Donahue JH. Hemorrhoidal banding: A warning. Dis Colon Rectum 1985; 28:291–293.
30. Wehrmann T, Riphaus A, Feinstein J, et al. Hemorrhoidal elastic band ligation with flexible videoendoscopes: A prospective, randomized comparison with conventional technique that uses rigid proctoscopes. Gastrointest Endosc 2004; 60(2):191–195.
31. Morgan J. Varicose state of saphenous hemorrhoids treated by the injection of tincture of persulphate of iron. Med Press Circular 1869:29–30.
32. Khoury GA, Lake SP, Lewis AA. A randomized trial to compare single with multiple phenol injection treatment for haemorrhoids. Br J Surg 1985; 72:741–742.
33. Walker AJ, Leicester RJ, Nicholls RJ, et al. A prospective study of infrared coagulation, injection and rubber band ligation in the treatment of haemorrhoids. Int J Colorectal Dis 1990; 5:113–116.
34. Nivatvongs S. Hemorrhoids. In: Gordon PH, Nivatvongs S, eds. Principles and Practice of Surgery for the Colon, Rectum and Anus, 2nd ed. St Louis: Quality Medical Publishing, 1999:193–215.
35. Goligher JC. Cryosurgery for hemorrhoids. Dis Colon Rectum 1976; 19:213–218.
36. Smith LE, Goodreau JJ, Fouty WJ. Operative hemorrhoidectomy versus cryodestruction. Dis Colon Rectum 1979; 22:10–16.
37. Neiger A. Hemorrhoids in everyday practice. Proctology 1979; 2:22.
38. Dennison A, Whiston RJ, Rooney S, et al. A randomized comparison of infrared photocoagulation with bipolar diathermy for the outpatient treatment of hemorrhoids. Dis Colon Rectum 1990; 33:32–34.
39. Johannes J, Bach S, Stubinger H, et al. Excision of thrombosed external hemorrhoid under local anesthesia. A retrospective evaluation of 340 patients. Dis Colon Rectum 2003; 46:1226–1231.
40. Johanson JF, Rimm A. Optimal nonsurgical treatment of hemorrhoids: A comparative analysis of infrared coagulation, rubber band ligation and injection sclerotherapy. Am J Gastroenterol 1992; 87:1601–1605.
41. MacRae HM, McLeod RS. Comparison of hemorrhoidal treatment modalities: A meta-analysis. Dis Colon Rectum 1995; 38:687–694.
42. MacRae HM, Temple LKF, McLeod RS. A meta-analysis of hemorrhoidal treatments. Seminars Colon Rectal Surg 2002; 13:77–83.

7 Hemorrhoids: Surgical Treatment

David J. Maron
Department of Colon and Rectal Surgery, University of Pennsylvania School of Medicine, Philadelphia, Pennsylvania, U.S.A.

Steven D. Wexner
Department of Colorectal Surgery, Cleveland Clinic Florida, Weston, Florida; Ohio State University Health Sciences Center, Columbus, Ohio; University of South Florida College of Medicine, Tampa, Florida, U.S.A.

INTRODUCTION

Surgical treatment of hemorrhoids should be considered for (1) symptomatic combined internal and external hemorrhoids, (2) hemorrhoids that are severely prolapsed requiring manual reduction, (3) hemorrhoids that have failed conservative, nonoperative therapy, and (4) hemorrhoids that are associated with other anorectal pathology, including fissure, fistula, ulceration, and large hypertrophied anal papilla.

Surgical treatment of hemorrhoids can be divided into two categories: conventional excisional hemorrhoidectomy and stapled hemorrhoidopexy. Conventional hemorrhoidectomy entails excision of the hemorrhoidal tissue (either with the use of scissors, scalpel, bipolar cautery, ultrasonic energy electrocautery, or laser), while the stapled hemorrhoidopexy causes a reduction of the prolapsed hemorrhoids with a concurrent disruption of the blood supply to the hemorrhoidal tissue. Each of these two major techniques will be discussed in detail.

Hemorrhoidectomy can be performed with general, regional, or local anesthesia; the choice of anesthesia should be individualized to each patient. The patient may be positioned in the lithotomy position, Sims (left lateral decubitus) position, or the prone jackknife position; the authors prefer the latter positioning. Read et al. (1) reviewed the anesthetic technique and positioning in 413 consecutive patients undergoing anorectal procedures at two institutions. They found that 94% of the procedures were performed in the prone position, with the majority (67%) of patients receiving intravenous sedation with local anesthesia, while 32% received regional anesthesia. Discharge from the recovery room was significantly quicker in patients receiving local anesthesia. The authors concluded that intravenous sedation with local anesthesia in the prone position is safe and effective, and may offer a potential cost savings by decreasing recovery room time for outpatient procedures.

The patient is given two sodium phosphate enemas (Fleet, Lynchburg, Virginia, U.S.A.) in the morning prior to the operation. Prophylactic antibiotics are not administered except in those patients who are at high risk (e. g., prosthetic valves, history of endocarditis) (2).

CONVENTIONAL HEMORRHOIDECTOMY

As mentioned, the goal of the conventional hemorrhoidectomy is the complete excision of the hemorrhoidal tissue. Although most patients will have enlarged hemorrhoids in the left lateral, right anterior, and right posterior positions, the surgeon must be prepared to excise any and all hemorrhoidal tissue within the anal canal taking care to preserve a bridge of normal mucosal or skin between the excision sites to prevent postoperative stenosis formation. This measure is especially true in cases of edematous or gangrenous hemorrhoids. Numerous procedures have been described for the surgical excision of hemorrhoids, including those operations detailed by Ferguson, Fansler, Milligan and Morgan, Parks, and Whitehead (3–7). The authors' preferred procedure for excisional hemorrhoidectomy is the modified closed Ferguson technique.

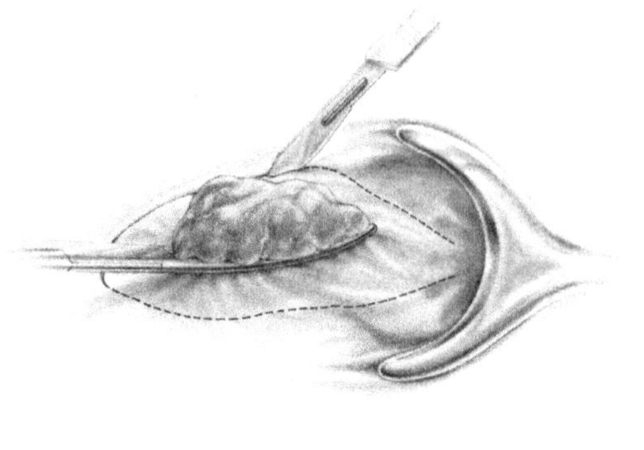

Figure 1 A Hill–Ferguson retractor is used to expose the hemorrhoidal bundle. *Source*: From Corman, ML. Colon and Rectal Surgery, Fifth Edition. 2005, Lippincott Williams and Wilkins, Philadelphia, Pennsylvania, U.S.A.

CLOSED FERGUSON TECHNIQUE

The patient is placed in the prone jackknife position with the buttocks taped apart. The anus is prepared with a providone–iodine solution. The anal submucosa is infiltrated with 0.5% bupiricaine Lidocaine with 1:200,000 epinephrine to help minimize bleeding and to help develop the plane between the hemorrhoids and the underlying internal anal sphincter muscle. An examination then confirms the preoperative findings and determines the number of hemorrhoidal bundles to be excised.

A Hill–Ferguson or Fansler retractor is placed in the anus to expose the hemorrhoidal bundle. An elliptical incision is begun on the perianal skin and is continued onto the anal mucosa to include both the external and internal hemorrhoids. Excision of the hemorrhoid can be undertaken with the use of a scalpel, scissors, electrocautery bipolar electrocautery, ultrasonic, shears or laser (Figs. 1 and 2). Dissection in the proper plane results in elevation of all of the varicosities (vertical fibers) with the specimen, while the internal sphincter muscle (transverse fibers) remains in its normal anatomical position. Bleeding typically means that the proper plane has not been dissected.

Once the entire hemorrhoidal bundle has been mobilized, the vascular pedicle at the superior edge is suture ligated with an absorbable suture (3–0 Vicryl, Ethicon Endosurgery, Cincinnati, Ohio, U.S.A.) and the hemorrhoid is removed (Fig. 3). Any small residual hemorrhoidal veins should be removed with the use of scissors or electrocautery, thereby limiting the chance of subsequent symptoms related to retained hemorrhoidal tissue. The mucosal edges are then approximated with the use of the same absorbable suture used to ligate the pedicle. The wound is closed using a running locking suture incorporating a superficial bite of the internal sphincter in order to eliminate any potential dead space (Fig. 4). At the mucocutaneous junction, the suture is no longer locked and the skin is closed in a simple running manner. At the outer edge, the suture is loosely tied to itself to provide an outlet should any postoperative hematoma develop. The other hemorrhoidal bundles are handled in a similar manner. Again, it is important to preserve bridges of anoderm between the excision sites and maintain the dentate line in its normal anatomic position. The ability to close all the incisions and maintain the retractor in place implies that the anal canal opening is adequate and the chance of postoperative stenosis is low.

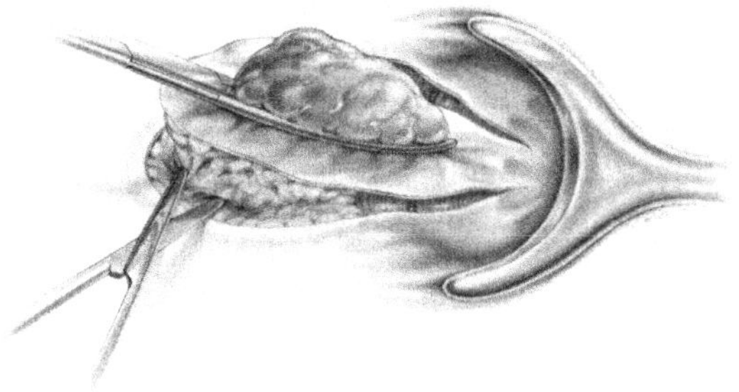

Figure 2 Using scissors or electrocautery, the hemorrhoid is dissected off the underlying internal sphincter muscle. *Source*: From Corman, ML. Colon and Rectal Surgery, Fifth Edition. 2005, Lippincott Williams and Wilkins, Philadelphia, Pennsylvania, U.S.A.

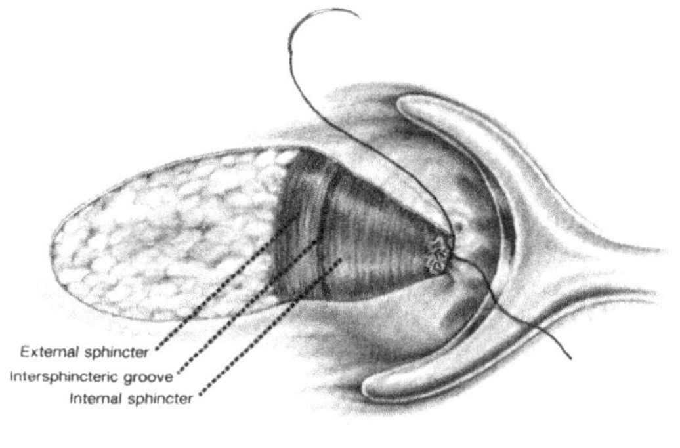

Figure 3 Open wound following excision of the hemorrhoid. *Source*: From Corman, ML. Colon and Rectal Surgery, Fifth Edition. 2005, Lippincott Williams and Wilkins, Philadelphia, Pennsylvania, U.S.A.

Some authors have suggested that the addition of an internal sphincterotomy in the lateral hemorrhoidal excision site reduces postoperative pain (8,9). Asfar et al. (8) evaluated anal stretch and lateral internal sphincterotomy in reducing posthemorrhoidectomy pain in a prospective randomized study. They found that only 18% of patients undergoing concomitant sphincterotomy required narcotic medications in the first 24 hours, compared with 100% of those patients who underwent anal stretch (8). In addition, only 6% of patients in the sphincterotomy group reported pain with the first bowel movement, compared with 96% in the anal stretch group. Amorotti et al. (9) similarly found that patients who underwent surgical sphincterotomy at the time of hemorrhoidectomy had less postoperative pain than patients who underwent chemical sphincterotomy or no other treatment. Khubchandani (10), however, found no statistically significant difference in pain between patients undergoing hemorrhoidectomy with and without sphincterotomy at four hours, at the time of the first bowel movement, and four days following surgery. It is not the practice of the authors to perform internal sphincterotomy at the time of hemorrhoidectomy, unless the patient has a chronic posterior midline anal fissure. The potential risk of compromise in continence seems to outweigh any theoretical benefits.

OPEN MILLIGAN MORGAN TECHNIQUE

This procedure was originally described by Frederick Salmon, the founder of St. Marks Hospital in London in the 1830s (11) and popularized by Milligan and Morgan (5). This procedure may be indicated when hemorrhoids are gangrenous or circumferential. The procedure begins with gentle dilatation of the anal canal with two to three fingers. Forceps are placed on the perianal skin just beyond the mucocutaneous junction and the hemorrhoid is everted. A second pair of forceps is placed on the internal component at the level of the anorectal ring and the hemorrhoidal bundle is excised off the underlying sphincter muscle. The hemorrhoidal pedicle is then suture ligated with absorbable suture and the hemorrhoid is removed. Hemostasis is obtained with the electrocautery and the wound is left open (Fig. 5). The surgeon must be careful to leave adequate bridges of anoderm to prevent postoperative anal stenosis with healing of the open hemorrhoid wounds (12). Although the authors usually perform Ferguson hemorrhoidectomy, they occasionally utilize the Milligan-Morgan technique.

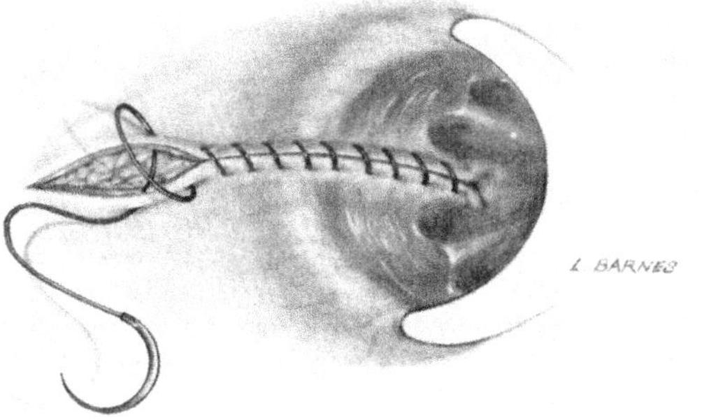

Figure 4 Closure of the mucosal defect. *Source*: From Corman, ML. Colon and Rectal Surgery, Fifth Edition. 2005, Lippincott Williams and Wilkins, Philadelphia, Pennsylvania, U.S.A.

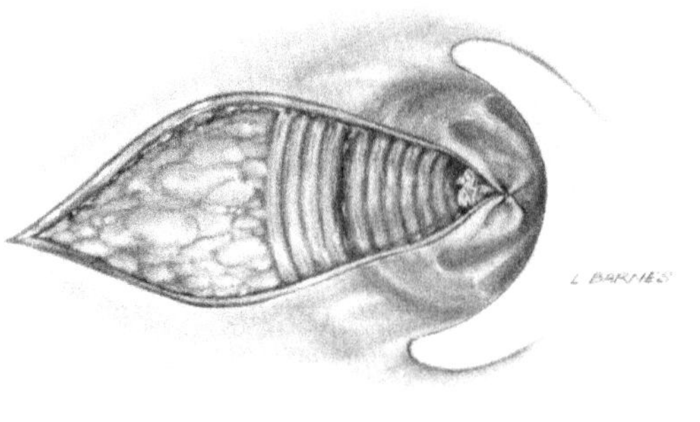

Figure 5 Completed open Milligan–Morgan Hemorrhoidectomy. *Source*: From Corman, ML. Colon and Rectal Surgery, Fifth Edition. 2005, Lippincott Williams and Wilkins, Philadelphia, Pennsylvania, U.S.A.

SUBMUCOSAL PARKS' HEMORRHOIDECTOMY

The submucosal hemorrhoidectomy was described by Parks (13) and involves incising the mucosa of the anal canal and removing the underlying hemorrhoidal tissue (Fig. 6). The purported advantage to this technique is that the wounds heal faster with less scarring and therefore a lower incidence of postoperative anal stenosis. A solution of 0.5% or 1% Lidocaine with 1:100,000 Epinephrine is injected into the submucosa and hemorrhoidal tissue. The skin incision begins outside the anus and involves a V-shaped cruciate incision with the removal of a minimal amount of anal mucosa. The anal mucosa is elevated off the hemorrhoidal tissue with the use of scissors. The hemorrhoidal plexus is then elevated off the internal sphincter muscle to the level of the pedicle, which is then ligated and the hemorrhoid removed. The flaps of the mobilized anal mucosa are then reapproximated with an absorbable suture, incorporating a superficial bite of the internal sphincter in order to eliminate any potential dead space; the skin may be

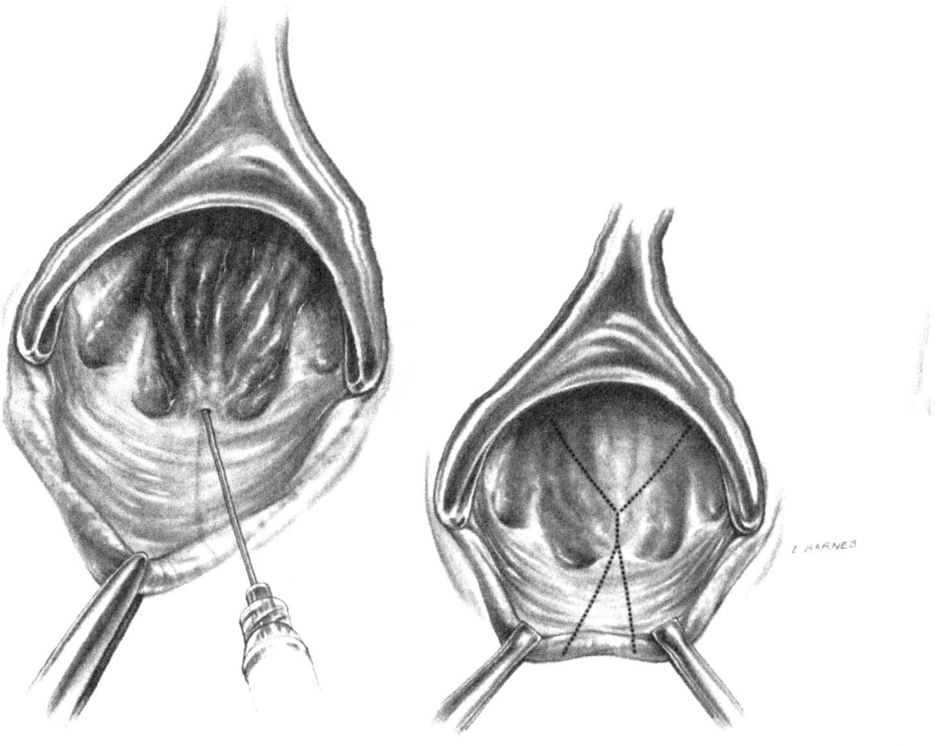

Figure 6 Parks' submucosal hemorrhoidectomy: (**A**) lidocaine with epinephrine is injected for hemostasis, (**B**) a cruciate incision is made in the anoderm. *Source*: From Corman, ML. Colon and Rectal Surgery, Fifth Edition. 2005, Lippincott Williams and Wilkins, Philadelphia, Pennsylvania, U.S.A.

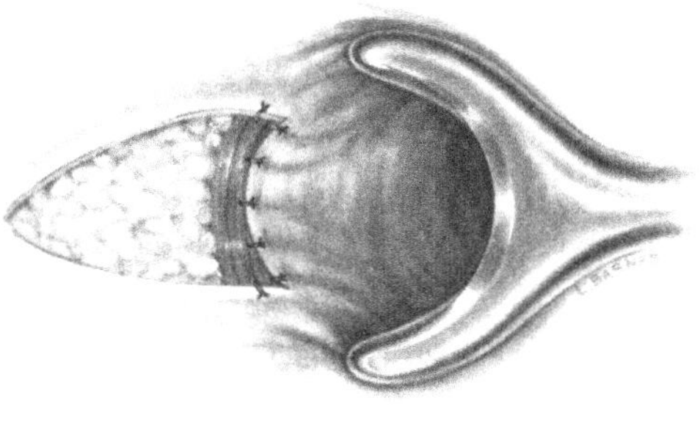

Figure 7 Modified Whitehead hemorrhoidectomy. *Source*: From Corman, ML. Colon and Rectal Surgery, Fifth Edition. 2005, Lippincott Williams and Wilkins, Philadelphia, Pennsylvania, U.S.A.

left open or closed. The authors have occasionally combined this technique with the Ferguson hemorrhoidectcomy, especially when a fourth quadrant is enlarged.

MODIFIED WHITEHEAD HEMORRHOIDECTOMY

This technique was described by Whitehead in 1882 (7), but it is very rarely performed by surgeons today. The modified Whitehead hemorrhoidectomy involves a circumferential incision at the level of the dentate line with excision of the submucosal and subdermal hemorrhoidal tissue. The redundant rectal mucosa is then excised and the proximal rectal mucosa is sutured circumferentially to the anoderm (Fig. 7). Although Whitehead reported good outcomes following this technique, many surgeons have encountered problems (14). Complications including stricture, loss of anal sensation, and development of mucosal ectropion (also referred to as "wet anus" or "Whitehead deformity") are often challenging to correct and have therefore caused this technique to fall out of favor (Fig. 8).

Several authors have reported favorable outcomes following Whitehead hemorrhoidectomy (15,16). Barrios and Khubchandani (15) reported good outcomes in 41 patients, however, late complications developed in 10% of the patients. These complications included anal stenosis, mucosal ectropion, and fecal incontinence. Wolff and Culp (16) examined the outcome of 484 patients following the Whitehead technique. They reported complications including fistula or abscess in 1%, flap loss in 7%, and a nonhealing wound in one patient. They reported no occurrences of mucosal ectropion, and recommended that this be the procedure of choice for

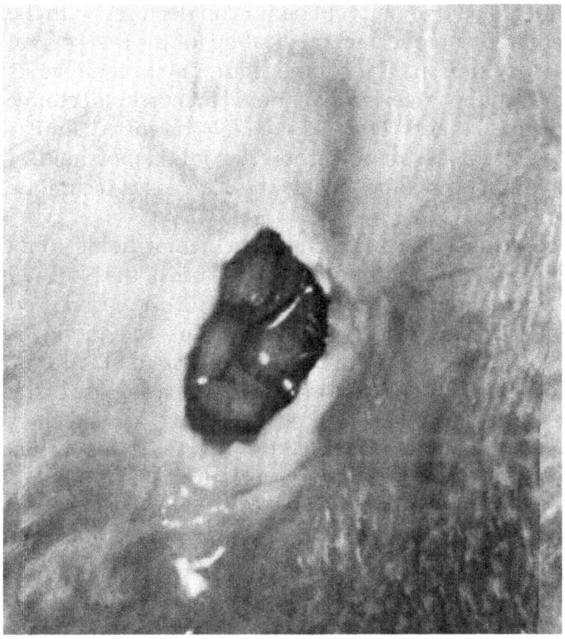

Figure 8 Whitehead deformity. *Source*: From Corman, ML. Colon and Rectal Surgery, Fifth Edition. 2005, Lippincott Williams and Wilkins, Philadelphia, Pennsylvania, U.S.A.

for circumferential prolapse and bleeding hemorrhoids (16). The authors do not employ this technique.

LIGASURE™ AND HARMONIC SCALPEL™ HEMORRHOIDECTOMY

Recently there has been interest in employing the use of the Ligasure diathermy (Valleylab, Boulder, CO) and Harmonic Scalpel (Ethicon Endosurgery, Cincinnati, Ohio, U.S.A.) to excise hemorrhoidal tissue. Several randomized studies have been published comparing the use of Ligasure with conventional hemorrhoidectomy (17–20). Franklin et al. (19) reported a statistically significant decrease in the length of operative time, pain with first bowel movement, and pain at postoperative days 1 and 14. Similarly, Chung and Wu (18) found a reduction in operative time and a reduction in pain on postoperative days 1 and 2. In addition, Jayne et al. (20) found a statistically significant reduction in the amount of intraoperative blood loss with the use of the Ligasure as compared with conventional electrocautery.

Armstrong et al. (21) evaluated the postoperative complications in 500 consecutive hemorrhoidectomies using the Harmonic Scalpel. Complications occurred in 4.8% of patients with the most frequent complication being urinary retention in 2%. Postoperative hemorrhage requiring operative exploration occurred in three patients and fecal incontinence in one patient. Chung et al. (22) conducted a randomized prospective study comparing Harmonic Scalpel hemorrhoidectomy, bipolar scissors hemorrhoidectomy, and scissors hemorrhoidectomy. They reported no difference among the three groups with respect to operative time, hospital stay, time to first bowel movement, pain expectation score, wound healing, or time to return to work or normal activity. They did find a statistically significant reduction in blood loss and postoperative pain score in patients in the Harmonic Scalpel hemorrhoidectomy group, although there was no difference in the amount of narcotic use between the groups.

LASER HEMORRHOIDECTOMY

In addition to its use in the treatment of colorectal polyps and carcinomas, laser therapy has been advocated by some authors in the treatment of hemorrhoids. Lasers which have been employed include argon, carbon dioxide, and neodymium:yttrium–aluminum garnet (Nd:YAG). Yu and Eddy (23) reported their experience in 134 patients who underwent hemorrhoidectomy with the use of the Nd:YAG laser. Patients typically required narcotic pain medication for the first several days and healing was generally complete by one month. The complication rate in their series did not differ significantly from accepted complication rates of conventional hemorrhoidectomy, although anal stenosis did develop in 2% of the patients. Iwagaki et al. (24) reported similar encouraging results in 1816 consecutive patients treated with carbon dioxide hemorrhoidectomy. Other authors have also reported favorable outcomes using the CO_2 laser technique (25,26).

Several randomized studies have been published comparing laser hemorrhoidectomy with conventional hemorrhoidectomy (26–29). Wang et al. (28) compared the use of the Nd:YAG laser to the closed Ferguson technique in 88 patients. Patients treated with the laser used significantly less narcotics and had a lower incidence of postoperative urinary retention (7% vs. 39%). Senagore et al. (29), however, failed to show any significant difference in blood loss, operative time, postoperative analgesia use, or time to return to work when comparing use of the Nd:YAG laser to conventional hemorrhoidectomy. The only significant difference was a greater degree of wound inflammation and dehiscence in the laser group at the 10 day postoperative visit. In addition, the use of the Nd:YAG laser added $480.00 per case, leading the authors to conclude that the use of lasers in the treatment of hemorrhoids could not be supported. Similarly, Leff (27) compared 170 patients who underwent outpatient CO_2 laser hemorrhoidectomy with 56 patients who underwent conventional closed hemorrhoidectomy. There were no observed differences in postoperative pain, wound healing, or complication rates. The authors do not use or recommend the laser to perform excisional hemorrhoidectomy.

OTHER SURGICAL TREATMENT OF HEMORRHOIDS

Several other surgical therapies in the treatment of hemorrhoids deserve mention. Anal stretch has been advocated by some authors in an attempt to decrease constriction of the anal canal, thereby reducing straining during defecation. This procedure, first described by Lord (30), involves dilation of the anus with the patient under anesthesia followed by continued outpatient dilation over the course of six months. While several trials have confirmed its efficacy (31,32), the Lord's procedure causes significantly lower anal pressures and can result in incontinence rates as high as 52% (33–35). The procedure has therefore fallen out of favor; however, some authors still recommend it for young male patients with thrombosed internal hemorrhoids (36).

Another technique which has become less frequently used is cryotherapy. This procedure involves the destruction of hemorrhoidal tissue by applying a cryoprobe cooled with either nitrous oxide or liquid nitrogen directly to the hemorrhoidal bundle in a circumferential manner. While initial studies reported favorable outcomes (37,38) other authors reported problems. Healing in one series frequently took more than six weeks (39). One report compared cryotherapy with closed hemorrhoidectomy and found that cryotherapy was associated with more prolonged pain as well as a foul-smelling discharge (40). In addition, a significant number of those patients treated with cryosurgery required further treatment of their hemorrhoids.

STAPLED HEMORRHOIDECTOMY

The stapled hemorrhoidopexy differs from conventional hemorrhoidectomy in that it causes a reduction of the prolapsed hemorrhoids with a concurrent disruption of the blood supply to the hemorrhoidal tissue rather than excision or destruction of the hemorrhoidal tissue. The circular stapling device used in the procedure was first introduced by Longo in 1998 (41). An international working party was convened to examine this procedure in 2001 and established criteria for performing the stapled hemorrhoidopexy (42).

Patients with prolapsing hemorrhoids requiring manual reduction or uncomplicated hemorrhoids which are irreducible by the patient but reducible at surgery are candidates for stapled hemorrhoidopexy. In addition, selected patients with spontaneously reducing hemorrhoids, patients with symptomatic hemorrhoids which have failed other office-based therapies, and patients with irreducible hemorrhoids at the time of surgery are also considered for this procedure (42). Stapled hemorrhoidectomy should not be performed in the presence of any perianal abscess or gangrene, as the operation does not remove the source of sepsis. In addition, patients with anal stenosis are not suitable for the procedure because the anus will not be able to accommodate the circular anal dilator (CAD). While the stapled hemorrhoidectomy reduces the prolapse of the hemorrhoidal tissue along with some redundant mucosa, full thickness rectal prolapse is not appropriately treated with this procedure (42).

While the treatment of other perianal conditions including anal fissure, fistulae, skin tags, hypertrophied anal papillae, and acute thrombosis can easily be accomplished during a conventional hemorrhoidectomy, the stapled hemorrhoidopexy does not involve incisions in the anoderm and therefore the surgeon must decide whether or not to treat these conditions concomitantly. If thrombosis is present, it is strongly recommended to incise and remove the thrombosed area at the time of the procedure (42). There has also been concern raised over stapled hemorrhoidopexy in patients with preexisting sphincter injury and those with anal incontinence. This concern relates to the use of the CAD leading to the further impairment of bowel control (42).

The most commonly used device for the stapled hemorrhoidopexy is the Proximate Hemorrhoidal Circular Stapler (Ethicon Endo-Surgery, Cincinnati, Ohio, U.S.A.) (Fig. 9). The procedure can be performed under local, regional, or general anesthesia. It is the authors' preference to perform this procedure in the prone position under general anesthesia. Following assessment of the hemorrhoids, the CAD is inserted into the anal canal and any external component is manually reduced (Fig. 10). The CAD is then secured to the skin with the use of a heavy silk suture. If the CAD cannot be inserted due to anal stenosis, the procedure is aborted. A purse-string suture is placed in the submucosa 3 to 4 cm above the dentate line using a 2-0 monofilament suture (Fig. 11). The bites should be placed close together and care should be taken not to involve the rectal musculature, particularly in the anterior quadrant in women. The fully opened stapler

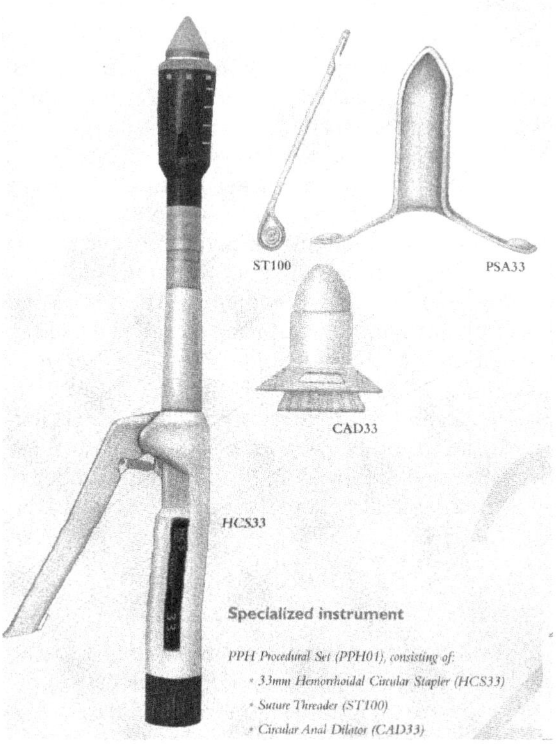

Figure 9 Proximate HCS—hemorrhoidal circular stapler—the PPH03 kit: A 33 mm hemorrhoidal circular stapler (HCS33), a suture threader (ST100), a circular anal dilator (CAD33) and a pursestring suture anoscope (PSA33). *Source*: From Ethicon Endo-Surgery, Inc., Cincinnati, Ohio, U.S.A.

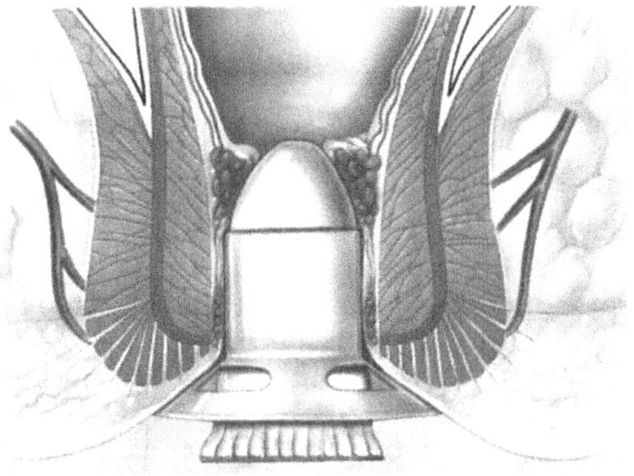

Figure 10 Insertion of the CAD into the anal canal. *Source*: From Person B, Wexner SD. Novel technology and innovations in colorectal surgery: the circular stapler for treatment of hemorrhoids and fibrin glue for treatment of perianal fistula. Surgical Innovation 2004; 11(4):241–252.

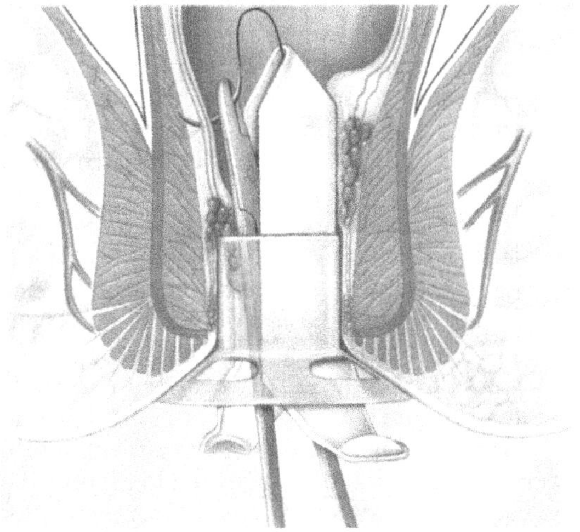

Figure 11 Placement of a submucosal pursestring suture above the dentate line. *Source*: From Person B, Wexner SD. Novel technology and innovations in colorectal surgery: the circular stapler for treatment of hemorrhoids and fibrin glue for treatment of perianal fistula. Surgical Innovation 2004; 11(4):241–252.

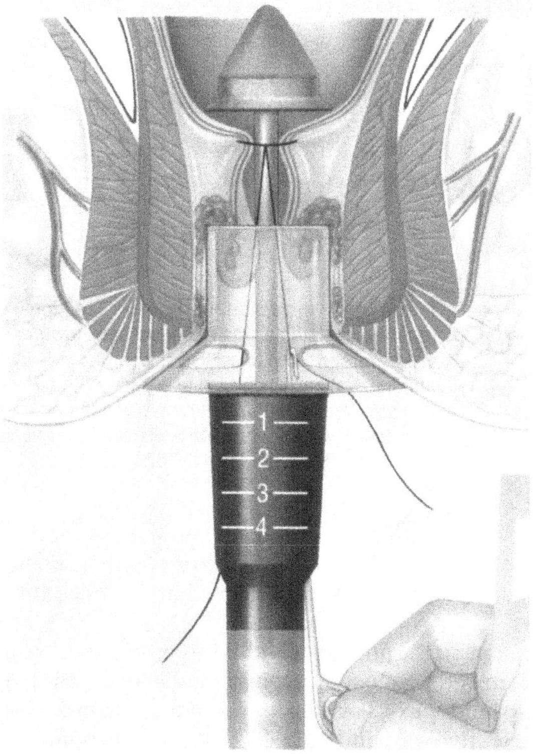

Figure 12 Insertion of the fully opened stapler with the anvil proximal to the pursestring. Tying down the suture around the stapler's shaft, and gently pulling the suture ends through the lateral channels of the stapler using the suture threader. *Source*: From Person B, Wexner SD. Novel technology and innovations in colorectal surgery: the circular stapler for treatment of hemorrhoids and fibrin glue for treatment of perianal fistula. Surgical Innovation 2004; 11(4):241–252.

is inserted such that the anvil is proximal to the purse string and the suture is tied down around the stapler's shaft. The ends of the suture are then passed through the lateral channels with the use of the stapler threader (Fig. 12). The ends of the suture are tied together to help facilitate traction while the stapler is being closed. The stapler is then aligned along the axis of the anal canal and closed while maintaining downward tension on the purse string (Fig. 13). The 4 cm mark on the stapler should be at the level of the anal verge once the stapler is fully closed. In female patients, the vagina is palpated to ensure that the vaginal wall has not been incorporated

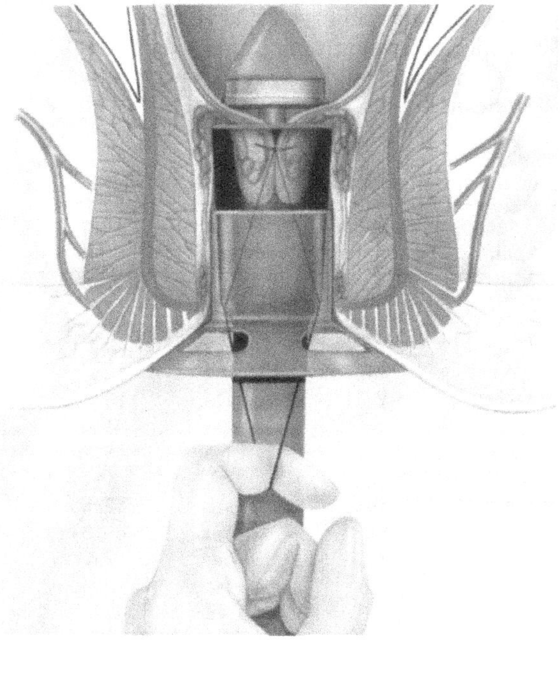

Figure 13 Closing the stapler while gently pulling on the suture. *Source*: From Person B, Wexner SD. Novel technology and innovations in colorectal surgery: the circular stapler for treatment of hemorrhoids and fibrin glue for treatment of perianal fistula. Surgical Innovation 2004; 11(4):241–252.

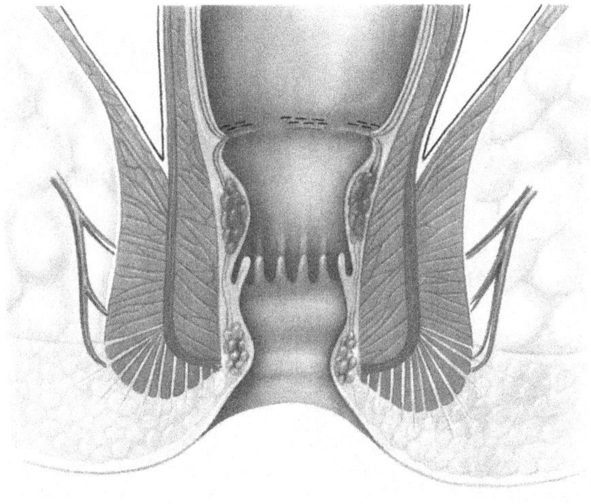

Figure 14 Inspection and suture reinforcement of the staple line as necessary. *Source*: From Person B, Wexner SD. Novel technology and innovations in colorectal surgery: the circular stapler for treatment of hemorrhoids and fibrin glue for treatment of perianal fistula. Surgical Innovation 2004; 11(4):241–252.

prior to firing the stapler. Following firing of the stapler, the head is opened and the stapler line is inspected (Fig. 14). Any bleeding at the staple line is reinforced with suture ligation using absorbable suture. The excised specimen should then be inspected to confirm that the procedure has been adequately performed.

The stapled hemorrhoidopexy avoids incision on the anoderm and is therefore associated with significantly less postoperative pain. Carriero and Longo (43) recently published a series of 1409 patients who underwent the stapled hemorrhoidopexy. Forty-three percent of patients had no pain, 61% had no pain by the second postoperative day, and only 4.7% of patients required strong pain medication for more than one week following surgery; 10 patients developed recurrence requiring a subsequent operation. Singer et al. (44) reported the results of 68 patients who underwent stapled hemorrhoidopexy at two institutions; 20% of patients returned to normal activity on the first postoperative day, and 99% within one week. Five patients had recurrence of their hemorrhoids requiring further therapy.

Senagore et al. (45) conducted a randomized, prospective trial comparing stapled hemorrhoidectomy with the closed Ferguson technique in 13 U.S. centers. Postoperative pain in the first two weeks, pain with first bowel movement, and need for postoperative analgesics were significantly reduced in the stapled hemorrhoidopexy group. Patients in the conventional hemorrhoidectomy group were more likely to present with new or worsening symptoms within the first six months, but after one year, the converse was observed. Other trials comparing stapled hemorrhoidectomy with conventional hemorrhoidectomy are presented in Table 1. Stapled hemorrhoidectomy is now the preferred method of the authors for the surgical treatment of internal hemorrhoids in the absence of a significant external component (46).

Table 1 Randomized Trials of Stapled Hemorrhoidopexy Compared with Conventional Hemorrhoidectomy

Author	Year	PPH *n*	Standard *n*	Reduced pain	Reduced hospital stay	Reduced recovery time	Duration of follow-up
Ho et al. (47)	2000	57	62	Yes	similar	Yes	–
Mehigan et al. (48)	2000	20	20	Yes	similar	Yes	1, 3, 6, 10 wk
Rowsell et al. (49)	2000	11	11	Yes	Yes	Yes	4 hr, 1 wk
Shalaby et al. (50)	2001	100	100	Yes	Yes	Yes	1 wk
Ganio et al. (51)	2001	50	50	Yes	Yes	No	16 mo
Boccasanta et al. (52)	2001	40	40	Yes	Yes	Yes	54 wk
Ortiz et al. (53)	2002	27	28	Yes	–	No	15.9 mo
Pavlidis et al. (54)	2002	40	40	Yes	Yes	–	–
Hetzer et al. (55)	2002	20	20	Yes	Yes	Yes	12 mo
Cheetham et al. (56)	2003	15	16	Yes	No	Yes	6–18 mo
Palimento et al. (57)	2003	37	37	Yes	No	Yes	17.5 mo
Kairaluoma et al. (58)	2003	30	30	Yes	No	No	12 mo
Racalbuto et al. (59)	2004	50	50	Yes	–	Yes	48 mo

THROMBOSED EXTERNAL HEMORRHOIDS

Thrombosed external hemorrhoids are a relatively common complication of hemorrhoidal disease. Their occurrence is often associated with physical exertion or straining such as heavy exercise, moving, or lifting furniture. Patients typically present with a painful, tender mass in the perianal area. The management of thrombosed external hemorrhoids depends on when in the course of the disease the patient presents (60). The pain associated with this condition typically peaks within 48 hours and normally begins to subside after four days. If left untreated, the clot in the thrombosed vessels will dissolve within several weeks or potentially may spontaneously drain through the thinned overlying skin. Following resolution, large thrombosed hemorrhoids may remain as skin tags.

Because this is a self-limiting condition, management is typically conservative and includes pain control with a mild analgesic, warm Sitz baths, and a bulk-producing agent containing fiber. If the patient presents within the first 48 hours, the procedure of choice is excision of the entire thrombosed hemorrhoid. This procedure may be performed in the office or emergency room. The area is anesthetized with a local anesthetic (0.5% bupivicaine with 1:200,000 epinephrine). Using scissors, the thrombosed hemorrhoid is excised with the underlying vein and a wedge of skin. It is important to excise the entire thrombus in order to prevent recurrence. The skin edges are then reapproximated with the use of a running absorbable suture (3-0 chromic).

COMPLICATIONS FOLLOWING SURGICAL HEMORRHOIDECTOMY

Common complications following surgical hemorrhoidectomy include pain, urinary retention, hemorrhage, and constipation. Postoperative pain is the patients' greatest fear and often prevents them from seeking therapy for hemorrhoids. Numerous methods of postoperative pain management have been attempted. Epidural morphine has been shown to provide excellent pain relief (61); however, this method is not applicable to outpatient surgery. Vinson-Bonnet et al. (62) assessed the efficacy of injection a long-acting local anesthetic (ropivicaine) following hemorrhoidectomy in a randomized, double-blind study. Patients in the ropivicaine group had less pain and required fewer doses of morphine in the immediate postoperative period. Others have found that injection of local anesthesia does not reduce the overall requirement of analgesics (63,64). Several authors have recommended the use of ketorolac tromethamine (Toradol) following anorectal surgery (65,66). O'Donovan et al. (65) found that pain control following direct injection of the internal sphincter muscle with Toradol at the time of surgery plus five days of oral therapy was equivalent to that of a subcutaneous morphine pump. Pain management with the use of transdermal fentanyl (67), nitroglycerin ointment (68,69), and botulinum toxin (70) have also been reported following surgical hemorrhoidectomy.

Urinary retention has been reported to occur in as many as 20% of patients following hemorrhoidectomy (71). Fluid overload is typically responsible, and limiting intravenous fluids during the intraoperative and postoperative period may reduce the incidence of retention. Bailey and Ferguson (72) found that only 3.5% of patients who were restricted to 250 cc of fluid postoperatively required urethral catheterization following hemorrhoidectomy. In contrast, 15% of patients who were offered unlimited oral liquids required placement of a Foley catheter (72). Hoff et al. (73) similarly reported a low incidence of urinary retention with perioperative fluid restriction. Prophylactic administration of bethanacol chloride (Urecholine) (74) and α-adrenergic blockers (75) have also been shown to be of benefit in the prevention of urinary retention.

Postoperative bleeding within 48 hours is almost always related to a technical error. Although treatment with submucosal injection with dilute epinephrine has been reported (76), most patients require a return to the operating room for inspection and suture ligation of any bleeding points. Delayed hemorrhage, which occurs beyond the initial 48 to 72 hours, has been reported in 0.8% to 2% of hemorrhoidectomies (71,77) and is likely related to erosion of the suture. Management varies from observation to packing with Gelfoam to operative inspection with suture ligation. Intraoperative suture ligation of all suture lines under general anesthesia is generally the best approach.

Constipation following hemorrhoidectomy may be related to a number of factors, including the effects of narcotic pain medications, anesthesia, and the surgical alteration of the anal canal, as well as the patient's fear of a painful bowel movement. This complication can be prevented with the use of a bulk-forming agent or gentle laxative. Johnson et al. (78) found that patients who received fiber postoperatively had less painful bowel movements and less discharge and soiling as compared to patients taking a regimen of sterculia, magnesium sulfate, and mineral oil. The postoperative use of senna has also been shown to prevent constipation following hemorrhoidectomy (79).

Complications following stapled hemorrhoidopexy are similar to those following conventional hemorrhoidectomy. There have been reports, however, of complications specific to the stapled technique. An increased rate of pelvic sepsis has been reported (80,81), and there have been published reports of rectal perforation (82). In addition, stricture development at the staple line has been reported at an incidence of 0.8% to 1.6% (83–85). Stricture following stapled hemorrhoidopexy can typically be treated with dilatation alone. Severe cases of stenosis or stricture may require operative dilatation or even anoplasty (86).

CONCLUSION

When dietary modifications and nonoperative treatments fail to improve symptoms related to hemorrhoids, operative therapy should be considered. Operative therapy has traditionally been in the form of surgical excision of the hemorrhoidal tissue, but stapled hemorrhoidopexy now offers an excellent alternative method of surgical treatment of hemorrhoids in the United States. Good outcomes require that the surgeon be skilled at more than one procedure and that treatment be tailored to the individual patient.

REFERENCES

1. Read TE, Henry SE, Hovis RM, et al. Prospective evaluation of anesthetic technique for anorectal surgery. Dis Colon Rectum 2002; 45:1553–1558.
2. The Standards Task Force. The American Society of Colon and Rectal Surgeons. Practice parameters for antibiotic prophylaxis to prevent infective endocarditis or infected prosthesis during colon and rectal endoscopy. Dis Colon Rectum 2000; 43:1193.
3. Ferguson JA, HeatonJR. Closed hemorrhoidectomy. Dis Colon Rectum 1959; 2: 176–179.
4. Fansler WA, Anderson JK. A plastic operation for certain types of hemorrhoids. J Am Med Assoc 1933; 101:1064.
5. Milligan ETC, Morgan, CN, Jones LE, et al. Surgical anatomy of the anal canal, and operative treatment of haemorrhoids. Lancet 1937; 2:1119.
6. Parks AG. Hemorrhoidectomy. Adv Surg 1971; 5:1–50.
7. Whitehead W. The surgical treatment of hemorrhoids. Br J Med 1882; 1:148.
8. Asfar SK, Juma TH, Ala-Edeen T. Hemorrhoidectomy and sphincterotomy. A prospective study comparing the effectiveness of anal stretch and sphincterotomy in reducing pain after hemorrhoidectomy. Dis Colon Rectum 1988; 31:181–185.
9. Amorotti C, Mosca D, Trenti C, et al. [Usefulness of lateral internal sphincterotomy combined with hemorrhoidectomy by the Milligan–Morgan's technique: results of a prospective randomized trial]. Chir Ital 2003; 55:879–886.
10. Khubchandani IT. Internal sphincterotomy with hemorrhoidectomy does not relieve pain: a prospective, randomized study. Dis Colon Rectum 2002; 45:1452–1457.
11. Allingham HW. The Diagnosis and Treatment of Disease of the Rectum. 7th ed. London: Bailliere, Tindall, & Cox, 1901.
12. Mazier WP. Hemorrhoids. In: Mazier WP, Levin, D. H., Luchtefeld, M. A., Senagore, A. J., eds. Surgery of the Colon, Rectum, and Anus. Philadelphia: W.B. Saunders, 1995:229–254.
13. Parks AG. The surgical treatment of haemorrhoids. Br J Surg 1956; 43:337–351.
14. Bonello JC. Who's afraid of the dentate line? The Whitehead hemorrhoidectomy. Am J Surg 1988; 156:182–186.
15. Barrios G, Khubchandani M. Whitehead operation revisited. Dis Colon Rectum 1979; 22:330–332.
16. Wolff BG, Culp CE. The Whitehead hemorrhoidectomy. An unjustly maligned procedure. Dis Colon Rectum 1988; 31:587–590.

17. Palazzo FF, Francis DL, Clifton MA. Randomized clinical trial of Ligasure versus open haemorrhoidectomy. Br J Surg 2002; 89:154–157.
18. Chung YC, Wu HJ. Clinical experience of sutureless closed hemorrhoidectomy with LigaSure. Dis Colon Rectum 2003; 46:87–92.
19. Franklin EJ, Seetharam S, Lowney J, et al. Randomized, clinical trial of Ligasure vs conventional diathermy in hemorrhoidectomy. Dis Colon Rectum 2003; 46: 1380–1383.
20. Jayne DG, Botterill I, Ambrose NS, et al. Randomized clinical trial of Ligasure versus conventional diathermy for day-case haemorrhoidectomy. Br J Surg 2002; 89:428–432.
21. Armstrong DN, Frankum C, Schertzer ME, et al. Harmonic scalpel hemorrhoidectomy: five hundred consecutive cases. Dis Colon Rectum 2002; 45:354–359.
22. Chung CC, Ha JP, Tai YP, et al. Double-blind, randomized trial comparing Harmonic Scalpel hemorrhoidectomy, bipolar scissors hemorrhoidectomy, and scissors excision: ligation technique. Dis Colon Rectum 2002; 45:789–794.
23. Yu JC, Eddy HJ. Laser, a new modality for hemorrhoidectomy. Am J Proctol Gastroenterol Colon Rectal Surg 1985; 36:9–13.
24. Iwagaki H, Higuchi Y, Fuchimoto S, et al. The laser treatment of hemorrhoids: results of a study on 1816 patients. Jpn J Surg 1989; 19:658–661.
25. Chia YW, Darzi A, Speakman CT, et al. CO2 laser haemorrhoidectomy—does it alter anorectal function or decrease pain compared to conventional haemorrhoidectomy? Int J Colorectal Dis 1995; 10:22–24.
26. Hodgson WJ, Morgan J. Ambulatory hemorrhoidectomy with CO2 laser. Dis Colon Rectum 1995; 38:1265–1269.
27. Leff EI. Hemorrhoidectomy—laser vs. nonlaser: outpatient surgical experience. Dis Colon Rectum 1992; 35:743–746.
28. Wang JY, Chang-Chien CR, Chen JS, et al. The role of lasers in hemorrhoidectomy. Dis Colon Rectum 1991; 34:78–82.
29. Senagore A, Mazier WP, Luchtefeld MA, et al. Treatment of advanced hemorrhoidal disease: a prospective, randomized comparison of cold scalpel vs. contact Nd:YAG laser. Dis Colon Rectum 1993; 36:1042–1049.
30. Lord PH. A new regime for the treatment of haemorrhoids. Proc R Soc Med 1968; 61:935–936.
31. Fussell K. Follow up of Lord's procedure for haemorrhoids. Proc R Soc Med 1973; 66:246–247.
32. Anscombe AR, Hancock BD. A clinical trial of the treatment of haemorrhoids by operation and the Lord procedure. Lancet 1974; 2(7875):250–253.
33. Creve U, Hubens A. The effect of Lord's procedure on anal pressure. Dis Colon Rectum 1979; 22:483–485.
34. Oritz H, Marti J, Jaurrieta E, et al. Lord's procedure: a critical study of its basic priniciple. Br J Surg 1978; 65:281–284.
35. Konsten J, Baeten CG. Hemorrhoidectomy vs. Lord's method: 17-year follow-up of a prospective, randomized trial. Dis Colon Rectum 2000; 43:503–506.
36. Williams NS. Haemorrhoidal disease. In: Williams NS, Keighley, M.R., eds. Surgery of the Anus, Rectum, and Colon. London: WB Saunders, 1993:295–364.
37. Savin S. Hemorrhoidectomy—how I do it: results of 444 cryorectal surgical operations. Dis Colon Rectum 1977; 20:189–196.
38. O'Callaghan JD, Matheson TS, Hall R. Inpatient treatment of prolapsing piles: cryosurgery versus Milligan–Morgan haemorrhoidectomy. Br J Surg 1982; 69:157–159.
39. Goligher JC. Cryosurgery for hemorrhoids. Dis Colon Rectum 1976; 19:213–218.
40. Smith LE, Goodreau JJ, Fouty WJ. Operative hemorrhoidectomy versus cryodestruction. Dis Colon Rectum 1979; 22:10–16.
41. Longo A. Treatment of hemorrhoid disease by reduction of mucosa and hemorrhoid prolapse with a circular suturing device: a new procedure. Proc 6th World Cong Endosc Surg 1998: 777–784.
42. Corman ML, Gravie JF, Hager T et al. Stapled haemorrhoidopexy: a consensus position paper by an international working party: indications, contra-indications and technique. Colorectal Dis 2003; 4:304–310.
43. Carriero A, Longo A. Intraoperative, perioperative, and postoperative complications of stapled hemorrhoidopexy. Osp Ital Chir 2003; 9:333–340.
44. Singer MA, Cintron JR, Fleshman JW, et al. Early experience with stapled hemorrhoidectomy in the United States. Dis Colon Rectum 2002; 45:360–367.
45. Senagore AJ, Singer MA, Abcarian H, et al. A prospective, randomized, controlled, multicenter trial comparing stapled hemorrhoidopexy and Ferguson hemorrhoidectomy: perioperative and one year results. Dis Colon Rectum 2004; 47:1824–1836.
46. Wexner SD. The quest for painless surgical treatment of hemorrhoids continues. J Am Coll Surg 2001; 193:174–178.

47. Ho YH, Cheong WK, Tsang C, et al. Stapled hemorrhoidectomy-cost and effectiveness. Randomized, controlled trial including incontinence scoring, anorectal manometry, and endoanal assessments at up to three months. Dis Colon Rectum 2000; 43:1666–1675.
48. Mehigan BJ, Monson JR, Hartley JE. Stapling procedure for haemorrhoids versus Milligan–Morgan haemorrhoidectomy: randomized controlled trial. Lancet 2000; 355:782–785.
49. Roswell M, Bello M, Hemingway DM. Circumferential mucosectomy (stapled haemorrhoidectomy) versus conventional haemorrhoidectomy: randomized controlled trial. Lancet 2000; 355:779–781.
50. Shalaby R, Desoky A. Randomized clinical trial of sapled versus Milligan–Morgan haemorrhoidectomy. Br J Surg 2001; 88:1049–1053.
51. Ganio E, Altomare DF, Gabrielli F, et al. Prospective, randomized, multicentre trial comparing stapled with open haemorrhoidectomy. Br J Surg 2001; 88:669–674.
52. Boccasanta P, Capretti, PG, Venturi M, et al. Randomized controlled trial between stapled circumferential mucosectomy and conventional circular hemorrhoidectomy in advanced hemorrhoids with external mucosal prolapse. Am J Surg 2001; 182:64–68.
53. Ortiz H, Marzo J, Armendariz P. Randomized clinical trial of stapled haemorrhoidopexy versus conventional diathermy haemorrhoidectomy. Br J Surg 2002; 89:1376–1381.
54. Pavlidis T, Papziogas B, Souparis A, et al. Modern stapled Longo procedure vs. conventional Milligan–Morgan hemorrhoidectomy: a randomized controlled trial. Int J Colorectal Dis 2002; 17:50–53.
55. Hetzer FH, Demartines N, Handschin AE, et al. Stapled vs excision hemorrhoidectomy: long-term results of a prospective randomized trial. Arch Surg 2002; 137:337–340.
56. Cheetham MJ, Cohn CR, Kamm MA, et al. A randomized, controlled trial of diathermy hemorrhoidectomy vs. stapled hemorrhoidectomy in an intended day-care setting with longer-term follow-up. Dis Colon Rectum 2003; 46:491–497.
57. Palimento D, Picchio M, Attanasio U, et al. Stapled and open hemorrhoidectomy: randomized controlled trial of early results. World J Surg 2003; 27:203–207.
58. Kairaluoma M, Nuorva K, Kellokumpu I. Day-case stapled (circular) vs. diathermy hemorrhoidectomy: a randomized, controlled trial evaluating surgical and functional outcome. Dis Colon Rectum 2003; 46:93–99.
59. Racalbuto A, Aliotta I, Corsaro G, et al. Hemorrhoidal stapler prolapsectomy vs. Milligan–Morgan hemorrhoidectomy: a long-term randomized trial. Int J Colorectal Dis 2004; 19:239–244.
60. Beck DE. Hemorrhoids. In: Beck DE, ed. Handbook of Colorectal Surgery. St. Loius: Quality Medical Publishing, 1997:299–311.
61. Kuo RJ. Epidural morhpine for post-hemorrhoidectomy pain analgesia. Dis Colon Rectum 1984; 27:529–530.
62. Vinson-Bonnet B, Coltat JC, Fingerhut A, et al. Local infiltration with ropivicaine improves immediate postoperative pain control after hemorrhoidal surgery. Dis Colon Rectum 2002; 45:104–108.
63. Chester JF, Stanford BJ, Gazet JC. Analgesic benefit of locally injected bupivicaine after hemorrhoidectomy. Dis Colon Rectum 1990; 33:487–489.
64. Pryn SJ, Crosse MM, Murison MS, McGinn FP. Postoperative analgesia for hemorrhoidectomy. Anaesthesia 1989; 44:964–966.
65. O'Donovan S, Ferrara A, Larach S, Williamson P. Intraoperative use of Toradol facilitates outpatient hemorrhoidectomy. Dis Colon Rectum 1994; 37:793–799.
66. Richman IM. Use of Toradol in anorectal surgery. Dis Colon Rectum 1993; 36:295–296.
67. Kilbride M, Morse M, Senagore A. Transdermal fentanyl improves management of postoperative hemorrhoidectomy pain. Dis Colon Rectum 1994; 37:1070–1072.
68. Wasvary HJ, Hain J, Mosed-Vogel M, et al. Randomized, prospective, double-blind, placebo-controlled trial of effect of nitroglycerin ointment on pain after hemorrhoidectomy. Dis Colon Rectum 2001; 44:1069–1073.
69. Coskun A, Duzgun SA, Uzunkoy A, et al. Nitroderm TTS band application for pain after hemorrhoidectomy. Dis Colon Rectum 2001; 44:680–685.
70. Davies J, Duffy D, Boyt N, et al. Botulinum toxin (botox) reduced pain after hemorrhoidectomy: results of a double-blind, randomized study. Dis Colon Rectum 2003; 46:1097–1102.
71. Bleday R, Pena JP, Rothenberger DA, et al. Symptomatic hemorrhoids: current incidence and complications of operative therapy. Dis Colon Rectum 1992; 35:477–481.
72. Bailey HR, Ferguson JA. Prevention of urinary retention by fluid restriction following anorectal oprations. Dis Colon Rectum 1976; 19:250–252.
73. Hoff SD, Bailey HR, Butts DR, et al. Ambulatory surgical hemorrhoidectomy—a solution to postoperative urinary retention? Dis Colon Rectum 1994; 37:1242–1244.
74. Gottesman L, Milsom JW, Mazier WP. The use of anxiolytic and parasympathomimetic agents in the treatment of postoperative urinary retention following anorectal surgery. Dis Colon Rectum 1989; 32:867–870.
75. Caraldo PA, Senagore AJ. Does alpha sympathetic blockade prevent urinary retention following anorectal surgery? Dis Colon Rectum 1991; 34:1113–1116.

76. Nyam DC, Seow-Choen F, Yo YH. Submucosal adrenaline injection for posthemorrhoidectomy hemorrhage. Dis Colon Rectum 1995; 38:776–777.
77. Rosen L, Sipe P, Stasik JJ, et al. Outcome of delayed hemorrhage following surgical hemorrhoidectomy. Dis Colon Rectum 1993; 36:743–746.
78. Johnson CD, Budd J, Ward AJ. Laxatives after hemorrhoidectomy. Dis Colon Rectum 1987; 30:780–781.
79. Corman ML. Management of postoperative constipation in anorectal surgery. Dis Colon Rectum 1979; 22:149–151.
80. Molloy RG, Kingsmore D. Life threatening pelvic sepsis after stapled hemorrhoidectomy. Lancet 2000; 355:810.
81. Maw A, Eu KW, Seow-Choen F. Retroperitoneal sepsis complicating stapled hemorrhoidectomy: report of a case and review of the literature. Dis Colon Rectum 2002; 45:826–828.
82. Ripetti V, Caricato M, Arullani A. Rectal perforation, retropneumoperitoneum, and pneumomediastinum after stapling procedure for prolapsed hemorrhoids: report of a case and subsequent considerations. Dis Colon Rectum 2002; 45:268–270.
83. Ravo B, Amato A, Bianco V, et al. Complications after stapled hemorrhoidectomy: can they be prevented? Tech Coloproctol 2002; 6:83–88.
84. Pescatori M. Management of post-anopexy rectal stricture. Tech Coloproctol 2002; 6:125–126.
85. Oughriss M, Yver R, Faucheron JL. Complications of stapled hemorrhoidectomy: a French multicentric study. Gastro Clin Bio 2005; 29:429–433.
86. Beck DE. Hemorrhoids. In: Beck DE, Wexner SD, eds. Fundamentals of Anorectal Surgery. 2nd ed. Philadelphia: W.B. Saunders, 1998:237–253.

8 Anal Fissure

Miguel del Mazo and Laurence R. Sands
University of Miami Medical Center, Miami, Florida, U.S.A.

INTRODUCTION

By definition, an anal fissure is a linear tear, usually painful, in the anoderm. Acute anal fissures are generally limited to the mucosa, while chronic anal fissures may extend into the submucosa and expose the internal anal sphincter (IAS). Chronic anal fissures may develop into anal ulcers and are usually associated with a sentinel pile, or skin tag. The majority of anal fissures occur in the posterior midline in both sexes (approximately 85%–90%), although anterior-based fissures occur more commonly in females (1).

PHYSIOLOGY

Anal fissures are the result of high-pressure dilation of the anal canal and are usually associated with severe constipation, the passage of a large hard stool, or repeated episodes of diarrhea. This dilation causes a physical tear in the anoderm that exposes the IAS. The exposed IAS spasms in response, causing pain, an increase in the resting tone of the IAS, decreased perfusion of the anoderm, and further tearing with an inability to adequately heal. It is suggested by anatomical cadaver data that a relative paucity of end arterioles in the posterior midline is responsible for this location having an increased association with anal fissure, suggesting an ischemic etiology of this entity (2). Repeated difficulties with evacuation can exacerbate this problem and result in poorly healing tissue and a chronic anal fissure.

CLINICAL HISTORY

The clinical history is the cornerstone of accurate diagnosis of anal fissures. Patients presenting with an acute anal fissure will complain of a tearing pain upon defecation associated with spots of fresh red blood. Patients often do not describe rectal hemorrhage or melena with their bowel movements. These presentations are associated with other potentially more serious problems. The anal pain may last for hours, but is most intense upon defecation. Some patients will develop avoidance behaviors leading to constipation, more forceful bowel movements, and a worsening of the cycle causing the anal fissure. Acute anal fissures are typically a self-resolving process when treated with conservative medical regimens. When the fissure remains persistent, an associated sentinel pile develops indicating signs of chronicity.

DIAGNOSIS

The physical examination will confirm the diagnosis that is often suspected after an accurate history is obtained. Upon retraction of the buttocks, a midline tear in the anoderm distal to the dentate line should be notable. Chronic anal fissures develop ulcers with raised edges and allow for visualization of the IAS. As mentioned earlier, most fissures are found in the posterior midline, while far fewer are found in the anterior midline. Fissures off the midline are concerning for an alternate process including malignancy, infection, or inflammatory bowel disease. Many patients will not tolerate complete digital rectal exam, anoscopy, or sigmoidoscopy, but limited anorectal examination is necessary to confirm the IAS spasm characteristic of anal fissures. Upon resolution of the patient's anal fissure and symptoms, the diligent practitioner is obligated to complete the full physical examination in order to fully assess for alternate pathologies. This may require examination under anesthesia in some cases.

Laboratory and imaging studies play no role in the diagnosis of anal fissure, although they may be of use when concomitant colorectal disease is present.

ALTERNATIVE PATHOLOGIES

There are many other alternative diagnoses that may mimic anal fissure. Some of these include perianal Crohn's disease, mucosal ulcerative colitis, anal cancer, human immunodeficiency virus with associated perianal sepsis and anal ulcerations, tuberculosis, syphilis, and myeloproliferative disorders including leukemia. Fissures may be present as a result of these other conditions and are often referred to as secondary fissures. For example, syphilitic chancre may resemble an anal fissure. These lesions however, are often painless and may be associated with inguinal lymphadenopathy. A sample of the discharge of these atypical lesions should reveal spirochetes on dark field microscopy. These patients may have concomitant anal condyloma at the time of diagnosis, possibly suggesting the alternative diagnosis. If suspected, antibiotic therapy should be instituted to treat perianal syphilis.

Anal malignancy usually presents with a deep-seated pain with an associated mass that has been present for some length of time. If malignancy is suspected, a biopsy is usually confirmatory; this may be performed in the office setting. The most common tumors seen in this region are epidermoid cancers.

Fissures may also be associated with pruritus ani. These fissures are often multiple and are typically a result of the trauma produced by constant perianal scratching. They typically occur at the anal margin rather than the anal canal where primary anal fissure is typically seen.

TREATMENT

Once the history and physical examination have established the diagnosis of primary anal fissure, the patient is initially treated with conservative medical and local therapy and given a follow-up appointment in four to six weeks. If there are any concerning signs on the initial examination, or if the history is not consistent with anal fissure, the practitioner should consider a biopsy of the fissure base at the time of the initial evaluation in order to rule out malignancy or leukemic infiltrates. The follow-up appointment is given to the patient to ensure adequate treatment of the fissure.

Conservative Treatment

Therapy is aimed at disrupting the cycle of recurrent pain, spasm, tearing, and poor wound healing that allows the fissure to persist. Conservative medical measures are usually first-line therapy (3). In order to reduce the trauma associated with hard stools, bulking agents or stool softeners are used. Warm sitz baths may help to relax the IAS and reduce the spasm associated with anal fissures, as well as provide a medium to allow anal vasodilatation with hopes of increasing the blood flow to the fissure base and allow healing of the fissure. Conservative therapy is often successful for acute anal fissure. However, success will diminish significantly once the fissure shows signs of chronicity.

OTHER MEDICAL THERAPY

Other types of medical therapy include anal nitroglycerin preparations, topical diltiazem ointment, and botulinum toxin injections. Nitrogen donors such as 0.2% nitroglycerin ointment or 0.2% to 0.8% glyceryl trinitrate cream may be used locally to allow anal vasodilatation to improve anal blood flow and reduce anal ischemia. However, this therapy has been associated with severe headaches and may be poorly tolerated. A recent study of 34 patients comparing 0.2% glyceryl trinitrate suppositories with placebo in a double-blind fashion revealed a statistically significant healing rate of 57% in the glyceryl trinitrate group compared to 38% in the placebo group (4). One of the more comprehensive reviews on the use of anal nitroglycerin was a double-blind multicenter prospectively randomized trial that compared placebo 0.1%, 0.2%, and 0.4% in both twice daily and three times daily dosing regimens. While all the groups reported healing rates of 50% including the placebo group, there was a 21% reduction in average pain associated with the 0.4% nitroglycerin group. Headaches were again the primary adverse event in the anal nitroglycerin groups and were noted to be dose related (5). There is currently no FDA-approved nitroglycerin ointment preparation available in the United States, and those receiving these ointments need to have them compounded by various pharmacies. The recommended dosing is a 0.4% nitroglycerin ointment to be administered twice daily.

The calcium-channel blockers, diltiazem and nifedipine, have been used topically to relax the IAS in hopes of healing and relieving the pain associated with anal fissure (6). In addition, oral diltiazem has been used and compared to the topical formulations. The topical ointments have shown greater efficacy in terms of healing with fewer side effects than a 60 mg dose of oral diltiazem (7). A study from India comparing 90 patients divided into groups receiving either 0.2% glyceryl trinitrate or 2% topical diltiazem ointment revealed superior results in terms of pain relief, late recurrence, and fewer side effects in the group receiving the diltiazem ointment (8). A meta-analysis comparing the topical glyceryl trinitrate with topical diltiazem ointment reviewed five studies, only two of which were control randomized studies and thus included in the meta-analysis. These 103 patients, 50 of whom received the glyceryl trinitrate, revealed that the two therapies were equally effective in terms of the recurrence and healing rates of the fissure. However, the glyceryl trinitrate was associated with greater side effects and a higher rate of headaches. This review concluded that topical diltiazem was preferred over the glyceryl trinitrate (9).

Alternatively, botulinum toxin injection has long been used to treat anal fissure (10). The mechanism of action is such that the toxin interferes with the release of acetylcholine from presynaptic nerve terminals resulting in a temporary paralysis of the IAS muscles. The muscle returns to function within several months, but this period of improved perfusion, decreased spasm, and less frequent tearing is often sufficient to allow healing. (11,12). A meta-analysis of four prospective randomized trials including 279 patients with chronic anal fissure compared results of chemical sphincterotomy with botox with surgical sphincterotomy. This analysis revealed both a higher complication and transient fecal incontinence rate associated with surgical sphincterotomy. However, it also showed a lower incidence of recurrence and a higher healing rate in the surgical sphincterotomy group. They concluded that as long as the patient is willing to cope with the transient incontinence associated with surgery, the patient is better served with surgical therapy (13). Although not a common side effect of botox injections, a case of Fournier's gangrene has recently been reported in a 77-year-old diabetic male who received botulinum toxin injection for anal fissure (14).

SURGICAL INTERVENTION

Lateral Internal Sphincterotomy

Patients with anal fissures who fail conservative medical therapies mentioned above would alternatively require surgical correction. Lateral internal anal sphincterotomy (LIS) is the most common surgical procedure for the treatment of anal fissure. It may be performed either through an open incision or via a closed technique in the outpatient setting. While some surgeons have performed this procedure in the office setting, the majority will do this under local anesthesia with some intravenous conscious sedation or under regional anesthesia with the patient in either the prone jackknife or lithotomy position. The goal is to divide a portion of the IAS in order to disrupt the spasms responsible for the pain related to the fissure, and possibly allow greater blood flow to the anal canal and thereby heal the fissure.

The open procedure is performed using a lateral circumferential perianal incision and then developing both the intersphincteric and submucosal planes. The IAS muscle is then identified and cut up to the level of the dentate line. Concomitant fissurectomy is often performed in order to cleanse the base of the fissure and promote healthy tissue for healing. A closed sphincterotomy accomplishes the same goal but without the direct visualization of the muscle fibers that are being cut. Comparison between the two techniques has not shown any significant differences in incontinence rates or in postoperative pain (15). Studies have been performed assessing the exact length of IAS muscle that should be cut during this procedure. A recent publication suggests that a controlled sphincterotomy cutting a little less muscle is associated with quicker pain relief, a lower incidence of fecal incontinence, and a negligible difference in healing of the fissure (16).

Complications from lateral internal sphincterotomy are rare but do include bleeding, delayed wound healing, urinary retention, pain, abscess, and fistula formation. More disturbingly, various studies have reported incontinence rates to flatus that are as high as 30% that may be persistent (17). Surgical therapy, however, is often associated with quicker time to symptomatic relief, faster rates of healing, and lower rates of recurrence and is successful in greater than 95% of patients (18). Other surgical options include anal dilation and flap advancement.

Failed sphincterotomy and fissure recurrence should be investigated by ruling out other anorectal conditions initially. It is important to exclude malignancy, infectious etiologies, or inflammatory bowel disease. Once these entities have been eliminated, the patient is generally studied with an anal ultrasound to assess adequacy of the previous internal sphincterotomy and anal manometry to assess the resting and squeeze pressures of the anal canal. If the ultrasound reveals an inadequate internal sphincterotomy with normal to high resting pressure within the anal canal, it is recommended that the patient undergo repeat internal sphincterotomy on the opposite side. If, however, the ultrasound demonstrates the previous internal sphincterotomy to be adequate and the resting pressures are already low within the anal canal, then one should consider some of the medical therapies described above or surgical flap advancement for fissure coverage in order not to cut additional anal sphincter muscle and risk incontinence.

Anal Dilatation

Anal dilation has been described for years but has concerned most surgeons due to the unpredictable nature of sphincter damage and associated fecal incontinence. This dilation has been described using either manual finger dilation or a pneumatic balloon technique (19). A prospective randomized study of 108 patients comparing sphincterotomy to anal dilation revealed higher rates of incontinence and recurrence in patients undergoing anal dilation. Therefore, these authors suggested that lateral internal sphincterotomy remains the surgical procedure of choice for chronic anal fissure (20).

Advancement Flap

In patients suffering from anal fissure with low resting pressure and some degree of incontinence, an advancement flap may be considered. This procedure will completely spare the muscle and therefore will not alter fecal control. In a series of 21 patients with chronic anal fissure who failed medical therapy and were treated by rotational advancement flap technique, 17 patients had complete resolution of their symptoms (21).

SUMMARY

The options available today for anal fissure are quite varied. In addition, there have been many publications on the various techniques. The internet has also allowed patients to become better informed regarding their medical conditions and treatment options. Patients now present to the physician's office fearful of what they have read regarding incontinence associated with sphincterotomy. While the patient needs to be well informed, it is also the physician's responsibility to provide proper counseling as to the best treatment options for the patient. When conservative options have been exhausted, surgical options need to be considered. Lateral internal sphincterotomy continues to be the procedure of choice for chronic anal fissure and may be performed with excellent overall results.

REFERENCES

1. Steele SR, Madoff RD. Systematic review: The treatment of anal fissure aliment. Pharmacol Ther 2006; 24(2):247–257.
2. Klosterhalfen B, Vogel P, Rixen H, et al. Topography of the inferior rectal artery: A possible cause of chronic, primary anal fissure. Dis Colon Rectum 1989; 32:43–52.

3. Sileri P, Mele A, Stolfi VM, et al. Medical and surgical treatment of chronic anal fissures: a prospective study. J Gastrointest Surg 2007; 11(11):1541–1548.
4. Emami MH, Sayedyahossein S, Aslani A. Safety and efficacy of new glyceryl trinitrate suppository formula: First double blind placebo-controlled clinical trial. Dis Colon Rectum May 2008(epub ahead of print).
5. Bailey HR, Beck DE, Billingham RP, et al. Fissure Study Group. A study to determine the nitroglycerin ointment dose and dosing interval that best promote the healing of chronic anal fissures. Dis Colon Rectum 2002; 45(9):1192–1199.
6. Griffen H. The role of topical diltiazen in the treatment of chronic anal fissures that have failed glyceryl trinitrate therapy. Colorectal Dis 2002; 4(6):430–435.
7. Jonas M, Neal KR, Abercrombie JF, et al. A randomized trial of oral vs. topical diltiazem for chronic anal fissures. Dis Colon Rectum 2001; 44(8):1074–1078
8. Shrivastava UK, Jain BK, Kumar P, et al. A comparison of the effects of diltiazem and glyceryl trinitrate ointment in the treatment of chronic anal fissure: A randomized clinical trial. Surg Today 2007; 37(6):482–485.
9. Sajid MS, Rimple J, Cheek E, et al. The efficacy of diltiazem and glyceryltrinitrate for the medical management of chronic anal fissure: A meta-analysis. Int J Colorectal Dis 2008; 23(1):1–6.
10. Lysy J, Israeli E, Levy S, et al. Long-term results of 'chemical sphincterotomy' for chronic anal fissure: A prosepective study. Dis Colon Rectum 2006; 459(6):858–864.
11. Collison RJ, Mortensen NJ. Is botulinum toxin injection a better treatment than nitroglycerin ointment for patients with chronic anal fissure? Nat Clin Pract Gastroenterol Hepatol. 2007; 4(11):598–599.
12. Collins EE, Lund JN. A review of chronic anal fissure management techniques. Coloproctol 2007; 11(3):209–223.
13. Sajid MS, Hunte S, Hippolyte S, et al. Comparison of surgical vs. chemical sphincterotomy using botulinum toxin for the treatment of chronic anal fissure: A meta-analysis. Colorectal Dis 2007 (epub ahead of print).
14. Mallo-González N, López-Rodríguez R, Fentes DP, et al. Fournier's gangrene following botulinum toxin injection. Scand J Urol Nephrol 2008; 42(3):301–303.
15. Wiley M, Day P, Rieger N, et al. Open vs. closed lateral internal sphincterotomy for idiopathic fissure-in-ano: A prospective, randomized, controlled trial. Dis Colon Rectum 2004; 47(6):847–852.
16. Menteş BB, Güner MK, Leventoglu S, et al. Fine-tuning of the extent of lateral internal sphincterotomy: Spasm-controlled vs. up to the fissure apex. Dis Colon Rectum 2008; 51(1):128–133.
17. Casillas S, Hull TL, Zutshi M, et al. Incontinence after a lateral internal sphincterotomy: Are we underestimating it? Dis Colon Rectum 2005; 48(6):1193–1199.
18. Sileri P, Mele A, Stolfi VM, et al. Medical and surgical treatment of chronic anal fissure: A prospective study. J Gastrointest Surg 2007; 11(11):1541–1548.
19. Renzi A, Izzo D, Di Sarno G, et al. Clinical, manometric, and ultrasonographic results of pneumatic balloon dilatation vs. lateral internal sphincterotomy for chronic anal fissure: A prospective, randomized, controlled trial. Dis Colon Rectum 2008; 51(1):121–127.
20. Ram E, Vishne T, Lerner I, et al. Anal dilatation versus left lateral sphincterotomy for chronic anal fissure: A prospective randomized study. Tech Coloproctol 2007 (epub ahead of print).
21. Singh M, Sharma A, Gardiner A, et al. Early results of a rotational flap to treat chronic anal fissures. Int J Colorectal Dis 2005; 20(4):339–342.

9 Fecal Incontinence: Evaluation

Jaime L. Bohl and Roberta L. Muldoon

Department of Surgery, Colon and Rectal Surgery Program, Vanderbilt University, Nashville, Tennessee, U.S.A.

INTRODUCTION

Anal incontinence is the involuntary loss of solid or liquid feces or flatus from the anal canal. The individual with anal incontinence suffers a heavy physical and psychological burden. Since patients with anal incontinence do not spontaneously report symptoms to medical providers (1), the impact on society as a whole is difficult to measure. Surveys of different populations measure a wide range of prevalence. In a community-based population, solid and liquid fecal incontinence ranges from 0.8% in men 15 to 60 years of age to 6.2% in women >60 years (2). While anal incontinence clearly increases with age, gender has not been found to significantly increase risk (2).

Fecal continence is dependent on the integrated function of multiple organ systems. The gastrointestinal system determines fecal consistency and allows for fecal storage. An intact neuromuscular system is necessary for anorectal sensation, rectal compliance, and anal sphincter function. Finally, the patient must have the cognitive capacity to voluntarily control defecation and the physical ability to locate a toilet. Breakdown in any one component can lead to symptoms of incontinence with increased symptom severity if several determinants of continence are impaired.

Evaluation of a patient with symptoms of fecal incontinence can involve multiple diagnostic techniques. To make optimal use of each diagnostic modality, the examiner should have a thorough understanding of the risk factors and etiology of fecal incontinence (Table 1). The assessment should start with a detailed history. A physical examination should be performed with emphasis on the anorectal examination. Based on findings from the history and physical examination, a preliminary diagnosis and etiology can be determined and treatment initiated. If the patient does not respond to conservative measures and alternative treatments are being considered, then the patient should undergo additional imaging and neuromuscular testing. Imaging techniques may include endoanal ultrasound (EAUS), magnetic resonance imaging (MRI), and defecography. Neuromuscular testing can involve anorectal manometry, anorectal sensory and compliance testing, external anal sphincter electromyography (EMG), and pudendal nerve terminal motor latency (PNTML) testing. The majority of patients with symptoms of fecal incontinence can be managed initially in the ambulatory setting with conservative treatment. If the patient fails to respond to conservative measures, then referral for additional diagnostic testing may be necessary. Diagnostic testing may require referral to specialty facilities for equipment and expertise in test administration and interpretation.

HISTORY

History taking should begin with characterization of the patient's incontinence. The type (gas, liquid, mucus, or solid), frequency, and severity (volume) of incontinence should be assessed. The patient's incontinence can also be characterized as passive (without the patient's knowledge), urge (with patient's awareness but lack of control to defer defecation), stress (with coughing or straining), or post defecatory (loss of stool immediately after defecation with no loss at other times). These types of incontinence have been shown to correlate with specific sphincter defects. For example, passive incontinence is related to internal anal sphincter defects while urge incontinence is related to external anal sphincter defects (3,4). Patients should be asked about their pad usage. The number of pads may help to clarify the volume and frequency of the patient's incontinence. Associated bowel symptoms and habits should be elicited. The patient should be asked about frequency of defecation, stool consistency, and if there is

Table 1 Causes of Fecal Incontinence

Anatomic	
	Prior anorectal surgery
	Obstetric injury
	Trauma (pelvic fractures)
	Rectal prolapse
Neurologic	
	Diabetes mellitus
	Multiple sclerosis
	Spinal cord trauma
	Cerebrovascular disorders
	Neoplasms
Gastrointestinal	
	Inflammatory bowel disease
	Diarrheal illnesses
	Malabsorption
	Radiation enteritis/proctitis
	Fecal impaction/overflow incontinence

associated straining with bowel movements. Symptoms of bloating, cramping, or abdominal pain may suggest inflammatory bowel disease or irritable bowel syndrome. The patient's use of laxatives or bulking agents should be obtained. This detailed assessment of the patient's symptoms further defines the severity and quality of a patient's incontinence as well as associated symptoms.

Patient diaries and questionnaires have been developed to help standardize the evaluation of anal incontinence. Use of patient diaries has been advocated to remove recall bias from a patient's history. Diary completion requires the patient to record in real-time instances of bowel movement, any associated straining, incomplete emptying, leakage, type of leakage, change in pads or underclothes, and use of laxatives. In addition to diaries, self-administered questionnaires have been developed to standardize the measurement of incontinence. Type and frequency of incontinence are assigned a numeric score which indicates severity of incontinence. Numeric scoring of incontinence symptoms allows clinicians to measure changes in a patient's symptoms and make comparisons among patients (5). The three scales used most commonly in research are the Cleveland Clinic Florida Fecal Incontinence (CCF-FI) scale (Table 2) (6); a modified version of the CCF-FI scale, the Vaizey scale (Table 3) (7); and the Fecal Incontinence Severity Index (FISI) (Table 4) (8). All three questionnaires assess type of incontinence (gas, mucus, liquid, or stool). For severity, the CCF-FI scale and Vaizey scale assign equal weight to gas, liquid, or solid fecal incontinence. Both scales also include an impact measure on patient activities or change in lifestyle (frequency of pad use, ability to defer defecation, and use of constipating medicines). In a small trial, these two scales were tested against others for reliability, correlation with clinical impression, and response to clinical intervention (7). On all three measures, the Vaizey scale scored the highest followed by the CCF-FI scale. In comparison, the FISI assigns subjective severity values to different types and frequency of incontinence. These values were assigned by both surgeons and patients and were comparable in most cases (5,8). In

Table 2 CCF-FI Grading Scale

	Frequency				
Type of incontinence	**Never**	**Rarely**	**Sometimes**	**Usually**	**Always**
Solid	0	1	2	3	4
Liquid	0	1	2	3	4
Gas	0	1	2	3	4
Wears pad	0	1	2	3	4
Lifestyle alteration	0	1	2	3	4

Total Score: 0 = Perfect continence; 20 = Complete incontinence.
Individual Item Score: Never = 0; Rarely = <1×/month; Sometimes = <1×/week, ≥1×/month; Usually = <1×/day, ≥1×/week; Always = ≥1×/day.
Source: From Ref. 6.

Table 3 Vaizey Scale

	Frequency				
Type of incontinence	**Never**	**Rarely**	**Sometimes**	**Weekly**	**Daily**
Solid	0	1	2	3	4
Liquid	0	1	2	3	4
Gas	0	1	2	3	4
Lifestyle alteration	0	1	2	3	4
				No	Yes
Need to wear a pad or plug				0	2
Taking constipating medications				0	2
Lack of ability to defer defecation for 15 min				0	4

Total Score: 0 = Perfect continence; 24 = Totally incontinent.
Individual Item Score: Never = no episodes in past 4 wk; Rarely = one episode in past 4 wk; Sometimes >1 episode in past 4 wk but <1 a week; Weekly = 1 or more episodes a week but <1 a day; Daily = 1 or more episodes a day.
Source: From Ref. 7.

this scale, there are four types of incontinence and five different frequencies (one to three times per month to two times per day). The overall possible score ranges from 0 to 61 with higher scores reflecting more severe incontinence. The inclusion of patient assigned severity scales increases the utility of the FISI. More research is needed to better assess how to incorporate the surgeon's and patient's perspective on severity. Additional tools are also needed to measure changes in score after treatment intervention. In summary, diaries may help reduce recall bias and questionnaires help standardize incontinence scores across multiple time points for each patient and among patients.

In order to obtain a complete patient history, additional medical, surgical, and medication history should be obtained after characterizing the type and frequency of incontinence. The examiner should focus on possible risk factors in each individual. In females, obstetrical trauma is the most recognized risk factor. Risk factors for sphincter injury during vaginal delivery include forceps delivery, episiotomy, parity, and advanced perineal tears (9). In males, a history of anorectal surgery as a cause of incontinence is more common than in females. In patients with incontinence after anorectal surgery, the internal anal sphincter is injured in a pattern specific to the original procedure while one-third of patients sustain injuries to their external anal sphincter (10). In older adults, risk factors include urinary incontinence, neurologic disease, poor mobility, cognitive decline, and advanced age (>70 years) (11). Patients should be questioned about earlier traumatic injuries, sexual history, earlier abdominal or perineal operations, and radiation treatments. Other medical conditions associated with incontinence include diabetes, cerebrovascular accidents, multiple sclerosis, Parkinson's disease, connective tissue disorders, and systemic infections (6). Finally, a review of all the patient's medications may reveal a pharmacologic cause of the patient's incontinence. Overall, incontinence is a symptom with many causes. A detailed history is necessary to completely evaluate the possible causes of an individual patient's incontinence.

Anal incontinence should also be characterized by its impact on the patient's quality of life. Indeed, the severity of fecal incontinence can be falsely underestimated if the patient has severely restricted social and physical activities in order to stay near the commode. Several scales have been used to assess impact of anal incontinence on patient well-being. The most widely used quality-of-life scale, which is not specific to incontinence, is the Short Form 36. This quality-of-life measure has been used in patients with anal incontinence but does not discriminate between patients with mild, moderate, or severe incontinence (12). A more specific scale, the Fecal Incontinence Quality of Life Scale (FIQL), measures changes in quality of life with regard to incontinence symptoms (Table 5). FIQL is a 29-item questionnaire with four subscales including lifestyle, coping/behavior, depression/self-perception, and embarrassment (13). Although the FIQL has reliability and validity, it has not been tested for responsiveness to change with treatment intervention. Other quality-of-life scales are available [Manchester Health Questionnaire (14) and Gastrointestinal Quality of Life Index] (15) and have been used in incontinent patients but are less specific and not as widely used. Most importantly, some assessment of the impact on quality of life should be made as symptom severity and effect on lifestyle are two different but very important measures.

Table 4 Fecal Incontinence Severity Index

For each of the following, please indicate on average *how often in the past month* you experienced any amount of accidental bowel leakage:	2 or more times a day		Once a day		2 or more times a week		Once a week		1 to 3 times a month		Never	
	Patient	**Surgeon**	**Patient**	**Surgeon**	**Patient**	**Surgeon**	**Patient**	**Surgeon**	**Patient**	**Surgeon**	**Patient**	**Surgeon**
Gas	12	9	11	8	8	6	6	4	4	2	0	0
Mucus	12	11	10	9	7	7	5	7	3	5	0	0
Liquid stool	19	18	17	16	13	14	10	13	8	10	0	0
Solid stool	18	19	16	17	13	16	10	14	8	11	0	0

For calculation of FISI scores, a higher score indicates greater severity. For individual items, patients and surgeons have coded a severity of that event from 1 to 20, with 1 = least severe condition and 20 = most severe condition.

Total score is the sum of responses to each line item.

Source: From Ref. 8.

Table 5 Fecal Incontinence Quality of Life Scale

Q1: In general, would you say your health is:

1. Excellent
2. Very good
3. Good
4. Fair
5. Poor

Q2: For each of the items, please indicate how much of the time the issue is a concern for you *due to accidental bowel leakage*.
!(If it is a concern for you for reasons other than accidental bowel leakage, then check the box under Not Apply, N/A).

Q2. Due to accidental bowel leakage:	Most of the time	Some of the time	A little of the time	None of the time	N/A
a. I am afraid to go out	1	2	3	4	[]
b. I avoid visiting friends	1	2	3	4	[]
c. I avoid staying overnight away from home	1	2	3	4	[]
d. It is difficult for me to get out and do things like going to a movie or to church	1	2	3	4	[]
e. I cut down on how much I eat before I go out	1	2	3	4	[]
f. Whenever I am away from home, I try to stay near a restroom as much as possible	1	2	3	4	[]
g. It is important to plan my schedule (daily activities) around my bowel pattern	1	2	3	4	[]
h. I avoid traveling	1	2	3	4	[]
i. I worry about not being able to get to the toilet in time	1	2	3	4	[]
j. I feel I have no control over my bowels	1	2	3	4	[]
k. I can't hold my bowel movement long enough to get to the bathroom	1	2	3	4	[]
l. I leak stool without even knowing it	1	2	3	4	[]
m. I try to prevent bowel accidents by staying very near a bathroom	1	2	3	4	[]

Q3: Due to accidental bowel leakage, indicate the extent to which you AGREE or DISAGREE with each of the following items. (If it is a concern for you for reasons other than accidental bowel leakage, then check the box under Not Apply, N/A).

Q3. Due to accidental bowel leakage:	Strongly agree	Somewhat agree	Somewhat disagree	Strongly disagree	N/A
a. I feel ashamed	1	2	3	4	[]
b. I cannot do many of things I want to do	1	2	3	4	[]
c. I worry about bowel accidents	1	2	3	4	[]
d. I feel depressed	1	2	3	4	[]
e. I worry about others smelling stool on me	1	2	3	4	[]
f. I feel like I am not a healthy person	1	2	3	4	[]
g. I enjoy life less	1	2	3	4	[]
h. I have sex less often than I would like to	1	2	3	4	[]
i. I feel different from other people	1	2	3	4	[]
j. The possibility of bowel accidents is always on my mind	1	2	3	4	[]
k. I am afraid to have sex	1	2	3	4	[]
l. I avoid traveling by plane or train	1	2	3	4	[]
m. I avoid going out to eat	1	2	3	4	[]
n. Whenever I go someplace new, I specifically locate where the bathrooms are	1	2	3	4	[]

(*continued*)

Table 5 Fecal Incontinence Quality of Life Scale (*Continued*)

Q4: During the past month, have you felt so sad, discouraged, hopeless, or had so many problems that you wondered if anything was worthwhile?

1. Extremely so—to the point that I have just about given up
2. Very much so
3. Quite a bit
4. Some—enough to bother me
5. A little bit
6. Not at all

Fecal Incontinence Quality of Life Scoring.
Scales range from 1 to 5, with 1 indicating a lower functional status of quality of life.
Scale scores are the average (mean) response to all items in the scale. (e. g., add the responses to all questions in a scale together and then divide by the number of items in the scale. Not Apply is coded as a missing value in the analysis for all questions.)
Scale 1. Lifestyle, 10 items: Q2a, Q2b, Q2 c, Q2 d, Q2e, Q2 g, Q2h, Q3b, Q31, and Q3m.
Scale 2. Coping/Behavior, 9 items: Q2f, Q2i, Q2j, Q2k, Q2 m, Q3d, Q3h, Q3j, and Q3n.
Scale 3. Depression/Self Perception, 7 items: Q1, Q3d, Q3f, Q3g, Q3i, Q3k, and Q4, (Question 1 is reverse coded.)
Scale 4. Embarrassment, 3 items: Q21, Q3a, and Q3e.
Source: From Ref. 13.

PHYSICAL EXAMINATION

A complete physical examination is necessary in the incontinent patient. This allows for the diagnosis of comorbid conditions, which contribute to or cause incontinence, and other conditions or symptoms which can be mistaken for incontinence. Once complete, emphasis should be placed on the anorectal examination, which is ideally performed in the prone jackknife position, although the left lateral position can be used in debilitated and pregnant patients. This begins with inspection for perineal soiling, excoriation, or scarring. The presence of other anorectal pathology should be documented (hemorrhoids, fistula, fissure, skin tags, condyloma, or ulceration). The examiner should note the degree of anal closure as a patulous or gaping anal orifice has been associated with rectal prolapse, sphincter defects, and neurologic disorders. A thinned or deformed perineal body may indicate neurologic deficits or obstetrical trauma. A keyhole deformity in the posterior midline is suggestive of earlier fissure surgery. After inspection, the examiner should ask the patient to perform a Valsalva maneuver to observe perineal descent. Ballooning of the perineum with straining suggests descending perineum syndrome or pelvic floor denervation. In addition, straining will reproduce mucosal or complete rectal prolapse when present. Finally, the examiner can assess anal wink or the reflex of the perineal skin to pin prick. Absence of external sphincter contraction to this stimulation suggests a neuropathic etiology. Next, the examiner should perform a digital rectal examination. The presence and consistency of stool should be noted. The resting anal tone as well as squeeze pressure should be assessed as these correlate with internal and external sphincter defects, respectively (16,17). The puborectalis can be palpated laterally and posteriorly and should flatten with Valsalva. In male patients, the prostate is palpated. In female patients, a bimanual examination with the thumb in the vagina and forefinger in the rectum is used to palpate a rectocele, cystocele, or enterocele. Additionally, bimanual examination of the anterior perineal body may be suggestive of an obstetrical injury. Finally, scars and masses can be palpated within the anal canal. The size, location, and mobility of the mass should be documented. The physical examination can be complimented with an endoscopic examination. A limited endoscopic examination of the rectum and anal canal is helpful for identifying other causes of incontinence including inflammation (proctitis, colitis, or scarring), neoplasm, fecal impaction, and fistulas. The anorectal examination in a patient with anal incontinence is important for the identification of anatomic causes. If the anorectal examination is suggestive of neurologic or muscular dysfunction, then additional diagnostic studies are warranted.

DIAGNOSTIC TESTING

There are multiple studies in the literature which attempt to assess whether additional diagnostic testing is necessary for patients with anal incontinence who have already undergone a thorough history and physical examination. In one study, 20% of initial diagnoses made after history and physical examination by two colon and rectal surgeons were found to be incorrect after additional diagnostic testing was obtained (18). Correct diagnosis of the etiology of the incontinence obtained from this additional testing resulted in a change in the treatment plan for 16% of patients. In another study, 10% of patients had a change in treatment plan after performance of diagnostic studies (19). Transanal ultrasound was most likely to alter diagnosis and treatment plan while manometry and PNTML results did not change diagnosis or treatment plans, in any patients. Experts agree that additional diagnostic testing is useful for identification of sensory and motor neuropathy as a cause for incontinence, as this is poorly discriminated on history and physical examination (20). They also agree that testing is necessary before surgical intervention. Overall, the need for diagnostic testing should be guided by patient's age, symptom severity, response to conservative therapy, and plans for surgical treatment.

IMAGING

Endoanal Ultrasound

EAUS is a popular office-based procedure that can be used to assess anal canal musculature in patients with fecal incontinence. To perform an EAUS, the patient is placed in the prone jackknife or left lateral position and a rotating endoprobe is introduced into the anal canal. The sphincter muscle is visualized in the proximal, middle, and distal anal canal. The internal anal sphincter appears as a hypoechoic or dark ring while the external anal sphincter appears as a hyperechoic or bright ring which surrounds the internal anal sphincter. Defects in either anatomic sphincter will appear as disruptions of the ring's smooth architecture with mixed echogenicity (21). Sphincter defects are described by their location and the size of the defect. In one study, EAUS was used dynamically to measure puborectalis function and anorectal angle at rest and with maximal voluntary contraction (22). A large anorectal angle at rest or with contraction was associated with incontinence symptoms. EAUS is used to visualize sphincter defects, define the surrounding anatomy, and evaluate the integrated function of anorectal musculature.

EAUS is dependent on technologist experience when used to visualize and diagnose sphincter injuries. In one study, clinicians were able to use EAUS to identify anterior anal sphincter defects with 100% accuracy when a defect was present (23). However, there was a false positive rate of 65% secondary to misidentification of puborectalis thinning in the proximal anterior canal. False positive rates were decreased when real-time ultrasound was used and sphincter defects were located in the distal anal canal. In order to decrease missed sphincter defects, some clinicians have incorporated the use of perineal body measurement (24,25). The perineal body is the distance between the internal anal sphincter and an ultrasonographer's finger on the posterior vaginal wall. It has been shown that a sphincter defect is more likely if the perineal body measurement is <10 mm. In addition, understanding of normal anatomic variants will help avoid misdiagnosis. For instance, defects in the external anal sphincter may be difficult to discriminate from perianal fat. In women, there is a natural gap or asymmetry in the proximal, anterior external anal sphincter, which can be mistaken for a sphincter injury (26,27). Overall, the experienced clinician understands anatomic pitfalls and uses techniques which allow improved visualization making EAUS a highly accurate tool in the identification of sphincter defects in incontinent patients.

Defecography

Defecography is a dynamic fluoroscopic examination that evaluates anatomical and structural abnormalities of the anorectum and pelvic floor during defecation. Dynamic images can reveal changes in anorectal angle, perineal descent, and anal canal length with rest, squeeze, strain, and evacuation. In addition, defecography assesses the adequacy of rectal emptying and is useful for the diagnosis of rectocele, enterocele, anismus, and megarectum. The anorectal angle should change with defecation (28). The anorectal angle during rest, squeeze, and evacuation has been found to be significantly larger in incontinent patients compared to continent patients (29). Overall, tonic activity of the puborectalis is important for continence and widening of the anorectal angle is associated with weakness of the pelvic floor musculature and anal sphincters. Perineal descent is the caudal movement of the pelvic floor during straining (28). Anal canal length and width is also measured with defecography. Efficiency of rectal emptying can also be measured with >90% evacuation considered normal. Images may reveal a structural defect such as a rectocele, cystocele, or megarectum, which can result in incomplete evacuation and future soiling (28). For the evaluation of fecal incontinence, defecography is most useful when obstructed defecation is suspected as a cause of the patient's leakage (30). When mechanical obstruction is not suspected as the cause of fecal incontinence, defecography is generally not recommended as a helpful diagnostic tool.

Magnetic Resonance Imaging

MRI has been recently introduced as a diagnostic alternative to EAUS and traditional defecography in the evaluation of fecal incontinence. Endoanal MRI requires the introduction of an endocoil into the anal canal. For the evaluation of external anal sphincter defects, MRI is thought to offer improved visualization secondary to a large contrast difference between the sphincter muscle and surrounding fat (31). In a prospective multicenter trial, endoanal MRI was compared to EAUS for the detection of external anal sphincter defects in incontinent patients (32). There was no difference in the detection of an external anal sphincter (EAS) defect between these two imaging modalities. Overall, the sensitivity and positive predictive value for the detection of EAS defects was 81% and 89% for endoanal MRI and 90% and 85% for EAUS. The advantage of endoanal MRI may be the identification of external anal sphincter atrophy and thinning. This may have functional significance for incontinent patients undergoing surgical correction with EAS thinning resulting in poorer functional outcome (31). Endoanal MRI may have a slight advantage for the detection and characterization of internal anal sphincter defects. When compared to EAUS, the accuracy for endoanal MRI was 77% versus 68%. Despite the increased potential accuracy of endoanal MRI, it is still expensive, not as widely available, and there is less experience with this modality as compared to EAUS.

Dynamic MRI allows for evaluation of the pelvic floor during defecation. Images of the sphincter and pelvic floor are taken at rest, squeeze, strain, and defecation. In one study, MRI defecography led to changes in the surgical treatment of 67% of incontinent patients (33). However, fluoroscopic defecography was not performed in this study, so it is difficult to ascertain if dynamic MRI offers any advantage over traditional defecography. Overall, the same criticisms of traditional defecography can be made of MRI defecography. Namely, it has limited utility in the evaluation of the incontinent patient since most diagnoses can be made with physical examination or other less expensive, more readily available imaging techniques.

NEUROMUSCULAR FUNCTION

Anorectal Manometry

Anal manometry is the measurement of pressures within the anal canal at rest and with voluntary contraction or squeeze. At rest, anal canal pressure is generated by the internal and external anal sphincter baseline tonicity. When the anal canal is voluntarily contracted, squeeze pressures (the increase in pressure over basal pressure) indicate external anal sphincter function. There are multiple systems for transducing anal pressures including water perfusion catheters, solid-state transducers, or balloon tip catheters. Currently, there is no standardization of equipment or methods of measurement. However, in a comparison of techniques, investigators found that values obtained with different manometric systems are similar enough to allow comparison of values (34). Investigators have attempted to identify a threshold value for resting and squeeze pressures which correlate with symptoms of incontinence. Unfortunately, there is broad overlap between continent and incontinent populations so that accuracy remains low. In one study, a maximum basal pressure above 40 mm Hg and squeeze pressure above >92 mm Hg was 96% accurate in identifying continent patients while values below these thresholds had an 88% accuracy in identifying incontinent patients (35). Resting and squeeze pressures have also been found to vary with age and gender. Therefore a wide degree of variance within a population is expected regardless of continence (36). In addition, severity of incontinence symptoms has not been shown to correlate with manometric pressures or predict postoperative results (19). Despite the poor accuracy of anal manometry for the diagnosis of fecal incontinence, the poor discrimination for cause of incontinence and no predictive value for treatment response, anal manometry continues to be used as a correlate with other diagnostic tests of incontinence. Anal manometry is also recommended for the diagnostic evaluation of fecal incontinence by the American Gastroenterological Association (36).

Rectal and Anal Sensory Testing

Rectal sensation or sensitivity to distention is necessary for voluntary control of defecation. Rectal distention causes tonic inhibition of the internal anal sphincter such that contraction of the external anal sphincter and puborectalis is necessary to maintain continence (i.e., the recto-anal inhibitory reflex). Without such feedback, there is involuntary loss of rectal contents. Measurements of rectal sensation are achieved with balloon distention of the rectum using continuous or phasic inflation. Measurements of the rectal sensory threshold or first detectable sensation, urge to defecate, and maximum tolerable volume can be determined. In patients with neurogenic fecal incontinence, biofeedback may improve the ability to perceive rectal distention with improvement in incontinence symptoms while absent rectal sensation on testing makes response to treatment unlikely (37). Decreased maximal rectal distention before the sensation of pain may be correlated with decreased rectal compliance. Reduced rectal compliance may lead to impaired reservoir function of the rectum with subsequent inability to defer defecation. Impaired reservoir function may be present in patients with urge incontinence secondary to previous rectal surgery or inflammation and fibrosis (38). Further standardization and refinement of rectal sensation measurement techniques along with classification of incontinence patients into subgroups (urge vs. passive) may make these diagnostic tests more clinically applicable.

Sensation within the anal canal allows better discrimination between stimuli compared to the rectum. Anal canal sensation is important for the sampling reflex whereby spontaneous relaxation of the internal anal sphincter allows exposure of the anal canal to rectal contents. Anal sensation is measured with bipolar electrodes inserted into the anal mucosa. The sensory threshold is measured by increasing the current from 1 to 20 mA until sensation is reached. Anal sensation is distinct from rectal sensation with poor correlation between the two values (36). Decreased anal sensation has been measured in patients with multiple anorectal disorders (hemorrhoids, prolapse, constipation, incontinence, and sphincter defects) (39). Although patients with fecal incontinence require a greater stimulus for anal sensation, investigators have found this measure to be of little value in the differentiation of incontinent patients from patients with other anorectal complaints.

Electromyography

EMG of the external anal sphincter and striated pelvic floor muscles can be performed in the evaluation of patient with fecal incontinence. EMG can be performed with concentric or single needle electrodes or surface electrodes. Concentric needle electrodes stimulate a large number of motor units simultaneously. Motor unit potentials with specific amplitude, duration, and shape are measured. Amplitude of the motor potential correlates with the number of motor units discharging. Higher amplitude corresponds to a greater number of motor units. The duration of a motor potential will increase with age and denervation secondary to greater motor potential dispersion. Finally, the shape of motor potential units is typically bi- or triphasic. Myopathic disorders will result in short duration polyphasic potentials while regeneration of denervated muscle leads to long duration polyphasic signals. In contrast, EMG can be performed with a single needle electrode that measures motor potentials of a single motor unit. This allows for the determination of fiber density, which is increasing in repaired, denervated muscle. Finally, EMG can be measured using surface electrodes. This method is more comfortable for the patient but limits the measure to gross motor activity within a larger number of motor units (28). The purpose of these studies is threefold: to map the external sphincter and identify an area of injury, to measure muscle contraction and relaxation, and to determine the integrity of external anal sphincter innervation (36). The role of EMG in the mapping of external anal sphincter defects has been largely replaced by EAUS (40). However, EMG may still be useful for the identification of neuronal injury and regeneration as well as the measurement of muscle contraction and relaxation during biofeedback therapy. In addition, EMG of the external anal sphincter may be predictive of functional outcome in patients who are treated with sacral nerve modulation (41).

Pudendal Nerve Terminal Motor Latency

PNTML measures the integrity of the pudendal nerve by measuring the latency of external anal sphincter motor response to electrical stimulation. Measurements using this technique are highly operator dependent as nerve latency is dependent on proximity of a fingertip-mounted electrode to the pudendal nerve at the ischial spine. Studies have also shown that there is a significant overlap of pudendal nerve latency in patients with functional anorectal disorders (42). In addition, PNTML may be normal in a patient with pudendal neuropathy since only the fastest action potential is measured in PNTML as compared to EMG measurements. Therefore, only bilateral prolongation of PNTML has been shown to correlate with decreased resting and squeeze pressures on manometry and clinical severity of incontinence (43). Due to the poor sensitivity and specificity of PNTML, it adds little additional diagnostic information.

CONCLUSIONS

Fecal incontinence is a symptom with many causes. For the evaluation of fecal incontinence, the clinician should take a thorough history and perform a complete physical examination. History taking should focus on known risk factors for fecal incontinence. The physical examination should focus on the anorectal examination and seek to rule out anatomic or functional causes for incontinence. With an initial diagnosis of the cause of incontinence, the clinician can then institute conservative outpatient therapy. If the etiology of the incontinence cannot be determined by history and physical examination or if the patient does not respond to conservative treatment, additional diagnostic studies may be warranted. The most useful diagnostic tools include EAUS and anal manometry. Suspicion of specific causes of incontinence should guide whether other studies such as MRI, defecography, rectal and anal sensory testing, and EMG will be beneficial.

REFERENCES

1. Leigh RJ, Turnberg LA. Faecal incontinence: The unvoiced symptom. Lancet 1982;1(8285):1349–1351.
2. Pretlove SJ, Radley S, Toozs-Hobson PM, et al. Prevalence of anal incontinence according to age and gender: A systematic review and meta-regression analysis. Int Urogynecol J 2006; 17: 407–417.
3. Engel AF, Kamm MA, Bartram CI, et al. Relationship of symptoms in faecal incontinence to specific sphincter abnormalities. In J Colorect Dis 1995; 10:152–155.
4. Shafnik A, El Sibai O, Shafik IA, et al. Stress, urge and mixed types of partial fecal incontinence: Pathogenesis, clinical presentation, and treatment. Am Surg 2007; 73:6–9.
5. Baxter NN, Rothenberger DA, Lowry AC. Measuring fecal incontinence. Dis Colon Rectum 2003; 46:1591–1605.
6. Jorge WM, Wexner SD. Etiology and management of fecal incontinence. Dis Colon Rectum 1993; 36:77–97.
7. Vaizey CJ, Carapeti E, Cahill JA, et al. Prospective comparison of faecal incontinence grading systems. Gut 1999; 44:77–80.
8. Rockwood TH, Church JM, Fleshman JW, et al. Patient and surgeon ranking of the severity of symptoms associated with fecal incontinence: The fecal incontinence severity index. Dis Colon Rectum 1999; 42(12):1525–1532.
9. Fitzgerald MP, Weber AM, Howden N, et al. Risk factors for anal sphincter tear during vaginal delivery. Ostet Gynecol 2007; 109:29–34.
10. Lindsey I, Jones OM, Smilgin-Humphreys MM, et al. Patterns of fecal incontinence after anal surgery. Dis Colon Rectum 2004; 47:1643–1649.
11. Chassagne P, Landrin I, Neveu C, et al. Fecal incontinence in the institutionalized elderly: Incidence, risk factors and prognosis. Am J Med 1999; 106:185–190.
12. Bordeianou L, Rockwood T, Baxter N, et al. Does incontinence correlate with quality of life? Prospective analysis of 502 consecutive patients. Colorectal Dis 2008; 10(3):273–279.
13. Rockwood TH, Church JM, Fleshman JW, et al. Fecal Incontinence Quality of life scale: Quality of life instrument for patients with fecal incontinence. Dis Colon Rectum 2000; 43:9–16.
14. Kwon S, Visco AG, Fitzgerald MP, et al. Validity and reliability of the modified Manchester health questionnaire in assessing patients with fecal incontinence. Dis Colon Rectum 2005; 48: 323–334.
15. Sailer M, Bussen D, Debus ES, et al. Quality of life in patients with benign anorectal disorders. Br J Surg 1998; 85:1716–1719.
16. Hill J, Corson RJ, Brandon H, et al. History and physical examination in the assessment of patients with fecal incontinence. Dis Colon Rectum 1994; 37:473–477.

17. Dobben AC, Terra MP, Deutekom M, et al. Anal inspection and digital rectal examination compared to anorectal physiology tests and endoanal ultrasonography in evaluating fecal incontinence. Int J Colorectal Disease 2007; 22:783–790.
18. Keating JP, Stewart PJ, Eyers AA, et al. Are special investigations of value in the management of patients with fecal incontinence? Dis Colon Rectum 1997; 40:896–901.
19. Liberman H, Faria J, Ternent CA, et al. A prospective evaluation of the value of anorectal physiology in the management of fecal incontinence. Dis Colon Rectum 2001; 44(11):1567–1574.
20. Bharucha AE, Wald A, Rao SSC. Anorectal manometry and imaging are necessary in patients with fecal incontinence. Am J Gastroenterol 2006; 101:2679–2684.
21. Hill K, Fanning S, Fennerty MB, et al. Endoanal ultrasound compared to anorectal manometry for the evaluation of fecal incontinence: A study of the effect these tests have on clinical outcome. Dig Dis Sci 2006; 51:235–240.
22. Pittman JS, Benson JT, Sumners JE. Physiologic evaluation of the anorectum: A new ultrasound technique. Dis Colon Rectum 1990; 33:476–478.
23. Sentovich SM, Wong WD, Blatchford GJ, et al. Accuracy and reliability of transanal ultrasound for anterior anal sphincter injury. Dis Colon Rectum 1998; 41:1000–1004.
24. Zetterstrom JP, Mellgren A, Madoff RD, et al. Perineal body measurement improves evaluation of anterior sphincter lesions during endoanal ultrasonography. Dis Colon Rectum 1998; 41:705–713.
25. Oberwalder M, Thaler K, Baig MK, et al. Anal ultrasound and endosonographic measurement of perineal body thickness. Surg Endosc 2004; 18:650–654.
26. Bollard RC, Gardiner A, Lindlow S, et al. Normal female anal sphincter: Difficulties in interpretation explained. Dis Colon Rectum 2002; 45:171–175.
27. Felt-Bersma RJF, van Baren R, Koorevaar M, et al. Unsuspected sphincter defects shown by anal endosonography after anorectal surgery: A prospective surgery. Dis Colon Rectum 1995; 38:249–253.
28. Smith LE, Blatchford GJ. Physiologic testing. In: Wolff BG, Fleshman JW, Beck DE, et al., eds. The ASCRS Textbook of Colon and Rectal Surgery. 1 st ed. New York: Springer, 2007:40–56.
29. Pilioni V, Fioravanti P, Spazzafumo L, et al. Measurement of anorectal angle by defecography for the diagnosis of incontinence. Int J Colorect Dis 1999; 14:131–135.
30. Dobben AC, Wiersma TG, Janssen LWM, et al. Prospective assessment of interobserver agreement for defecography in fecal incontinence. Am J Radiol 2005; 5:1166–1172.
31. Stoker J, Rociu E, Wiersma TG, et al. Imaging of anorectal disease. Br J Surg 2000; 87:10–27.
32. Dobben AC, Terra MP, Slors JF, et al. External anal sphincter defects in patients with fecal incontinence: Comparison of endoanal MR imaging and endoanal US. Radiology 2007; 242(2):463–471.
33. Hetzer FH, Andreisek G, Tsagari C, et al. MR defecography in patients with fecal incontinence: Imaging findings and their effect on surgical management. Radiology 2006; 240:449–457.
34. Simpson RR, Kennedy ML, Nguyen MH, et al. Anal manometry: A comparison of techniques. Dis Colon Rectum 2006; 49:1033–1038.
35. Hiltunen KM. Anal manometric findings in patients with anal incontinence. Dis Colon Rectum 1985; 28:925–928.
36. Diamant NE, Kamm MA, Wald A, et al. American gastroenterological association medical position statement on anorectal testing techniques. Gastroenterology 1999; 116:732–760.
37. Wald A, Tunuguntla AK. Anorectal sensorimotor dysfunction in fecal incontinence and diabetes mellitus: Modification with biofeedback therapy. N Engl J Med 1984; 310:1282–1287.
38. Salvioli B, Bharucha AE, Rath-Harvey D. Rectal compliance, capacity, and rectoanal sensation in fecal incontinence. Am J Gastroeneterol 2001; 96:2158–2168.
39. Felt-Bersma RJF, Poen AC, Cuesta MA, et al. Anal sensitivity test: What does it measure and do we need it? Cause or derivative of anorectal complaints? Dis Colon Rectum 1997; 40(7):811–816.
40. Tjandra JJ, Milsom JW, Schroeder T, et al. Endoluminal ultrasound is preferable to electromyography in mapping anal sphincter defects. Dis Colon Rectum 1993; 36:689–692.
41. Altomare DF, Rinaldi M, Petrolino M, et al. Reliability of electrophysiologic anal tests in predicting outcome of sacral nerve modulation for fecal incontinence. Dis Colon Rectum 2004; 47:853–857.
42. Pfeifer J, Salanga VD, Agachan F, et al. Variation in pudendal nerve terminal motor latency according to disease. Dis Colon Rectum 1997; 40:79–83.
43. Riccardi R, Mellgren AF, Madoff RD, et al. The utility of pudendal nerve motor latencies in idiopathic incontinence. Dis Colon Rectum 2006; 49:852–857.

10 Fecal Incontinence: Office-Based Management

Tisha Lunsford
Division of Gastroenterology and Hepatology, Mayo Clinic Arizona, Scottsdale, Arizona, U.S.A.

Jonathan Efron
Division of Colorectal Surgery, Mayo Clinic Arizona, Scottsdale, Arizona, U.S.A.

INTRODUCTION

The key to successful office-based management of fecal incontinence is appropriate characterization of the incontinence and a subsequent tiered approach to treatment. If possible, it is imperative to classify the underlying pathophysiology of the patient's fecal incontinence as this will direct treatment strategies and may predict outcomes. The differential diagnosis of fecal incontinence is vast (Table 1) (1–3). Moreover, as the development of fecal incontinence is multifactorial, it is important that the clinician carefully extract and isolate which pathophysiologic factors are responsible for the incontinence. Improvement in any single factor may provide significant clinical improvements.

The four crucial components to maintaining continence include (a) sensory, (b) motor, (c) structural, and (d) cognitive or behavioral mechanisms. Incontinence occurs when one or more of these components are disrupted to an extent that the other components cannot compensate. A practical example would be that of a patient who has suffered from obstetric trauma resulting in damage to the external anal sphincter and pudendal nerve in her early twenties, but did *not* experience incontinence until she developed microscopic colitis in middle age. While the sphincter defect and nerve injury are consistent with a disruption in sensory and structural mechanisms that are important for maintaining continence, the development of increased intestinal motility and decreased stool transit time results in further insult by altering motor control mechanisms. In this case, it is crucial that the microscopic colitis is diagnosed and treated, as any intervention to restore an intact sphincter would be unlikely to provide significant relief from incontinence. This case emphasizes the key role that a thorough clinical history and physical examination play in the development of treatment strategies tailored to meet the specific needs of the incontinent patient.

It is also critical to characterize the subtype of incontinence. Clinically, there are three subtypes (a) passive incontinence—the involuntary discharge of stool or gas without awareness; (b) urge incontinence—the discharge of fecal matter in spite of active attempts to retain bowel contents; and (c) fecal seepage—the passive leakage of stool usually following an otherwise normal evacuation; fecal seepage may also occur in patients with abnormal bowel function and may also be purely functional in nature (3,4). Evaluation of the severity of incontinence and the effect of incontinence on the patient's daily function is also important in planning treatment strategies. This can be simply and objectively measured using the Cleveland Clinic Florida Fecal Incontinence (CCF-FI) scale and patient symptom diaries (Tables 2 and 3) (5–7). Once the multifactorial mechanisms, severity, type, and impact of incontinence have been assessed, tailored treatment strategies may then effectively be implemented.

In the outpatient setting, a deranged bowel habit is the most likely culprit underlying a patient's complaint of incontinence. Diarrhea and constipation are two of the most common conditions precipitating or exacerbating fecal incontinence. Therefore, the majority of the ensuing discussion will focus on an effort to evaluate and treat altered bowel habits and their associated incontinence, known as functional fecal incontinence (8,9).

ALTERED BOWEL HABITS AND FECAL INCONTINENCE (FUNCTIONAL FECAL INCONTINENCE)

Functional fecal incontinence is defined as recurrent uncontrolled passage of fecal material for at least one month in an individual who has no evidence of neurologic or structural etiologies.

Table 1 Differential Diagnosis of Fecal Incontinence

Anatomic derangements	
Congenital abnormalities of the anorectum	
Fistula	
Rectal prolapse	
Anorectal trauma	Trauma Obstetric trauma Surgery (hemorrhoidectomy, anal dilation)
Inflammation	IBD, radiation injury, prolapse
Neurologic diseases	
Central nervous system processes	CVA, dementia, brain tumors, multiple sclerosis, tabes dorsalis, spinal cord lesions, iatrogenic sedation, mental retardation
Peripheral nervous system processes	Cauda equina lesions Polyneuropathies (diabetes mellitus, Shy-Drager syndrome, toxic neuropathy)
Traumatic neuropathy	Perineal descent (perhaps from excessive strain) Obstetric injury
Altered rectal sensation	Fecal impaction Chronic constipation
Skeletal muscle disease	Myasthenia gravis Myopathies, muscular dystrophy
Smooth muscle dysfunction	
Abnormal rectal compliance	IBD releated proctitis, radiation proctopathy, rectal ischemia, fecal impaction
Internal anal sphincter weakness	Radiation proctopathy, diabetes mellitus, childhood encopresis
Miscellaneous	Severe diarrhea, IBS, temporary decrease in mobility, functional fecal incontinence, fecal seepage

Source: Adapted from Ref. 1.

Functional fecal incontinence can occur in any patient with a deranged bowel habit. Table 4 outlines the diagnostic Rome III for fecal incontinence.

Common etiologies of diarrhea include irritable bowel syndrome (IBS), lactose or fructose intolerance, inflammatory bowel disease (IBD), small-bowel bacterial overgrowth, short bowel syndrome, bile acid malabsorption (either after cholecystectomy or small-bowel IBD), celiac sprue, microscopic colitis, and diabetic-associated diarrhea. Common etiologies of constipation also include IBS, lack of dietary fiber, immobility, medications, neurogenic disorders, slowed colonic transit, and functional defecation disorders (FDD). Constipation may precipitate fecal incontinence by causing fecal impaction with subsequent overflow incontinence. Diminished rectal sensations and increased rectosigmoid compliance can reduce the ability of the rectum to

Table 2 Fecal Incontincence Severity Score

Incontinence type	Frequency				
	None (never)	Less than once per month (rarely)	Once or more per month, less than once per week (sometimes)	Once or more per week, less than oncer per day (usually)	Once or more per day (always)
Accidental leakage of solid stool?					
Accidental leakage of liquid stool?					
Accidental leakage of gas?					
Do you wear a pad or undergarment?					
Do you alter your lifestyle due to bowel leakage?					

Score: 0 = perfect continence, 20 = complete incontinence, "never" scores 0 points.
Source: Adapted from Ref. 6.

Table 3 Sample from the Gastrointestinal Health Diary

Date/ time	GI Medications (glycolax, hyocyamine, dicyclomine, OTC laxatives)	Fiber supplement (how much, what type?)	Enema required? Tap water, other?	Type of BM? (1–7)[a]	Degree of strain? (1–10)[b]	Accidents yes/no	Type? Aware? Mucus? Stain?	Additional comments

[a]Type of BM (Patient directed to diary page with stool pictorials and descriptions adapted from the Bristol Stool Scale.
[b]Strain (On 1–10 scale, with 1 being minimal strain and 10 being maximal strain):
1–3 = minimal strain, 4–6 = moderate strain, 7–10 = maximal stain.

perform its reservoir function and reduce the patient's perception of stool or flatus within the rectum. Altered sensation, coupled with sphincter dysfunction, may result in anal incontinence. Treatment of the altered bowel habit is crucial to providing symptomatic relief.

PATIENTS WITH FECAL INCONTINENCE AND DIARRHEA

After an appropriate work-up has excluded organic disease, the first step in treatment is the initiation of bulking agents such as psyllium or methylcellulose (Metamucil® or Citrucel®), partially hydrolyzed guar gum (Benefiber®), and previously attapulgite (Kaopectate®). Due to concerns of high lead levels, the makers of Kaopectate have recently reformulated the drug so that its primary ingredient is bismuth salicylate (the primary ingredient in Pepto Bismal®). When using bulking agents, modifying stool consistency is the primary goal because formed stool is much easier to control than loose stool. The formulations of psyllium, methylcellulose and guar gum are available in both powder and tablet form. Tablets, in a recommended dose of one to two tablets twice daily, are preferred in the case of loose or diarrheal stools, as fiber may

Table 4 Rome III Criteria for Functional Fecal Incontinence

1. Recurrent uncontrolled passage of fecal material in an invidual with a developmental age of at least 4 years and one or more of the following:
   a. Abnormal functioning of normally innervated and structurally intact muscles.
   b. Minor abnormalities of sphincter structure and/or innervation; and/or
   c. Normal or disordered bowel habits (fecal retention or diarrhea); and/or
   d. Psychological causes

And

2. Exclusion of all of the following:
   a. Abnormal innervation caused by lesion(s) within the brain (e.g., dementia, spinal cord or sacral nerve roots or mixed lesions (e.g., multiple sclerosis), or as part of a generalized peripheral or autonomic neuropathy (e.g., owing to diabetes)
   b. Anal sphincter abnormalities associated with a multisystem disease (e.g., scleroderma)
   c. Structural or neurogenic abnormalities believed to be the major or primary cause of FI

Source: From Ref. 10.

Table 5 Guidelines for Use of Common Antidiarrheal Medications in Fecal Incontinence AQ5

Medication	Precautions	Adult dosing	Adverse effects
Fiber supplementation	May interfere with absorption of other medications, therefore very specific dosing guidelines must be outlined for patients May reduce insulin requirement in diabetic patients	Begin 1–2 tablets of preferred formulation BID with *sips* of water only	Flatulence, bloating, abdominal pain, anorexia, asthma reactions, esophageal/intestinal obstruction
Loperamide	Use cautiously in patients with active inflammatory disease of the colon or with infectious diarrhea	Begin at 2 mg PO BID Okay to titrate to 4 mg PO BID, as needed If larger doses are needed (often are in patients with IBS-D) titrate up slowly May increase resting anal sphincter tone	Central nervous system (CNS) depression, paralytic ileus, rash, dizziness, fatigue, cramping, constipation, dry mouth, nausea and vomiting
Diphenoxylate/Atropine	Use cautiously in patients with active inflammatory disease of the colon or with infectious diarrhea	Begin at 2 tablets of diphenoxylate 2.5 mg/atropine 0.025 mg PO daily Titrate up slowly to a maximum dose of 2 tablets PO QID	Toxic megacolon, CNS effects Atropine may cause anticholinergics effects (dry mouth, blurred vision), drowsiness, tachycardia, abdominal pain, pruritis and urinary retention
Alosetron	Reintroduced/approved by the Food and Drug Administration (FDA) as unlabeled investigational agent for managing diarrhea in women with irritable bowel syndrome	Prescribing limited to physicians enrolled in GlaxoSmithKline program Begin 0.5 mg PO daily; may be increased to 0.5 mg PO BID if no response in 4 wk Maximum daily dose 1 mg PO BID Discontinue if no improvement at 1 mg twice/day for 4 wk	Constipation, ischemic colitis severe enough to be fatal
Clonidine	Use cautiously in patients with coronary artery or cerebrovascular disease, patients on other anti-hypertensive agents, impaired liver or renal function	Begin 0.1 mg PO BID May increase to 0.3 mg PO BID. Wean off slowly if ineffective	Severe rebound hypertension, dry mouth, drowsiness, CNS effects, constipation, sedation, orthostatic hypotension, headache, rash, nausea, anorexia, joint pain, impotence, leg cramps, edema, dry eyes
Cholestyramine	Use cautiously in patients with coronary artery disease May interfere with absorption of other medications, therefore very specific dosing guidelines must be outlined for patients Contraindicated in patients with biliary obstruction	Begin 4 g PO daily Practical dosing is usually 4 g PO BID; however, maximum daily dosing is 24 g	Flatulence, nausea, dyspepsia, abdominal pain, anorexia, sour taste, headache, rash, hematuria, fatigue, bleeding of gums, weight loss

Table 5 (*Continued*)

Medication	Precautions	Adult dosing	Adverse effects
Colestipol	May interfere with vitamin absorption May interfere with absorption of other medications, therefore very specific dosing guidelines must be outlined for patients	Begin 2 g (2, 1 g tablets) PO daily Increase to BID or 2–4 g PO every 1–2 mo to a maximum of 16 g/day	Gastrointestinal bleeding, abdominal pain, bloating, flatulence, dyspepsia, liver dysfunction, musculoskeletal pain, rash, chest pain, headache, anorexia, dry skin
Probiotics	Avoid use in immunocompromised or septic patients Formulations are highly variable and are not subject to FDA approval	Variable; usually dose is titrated to number of stools patient is having per day Formulations containing *Bifidobacterium* have been shown to be clinically useful	None currently known
Tincture of Opium	Use cautiously in the elderly, patients with seizure disorder, head injury, increased intracranial pressure, asthma, Chronic Obstructive Pulmonary Disease (COPD), biliary disease, urethral stricture, prostatic hypertrophy, impaired renal/liver function, Addison's disease and in patients with substance abuse history	Begin 1–2 drops PO BID Slowly titrate up to a maximum dose on 12 drops PO BID	Lightheadedness, dizziness, sedation, nausea, vomiting, sweating, dry mouth, anorexia, urinary hesitancy/retention, weakness, flushing, pruritus, headache, rash, CNS effects/depression, hypotension, bradycardia, syncope, shock, cardiac arrest, increased intracranial pressure, seizures, respiratory depression, abuse/dependency, withdrawal if abrupt discontinuation, dysphoria/euphoria, biliary spasm, anaphylactoid reaction
Amitriptyline	Contraindicated with MAO inhibitor use within past 14 days, recent myocardial infaction Use caution in the elderly, patients with coronary artery disease, genitourinary obstruction, urinary retention, prostatic hypertrophy, narrow-angle glaucoma, increase intraocular pressure, seizure disorder, thyroid disease, diabetes mellitus, asthma, Parkinson's disease, impaired liver function, schizophrenia, bipolar disorder, history of alcohol abuse or suicide risk	Begin 10 mg PO QHS May increase to 25 mg PO daily and then increase by 25 mg increments to a daily maximum of 150 mg May give in divided doses	Sedation, nausea, vomiting, increased appetite, weight gain, orthostatic hypotension, hypertension, syncope, severe cardiac effects, CNS effects, increased intraocular pressure, hematologic effects, suicidality, angioedema, anticholinergic effects (dry mouth, blurred vision), urinary retention/frequency, pruritus, libido changes, gynecomastia, galactorrhea, tremor, impotence
Cilansetron	Currently unknown	Currently not FDA approved; In phase III clinical development	Currently unknown

Source: Adapted from Ref. 2.

procure more benefit as a bulking agent when taken with only sips of a noncaffeinated clear beverage. Bismuth salicylate may also be used; however, unlike the fiber formulations, this medication should only be used for temporary relief of symptoms. Pharmacotherapy with agents such as loperamide, diphenoxylate/atropine, alosetron, clonidine, cholestyramine, colestipol, probiotics, tincture of opium, and amytriptyline are usually reserved for patients with more persistent diarrhea that does not respond to conservative bulking agents. Intuitively, the subsequent decreased stool frequency produced by these agents should lessen the frequency of incontinent episodes. Applications and dosing guidelines for the aforementioned pharmacologic agents are outlined in Table 5. However, special concerns may arise in patients with IBS-Diarrhea (IBS-D) predominant as conservative fiber therapy may exacerbate abdominal bloating and discomfort and may precipitate poor compliance. If these bothersome symptoms do not abate after 7 days of use, initiation of pharmacotherapy, including loperamide, amytriptyline, probiotics (specifically those that contain Bifidobacterium), alosetron (limited to certified prescribers), or cilansetron (currently in phase III clinical development), may provide more effective relief for the subset of patients with IBS-D (11–17).

PATIENTS WITH FECAL INCONTINENCE AND CONSTIPATION

Constipation is more difficult to define but is best divided into three subtypes (a) normal-transit constipation (functional constipation or IBS), (b) slow-transit constipation, and (c) functional defecation disorder (FDD) (18). Slow-transit or FDD may precipitate incomplete evacuation, megarectum, and/or decreased rectal sensation. Most cases of fecal incontinence with underlying constipation involve patients who suffer from chronic constipation as opposed to transient bouts of constipation that can be attributed to decreased mobility, decreased fiber or fluid intake, or use of medications such as narcotic analgesics. Constipation is generally defined as three or less bowel movements per week; however, patients most often use the term "constipation" to refer to difficult defecation. Chronic constipation may predispose a patient to increased rectal capacity and decreased rectal sensitivity, thereby placing the patient at risk for overflow incontinence. Subsequently, a patient may actually report that they have diarrhea due to frequent liquid bowel movements and liquid incontinence. It is important for the practitioner to clarify the volume and consistency of incontinent episodes, as overflow incontinence will most likely be associated with small volume, liquid or soft stool loss without a preceding normal bowel movement. This is in opposition to fecal seepage, which usually follows a normal bowel movement although it can certainly also occur in the setting of an abnormal bowel habit. Importantly, constipation may predispose the patient to hemorrhoids or rectal prolapse, which may result in soiling of undergarments with mucus or blood instead of true incontinence; however, the patient may report the staining of undergarments as incontinence. Once constipation has been identified as the underlying etiology for the patient's incontinence, a work-up should ensue to define the subtype of constipation. The work-up may include endoscopic evaluation, anorectal manometry, defecography, dynamic pelvic floor magnetic resonance imaging (MRI), and/or a colonic transit studies. Results from the diagnostic evaluation should help guide appropriate intervention strategies. A common algorithm for diagnostic and treatment strategies is presented in Figure 1. Once the subtype of constipation has been determined, appropriate treatments can be initiated (18). Dosing guidelines for common pharmacologic therapies used in constipation are outlined in Table 6. As with diarrhea, dietary fiber is the first line of therapy in constipation associated with fecal incontinence. However, in patients suffering from constipation or desiccated stool, adequate water ingestion of at least 64 ounces per day is encouraged. Again, caution is advised when initiating fiber therapy in patients who suffer with IBS as abdominal bloating and discomfort may prevent successful use of the supplement. Fiber should always be initiated in low doses and titrated up to 10 to 15 g of fiber supplementation per day, as tolerated. This supplementation is an adjunct to the usual 10 to 15 g of soluble and insoluble fiber contained in the average Western diet. Pharmacologic agents should be reserved for patients who do not respond to or do not tolerate conservative interventions. However, when using certain laxatives, the practitioner must be careful not to precipitate excess gas production and subsequent incontinence of flatus. Nonabsorbable sugars (lactulose, sorbitol, and glycerin) draw water osmotically into the intestinal lumen, stimulate colonic motility, and may cause initial abdominal discomfort, distention or flatulence within the first 48 hours. These aggravating symptoms usually abate

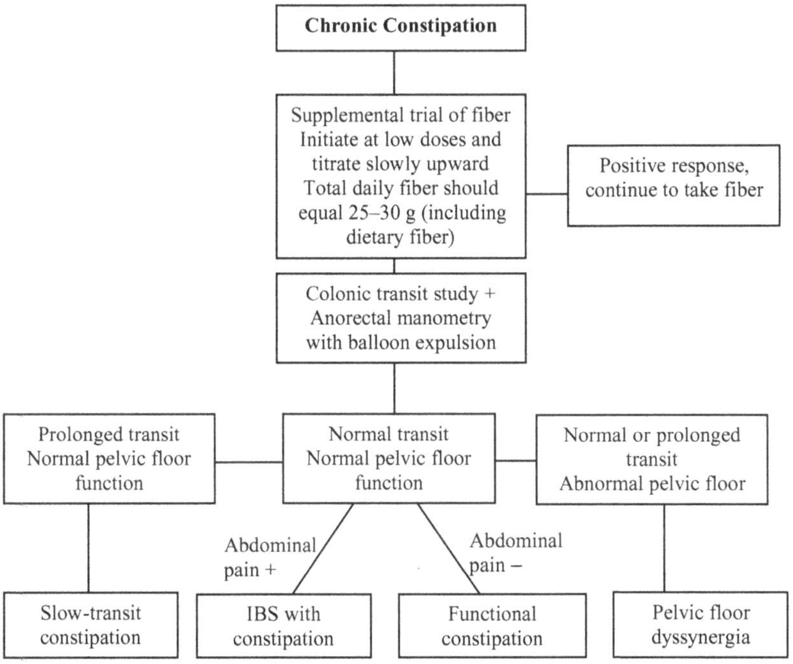

Figure 1 Diagnostic algorithm for determining chronic constipation subtypes. *Source*: From Ref. 18.

with ongoing treatment. Alternatives to laxatives include Amitiza® (lubiprostone), a chloride channel activator indicated for the treatment of chronic idiopathic constipation in adults and treatment of irritable bowel syndrome with constipation in women = 18 years of age. Others include polyethylene glycol, saline laxatives (sodium phosphate, magnesium sulfate, magnesium citrate, and magnesium hydroxide), enemas (sodium phosphate, bisacodyl, mineral oil, or tap water), and suppositories (glycerin or bisacodyl) (19). Creative medication usage may also help, such as utilizing "adverse" side effects of certain medications to achieve a desired bowel habit. For instance, Arthrotec®, a combination of diclofenac and misoprostol (prostaglandin E, 1-an agent used in peptic ulcer disease (PUD) prophylaxis), has the "adverse" side effect of loose stools or diarrhea. For patients who require chronic NSAIDs for analgesia, the use of Arthrotec may replace the use of another NSAID and a separate PPI used for PUD prophylaxis, while simultaneously relieving the constipation. In patients who suffer with depression and/or anxiety and IBS-C, use of some selective serotonin reuptake inhibitors, such as Zoloft®, may help relieve the psychological symptoms and visceral hypersensitivity while also predisposing them to the "side effect" of loose stools or diarrhea (20).

PATIENTS WITH FECAL INCONTINENCE AND FUNCTIONAL DEFECATION DISORDERS INCLUDING DYSSYNERGIC DEFECATION AND/OR INADEQUATE DEFECATORY PROPULSION WITH INCOMPLETE EVACUATION

The mainstay of treatment in patients who report symptoms of dyssynergic defecation (significant straining, sensation of incomplete evacuation) is biofeedback therapy (21). However, it is imperative that biofeedback be reserved for the specific subset of patients with paradoxical pelvic floor contractions and those who meet the Rome III criteria for FDD (Table 7).

One of the likely weaknesses of the majority of behavioral intervention studies on dyssynergia is that many of the patients in these studies probably did not have true dyssynergia and were poor candidates for biofeedback. Biofeedback therapy (for both FDD and fecal incontinence) will be discussed below. If biofeedback is not indicated or further relief in addition to biofeedback is desired, instruction in clearing the rectal vault of its contents during scheduled intervals may also prove beneficial. Methods for keeping the rectal vault clear include suppositories, retrograde enemas, and the pharmacologic therapies used in chronic constipation. Rectally

Table 6 Guidelines for Use of Medications for Constipation in Fecal Incontinence

Medication	Precaution	Adult dosing	Adverse effects
Fiber supplementation	May interfere with absorption of other medications, therefore very specific dosing guidelines must be outlined for patients May reduce insulin requirement in diabetic patients	Begin 4 g preferred preparation daily Titrate up to BID dosing slowly for an optimal daily dose of 16 g supplemental fiber daily Emphasis on adequate fluid intake is paramount for success of treatment	Flatulence, bloating, abdominal pain, anorexia
Nonabsorbable sugars (lactulose, sorbitol)	Use cautiously in patients with diabetes mellitus, galactosemia	15–30 cc PO daily Maximum dose: 60 cc/daily	Lactic acidosis, hypernatremia, flatulence, bloating, abdominal pain, anorexia, nausea, vomiting, electrolyte disorders
Saline laxatives (sodium phosphate, magnesium sulfate, magnesium citrate and magnesium hydroxide)	Use cautiously in the elderly Contraindicated in patients with congestive heart failure or renal dysfunction	Variable	Flatulence, bloating, abdominal pain, anorexia, nausea, vomiting, electrolyte disorders
Amitza® (lubiprostone)[a]	It may be teratogenic and must be used cautiously in patients with a history of small bowel obstruction	The dose is 24 mg PO BID with food and water for chronic constipation and 8 mg PO BID with food and water for IBS–C	Nausea, diarrhea, abdominal pain, and teratogenicity
Enemas	Use cautiously in patients with known inflammatory conditions of the rectum	Variable	Hematochezia, rectal burning or stinging
Suppositories (glycerin or bisacodyl)	Use cautiously in patients with known inflammatory conditions of the rectum	Variable	Hematochezia, rectal burning or stinging

[a]All women of child-bearing age should have a negative pregnancy test prior to beginning treatment and counseled.
Source: Adapted from Ref. 2.

administered therapies are usually preferred in dyssynergic patients as oral laxation can be both unpredictable and create unwanted abdominal cramping and loose stools with faster colonic transit. Glycerin suppositories are composed of a trihydroxy alcohol, which, when placed in direct contact with rectal mucosa, promotes water movement into the distal bowel, stimulates peristalsis, and generally results in a bowel movement within an hour. Tap water enemas are also a very safe alternative, as they contain no irritant chemicals that may result in rectal discomfort, burning or bleeding. These agents should be used by the dyssynergic patient after an unsatisfactory bowel movement or at scheduled times every day or every other day. For those

Table 7 Diagnostic Criteria for Functional Defecation Disorders

1. The patient must satisfy diagnostic criteria for functional constipation
2. During repeated attempts to defecate must have at least 2 of the following;
   a. Evidence of impaired evacuation, based on balloon expulsion test or imaging
   b. Inappropriate contraction of the pelvic floor muscles (i.e., anal sphincter or puborectalis) or less than 20% relaxation of basal resting sphincter pressure by manometry, imaging or EMG
   c. Inadequate propulsive forces assessed by manometry or imaging

patients who fail these standard therapies, further evaluation for rare internal hernias with dynamic pelvic floor MRI or referral to a surgeon who performs puborectalis intramuscular injection of botulinum toxin may be necessary. However, most patients will have a marked improvement with instruction in ways to stimulate defecation at scheduled intervals to keep the rectum clear in addition to biofeedback behavioral treatment (22,23).

PATIENTS WITH FECAL SEEPAGE

Fecal seepage is distinctly different from fecal incontinence in that it usually involves the loss of a small amount of liquid or soft stool after a normal bowel movement (3,24). However, patients may report an abnormal bowel habit or may report symptoms more consistent with anal sphincter dysfunction which is not appreciated as a physiologic abnormality on objective anorectal testing. Interestingly, fecal seepage is more prevalent in men and in those patients with preserved anal sphincter function and rectal reservoir capacity. Similar to patients with disordered defecation, patients with fecal seepage have been shown to demonstrate dyssynergia with impaired balloon expulsion during anorectal manometry testing when compared with other incontinent patients. Similar to patients with dyssynergia, administration of rectal agents and bowel hygiene training (perhaps as a counseling component of biofeedback) are the mainstay of treatment. However, in patients with fecal seepage, clearance of the rectal vault should be performed at a scheduled time each day, regardless of urge to defecate. Ideally, the designated time should be within 30 minutes after a meal to take advantage of the gastrocolic reflex although any time that the patient has specifically set aside for defecation is likely to be beneficial.

THE ROLE OF BIOFEEDBACK TRAINING

Biofeedback Therapy

Biofeedback therapy is a form of operant conditioning or instrumental learning in which information about a physiological process which would otherwise be unconscious is presented to a subject with the aim of having the subject modify that process consciously. For patients with fecal incontinence, the process involves brisk external anal sphincter contraction in response to rectal distention, while for patients with dyssynergic defecation, the process focuses on improvement in abdominopelvic coordination. Biofeedback has long been advocated as first-line therapy for patients whose symptoms are mild-to-moderate due to its safety, affordability, and perceived efficacy. Although often playing a pivotal role in the treatment of fecal incontinence, the recently published Cochrane systematic review of controlled clinical trials on biofeedback has indicated that the combination of a limited number of identified trials and methodological weaknesses would not allow for reliable assessment of the role of biofeedback therapy in the management of patients with fecal incontinence (25–33). Moreover, a recent study conducted by a leader in the field suggested that patient–therapist interaction and patient coping strategies may be more important in improving symptoms than performing exercises or receiving physiological feedback on sphincter function (29). However, as mentioned above, the majority of behavioral intervention studies on fecal incontinence included patients who did not meet the Rome II criteria for dyssynergia (see above) and/or did not have a physiologically proven abnormality of their anal sphincter. This factor alone may explain less than optimal clinical outcomes. However, despite the lack of sound experimental methodology, appropriate control groups and validated outcome measures, reports from centers experienced with the technique suggest that in 60 to 70% of a select group of patients, biofeedback may eliminate symptoms in up to one half of patients and decrease symptoms and improve quality of life in up to two thirds. Excellent results can be anticipated if the correct subset of patients are chosen for treatment. Although there is insufficient evidence with which to select patients suitable for anorectal biofeedback training, most experts agree that the appropriate patient for referral should have physiological evidence of anal dysfunction, be able to cooperate, be well motivated, and possess some degree of perception of rectal distention and the ability to contract the external anal sphincter. The presence of severe fecal incontinence, pudendal neuropathy, and underlying neurologic problems has been associated with a suboptimal prognosis. Moreover, in patients less than 55 years of age with concurrent dyssynergic defecation, defecatory dysfunction must be corrected prior to strength training, as they have been shown to have poor treatment outcomes (34–37). Chapter 5 discussed biofeedback therapy in more detail.

Cognitive Behavioral Therapy

Cognitive behavioral therapy (CBT) is an action-oriented form of psychosocial therapy that assumes that maladaptive, or faulty, thinking patterns cause maladaptive behavior and negative emotions. Maladaptive behavior is defined as behavior that is counterproductive or interferes with everyday living. CBT focuses on changing an individual's thoughts (cognitive patterns) in order to change behavior and emotional status. Although CBT has less systematic support than biofeedback therapy, some leaders in the field believe that it may improve outcomes (38). Currently, objective evidence evaluating CBT is limited to six controlled trials, four of which had positive results for treatment. Its use is based on evidence that it is helpful in patients who suffer from functional gastrointestinal disorders such as IBS, rumination syndrome, and functional fecal incontinence. Currently, there are no recommendations as to which patients would most benefit from CBT. The success of CBT is highly dependant upon the availability of CBT therapy and the patient's openness to therapy. Patients who are candidates for CBT should be referred to a certified specialist in this area; therefore, no further discussion of CBT will ensue.

OTHER TREATMENT OPTIONS FOR FECAL INCONTINENCE

Phenylephrine Gel

Phenylephrine gel is currently being tested in clinical trials and is believed to act locally by increasing anal sphincter tone and improving anal canal resting pressure. Therefore, this agent may be useful for those patients who suffer from mild passive fecal incontinence with intact internal anal sphincter muscles but a low resting anal sphincter pressure. In experiments, which were restricted to patients who were not pregnant and did not have ischemic heart disease, aortic aneurysm, IBD, or uncontrolled hypertension, a 2.5 cm application of 10% to 30% concentration had a therapeutic effect for most patients at one hour. Exact concentration appears to be more important to achieve initial effect as lesser concentrations have been shown to maintain therapeutic effect. Adverse effects included transient stinging or burning with higher concentrations (2,39).

Improvement of Hygiene in Fecal Seepage

Rectal prolapse or hemorrhoids may be the culprits behind fecal or mucoid seepage or undergarment soiling. Instruction in improved rectal hygiene, surgical treatment of the rectal prolapse, or medical/surgical or endoscopic treatment of hemorrhoids may provide symptomatic relief (3).

Anal Plug Devices

A pragmatic treatment for fecal seepage has been the use of an anal plug made of cotton wool. To expand this treatment option, a novel disposable anal continence plug was developed to temporarily occlude the rectum in the setting of fecal incontinence. The plug is attached to the rectum using a tape applied to the perineum. However, subsequent clinical assessment of the plug has shown that it is not well tolerated and may be most useful in those patients with impaired rectal sensation (3).

Electrical Stimulation

Results after application of electric current to the anal canal to stimulate muscle contraction have thus far been disappointing. However, treatment with sacral nerve stimulation (SNS), a treatment currently utilized in urinary incontinence, may hold promise for patients who suffer from severe fecal incontinence. More investigation is needed into these devices before they can be used in the treatment of fecal incontinence (3).

OFFICE OR AMBULATORY PROCEDURES FOR MANAGEMENT OF FECAL INCONTINENCE

While the primary office-based management of fecal incontinence involves the previously described techniques, there are several new minimally invasive interventions for fecal incontinence that can be performed in the office, endoscopy suite, or ambulatory surgery center. Some of these techniques are still experimental and under investigation, while other have FDA approval and are currently available for clinical use. The benefits seen with these techniques are primarily in patients with mild-to-moderate fecal incontinence.

Injectables

Two separate substances have been developed for injection in and around the anal canal for the management of fecal incontinence; both substances are still under investigation and are not yet widely available. Bioplastique™ (Uroplasty BV Inc., The Netherlands) is an injectable form of silicone and Durasphere™ (Boston Scientific, Natick, Massachusetts, U.S.A.) and is a slurry suspension of small carbon coated beads. Both injectables have been primarily used in patients with intact external sphincters who are thought to have incontinence secondary to internal sphincter dysfunction.

Kenefick et al. (40) described a pilot study of six patients who had silicone injected transphincterically into three separate locations at or above the dentate line. The silicone was thought to act as a passive barrier to the passage of liquid or solid stool. Anal manometry, ultrasound, fecal incontinence scores, and quality of life scores were measured before and after injection. Five of the six patients had significant subjective improvement. Fecal incontinence scores improved from a mean of 14 pre therapy to eight post injection. There was also significant improvement in SF-36 scores. There did seem to be an increase in resting and squeeze pressures, and no migration of the silicone was seen on ultrasound.

Durasphere utilizes carbon coated beads to enhance anal function. The beads originally were injected submucosally at and above the dentate line and therefore provide bulk and passive resistance to the passage of stool. Davis et al. (41) injected 18 patients in this manner during a pilot study. Mean follow-up after injection was 28.5 months and anal manometry and ultrasound, along with satisfaction and quality of life scores, were measured pre injection and at periodic points after injection. The authors documented a significant improvement in fecal incontinence scores and quality of life scores, but saw no change in anorectal physiology. Patients who improved maintained that benefit up to the 28.5 month mark. Complications resulting from the injection of Durasphere include infection, abscess formation, and bead extrusion.

To prevent bead extrusion, the method of injection has been modified. Weiss et al. (42) reported on seven patients that had some intersphincteric injections of the Durasphere beads in three separate locations around the anal canal. They saw significant improvement in incontinence and quality of life scores and subjective improvement in four of the seven patients. The current technique for injecting the Durasphere beads is an intersphincteric injection between the hemorrhoidal bundles in the left anterior, left posterior, and right lateral positions. There appears to be fewer problems with bead leakage after injection with this technique. Currently, a randomized prospective, blinded placebo trial is underway comparing injection of Durasphere to saline for fecal incontinence.

Radiofrequency (Secca™ Procedure)

The Secca procedure utilizes radiofrequency energy delivered to the lower rectum and anal canal to enhance continence. The procedure does require sedation and is therefore generally performed in an ambulatory surgery center or endoscopy suite. The procedure is performed with a specialized anoscope that delivers the radiofrequency energy to the desired locations around the lower rectum and anal canal. The patient is placed in either the prone jackknife, lithotomy, or left lateral position to perform the procedure. After positioning, local anesthetic is administered and the dentate line is marked in four different locations. This marking is useful to identify the dentate line during the procedure. Radiofrequency energy is then delivered to four separate quadrants in the anal canal and distal rectum starting 5 mm below the dentate line. Radiofrequency energy is delivered through needle electrodes that, when deployed, penetrate into the submucosa of the anal canal and distal rectum. The needles are temperature and impedance controlled and will automatically shut off if the submucosal temperature or mucosal temperature exceeds set limits to prevent excessive burning. The energy is delivered at five separate levels, 5 mm apart, in each quadrant. The entire procedure takes between 30 and 40 minutes.

The Secca procedure was originally described by Takahashi et al. (43) in 2002 in a pilot study of 10 patients. They found that treated patients had significant improvement in there fecal incontinence and quality of life scores. The improvement did not become evident until six weeks after the procedure had been completed and showed continued improvement until six months post procedure. At the two years follow-up, these patients demonstrated sustained improvement (44).

This initial success led to a five center prospective trial performed in the United States on 50 patients with six-month follow-up (45). Multiple exclusion criteria included a history of pelvic irradiation, history of inflammatory bowel diseases, the presence of infection or fistulas, and others. No changes were seen in any anorectal physiologic testing (manometry or anal ultrasound), but significant improvement was seen in fecal incontinence and quality of life scores. Significant complications included two patients who developed anal necrosis. These occurred early in the trial and resulted in modifications of the device and procedure and no further episodes were documented after these changes. The Secca procedure has been approved by the FDA for use in the United States and is currently available. A randomized controlled single-blinded placebo trial has been completed on 100 patients with one-year follow-up, but final publication is still pending.

Both the radiofrequency and the synthetic injectables are good options for patients with mild fecal incontinence who fail other methods of conservative management. Patients with external sphincter defects and incontinence who are operative candidates should undergo sphincter repair as a primary therapy. Those patients who have internal sphincter dysfunction, persistence incontinence after external sphincter repair, or idiopathic incontinence may respond well to one of these minimally invasive techniques.

REFERENCES

1. Schiller LR. Fecal incontinence. In: Feldman M, Scharschmidt BF, Sleisenger MH, eds. Sleisenger Fordtran's Gastrointestinal and Liver Disease. 6th ed: 1998;163.
2. Scarlett Y. Medical management of fecal incontinence. Gastroenterology 2004; 126:S55–S63.
3. Rao SSC. Diagnosis and management of fecal incontinence. Am J Gastroenterol 2004; 99(8): 1585–1604.
4. Rao SSC. Pathophysiology of adult fecal incontinence. Gastroenterology 2004; 126:S14–S22.
5. Crowell MD, Schettler-Duncan A, Brookhart K, et al. Fecal incontinence: Impact on psychosocial function and health-related quality of life. Gastroenterology 1998; 114:A738.
6. Jorge JM, Wexner SC. Etiology and management of fecal incontinence. Dis Colon Rectum 1993; 36:77–97.
7. Rockwood TH, Church JM, Fleshman JW, et al. Patient and surgeon ranking of the severity of symptoms associated with fecal incontinence: The fecal incontinence severity index. Dis Colon Rectum 199; 42(12):1525–1531.
8. Crowell MD, Lacy BE, Schettler VA, et al. Subtypes of anal incontinence associated with bowel dysfunction: Clinical, physiologic, and psychosocial characterization. Dis Colon Rectum 2004; 47(10):1627–1635.
9. Mavrantonis C, Wexner SD. A clinical approach to fecal incontinence. J Clin Gastroenterol 1998; 27(2):108–121.
10. Wald, A, Bharucha, Enck, P and Rao SSC. Functional anorectal disorders. In: Drossman, DA, Corazziari, E, Spiller, R, Thompson WG, Delvaux, M, Talley NJ, Whitehead, WE., 3rd eds. Rome III: The Functional Gastrointestinal Disorders, Third Ed. 2006; 639–686.
11. Camilleri M. Treating irritable bowel syndrome: Overview, perspective and future therapies. Br J Pharmacol 2004; 141:1237–1248.
12. Cann PA, Read NW, Holdsworth CD, et al. Role of loperaminde and placebo in management of irritable bowel syndrome (IBS). Dig Dis Sci 1984; 29:239–247.
13. Hallgren T, Fasth S, Belbro D, et al. Loperamide improves anal sphincter function and continence after restorative proctocolectomy. Dig Dis Sci 1994; 39:2612–2618.
14. Harford WV, Krejs GJ, Santa Ana C, et al.Acute affect of diphenoxylate with atropine (Lomotil) in patients with chronic diarrhea and fecal incontinence. Gastroenterology 1980; 78:440–443.
15. O'Mahony L, McCarthy J, Kelly P, et al. Lactobacillus and bifidobacterium in irritable bowel syndrome: Symptom responses and relationship to cytokine profiles. Gastroenterology 2005; 128:541–551.

16. Santoro GA, Eitan B, Pryde A, et al. Open study of low-dose amitriptyline in the treatment of patients with idiopathic fecal incontinence. Dis Colon Rectum 2000;43(12):1676–1682.
17. Sun W, Donnelly TC. Effects of loperamide oxide on gastrointestinal transit time and anorectal function in patients with chronic diarrhea and faecal incontinence. Scand J Gastroenterol 1997; 32:34–38.
18. Prather CM. Subtypes of constipation: Sorting out the confusion. Review in Gastroenterol Disorders 2004; 4(suppl 2):S11–S16.
19. DiPalma JA. Current treatment options for chronic constipation. Rev Gastroenterol Disord 2004; 4(suppl 2):S34–S41.
20. Crowell MD, Jones MP, Harris LA, et al. Antidepressants in the treatment of irritable bowel syndrome and visceral pain syndromes. Curr Opin Investig Drugs 2004; 5(7):736–742.
21. Rao SSC, Happel J, Welcher K. Obstructed defecation: a failure of recto-anal coordination. Am J Gastroenterol 1998; 93:1042–1050.
22. Thompson WG, Longstreth GF, Drossman DA, et al. Functional bowel disorders and fuctional abdominal pain. Gut 1999; 45(suppl 2):II43–II47.
23. Crowell MD. Pathogenesis of slow transit and pelvic floor dysfunction: From bench to bedside. Reviews in Gastroenterol Disorders 2004; 4(suppl 2):S17–S27.
24. Rao SSC. Investigation of the pathophysiology of fecal seepage. Am J Gastroenterol 2004; 99:2204–2209.
25. Enck P. Biofeedback training in disordered defecation: A critical review. Dig Dis Sci 1993; 38:1953–1960.
26. Glia A, Gylin M, Akerlund JE, et al. Biofeedback training in patients with fecal incontinence. Dis Colon Rectum 1998; 41(3):359–364.
27. Miner PB, Donnelly TC, Read NW. Investigation of the mode of action of biofeedback in treatment of fecal incontinence. Dig Dis Sci 1990; 35:1291–1298.
28. Norton C, Hosker G, Brazzelli M. Effectiveness of Biofeedback and/or Sphincter Exercises for the Treatment of Fecal Incontinence in Adults. [update of Cochrane Database Syst Rev 2000(2):CD002111;PMID:10796859] Cochrane Database of Systematic Reviews.3:CD002111, 2006.
29. Norton C, Chelvanayagam S, Wilson-Barnett J, et al. Randomized controlled trial of biofeedback for fecal incontinence. Gastroenterology 2003; 125:1320–1329.
30. Rao SSC. The technical aspects of biofeedback therapy for defecation. Gastroenterologist 1998; 6(2):86–103.
31. Wald A. Biofeedback therapy for fecal incontinence. Ann Intern Med 1981; 95:146–149.
32. Whitehead WE, Burgio KL, Engel BT. Biofeedback treatment of fecal incontinence in geriatric patients. J Am Geriatr Soc 1985; 33:320–324.
33. Norton C. Behavioral management of fecal incontinence in adults. Gastroenterology 2004; 126:S64–S70.
34. Fernandez-Fraga X, Azpiroz F, Aparici A, et al. Predictors of response to biofeedback treatment in anal incontinence. Dis Colon Rectum 2003; 46(9):1218–1224.
35. Palsson OS, Heymen S, Whitehead WE. Biofeedback treatment for functional anorectal disorders: A comprehensive efficacy review. Appl Psychophysiol Biofeedback 2004; 29(3):153–174.
36. Prather CM. Physiologic variables that predict the outcome of treatment for fecal incontinence. Gastroenterology 2004; 126:S135–S140.
37. Tries J. Protocol-and therapist-related variable affecting outcomes of behavioral interventions for urinary and fecal incontinence. Gastroenterology 2004; 126:S152–S158.
38. Drossman DA, Toner BB, Whitehead WE, et al. Cognitive-behavioral therapy versus education and desipramine versus placebo for moderate to severe functional bowel disorders. Gastroenterology 2003; 125:19–31.
39. Carapeti EA, Kamm M, Nicholls RJ. Randomized, controlled trial of topical phenylephrine for fecal incontinence in patients after ileoanal pouch construction. Dis Col Rectum 2000; 43(8):1059–1063.
40. Kenefick NJ, Vaizey CJ, Malouf AJ, et al. Injectable silicone biomaterial for feacal incontinence due to internal anal sphincter dysfunction. Gut 2002; 51(2):225–228.
41. Davis K, Kumar D, Poloniecki J. Preliminary evaluation of an injectable anal sphincter bulking agent (Durasphere) in the management of faecal incontinence. Aliment Pharmocol Ther 2003; 18(2):237–243.
42. Weiss EG, Efron JE, Nogueras JJ, et al. Submucosal injection of carbon-coated beads is a successful and safe office-based treatment for fecal incontinence [meeting abstract]. Dis Colon Rectum 2002; 45:A46.
43. Takahashi T, Garcia-Osogobio S, Valdovinos MA, et al. Radiofrequency energy delivery to the anal canal for the treatment of fecal incontinence. Dis Colon Rectum 2002; 44(4):A37.
44. Takahashi T, Valdovinos MA, Mass W, et al. Radiofrequency energy delivery for the treatement of fecal incontinence: Results of extended two year follow up. Dis Colon Rectum 2002; 45(4): A25.
45. Efron JE, Corman ML, Fleshman J, et al. Multi-center open label prospective trial evaluating the safety and effectiveness of temperature controlled radio frequency energy delivery to the anal canal (Secca procedure) for the treatment of fecal incontinence. Dis Colon Rectum 2003; 46(12):1606–1618.

11 Fecal Incontinence: Surgical Management

Juan J. Nogueras
Department of Colorectal Surgery, Cleveland Clinic Florida, Weston, Florida, U.S.A.

Anne Y. Lin
Department of Surgery, Division of Colorectal Surgery, Washington University, St. Louis, Missouri, U.S.A.

INTRODUCTION

Fecal incontinence is a devastating disorder, which can be associated with poor self-image and social isolation. The incidence of incontinence varies in published reports likely secondary to under-reporting of symptoms and variations in the sampling of populations. A community-based survey of approximately 7000 individuals reported a 2.2% incidence of fecal incontinence (1). Another review reported higher rates of 11% to 15% (2). One study on nursing home patients found that 45% of its patients had fecal incontinence (3).

Fecal incontinence is defined as involuntary loss of rectal contents through the anal canal. Normal continence involves coordinated activity of the internal and external anal sphincters, pelvic floor muscles, and neural input. When these factors are disrupted, fecal incontinence may result.

The majority of cases of fecal incontinence are acquired, predominantly from vaginal delivery, but also from anorectal surgery, and trauma. Vaginal delivery can cause direct sphincter injury as well as traction injury to the pudendal nerve. A thorough history should be obtained to elicit other possible causes of fecal incontinence such as fecal impaction with overflow incontinence, neurological disorders including diabetes mellitus or stroke, functional gastrointestinal tract disorders such as inflammatory bowel disease or infectious diarrhea, radiation exposure, and medication usage.

ASSESSMENT

Fecal incontinence is classified using objective scoring systems such as the Cleveland Clinic Fecal Incontinence (CCF-FI) score (Table 1) (4). This scale characterizes the degree of incontinence using factors such as (1) the frequency of incontinence to gas, liquid, and solid stool; (2) the degree of alteration in lifestyle; and (3) the use of pads. A score of zero indicates total control, whereas a score of 20 indicates complete incontinence. These scores have been validated for determining alteration in quality of life and subsequent referral for surgery (5). Additional history regarding quality of life can be obtained using the Fecal Incontinence Quality of Life (FIQOL) Scale questionnaire.

In addition to a thorough history, a complete physical examination includes examination of the perineal body, evaluation for rectal prolapse and fecal impaction, and assessment of sphincter tone and perianal sensation. Endoscopic evaluation is also useful to exclude an inflammatory condition, solitary rectal ulcer, villous adenoma, or mass. Anorectal physiology testing includes endoanal ultrasound for evaluation of sphincter anatomy and anal manometry for assessment of anal sphincter function. Measurements taken during manometry include anal resting and squeeze pressures, rectoanal inhibitory reflex, rectal compliance, and sensory thresholds with balloon distension. Neurophysiological testing includes either single-fiber electromyography or pudendal nerve terminal motor latency (PNTML) testing.

MEDICAL MANAGEMENT

The management of fecal incontinence includes first identifying and treating the causes of diarrhea, including exclusion of fecal impaction with overflow incontinence. Dietary modification

Table 1 Cleveland Clinic Florida Fecal Incontinence Score

	Frequency				
Type of incontinence	**Never**	**Rarely**	**Sometimes**	**Usually**	**Always**
Solid	0	1	2	3	4
Liquid	0	1	2	3	4
Gas	0	1	2	3	4
Wears pad	0	1	2	3	4
Lifestyle alteration	0	1	2	3	4

Never, 0; rarely, $<$1/mo; sometimes, $<$1/wk, 1/mo; usually, $<$1/day, 1/wk; always, 1/day.
0, perfect; 20, complete incontinence.

with fiber and bulking agents and medication such as loperamide, diphenoxylate, or bile acid binders can be useful for improving the consistency of liquid stool. Behavioral modification such as biofeedback therapy may be helpful for those motivated patients with pelvic floor dysynergia, in particular those with impairment in rectal sensation or with external anal sphincter weakness (7).

SURGICAL MANAGEMENT

Anterior Sphincteroplasty

When medical management fails, surgical intervention may be an alternative. If a sphincter injury is present on endoanal ultrasound imaging, an overlapping sphincteroplasty procedure is a viable surgical option. Mechanical bowel preparation and parenteral antibiotics are given preoperatively. A Foley catheter is inserted and the patient is placed in the prone jackknife position. A curved incision is made along the perineal body between the anus and the vagina. The dissection begins laterally with identification of the retracted ends of the external anal sphincter and mobilization of the external sphincter from the surrounding ischiorectal fossa fat. Care is taken to limit dissection to less than half the circumference of the anal canal to avoid damaging the posterolateral nerves. The dissection then proceeds medially, opening up the space between the distal rectum and the vagina. The intersphincteric space is identified, and the anterior levator muscle plate is grasped for suture plication. The scar tissue in the retracted ends of the external anal sphincter is preserved to facilitate suture repair. The sphincter muscle ends are then brought together either in an end-to-end or overlapping fashion with the use of sutures (Fig. 1). Anterior levatorplasty facilitates and eliminates tension of the external sphincter repair. The wound is then closed in a V–Y fashion with the central portion of the wound left open for drainage. Postoperative care includes close attention to regulation of bowel function.

The results of overlapping sphincteroplasty for fecal incontinence are mixed. As continence is a result of the interplay of rectal sensation, muscle strength, and nerve function, merely reapproximating the sphincter may not always hold the key to restoration of function.

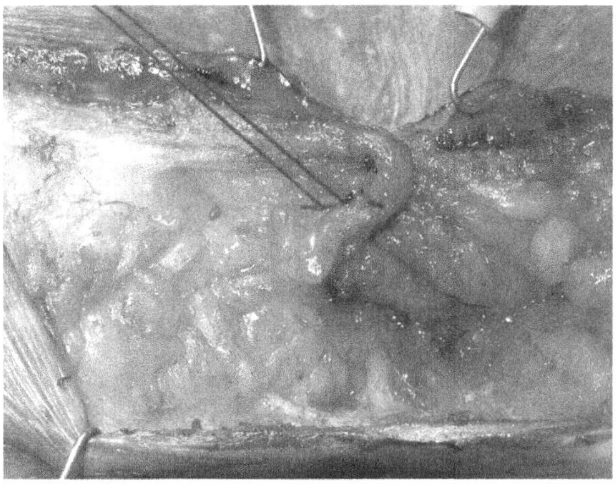

Figure 1 Overlapping sphincteroplasty.

There are no clear cut predictors of success. After review of 77 patients with a mean two-year follow-up, it was noted that neither age, parity, prior sphincteroplasty, cause or duration of incontinence, extent of electromyography damage, size of the endoanal ultrasound defect, nor any manometric parameter correlated with outcome. The only factor predictive of long-term success in this patient population was bilateral normal pudendal nerve terminal latency (8). Halverson and Hull (9) reviewed their results of 71 patients who underwent anterior overlapping sphincteroplasty and found that after a median follow-up of 69 months, greater than half of the patients were incontinent to solid or liquid stool. In a similar retrospective review, Barisic et al. (10) found that initially, the 65 patients in the study did well with a mean CCF-FI score of 3.6 at three months after surgery. This, however, deteriorated to a mean score of 6.3 with a longer follow-up. Although these studies showed less encouraging long-term results, recent studies have demonstrated sustained improvement in quality of life at a median follow-up of 84 months (11,12).

In patients without a sphincter defect, a variety of other surgical techniques may be beneficial.

Other Surgical Procedures

Artificial Bowel Sphincter

The Acticon Neosphincter® (American Medical Systems, Minnetonka, Minnesota, U.S.A.) is a synthetic device which replaces the function of the patient's sphincter. Adapted from the field of urology, the component consists of (1) an inflatable cuff which is implanted around the anus; (2) a control pump which activates and deactivates the device and which is placed in the scrotum of men and labia major of women; and (3) a pressure-regulating balloon, which is placed in the space of Retzius (Fig. 2). Constant cuff inflation is maintained by the pressure-regulating balloon, which keeps the anus closed. Pump activation allows fluid to egress from the cuff to the balloon, with resulting deflation of the cuff, which enables evacuation from the anus. The fluid then returns to the cuff. Report of a multi-center trial of 112 patients by Wong et al. (13) showed that 67% of patients at one-year follow-up had a functioning device. Significant improvement in incontinence scores and quality of life measures were found in 85% of patients. There were 384 complications in 99 patients (88%); 41 patients (37%) had their device explanted and 25% required surgical intervention related to infections. In a long-term follow-up, almost 50% of patients at a five-year follow-up had their device explanted (14). More recently, lower infection rates were noted in a series of 33 patients who had implantation of an artificial bowel sphincter. Seven devices were explanted with one patient having a successful reimplantation. Ultimately, 82% of the patients had a functioning device at a mean of 17-month follow-up (15).

Although the procedure has limitations, it is often one of a few remaining viable options for patients who may otherwise require a permanent stoma. For patients with little perineal tissue, graciloplasty may provide tissue bulk prior to implantation of the neosphincter. Improvements

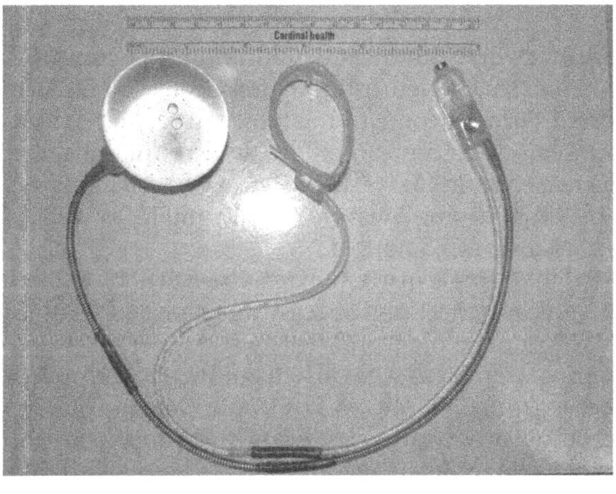

Figure 2 Artificial bowel sphincter.

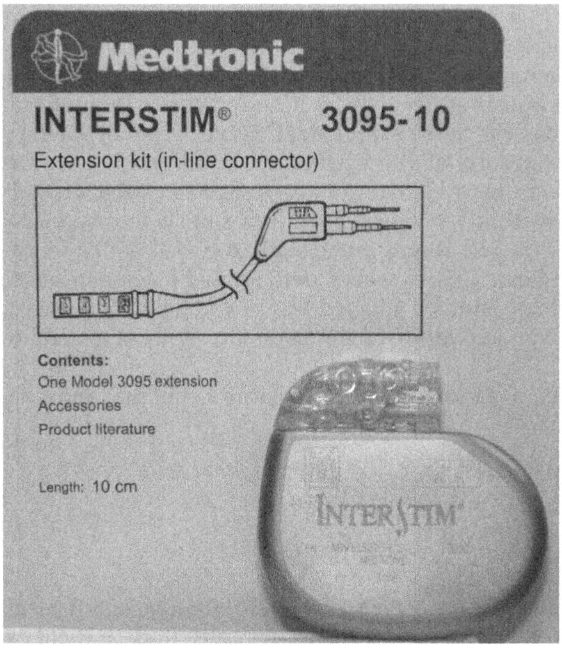

Figure 3 Sacral nerve stimulation.

in operative technique including changes to the antibiotic regimen may help to decrease the rate of infectious complications.

Sacral Nerve Stimulation

The applicability of sacral nerve stimulation (SNS) for fecal incontinence came about secondary to observations that patients treated by SNS for urinary incontinence with associated symptoms of fecal incontinence subsequently had improvement in both urinary and fecal incontinence. Patients with fecal incontinence alone are the focus of a multi-center trial in the United States. Neurostimulation is achieved with an electrode which is percutaneously placed in the third sacral foramina (Fig. 3). Temporary stimulation with a pacing wire extension is then undertaken to assess the response to stimulation and the effect on fecal incontinence. Once the patient displays success with treatment, a permanent generator is implanted.

It is postulated that sacral neuromodulation acts at the level of the efferent motor neuron with stimulation resulting in contraction of the pelvic floor and sphincter muscles. A less well understood mechanism of improved continence is through the sacral reflexes that regulate rectal sensitivity and contractility (16). The first report in the literature of permanent implantation of a SNS was published in The Lancet in 1995 (17). Three patients were implanted with symptomatic improvement attributed to increases in anal squeeze pressures. Conversely, Michelsen (18) found that SNS resulted in significant increases in rectal capacity and anal resting pressures with no significant change in squeeze pressures.

Since 1995, SNS has gained acceptance in several European countries and is currently under study in the United States. The Initial Italian Sacral Neurostimulation Group Experience has provided us with some insight into the mid-term outcome of this procedure (19). Sixteen patients were implanted with permanent stimulators. At a mean follow-up of 15 months, the number of incontinent episodes in 14 days decreased from 11.5 (±4.8) to 0.6 (±0.9). Manometric evaluation revealed an increase in the mean maximal resting pressure of 11.9 mmHg, as well as an increase in the mean maximal squeezing pressure of 15.3 mmHg.

Kenefick and Vaizey (20) recently reported their single institution results with SNS. Fifteen consecutive patients were implanted over a five-year period, and success was reported in all 15 patients at a median follow-up of 24 months. The number of incontinent episodes per one week period decreased from 11 to 0. The manometric parameters were also significantly improved as reflected by a mean resting pressure increase from 35 to 49 cm H_2O, and a mean squeeze pressure increase from 43 to 69 cm H_2O. Rectal sensitivity also significantly improved, as did the amount of time during which patients were able to defer the call to stool. Leroi et al. (21)

conducted the first double blind multi-center crossover study with 34 patients. They found that there was significant improvement in the severity of incontinence when the stimulator was on versus off. Most recently, SNS has been shown to improve quality of life and significantly lower the CCF-FI scores in a group of 44 patients with a 13-month (1–42) follow-up (22).

Stimulated Graciloplasty

The technique of stimulated graciloplasty most commonly used today involves transposition of the gracilis muscle around the anus with anchoring of the muscle to the contralateral ischial tuberosity. Stimulator and electrode implantation is also performed. Neuromuscular conditioning begins usually three days after implantation with increasing duration of muscle contraction. The fast twitch, easily fatigable gracilis muscle is converted to slow twitch, fatigue-resistant fibers with low electrical stimulation. A diverting stoma may also be added. Continence and quality of life were demonstrated by the Dynamic Graciloplasty Therapy Study Group to have improved significantly in approximately 60% of patients (23). In a two-year follow-up, this effect was shown to be durable with significant improvement noted in 62% of patients (24). The procedure, however, can be technically demanding with high complication rates including device failure or erosion, leg pain, and infection. These can usually be treated effectively without adverse functional outcome with the exception of infection. In a systematic review, the efficacy rate ranged from 42% to 85% with a reoperative rate of 0.14 to 1.07 per patient (25). This procedure is available in other countries, but not currently approved in the United States.

SUMMARY

The approach to a patient with fecal incontinence generally involves a systematic evaluation. This involves an assessment of patients' comorbidities, the causes of fecal incontinence, as well as interpretation of the results of anatomic and physiologic testing. It is important to evaluate for causes of fecal incontinence such as diarrhea, which may benefit from fiber and antimotility agents. A trial of biofeedback therapy for pelvic floor dysynergia may be appropriate. For surgical candidates with a sphincter defect, overlapping sphincteroplasty may be the best option. Patients with severe fecal incontinence who do not have a sphincter defect can be offered more advanced surgical options including SNS and artificial bowel sphincter. A permanent stoma also remains a viable alternative.

REFERENCES

1. Nelson R, Norton N, Cautley E, et al. Community-based prevalence of anal incontinence. JAMA 1995; 274(7):559–561.
2. Macmillan A, Merrie A, Marshall R, et al. The prevalence of fecal incontinence in community-dwelling adults: A systematic review of the literature. Dis Colon Rectum 2004; 47(8);1341–1349.
3. Nelson R, Furner S, Jesudason V, et al. Fecal incontinence in Wisconsin nursing homes: Prevalence and associations. Dis Colon Rectum 1998; 41(10):1226–1229.
4. Jorge JM, Wexner SD. Etiology and management of fecal incontinence. Dis Colon Rectum 1993; 36(1):77–97.
5. Rothbarth J, Bemelman W, Meijerink W, et al. What is the impact of fecal incontinence on quality of life? Dis Colon Rectum 2001; 44(1):67–71.
6. Rockwood TH, Church JM, Fleshman JW, et al. Fecal Incontinence Quality of Life Scale: Quality of life instrument for patients with fecal incontinence. Dis Colon Rectum 2000; 43(1):9–16.
7. Diamont NE. AGA technical review on anorectal testing techniques. Gastroenterology 1999; 116:735–760.
8. Gilliland R, Altomare DF, Moreira H Jr., et. al. Pudendal neuropathy is predictive of failure following anterior overlapping sphincteroplasty. Dis Colon Rectum 1998; 41(12):1516–1522.
9. Halverson AL, Hull TL. Long-term outcome of overlapping anal sphincter repair. Dis Col Rectum 2002; 45(3):345–348.
10. Barisic GI, Krivokapic ZV, Markovic VA, et. al. Outcome of overlapping anal sphincter repair after 3 months and after a mean of 80 months. Int J Colorectal Dis 2006; 21(1):52–56.
11. Maslekar S, Gardiner A, Duthie G, et al. Anterior anal sphincter repair for fecal incontinence: Good longterm results are possible. J Am Coll Surg 2007; 204:40–46.

12. Grey B, Sheldon R, Telford K, et al. Anterior anal sphincter repair can be of long term benefit: A 12-year case cohort from a single surgeon. BMC Surg 2007; 7:1.
13. Wong W, Congliosi S, Spencer M, et al. The safety and efficacy of the artificial bowel sphincter for fecal incontinence: Results from a multicenter cohort study. Dis Colon Rectum 2002; 45(9):1139–1153.
14. Mundy L, Merlin T, Maddern G, et al. Systematic review of safety and effectiveness of an artificial bowel sphincter for faecal incontinence. Br J Surg 2004; 91(6):665–672.
15. Melenhurst J, Koch SM, van Gemert WG, et al. The artificial bowel sphincter for fecal incontinence: A single centre study. Int J Colorectal Dis. 2008; 23(1):107–111.
16. Malouf AJ, Vaizey CJ, Nicholls RJ, et al. Permanent sacral nerve stimulation for fecal incontinence. Ann Surg 2000; 232(1):143–148.
17. Matzel KE, Stadelmaier U, Hohenfeller M, et al. Electrical stimulation of spinal nerves for treatment of fecal incontinence. Lancet 1995; 346:1124–1127.
18. Michelsen HB, Buntzen S, Krogh K, et. al. Rectal volume tolerability and anal pressures in patients with fecal incontinence treated with sacral nerve stimulation. Dis Col Rectum 2006; 49(7):1039–1044.
19. Ganio E, Ratto C, Masin, A, et al. Neuromodulation for fecal incontinence: Outcome in 16 patients with definitive implant. Dis Colon Rectum 2001; 44(7):965–970.
20. Kenefick NJ, Vaizey CJ, Cohen CG, et al. Medium-term results of permanent sacral nerve stimulation for fecal incontinence. Br J Surg 2002; 89:896–901.
21. Leroi AM, Parc Y, Lehur PA, et al. Efficacy of sacral nerve stimulation for fecal incontinence: Results of a multicenter, double blind crossover trial. Ann Surg 2005; 242(5):662–669.
22. Hetzer FH, Hahnloser D, Clavien PA, et. al. Quality of life and morbidity after permanent sacral nerve stimulation for fecal incontinence. Arch Surg 2007; 142:8–13.
23. Baeten C, Konsten J, Spaans F, et al. Safety and efficacy of dynamic graciloplasty for fecal incontinence: Report of a prospective, multicenter trial. Dynamic Graciloplasty Therapy Study Group. Dis Colon Rectum 2000; 43(6):743–751.
24. Wexner S, Baeten C, Bailey R, et al. Long-term efficacy of dynamic graciloplasty for fecal incontinence. Dis Colon Rectum 2002; 45(6):809–818.
25. Chapman A, Geerdes B, Hewett P, et al. Systematic review of dynamic graciloplasty in the treatment of faecal incontinence. Br J Surg 2002; 89(2):138–153.

12 Constipation: Evaluation and Management

Badma Bashankaev and Eric G. Weiss
Department of Colorectal Surgery, Cleveland Clinic Florida, Weston, Florida, U.S.A.

Marat Khaikin
Department of Surgery and Transplantation, Sheba Medical Center, Sackler School of Medicine, Tel Aviv, Israel

BACKGROUND

Constipation has been recognized as a medical condition as far back as primeval times. In ancient Egypt, one of Pharaoh's physician's titles was "Shepherd of the anus of the Pharaoh." The Ebers Papyrus (1550 BC) had already contained a "pathophysiologic" explanation of constipation caused by autointoxication (1,2). From that time until the second half of the 20th century, the "autointoxication" theory, including the necessity of daily bowel movements, was the dominant explanation of the condition (2). Changes in lifestyle, diet, increased daily stress, and increased length of life led to the common picture of modern constipation.

The modern definition of constipation is based on numerous different etiologies. Some etiologies are lifestyle related, such as diet, psychological factors, the amount of physical activity, social habits, and eating disorders such as bulimia/anorexia. Others are based on anatomic abnormalities including cancer, rectal prolapse, rectal intussusception, rectocele, and sigmoidocele. There are also functional disorders with lack of pelvic relaxation [paradoxical puborectalis contraction (PPC)], or impaired gastrointestinal motility which can cause constipation and, rarely, an infectious etiology like Chagas' disease (trypanosomiasis) is the cause. Finally, comorbidity-related constipation due to pharmacological, metabolic, endocrine, neurological, and systemic disorders can also occur.

Despite the modern medical view on constipation, society still has a strong belief in "auto-intoxication"; others, however, have dispelled this view as myth (3,4).

EPIDEMIOLOGY AND ECONOMICAL IMPACT

Although there is no worldwide study that uses any single criterion for constipation, data from single country surveys are available for extrapolation. A systematic review of the literature showed that the prevalence of constipation in North America ranges from 1.9% to 27.2% (with most studies reporting from 12% to 19%). Prevalence estimates by gender support a female:male ratio of 2.2:1 in most studies, but others show a very small female:male prevalence ratio (5). Recent studies from Sweden found that 4.3% females and 1.7% males reported less than 3 bowel movements per week (6). A New Zealand survey showed that 4.9% of responders were already using laxatives due to constipation, while another 26.2% increased fiber to avoid constipation (7). In addition, constipation tends to increase with age and the prevalence increases after the age of 65 (5,8).

The economical impact of constipation can easily be seen by the sale of over-the-counter laxatives. Sales have increased from $325 million in 1986 to $725 million in 1995 and $825 million in 2000 in the United States (9–11). According to Wald (12), only one-third of constipated patients seek medical help. Review of data from the 2001 National Ambulatory Medical Care Survey and the 2001 National Hospital Ambulatory Medical Care Survey showed that >5.7 million outpatient physician visits occurred in 2001 due to constipation-related problems. Constipation was the primary diagnosis in more than 2.4 millions visits to physician offices (44%), hospital outpatient clinics (51%), and emergency rooms (56%) in this review (13). The 2001 study of National Hospital Discharge Survey reported 282,161 (95% CI: 247,554–316,768) inpatient hospitalizations with a medical diagnosis of constipation, while 38,361 (95% CI: 30,647–46,075) had constipation as the primary diagnosis at discharge (13). In 1996, Rantis et al. (14) calculated the mean cost of only the diagnostic evaluation of chronic constipation to be $2752 ($1150–4792) per patient.

DEFINITIONS AND CRITERIA OF CONSTIPATION

The long-standing criteria define constipation as the frequency of bowel movements. Less than three bowel movements per week were considered a pathological finding. This definition was based on a 1965 publication in *British Medical Journal*, which showed that 99% of responders (factory workers) had three bowel movement per day to three bowel movements per week (15). More frequent than the number of bowel movements were the patient's complaints relative to hardness of stool, straining, and the feeling of incomplete evacuation.

In 1978, Manning (16) developed criteria to distinguish patients with IBS from those who had structural (organic) diseases of the gastrointestinal tract. These criteria were transformed and modified into Rome I, and subsequently Rome II criteria.

After 1999, all prior definitions of constipation were included in the Rome II criteria of functional gastrointestinal disorders, which describes functional constipation as at least 12 weeks of constipation, which need not be consecutive, in the preceding 12 months with two or more signs or symptoms of: (1) straining >25% of defecations, (2) lumpy or hard stools >25% of defecations, (3) sensation of incomplete evacuation >1/4 of defecations, (4) sensation of anorectal obstruction/blockage >25% of defecations, (5) manual maneuvers to facilitate >25% of defecations (e.g., digital evacuation, support of the pelvic floor), and/or (6) <3 defecations per week; loose stools are not a criterion for IBS (17,18).

Despite being described for almost decades, the Rome II criteria are not typically used by most physicians except gastroenterologists. In a study conducted at Vanderbilt University Medical Center, 166 physicians in various levels of training were enrolled, including 24 surgeons (13 general). Some surgical specialists were less familiar with the Rome II criteria than internists and gastroenterologists (19), only one of whom was using it. Physicians who used the criteria clinically included 12 of 18 gastroenterologists and 7 of 34 internists.

It was estimated that approximately 63 million Americans meet Rome II criteria for constipation (5). The average American consumes approximately 5 to 14 grams of fiber per day, which is only 16% to 50% of the recommended amount by American Dietetic Association (20). The majority of constipated Americans receive adequate treatment by primary care physicians and gastroenterologists. Typical recommendations include a healthy, well balanced diet with adequate fiber (about 20–30 g) adequate water intake (about 1/2 gallon or 2 liters or 8–10 glasses of liquid are required per day) and physical activity. Despite these basic maneuvers, many patients with constipation are referred to a variety of medical specialists or self-refer to specialist due to persistent symptoms.

EVALUATION AND INITIAL REPORT

The initial colorectal evaluation rules out secondary causes of constipation from primary functional constipation. Secondary causes are (1) structural in origin (cancer, strictures, Crohn's disease, and diverticular disease), (2) metabolic and/or endocrine disorders (hypothyroidism, hyperparathyroidism, diabetes, MEN IIb syndrome, and pregnancy), (3) psychoneurological pathologies (Parkinson's disease, multiple sclerosis, spinal cord post-traumatic damages and lesions, depression, herpes zoster, and individuals with intellectual disability), (21) (4) side effects of medication (antacids, anticonvulsants, anticholinergics, opioid analgesics, antidepressants, and calcium channel blockers).

Exclusion of these conditions is essential in determining whether a functional type of constipation exists.

The differential diagnosis of constipation is complex. Careful history taking is extremely important and includes in-depth social and psychological questioning. Specific questions regarding the presence or absence of multiple sclerosis, Parkinson's disease, hypothyroidism, history of sexual abuse, food intake, or a family history of constipation are important. Certain conditions can be ruled out based on history alone such as a long-standing condition (since childhood) may suggest Hirschsprung's disease. Young, urban woman with social and work-related stress and insomnia, with a recent onset of constipation and no other medical history may be indications of depression. A recent onset of constipation, associated with bleeding, mucous discharge, vomiting, crampy abdominal pain, weight loss, or melena, especially if the patient is above 50 years of age, should be suspect for cancer until proven otherwise. Patients should be queried about important factors such as dietary habits, medications (prescription and over-the-counter), and lifestyle. Utilization of the Rome II criteria is useful to help characterize constipation. Questions about assisted defecation, including digitation, manual support of the perineum, and digital posterior vaginal wall pressure, are useful to rule out outlet type of constipation.

Physical examination is extremely important. The abdominal examination may show abdominal masses, ascites, hernias, and other abnormalities. A perineal examination is mandatory. Examining the perineum using a Ritter table with the patient in the prone-jackknife position is our preferred method. This position is well tolerated by most patients and allows excellent visualization of the perineum, anus, distal rectum, and the vagina. A digital rectal examination can detect masses in the distal rectum, the presence of an anterior rectocele, loss of sensation in a specific dermatomal distribution, and the presence of excessive perineal descent, and allows for the evaluation of sphincter tone at rest and squeeze and the absence of puborectalis muscle relaxation. Prior to an anorectal examination, patients are asked to take two Fleet™ (Fleets phosphosoda, Lynchburg, Virginia, U.S.A.) enemas to empty the rectum of stool. While various types of anoscopes exist, we prefer the Henkle James SR anoscope—a side viewing slotted anoscope. Anoscopy should be performed in addition to digital rectal examination. If any abnormal findings are detected during the initial examination, further diagnostic testing may be ordered. Diagnostic colonoscopy is typically performed in all patients older than 30 years of age and based on severity of symptoms in younger patients as part of the initial workup for constipation.

Once a structural etiology of constipation is ruled out, a diagnosis of functional constipation is reasonable. Functional constipation can be divided into three major types: (1) constipation-predominant irritable bowel syndrome (IBS); (2) obstructive defecation, also known as pelvic floor dyssynergia, dyssynergic defecation, anismus, or outlet obstruction; and (3) "slow transit constipation" or "colonic inertia," which is characterized by a prolonged length of time for stool to pass through the entire colon (22,23).

In a study of 277 patients with constipation, only 11% were found to have "slow transit constipation," 13% had "pelvic floor dysfunction," and 5% had a combination of both. The vast majority of cases (71%) had IBS (24). Thus, the initial treatment of constipation should be to treat the patient's symptoms with lifestyle modifications, over-the-counter and prescription medications, and fiber and fluids.

The initial approach for treatment of constipation includes explaining to the patient the misconceptions related to defecation and constipation in an extensive and simplified form. This includes dispelling the ideas of "autointoxication" and the obligated bowel movement per day (3), encouraging physical activity, and advising patients not to neglect the call to stool. A dietary assessment with increased fiber intake with bulking agents (20–30 g/day dietary fiber with 8–10 glasses of water or other noncaffeinated liquid intake) as an initial treatment should be presented to the patient (25).

Specific attention should be paid to IBS-related constipation. A recent meta-analysis of 51 double-blind clinical IBS trials showed that the recommendation of fiber and bulking agents in the treatment of IBS constipation was weak. Supplemental fiber may be even worse than a normal diet and may aggravate symptoms such as pain and bloating. Abnormal bacterial fermentation of fiber, the absence of normal methanogenic flora and altered gas handling may induce bloating and abdominal pain with increased fiber. But bulking agents can be successfully used in non-IBS constipation (26,27).

The initial treatment of constipation is typically given for six months and, if therapy fails to improve, further investigational anorectal physiology studies are indicated. Investigation studies can be divided into several types based on methods of functional analysis (Table 1).

Anorectal Manometry

The principal purpose of anorectal manometry is to rule out adult-onset or short-segment Hirschsprung's disease (28). The protocol at Cleveland Clinic Florida, for example, is to perform anal manometry consisting of two parts: (1) estimating sphincter pressure, including resting, squeezing pressures, and the high pressure zone of the anal canal; and (2) sensation determination, including evaluation of the presence of the rectoanal inhibitory reflex, estimation of rectal first sensation volume, and maximum tolerable volume with pressure evaluation for rectal compliance calculations. See chapter 3 for specific instructions on performing anorectal manometry.

Table 1 Functional Analysis of Constipation

Methods estimating function:
Anal manometry (evaluating sphincters, rectum), including balloon expulsion test
Electromyography (evaluating sphincters)
Pudendal nerve terminal motor latency (examining pudendal nerve conductivity)
Direct visualizing function methods:
Cinedefecogram (which evaluates rectum, pelvic floor muscles)
Dynamic MRI defecography (rectum, pelvic floor muscles)
Single capsule Sitz-Mark study (slow colonic transit)
Indirect visualizing methods:
Breath hydrogen concentration test
Estimation of plasma sulfapyridine
Scintigraphic defecography

Balloon Expulsion Test

The balloon expulsion test was first described by Barnes as a diagnostic tool for obstructed defecation. This test can be performed at the time of manometry (See chap. 3). Normal individuals should be able to evacuate the balloon without difficulty. Failure to do so after five attempts is suggestive, but not diagnostic, of obstructed defecation.

Cinedefecography

The purpose of cinedefecography is to provide a dynamic characterization of the interaction between the anal sphincter complex, puborectalis muscle, and the rectum to help define abnormalities in the pelvic floor. Cinedefecography is a real-time video image of the patient defecating. It is a diagnostic tool of the functional origin of obstructed defecation. Obstructed defecation can be PPC (also known as nonrelaxing puborectalis syndrome, dyskinetic puborectalis, paradoxical puborectalis, and anismus). It is used to detect an anatomical (mechanical) origin of obstructed defecation such as anterior and posterior rectocele, sigmoidocele, enterocele, mucosal and full thickness rectal prolapse, intussusception, or solitary rectal ulcer.

Cinedefecography is one of the two tests (the other being electromyography (EMG), discussed later) capable of diagnosing PPC. Criteria to make this diagnosis include failure of the anorectal angle (ARA) to open, persistence of the puborectalis impression on the rectum, and incomplete or delayed rectal emptying. Other findings consistent with PPC include a capacious rectum on lateral X-ray film, a long and persistently closed anal canal, ballooning of the rectum, and the presence of a compensatory anatomic abnormality such as a rectocele.

Cinedefecography may show abnormalities which may or may not be clinically relevant. One must determine the role that these abnormalities play, if any, in the patient's symptoms. For example, for an anterior rectocele to be a significant factor in obstructed defecation, defecography will need to show on straining that the propulsive forces will be directed into the rectocele rather than toward the anus (redirection of forces) and, on postevacuation images, retained contrast in the rectocele (nonemptying rectocele).

Enteroceles and sigmoidoceles are diagnosed when a loop of small bowel or sigmoid colon descend into the pelvis during straining. Although these conditions are a common finding on dynamic defecography, they typically have no physiologic significance. In a few patients, the loop of small bowel or sigmoid colon will place pressure on the anterior, lateral, or posterior surface of the rectum, which can narrow the rectum or obliterate the anorectal outlet. Jorge et al. (29) were among the first to describe a sigmoidocele and proposed a classification system to determine their significance. Sigmoidoceles were found to be present in 5.2% of 463 consecutive cinedefecographies performed for constipation, half of which impaired rectal emptying. Internal intussusception or internal prolapse in some cases was associated with solitary rectal ulcers and constipation. Shorvon et al. (30) showed that a significant number of patients without any complaints of constipation or difficulty in defecation have this radiographic finding with straining.

The radiation exposure of this test is approximately 0.6 mSv for males and 3 to 7 mSv for females, which is three times less than that of a standard barium enema. Although the over all dose of radiation to the body is less, the local dose of radiation to the pelvis is higher for cinedefecography. This is important since the majority of patients being evaluated with

Table 2 Normal Values

Measurement	Normal values
Anorectal angle (degree)	
Resting	70–140
Squeezing	75–90
Pushing	100–180
Perineal descent (cm)	
Resting	3–4
Pushing	6–8
Puborectalis length (cm)	
Resting	14–16
Squeezing	12–15
Pushing	15–18

defecography are women and ovarian exposure to radiation is not trivial but acceptable when the test is indicated. Prior to defogram, women of childbearing age need to be assessed for pregnancy status, as with all radiographic studies. See chapter 3 for technique of performing cinedefecography.

Static defecography is used to measure the ARA, perineal descent, and puborectalis length at rest, squeeze, and pushing. The difference between rest and maximal push is calculated for each measurement to assess pelvic floor dynamics. The most common definition of the ARA is the angle between the axis of the anal canal and the distal half of the posterior rectal wall (31). Regardless of the technique used or the exact angle measured, the ARA becomes more acute during squeeze due to the contraction of the puborectalis to defer defecation and becomes more obtuse during relaxation of the puborectalis. It is not helpful to compare exact values among patients. More importantly, the test provides a basis for relative comparison of a dynamic process for each individual. Perineal descent is defined by measuring the vertical distance between the position of the ARA and a fixed plane, usually the pubococcygeal line (PCL). Table 2 shows normal values associated with cinedefecography.

Some centers have described four-contrast defecography known as "pelvic floor-oscopy" to help better delineate the pelvic anatomy (32,33). Although this type of defecography may better delineate the pelvic anatomy, no study comparing it to standard cinedefecography has been performed, thus it is unclear whether this truly adds any other clinically relevant information.

Dynamic Magnetic Resonance Imaging Defecography

An alternative to cinedefecography is dynamic magnetic resonance imaging (MRI) defecography. This is a new imaging modality using MRI. It has several advantages such as elimination of radiation exposure, examination of all pelvic floor compartments, precise relationship to bony landmarks, and reduction of interobserver variability. The disadvantage of this procedure is that the study is not truly dynamic. In closed MRI defecography, the patient is expelling contrast in the supine position, which is not the natural position for defecation. Also using an endorectal coil (3 cm in diameter) is not very comfortable and may alter defecation dynamics. There is also a tenfold increase in the cost of dynamic MRI compared to standard cinedefecography (34).

Electromyography

EMG is visual and auditory recording of the electrical activity of the external anal sphincter and puborectalis muscles. Currently, there are four techniques of anal EMG evaluation: concentric needle EMG, surface EMG, single-fiber EMG, and wire electrode EMG (35,36). EMG helps to diagnose altered patterns of anal sphincter and pelvic floor muscle contraction and relaxation associated with constipation including PPC. Chapter 3 outlines the techniques of performing the various types of EMG evaluation.

Pudendal Nerve Terminal Motor Latency

Approximately 25% of patients with constipation have a prolonged pudendal nerve terminal motor latency (PNTML), which is more characteristic in fecal incontinence. This test determines if chronic injury of the pudendal nerve is present. This is associated with chronic straining as a result of obstructed defecation (rectal prolapse, increased perineal descent, among others).

Knowledge of whether a neuropathy is present can help in therapeutic decision-making (35–37). PNTML evaluates the time (latency) from intrarectal stimulation of pudendal nerve to muscle response (compound muscle action potential). See chapter 3 for specific technique of performing PNTML.

Colonic Transit Study

Colonic transit study is used to diagnose slow colonic transit constipation. This single capsule Sitzmark™, which contains 24 radio-opaque markers and is ingested by the patient, is the most frequent colonic transit study used. In patients with normal motility, at least 80% of the markers will have passed through the entire colon and be found in the rectum or completely evacuated by day 5. If five or more radio-opaque markers have not reached the rectum by day 5, then the study results are consistent with an abnormal colonic transit study. If the majority of markers are in the distal colon and rectum, obstructed defecation should be suspected. See chapter 3 for the specific technique of performing colonic transit study.

Scintigraphic Defecography

Another method available to study colonic transit is scintigraphic defecography, using specially designed methacrylate-coated capsules (pH-sensitive coating—pH milleu of 7.2–7.4) containing 111In or 99mTc, which dissolve in the terminal ileum. In over 90% of cases, the radiolabeled pellets or charcoal are released as a bolus in the terminal ileum or right colon. The Mayo Clinic experience has shown a high correlation between this technique and the standard Sitzmark study in a highly selective group of patients. An advantage of scintigraphy, as demonstrated by multiple studies in the literature, is that in addition to colonic transit, gastric emptying and small bowel transit can be evaluated as part of the same test.

Breath Hydrogen Concentration Test

If any signs of a prolonged orocecal transit are noted (vomiting or nausea), constipation may be part of a diffuse gastrointestinal dysmotility disorder known as "pan-enteric inertia." Thus, the exclusion of delayed gastric emptying and abnormal small-bowel transit should be performed. Gastric emptying can be assessed with standard radiological means. Evaluation of small-bowel transit time is routinely done with the determination of a breath hydrogen concentration test. It measures the time required for the appearance of hydrogen peak in the expelled breath, after the oral intake of lactulose or baked beans, which are metabolized by colonic lactobacillus. Another test is based on the same principle—estimation of plasma sulfapyridine, a metabolite of orally administered salicylazosulfapyridine. This requires about 300 mL of blood with similar to breath hydrogen limitations.

In our institution, routine physiological studies in constipated patients include (1) anal manometry, (2) cinedefecography, (3) electromyography, and (4) single capsule Sitzmark study. If there are any signs of prolonged orocecal transit such as delayed gastric emptying or biliary dyskinesia, patients should also undergo breath hydrogen concentration test with lactulose to assess small-bowel transit time.

FAILURE OF CONSERVATIVE TREATMENT

If initial conservative treatment fails to resolve constipation, anorectal physiology evaluation should be performed. If these tests fail to find any pathological causes of constipation, this condition should be considered idiopathic. Conversely, functional or anatomic causes may be found.

Laxatives

Laxatives can be used as the next step in the conservative treatment scheme, starting with osmotic laxatives (magnesium and sodium derivatives, polyethylene glycol (PEG), and lactulose). The use of stimulant laxatives (senna and diphenylmethane derivates, castor oil, and docusates) should be limited due to their multiple side effects (38). One should be aware of possible myenteric plexus damage, melanosis coli, and possible neoplastic changes due to chronic abuse of the senna-based laxatives.

Pharmacotherapy

Pharmacotherapy of constipation still has relatively few safe medications. For example, a selective 5-HT_4 receptor agonist (tegaserod, Zelnorm) has shown efficacy in providing relief from the symptoms of chronic constipation, but was recently withdrawn from the U.S. market due to the related increase of heart attacks and strokes.

One of the novel agents that is available is lubiprostone (Amitiza), which is a bicyclic functional fatty acid that acts locally as a selective chloride channel (ClC-2) activator in the apical membrane of the intestinal epithelium causing an increase in water secretion and intestinal motility (39). Clinical trials did not demonstrate alteration of serum sodium or potassium concentrations (40).

Recent changes in the understanding of the pathogenesis of constipation-predominant IBS clarified success of selective low dose serotonin reuptake inhibitors or tricyclic antidepressants in the gastroenterologic practice (41,42). It is interesting to note that the desired effect is achieved at doses lower than those used to treat depression. Serotonin reuptake inhibitors play the most significant role in global symptoms and thus improving the quality of life in IBS patients (43). Although the common explanation of their effect is through the facilitation of endogenous endorphin release and the blockade of reuptake leading to enhancement of descending inhibitory pain pathways, the psychoform mechanism of action in IBS needs to be more thoroughly investigated (44,45).

There are reports in the literature citing the successful use of misoprostol (46,47) and colchicine (48,49). However, their role in the treatment of constipation is yet to be determined. In patients with both idiopathic constipation and functional/anatomical obstructed defecation, treatment should be combined with biofeedback. Failure of biofeedback along with progressively increasing complaints and a decreasing quality of life may result in a colectomy. As a last therapeutic option for patients, one may consider a permanent colostomy/ileostomy.

Biofeedback Therapy

Biofeedback therapy is aimed at "retraining" the anal sphincter and pelvic floor muscles physiologically using behavioral techniques. Biofeedback uses special external devices that demonstrate and alter "errors" of defecation with audio/visual feedback, which the patient sees; its principle is based on recognition of previously unrecognized body functions, which were thought to be uncontrolled. This recognition gives the patient the ability to practice defecation functions and improve the effectiveness of the defecation process. Biofeedback is associated with a high success rate ranging from 22% to 100% for obstructed defecation and 12% to 77.8% for idiopathic constipation with no reported morbidity (50,51).

The most common biofeedback technique uses either manometric or EMG instrumentation to monitor physiologic function. Manometric biofeedback uses an intrarectal balloon with pressure sensors, while the EMG method uses either surface electrodes attached to the perineal skin or intra-anal sensors. A computer display with light bars will convert these signals from sensors to feedback while the patient and biofeedback therapist can interpret the changes.

Nonstandard biofeedback training consists of 3 to 10, 1-hour sessions under the supervision of a trained biofeedback therapist. In addition, patients are instructed to keep a daily diary of bowel movements, medications, and the use of enemas, laxatives, or digitations, to aide in monitoring improvement of biofeedback therapy.

MANAGEMENT OF SPECIFIC FORMS OF CONSTIPATION

There are two types of constipation typically evaluated and treated by colorectal surgeons. Obstructive defecation, also known as pelvic floor dyssynergia, dyssynergic defecation, anismus or outlet obstruction, is one type; this type can be further subdivided into functional origin, such as nonrelaxing puborectalis syndrome (dyskinetic puborectalis, PPC) or anatomic (mechanical) origin, (anterior or posterior rectocele, sigmoidocele, enterocele, mucosal and full thickness rectal prolapse, intussusception, or solitary rectal ulcer). The latter is known as "slow transit constipation" or "colonic inertia" (22,23).

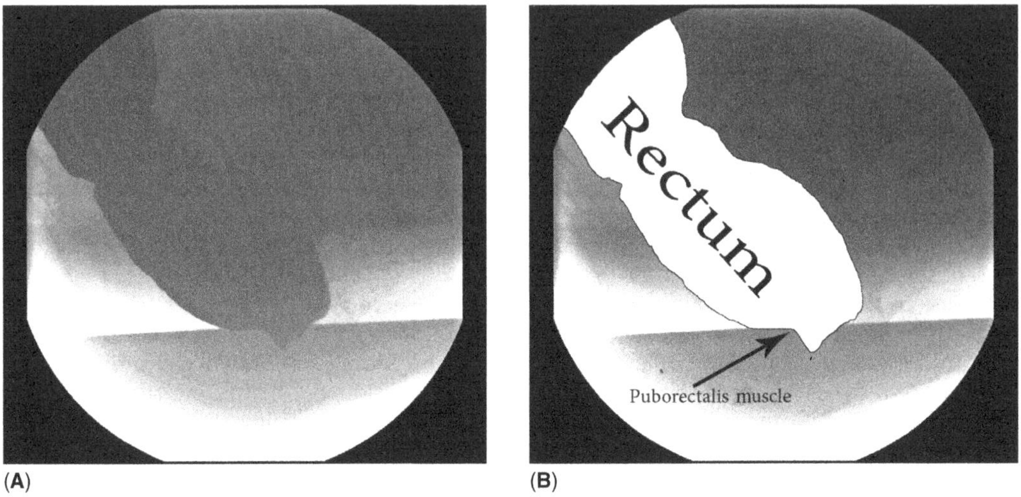

Figure 1 (**A**, **B**) Cinedefecography of PPC at rest.

Paradoxical Puborectalis Contraction

The puborectalis muscle is a striated U-shaped sling in the medial portion of the levator ani muscle. Its anterior-directed contraction is an important component of continence. In normal defecation, there is a voluntary relaxation of the external anal sphincter and the pelvic floor muscles, including the puborectalis muscle. Failure of the puborectalis to relax or paradoxical contraction of the muscle with further constipation can result in obstructed defecation. Although the etiology of PPC is unknown, many investigators feel it is one finding of a more generalized pelvic floor disorder with an associated significant psychological component. Patients with PPC typically complain of straining, splinting, the need to digitate during defecation, tenesmus, and the feeling of incomplete evacuation. They may also require suppositories and enemas to defecate. Digital rectal examination often reveals hypertonia or spasm of the puborectalis muscle. Anal manometry may show an increased length of the anal canal (>4 cm). The main diagnostic tool for PPC is cinedefecography (Figs. 1–6).

Although cinedefecography is superior to EMG in diagnosing PPC, ideally a combination of both tests should be used (52). Treatment of PPC includes standard initial conservative therapy with diet and lifestyle changes (success rate 55–100%). Subsequent treatment with biofeedback therapy in patients who fail initial conservative treatment is successful in 30% to 100% of patients (51). If biofeedback therapy fails, botulinum toxin type A injection into the puborectalis muscle

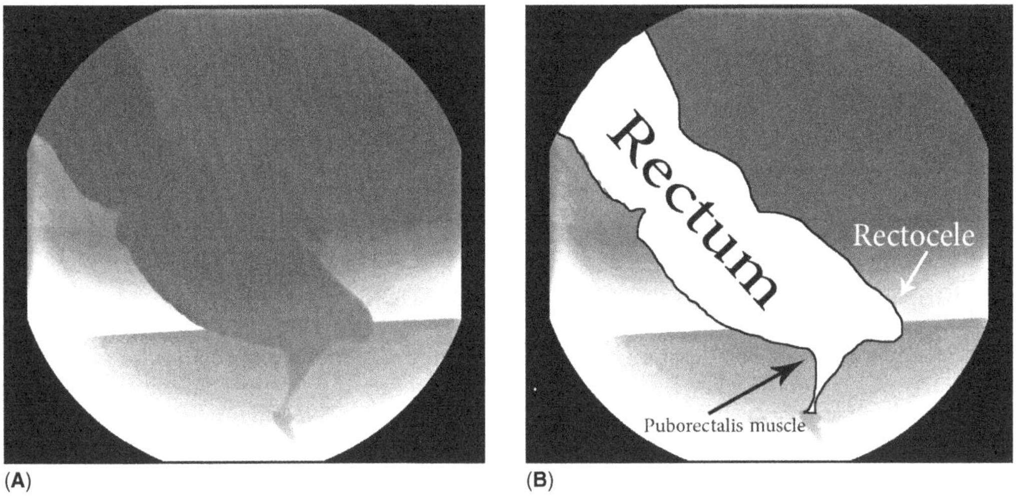

Figure 2 (**A**, **B**) Cinedefecography of PPC at push.

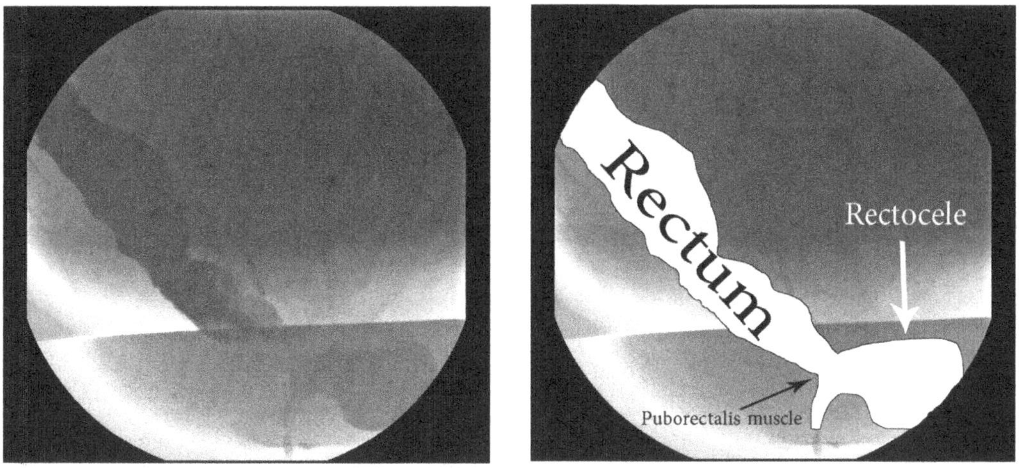

(A) (B)

Figure 3 (**A**, **B**) Cinedefecography of PPC at push showing the nonrelaxation of the pubeorectalis muscle and significant anterior rectocele.

and external anal sphincter may be performed with success rates ranging from 50% to 75% (53–55). Although surgical treatment has been used in the past, it is generally noneffective. Partial resection, posterior division, or simple anal dilation have all been associated with poor outcomes in patients with PPC.

Rectocele

Rectocele, an outpouching or protrusion of the rectal wall is very common in women with pelvic floor disorders and is commonly found in the asymptomatic patient; 17% of male patients with constipation have rectocele (56). The pathogenesis of the condition in males is related to rectal pressures that are higher than those in the vagina in females. Fascial defects of the rectovaginal septum after childbirth, constipation, or conditions that lead to increased abdominal pressure promote protrusion of rectal contents toward the vagina. In females, the typical clinical presentation is a protrusion of the rectum into the posterior vaginal wall (Figs. 7–10) (57).

The clinical significance of rectoceles is still debatable. Differences in terminology between a urogynecological and colorectal practice make this situation more confusing. Recent reviews have stressed the importance of standardizing the terminology; one author performed a methodological review of the gynecologic and colorectal literature on rectoceles (58). He concluded that

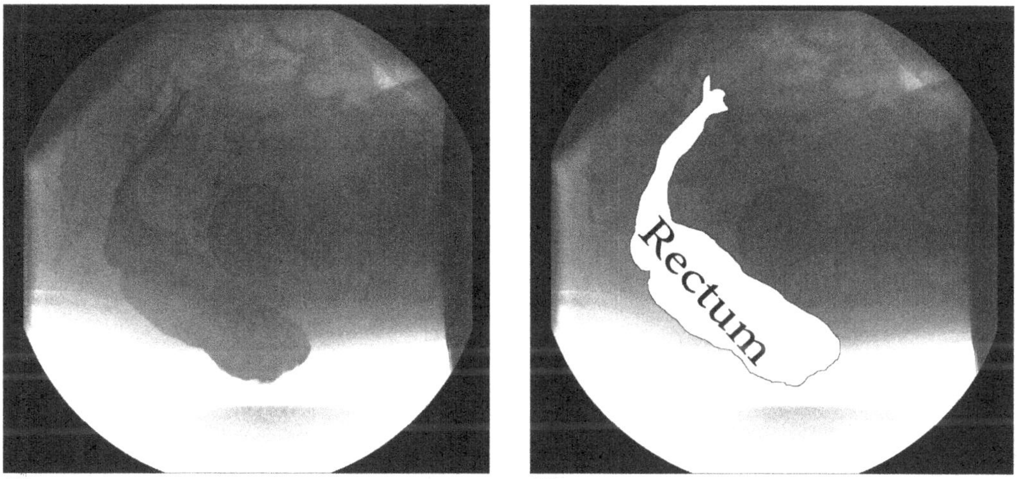

(A) (B)

Figure 4 (**A**, **B**) Cinedefecography of PPC at rest.

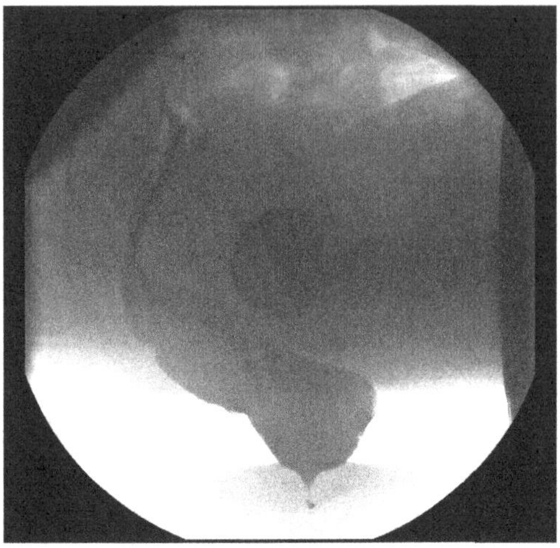

(A)

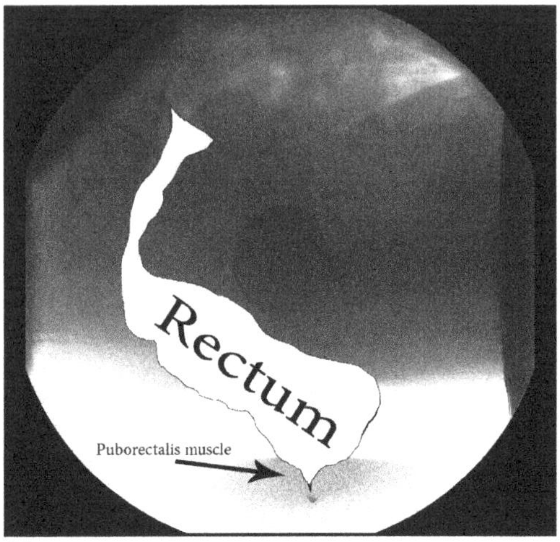

(B)

Figure 5 (A, B) Cinedefecography of PPC at push.

the terms "posterior colpocele" and "rectocele" are simply anatomical descriptive terms and that they need to be adopted when appropriate. These conditions are frequently asymptomatic findings. The terms cannot be adopted as synonyms of possible clinical problems that may be related to them such as vaginal bulging obstructed defecation and dyspareunia. The author noted that the patient's symptoms and quality of life, rather than the variability in terminology, should be the primary concern.

Rectoceles may cause mild-to-severe anorectal symptoms, such as perineal pressure, the sensation of a pouch in the vagina, or incomplete evacuation requiring rectal or vaginal digitations or perineal support. Additional evaluation by a gynecologist or a urologist may be requested if other pelvic floor abnormalities are noted. In some institutions, patients are selected for surgery according to the size of the rectocele (>3 cm), the inability to empty the rectocele at cinedefecography, or the use of digitation or perineal support provided in order to empty the rectum. Rectoceles can be repaired via a transvaginal, transrectal, or transperineal approach with or without the use of mesh. The choice of procedure and the route of procedure are typically based on the specialty, with colorectal surgeons using a transanal approach, while urogynecologists use a perineal/vaginal route (59). Overall success rates vary from 65% to 100% (Table 3) (60,61).

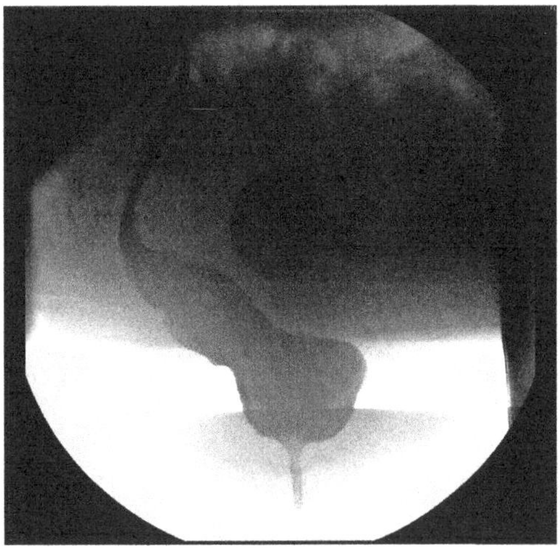

(A)

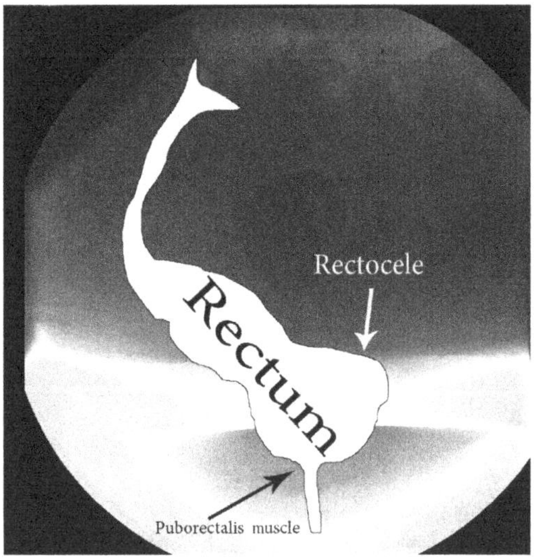

(B)

Figure 6 (A, B) Cinedefecography of PPC at push showing nonrelaxing puborectalis muscle "notch" above the anal canal.

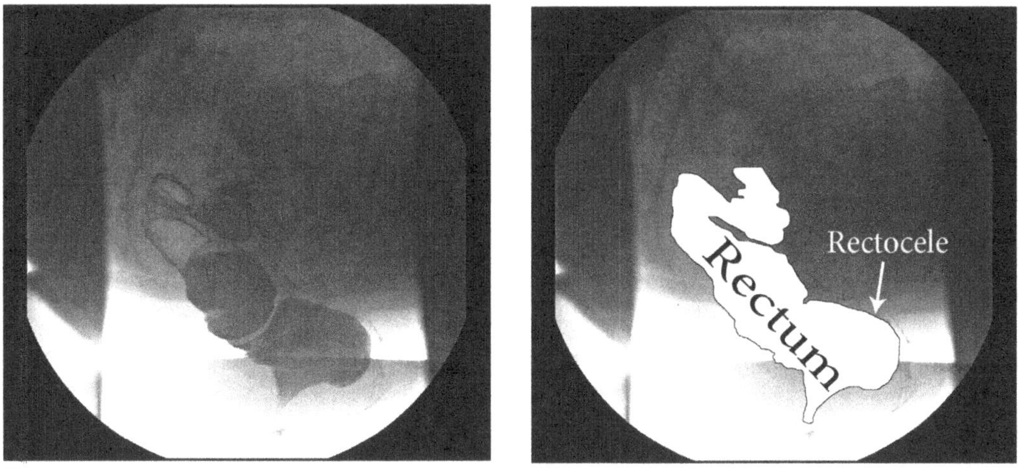

(**A**) (**B**)

Figure 7 (**A**, **B**) Cinedefecography of anterior rectocele at rest.

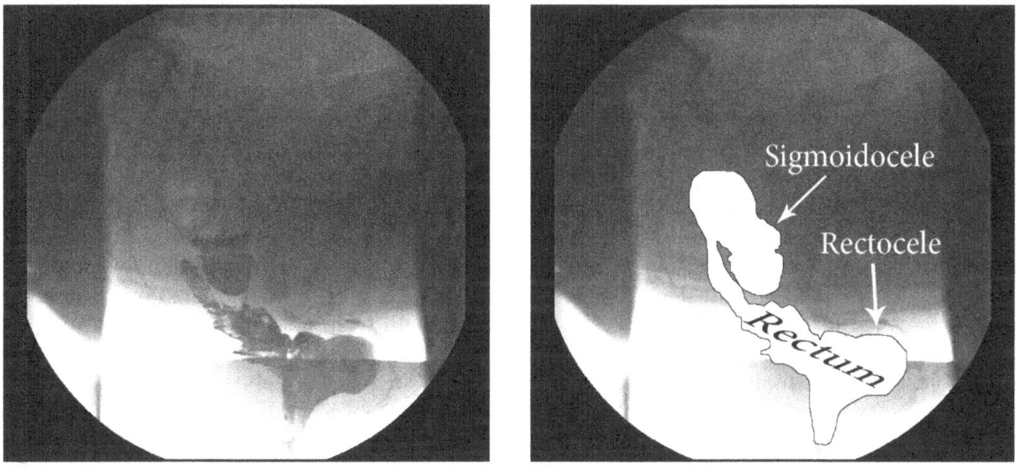

(**A**) (**B**)

Figure 8 (**A**, **B**) Cinedefecography of anterior rectocele postevacuatory, showing the significant rectocele, sigmoidocele 2 degree, and rectal intussusception.

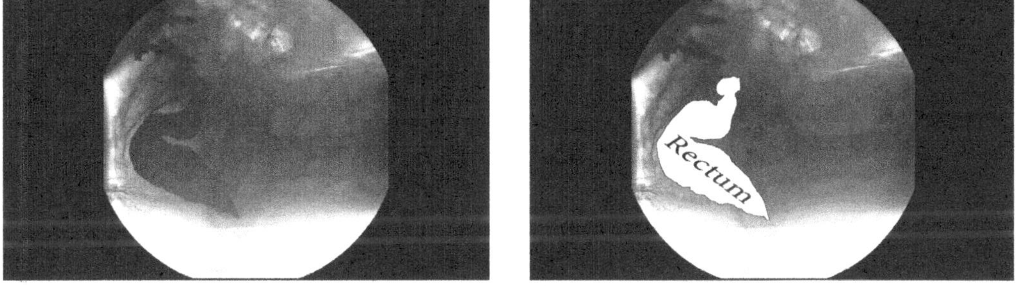

(**A**) (**B**)

Figure 9 (**A**, **B**) Cinedefecography of anterior rectocele at rest.

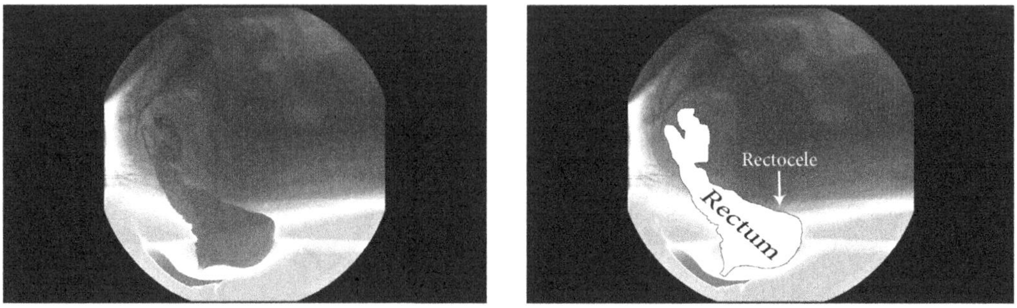

(A) (B)

Figure 10 (**A**, **B**) Cinedefecography of anterior rectocele postevacuatory.

Cul-De-Sac Hernias (Sigmoidocele and Enterocele)

Approximately 8.3% to 11% of constipated patients who undergo anorectal physiology tests have cul-de-sac hernias—also known as sigmoidoceles or enteroceles. A sigmoidocele is a protrusion of the peritoneum between the rectum and vagina that contains the sigmoid colon. An enterocele is a protrusion of the peritoneum between the rectum and vagina containing the small intestine (Figs. 11–14) (63).

These conditions are often diagnosed in females who have previously undergone hysterectomy and may coexist with other abnormalities of obstructed defecation (31,63).

Commonly used systems evaluating the degree of descent of the lowest portion of the sigmoid colon or small bowel in cinedefecography include first degree—intrapelvic, but not surpassing the PCL; second degree—below PCL, but above ischiococcygeal line (ICL); and third degree—below the ICL (29).

In our institution, a diagnosis of enterocele is made when the rectal outline with contrast is divided from the vaginal outline. First- and second-degree sigmoidoceles are often normal anatomic variants. A nonemptying sigmoidocele can be the cause of incomplete evacuation. Patients with first- and second-degree sigmoidocele can be conservatively treated with biofeedback therapy, while third-degree sigmoidoceles may benefit from operative therapy. When the symptoms of obstructed defecation impair the quality of life, surgical treatment, namely, sigmoid colectomy, is usually performed in an open or laparoscopic manner. Other procedures such as subtotal colectomy and rectopexy with or without obliteration of the Douglas pouch may also be used, as well as transvaginal repair (64,65).

Table 3 Rectocele Repair: Type of Procedure and Approach

Approach	Main step	Functional improvement (%)[a]	Dyspareunia (%)[a]	Recurrence of symptoms (%)[a]
Transvaginal				
Posterior colpoperineorrhaphy	Plication of levator muscles in the midline and redundant vaginal wall resection	60–90	9–50	7–33
Fascia defect repair	Discrete fascial defects repair	35–88	2–46	18–44
Transperineal				
Without mesh	Strengthening of rectovaginal septum with levators plication	64–100	NA	9–15
With mesh	Strengthening of rectovaginal septum with levators placation + mesh	80–100	5–69	6
Transrectal		38–100	NA	30–67

[a]Based on studies from the literature.

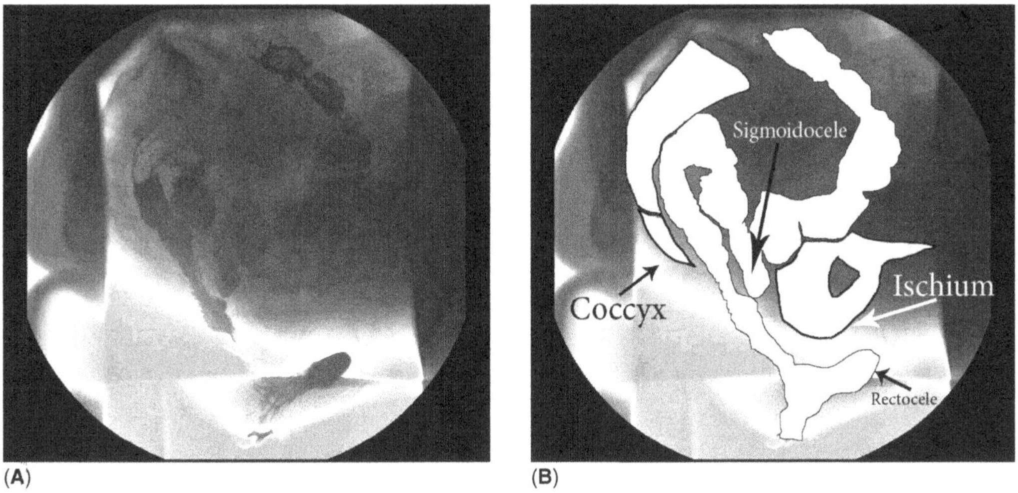

Figure 11 (**A**, **B**) Cinedefecography of sigmoidocele 2 degree.

Rectal Intussusception (Internal Rectal Prolapse, Internal Procidentia)

Rectal intussusception is a circumferential infolding of the midrectal wall into, but not beyond, the anal verge and occurs during defecation (67). Although rectal intussusception is a common finding in defecography in constipated patients, it can also be found in 1/3 of asymptomatic patients (Figs. 15–18) (67,68).

Treatment of intussusception is generally conservative. However, surgical repair is warranted when the intussusception progresses to full thickness rectal prolapse or, in some cases, when symptoms persist despite conservative therapy. One of the novel techniques established for repair of intussusception is the double stapled transanal rectal resection (STARR) procedure (69–74). The STARR procedure is based on the stapled hemorrhoidopexy technique Procedure for Prolapse and Hemorrhoids (PPH), originally presented by Antonio Longo in Italy (76). The STARR procedure requires two circular staplers that produce a circumferential transanal full-thickness resection of the rectal wall redundancy. Various authors have reported recurrence rates from 0% to 5% after 6 to 24 months of follow-up. There has been some data suggesting 33% recurrence rate after the STARR procedure (76) and there are also reports of rectovaginal fistulas related to this procedure (77,78).

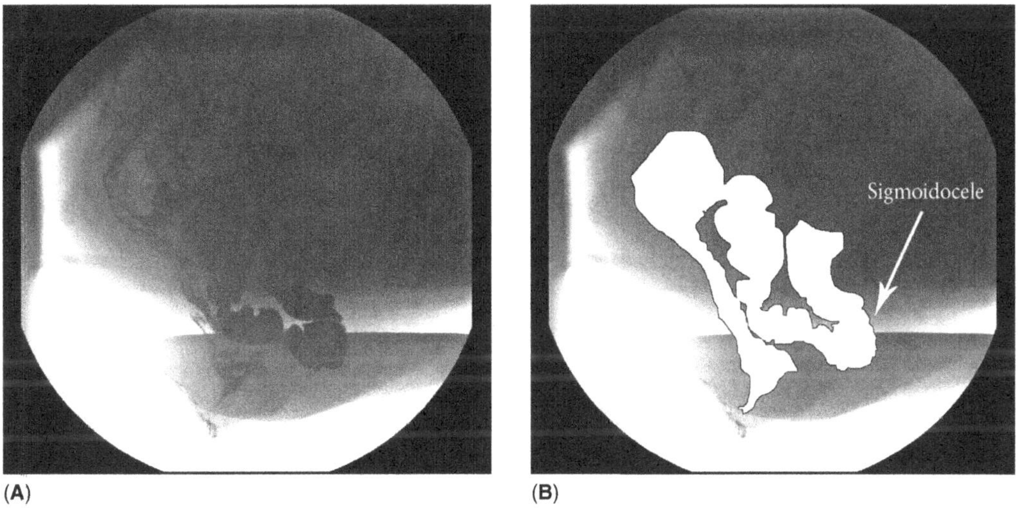

Figure 12 (**A**, **B**) Cinedefecography of sigmoidocele 3 degree.

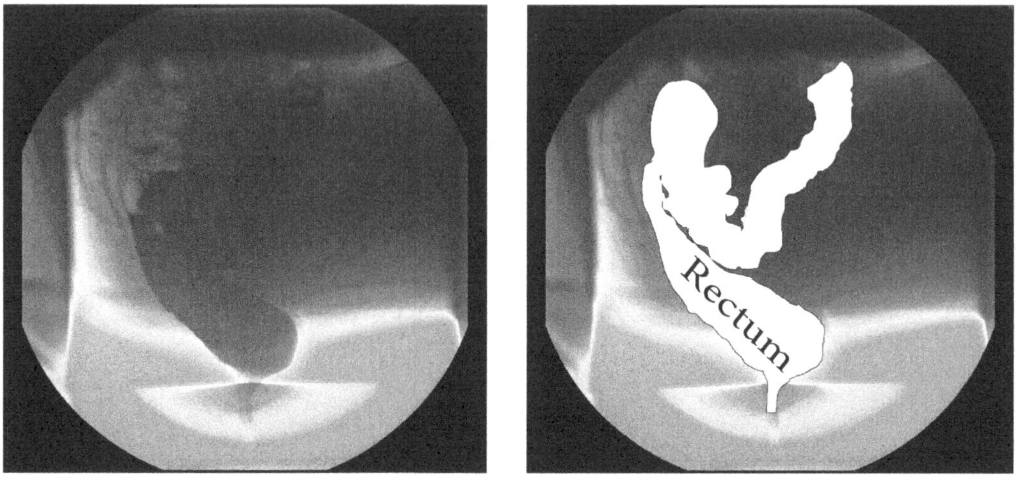

(A) (B)

Figure 13 (**A**, **B**) Cinedefecography of sigmoidocele 3 degree at rest.

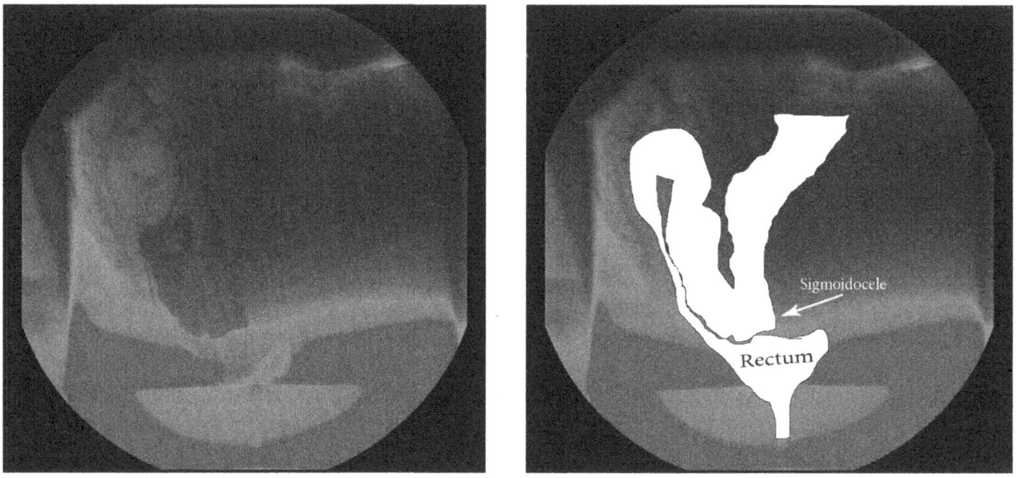

(A) (B)

Figure 14 (**A**, **B**) Cinedefecography of sigmoidocele 3 degree at push.

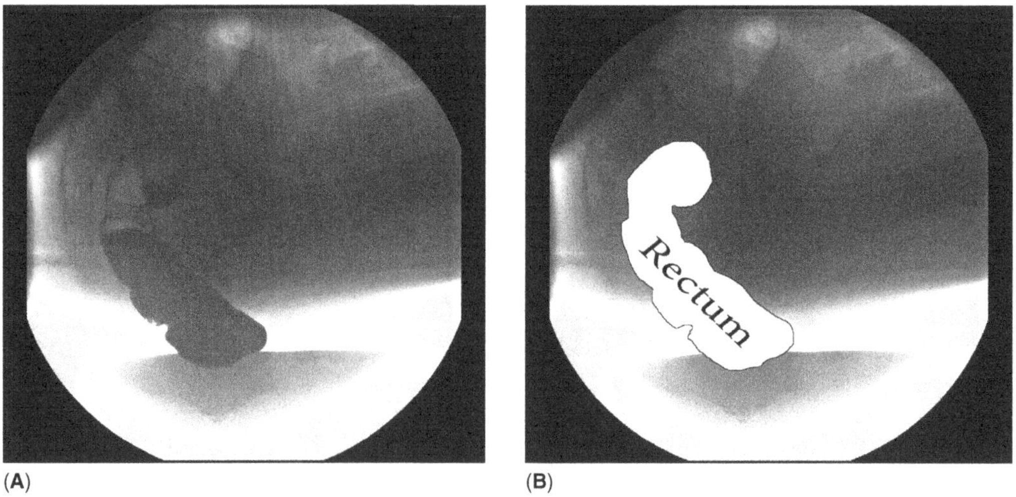

(A) (B)

Figure 15 (**A**, **B**) Cinedefecography of rectal intussusception at rest.

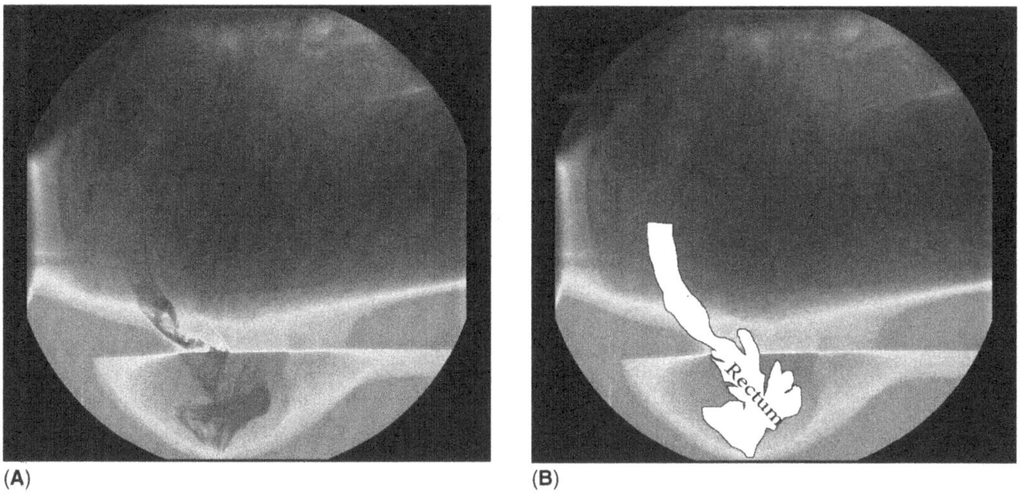

Figure 16 (**A**, **B**) Cinedefecography of rectal intussusception at push.

Rectal Prolapse

Similar to intussusception rectal prolapse is an infolding of the rectal wall that goes through the anus and presents outside the anus (Figs. 19–21). It is important to distinguish mucosal prolapse from full-thickness prolapse (procidentia). Physical examination, cinedefecography, and endorectal ultrasound can help in the evaluation. Full-thickness rectal prolapse is seen at the extreme ages, usually in pediatric and geriatric patients. In adults, there is no successful initial conservative treatment of full-thickness rectal prolapse and surgery is required. The Cochrane review in 2006 failed to demonstrate that which surgical procedures offered the most optimal results (79).

Surgical options for repair of prolapse include abdominal procedures, combining rectopexy with or without colonic resection as well as perineal procedures such as Delorme's operation (mucosectomy), and Altemeier's procedure (perineal rectosigmoidectomy) (Table 4).

Solitary Rectal Ulcer

Solitary rectal ulcer presents with either single or multiple ulcerations of the rectal mucosa (80). Since its appearance can mimic cancer, biopsies from the lesion should be performed to exclude a malignancy. The etiology of this rare condition is unknown; however, it is usually associated with intussusception, rectal prolapse, or PPC. The initial treatment of solitary rectal ulcer is conservative therapy consisting of high dietary fiber and adequate fluid intake, laxatives,

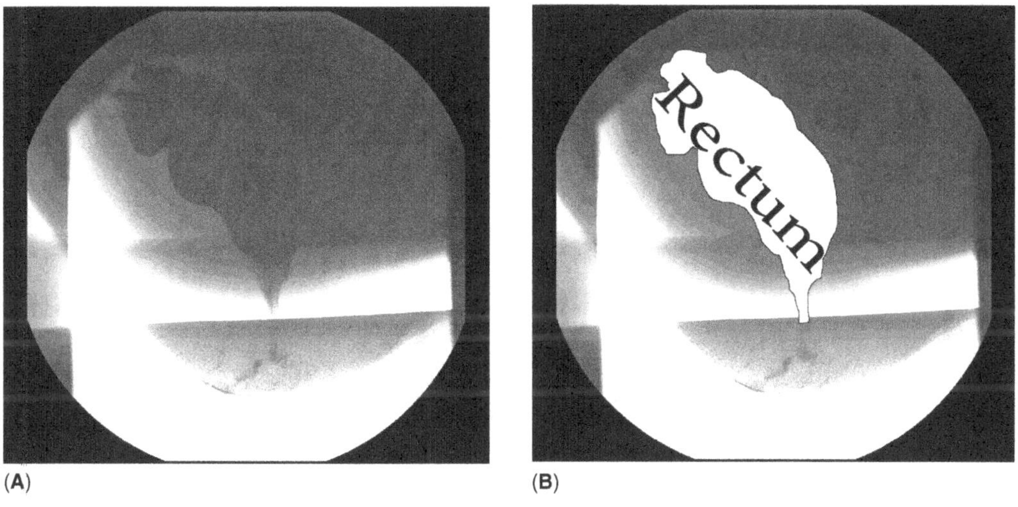

Figure 17 (**A**, **B**) Cinedefecography of rectal intussusception at rest.

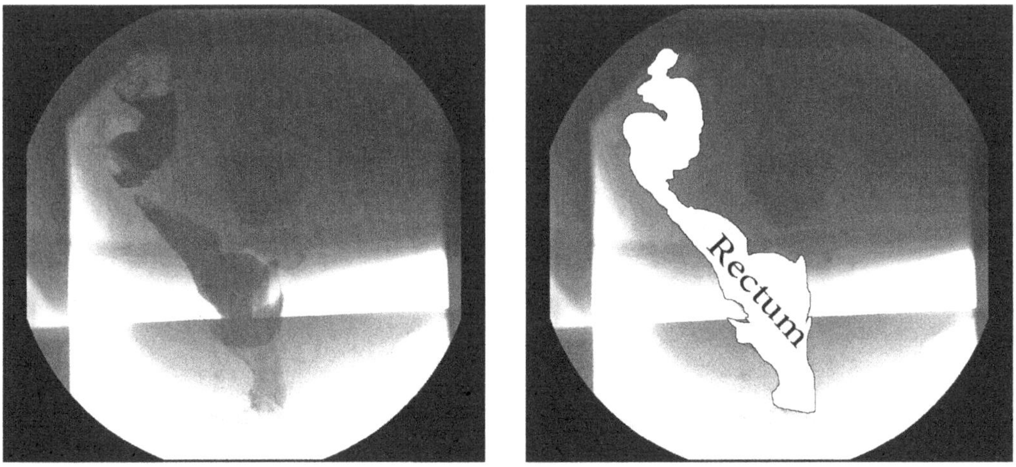

(**A**) (**B**)

Figure 18 (**A**, **B**) Cinedefecography of rectal intussusception at push.

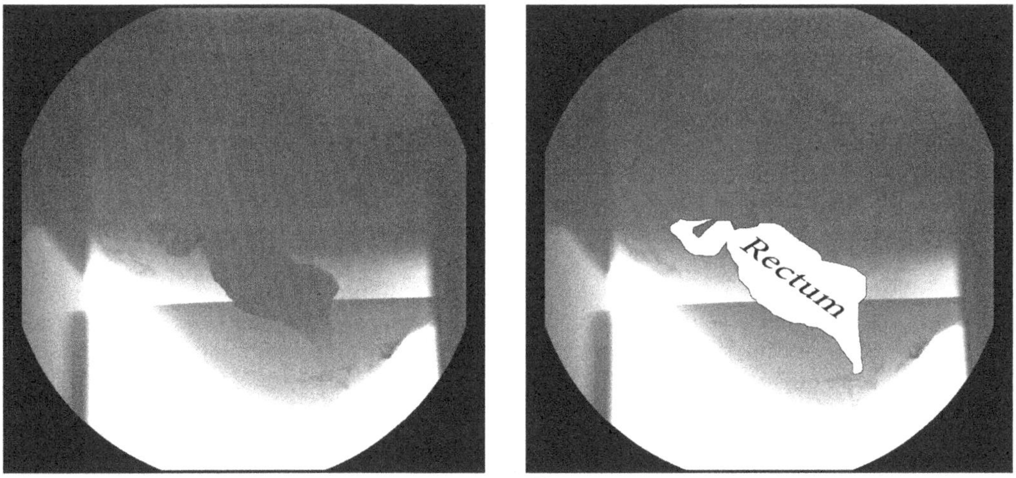

(**A**) (**B**)

Figure 19 (**A**, **B**) Cinedefecography of rectal prolapse at rest.

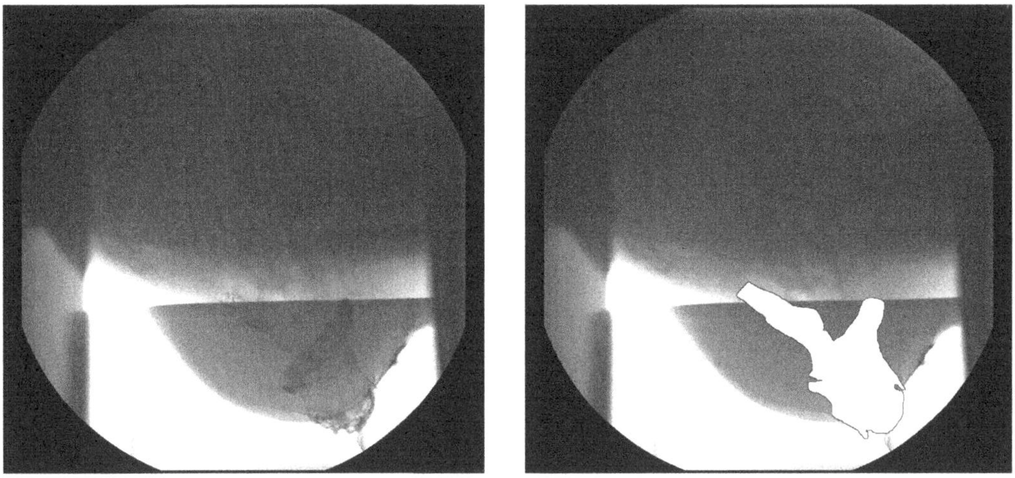

(**A**) (**B**)

Figure 20 (**A**, **B**) Cinedefecography of rectal prolapse at push.

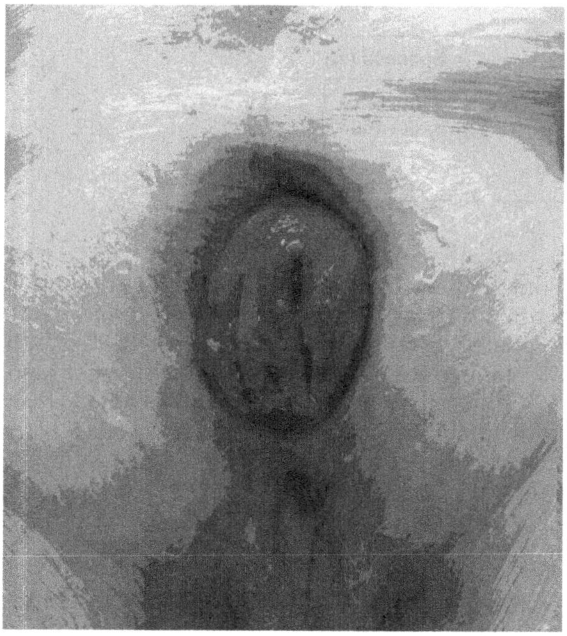

Figure 21 Clinical presentation of the rectal prolapse.

and suppositories. The role of biofeedback is also important in treatment. Theories explain the pathophysiology of solitary rectal ulcer through chronic repeated trauma of the rectal area and ischemia of the intussuscepted/prolapsed rectal wall. However, only 38% of patients in the study by Rao et al. (80) showed mucosal intussusception and only one had rectal prolapse. Additionally, other authors have detected increased rectal sensitivity ($p > 0.0007$), which lead them to hypothesize that rectal hypersensitivity may lead to a persistent desire to defecate and a feeling of incomplete evacuation. Over time, this may cause excessive straining and may lead to altered defecatory behavior, resulting in dyssynergia. This may further aggravate the feeling of incomplete evacuation and lead to the use of digital maneuvers to facilitate defecation. The excessive straining, mucosal intussusception, and digital maneuvers may cause rectal mucosal trauma and bleeding.

Supporting this data, behavioral treatment (biofeedback) resulted in complete healing in 36%, ≥50% healing in 18%, and <50% healing in 36% of patients. In addition, patients experienced decreased straining and stool frequency ($p < 0.05$) and an overall improved bowel satisfaction score ($p < 0.001$). In the study by Jarett et al. (81), subjective symptomatic improvement after biofeedback treatment was reported by 75% of patients. Biofeedback resulted in a significant improvement in rectal mucosal blood flow in patients who felt subjectively better after biofeedback ($p = 0.001$).

Table 4 Surgical Approach to Rectal Prolapse

Approach	Follow-up (months)	Recurrence (%)
Suture rectopexy for rectal prolapse		
Open	47–144	0–3
Laparoscopic	24–48	0–7
Posterior mesh rectopexy		
Open	12–84	0–6
Laparoscopic	8–30	0–4
Anterior sling rectopexy	12–83	0–12
Suture rectopexy with resection		
Open	17–98	0–5
Laparoscopic	12–62	0–2.5
Delorme Procedure	11–47	0–38
Perineal Rectosigmoidectomy	12–120	0–16

Table 5 Surgery for Solitary Rectal Ulcer Syndrome

Approach	Follow-up (months)	Success (%)
Delorme procedure	2–48	55–86
Rectopexy	12–90	50–100
Transanal local excision	NA	42
Laparoscopic rectopexy	71–106	86

Despite the success of biofeedback some patients require surgery for this condition. Surgery may result in clinical improvement in 5% to 86% of patients in short-term follow-up (82,83). In a study from the St. Mark's Hospital, long-term results, with a mean of 90-month follow-up, were worse. In 66 patients, 14 (30%) required a stoma (generally for constipation) and 8 (12%) required additional surgery. Only 50% had improvement, fewer with rectopexy than the Delorme's procedure (84). Seven year follow-up of mesh rectopexy for solitary rectal ulcer syndrome in 11 patients showed no endoscopic recurrence in 7 patients while 1 had recurrent symptoms where were not confirmed endoscopically (Table 5) (85).

Slow Transit Constipation

Initial treatment of this group of patients includes diet and lifestyle modifications. Medical therapy with a step approach is usually recommended starting with bulking agents (fiber supplements), then adding hyperosmolar agents (sorbitol, lactulose), and ultimately saline and stimulant laxatives (86). Biofeedback treatment has also shown symptomatic improvement in 63% of patients with slow colonic transit (87).

Patients who are unresponsive to conservative and behavioral therapy are candidates for surgery after the required tests to rule out concomitant obstructed defecation. Conditions when both abnormalities are present are highlighted in a study from Italy describing the "iceberg syndrome" in patients with combined slow colonic transit and obstructed defecation in which neglected "underwater rocks" or occult lesions may be the cause of surgical failure (88).

Subtotal colectomy with ileorectal anastomosis is the current procedure of choice for the surgical treatment of colonic inertia. Other alternatives include ileosigmoid anastomosis and cecorectal anastomosis. Careful selection of patients for slow colonic transit surgery may result in up to 85% to 100% patient satisfaction, while poor selection results in a success rate of only 5% (89).

In addition to the standard risks associated with surgery, informed consent should include the possibility of anastomotic leak, infection, bleeding, postoperative bowel obstruction, and specific problems related to colectomy for constipation. While the frequency of bowel movements will improve, the bloating, pain, nausea, and other functional symptoms may persist or even worsen. Some patients without these symptoms preoperatively may subsequently develop them following surgery. All patients should be consented that a permanent stoma may be the result of treatment in the long term (Table 6).

Table 6 Results of Surgical Treatment of Constipation

Author	Patients in the study	Operated (%)	Success (%)
Pemberton et al., 1991	277	14	100
Wexner et al., 1991	163	10	94
Sunderland et al., 1992	228	8	88
Mahendrarajah et al., 1994	19	47	88
Redmond et al., 1995	37	100	90
Nyam et al., 1997	131	39.6	85
Pikarsky et al., 2001	403	12	100
Simple et al., 2005	14	100	91
Zutshi et al., 2006	69	100	77
Ripetti et al., 2006	450	3.3	94

CONCLUSION

Constipation requires a thorough informative office visit with instruction to set patients on the right path of corrected diet, physical activity, fiber supplements, and adequate water intake. In case of failure of the initial treatment, results of anorectal physiology laboratory tests should be correlated with patients' complaints. Surgical treatment can be successful in a well-selected population with constipation. A multidisciplinary approach in patients with complex obstructed defecation may yield better results. Good clinical judgment as in all areas of medicine is paramount for good success in managing the constipated patient.

REFERENCES

1. Whorton J. Civilisation and the colon: Constipation as the "disease of diseases." BMJ 2000; 321(7276):1586–1589.
2. Whorton JC. Inner Hygiene: Constipation and the Pursuit of Health in Modern Society. New York: Oxford University Press, USA, 2000.
3. Wald A, Constipation in the primary care setting: Current concepts and misconceptions. Am J Med 2006; 119(9): 736–739.
4. Muller-Lissner SA, et al. Myths and misconceptions about chronic constipation. Am J Gastroenterol 2005; 100(1):232–242.
5. Higgins PD, Johanson JF. Epidemiology of constipation in North America: A systematic review. Am J Gastroenterol 2004; 99(4):750–759.
6. Johanson JF, Sonnenberg A, Koch TR. Clinical epidemiology of chronic constipation. J Clin Gastroenterol 1989; 11(5):525–536.
7. Walter S, et al. A population-based study on bowel habits in a Swedish community: Prevalence of faecal incontinence and constipation. Scand J Gastroenterol 2002; 37(8):911–916.
8. Lynch AC, et al. The prevalence of faecal incontinence and constipation in a general New Zealand population; a postal survey. N Z Med J 2001; 114(1142):474–477.
9. Curry CE. Laxatives. In: Llewellyn, R., ed. Handbook of Nonprescription Drugs. Washington, DC: American Pharmaceutical Association, 1986:75–97.
10. "Constipation - Pamphlet". Pamphlet by: National Institute of Diabetes & Digestive & Kidney Diseases. July 1995.
11. Rao SS. Constipation: evaluation and treatment. Gastroenterol Clin North Am 2003; 32(2):659–683.
12. Wald A. Constipation and constipation syndromes. In: Weinstein WM, Hawkey CJ, Bosch J, eds. Clinical gastroenterology and hepatology. Philadelphia: Elsevier, Mosby, 2005.
13. Martin BC, Barghout V. National estimates of office and emergency room constipation-related visits in the United States. Am J Gastroenterol 2004; 99(suppl):S244.
14. Rantis PC Jr, et al. Chronic constipation—is the work-up worth the cost? Dis Colon Rectum 1997; 40(3):280–286.
15. Connell AM, et al. Variation of bowel habit in two population samples. Br Med J, 1965; 2(5470):1095–1099.
16. Mearin F, et al. Splitting irritable bowel syndrome: From original Rome to Rome II criteria. Am J Gastroenterol 2004; 99(1):122–130.
17. Thompson WG, et al. Functional bowel disorders and functional abdominal pain. Gut 1999; 45(suppl 2):II43–II47.
18. Www.Romecriteria.Org/Documents/Rome_II_App_A.Pdf.
19. Charapata C, Mertz H. Physician knowledge of Rome symptom criteria for irritable bowel syndrome is poor among non-gastroenterologists. Neurogastroenterol Motil 2006; 18(3):211–216.
20. Bialostosky K, et al. Dietary intake of macronutrients, micronutrients, and other dietary constituents: United States 1988–1994. Vital Health Stat 11, 2002;(245):1–158.
21. Bohmer CJ, et al. The prevalence of constipation in institutionalized people with intellectual disability. J Intellect Disabil Res 2001; 45(Pt 3):212–218.
22. Ehrenpreis ED. Constipation-predominant irritable bowel syndrome. In : Wexner SD, Duthie GS, eds. Constipation: Etiology, Evaluation and Management. London: Springer-Verlag London Ltd, 2006.
23. Khaikin M, Wexner SD. Treatment strategies in obstructed defecation and fecal incontinence. World J Gastroenterol 2006; 12(20):3168–3173.
24. Pemberton JH, Rath DM, Ilstrup DM. Evaluation and surgical treatment of severe chronic constipation. Ann Surg 1991; 214(4):403–411; Discussion 411–413.
25. Sandler R, Person B, Raju R. Medical treatment of constipation. In: Wexner SD, Duthie GS, eds. Constipation: Etiology, Evaluation and Management. London: Springer-Verlag London Ltd, 2006.
26. Lesbros-Pantoflickova D, et al. Meta-analysis: The treatment of irritable bowel syndrome. Aliment Pharmacol Ther 2004; 20(11–12):1253–1269.

27. Chuwa EW, Seow-Choen F. Dietary fibre. Br J Surg 2006; 93(1):3–4.
28. Arce DA, Ermocilla CA, Costa H. Evaluation of constipation. Am Fam Physician 2002; 65(11):2283–2290.
29. Jorge JM, Yang YK, Wexner SD. Incidence and clinical significance of sigmoidoceles as determined by a new classification system. Dis Colon Rectum 1994; 37(11):1112–1117.
30. Shorvon PJ, et al. Defecography in normal volunteers: Results and implications. Gut 1989; 30(12):1737–1749.
31. Jorge JM, Habr-Gama A, Wexner SD. Clinical applications and techniques of cinedefecography. Am J Surg 2001; 182(1):93–101.
32. Altringer WE, et al. Four-contrast defecography: Pelvic "floor-oscopy." Dis Colon Rectum 1995; 38(7):695–699.
33. Saclarides TJ, et al. Clarifying the technique of four-contrast defecography. Dis Colon Rectum 1996; 39(7):826.
34. Matsuoka H, et al. A comparison between dynamic pelvic magnetic resonance imaging and video-proctography in patients with constipation. Dis Colon Rectum 2001; 44(4):571–576.
35. Lefaucheur JP. Neurophysiological testing in anorectal disorders. Muscle Nerve 2006; 33(3):324–333.
36. Wiesner A, Jost WH. EMG of the external anal sphincter: Needle is superior to surface electrode. Dis Colon Rectum 2000; 43(1):116–118.
37. Brindley GS. Electroejaculation: Its technique, neurological implications and uses. J Neurol Neurosurg Psychiatry 1981; 44(1):9–18.
38. Xing JH, Soffer EE. Adverse effects of laxatives. Dis Colon Rectum 2001; 44(8):1201–1209.
39. Johanson JF. Review of the treatment options for chronic constipation. Medgenmed 2007; 9(2):25.
40. Johanson JF, Ueno R. Lubiprostone, a locally acting chloride channel activator, in adult patients with chronic constipation: A double-blind, placebo-controlled, dose-ranging study to evaluate efficacy and safety. Aliment Pharmacol Ther 2007; 25(11):1351–1361.
41. Wald A. Irritable bowel syndrome. Curr Treat Options Gastroenterol 1999; 2(1):13–19.
42. Wald A. Psychotropic agents in irritable bowel syndrome. J Clin Gastroenterol 2002; 35(1 suppl):S53–S57.
43. Spiller R, et al. Guidelines on the irritable bowel syndrome: Mechanisms and practical management. Gut 2007; 56(12):1770–1798.
44. Clouse RE, Lustman PJ. Use of psychopharmacological agents for functional gastrointestinal disorders. Gut 2005; 54(9):1332–1341.
45. North CS, Hong BA, Alpers DH. Relationship of functional gastrointestinal disorders and psychiatric disorders: Implications for treatment. World J Gastroenterol 2007; 13(14):2020–2027.
46. Roarty TP, et al. Misoprostol in the treatment of chronic refractory constipation: Results of a long-term open label trial. Aliment Pharmacol Ther 1997; 11(6):1059–1066.
47. Soffer EE, Metcalf A, Launspach J. Misoprostol is effective treatment for patients with severe chronic constipation. Dig Dis Sci 1994; 39(5):929–933.
48. Frame PS, et al. Use of colchicine to treat severe constipation in developmentally disabled patients. J Am Board Fam Pract 1998; 11(5):341–346.
49. Verne GN, et al. Colchicine is an effective treatment for patients with chronic constipation: An open-label trial. Dig Dis Sci 1997; 42(9):1959–1963.
50. Jorge JM, Habr-Gama A, Wexner SD. Biofeedback therapy in the colon and rectal practice. Appl Psychophysiol Biofeedback 2003; 28(1):47–61.
51. Vickers D. Biofeedback for constipation. In : Wexner SD, Duthie GS. eds. Constipation: Etiology, Evaluation and Management. London: Springer-Verlag London Ltd, 2006.
52. Jorge JM, et al. Cinedefecography and electromyography in the diagnosis of nonrelaxing puborectalis syndrome. Dis Colon Rectum 1993; 36(7):668–676.
53. Ron Y, et al. Botulinum toxin type-a in therapy of patients with anismus. Dis Colon Rectum 2001; 44(12):1821–1826.
54. Joo JS, et al. Initial North American experience with botulinum toxin type a for treatment of anismus. Dis Colon Rectum 1996; 39(10):1107–1111.
55. Maria G, et al. Experience with type a botulinum toxin for treatment of outlet-type constipation. Am J Gastroenterol 2006; 101(11):2570–2575.
56. Chen HH, et al. Associations of defecography and physiologic findings in male patients with rectocele. Tech Coloproctol 2001; 5(3):157–161.
57. Dietz HP, Korda A. Which bowel symptoms are most strongly associated with a true rectocele? Aust N Z J Obstet Gynaecol 2005; 45(6):505–508.
58. Soligo M. Posterior pelvic floor dysfunction: There is an immediate need to standardize terminology. Int Urogynecol J Pelvic Floor Dysfunct 2007; 18(4):369–371.
59. Pollak J, Davilla GW. Rectocele repair: The gynecologic approach. Clin Colon Rectal Surg 2003; 16:061–070, DOI: 10.1055/S-2003-39038.
60. Maher C, Baessler K. Surgical management of posterior vaginal wall prolapse: An evidence-based literature review. Int Urogynecol J Pelvic Floor Dysfunct 2006; 17(1):84–88.

61. Zbar AP, et al. Rectocele: Pathogenesis and surgical management. Int J Colorectal Dis 2003; 18(5):369–384.
62. Lowry AC, et al. Consensus Statement of Definitions for Anorectal Physiology and Rectal Cancer: Report of the Tripartite Consensus Conference On Definitions for Anorectal Physiology and Rectal Cancer, Washington, DC, May 1, 1999. Dis Colon Rectum 2001; 44(7):915–919.
63. Takahashi T, et al. Enterocele: What is the clinical implication? Dis Colon Rectum 2006; 49(10 suppl):S75–S81.
64. Farrell SA. Vaginal repair of a sigmoidocele. Int Urogynecol J Pelvic Floor Dysfunct 2000; 11(5):325–327.
65. Raz S, VW Nitti, Bregg KJ. Transvaginal repair of enterocele. J Urol 1993; 149(4):724–730.
66. Tsiaoussis J, et al. Rectoanal intussusception: Presentation of the disorder and late results of resection rectopexy. Dis Colon Rectum 2005; 48(4):838–844.
67. Dvorkin LS, et al. Rectal intussusception in symptomatic patients is different from that in asymptomatic volunteers. Br J Surg 2005; 92(7):866–872.
68. Dvorkin LS, et al. Rectal intussusception: Characterization of symptomatology. Dis Colon Rectum 2005; 48(4):824–831.
69. Lahr SJ, et al. Operative management of severe constipation. Am Surg 1999; 65(12):1117–1121; Discussion 1122–1123.
70. Ommer A, et al. Stapled transanal rectal resection (STARR): A new option in the treatment of obstructive defecation syndrome. Langenbecks Arch Surg 2006; 391(1):32–37.
71. Von Papen M, et al. Functional results of laparoscopic resection rectopexy for symptomatic rectal intussusception. Dis Colon Rectum 2007; 50(1):50–55.
72. D'Hoore A, Penninckx F. Laparoscopic ventral recto(Colpo) pexy for rectal prolapse: Surgical technique and outcome for 109 patients. Surg Endosc 2006; 20(12): 1919–1923.
73. Ashari LH, et al. Laparoscopically-assisted resection rectopexy for rectal prolapse: Ten years' experience. Dis Colon Rectum 2005; 48(5):982–987.
74. Madiba TE, MK Baig, Wexner SD. Surgical management of rectal prolapse. Arch Surg 2005; 140(1):63–73.
75. Jayne DG, Finan PJ. Stapled transanal rectal resection for obstructed defaecation and evidence-based practice. Br J Surg 2005; 92(7):793–794.
76. Binda GA, Pescatori M, Romano G. The dark side of double-stapled transanal rectal resection. Dis Colon Rectum 2005; 48(9):1830–1831; Author Reply 1831–1832.
77. Pescatori M, et al. Rectovaginal fistula after double-stapled transanal rectotomy (STARR) for obstructed defaecation. Int J Colorectal Dis 2005; 20(1):83–85.
78. Bassi R, Rademacher J, Savoia A. Rectovaginal fistula after STARR procedure complicated by haematoma of the posterior vaginal wall: Report of a case. Tech Coloproctol 2006; 10(4):361–363.
79. Bachoo P, Brazzelli M, Grant A. Surgery for complete rectal prolapse in adults. Cochrane Database Syst Rev 2000; (2):CD001758.
80. Rao SS, et al. Pathophysiology and role of biofeedback therapy in solitary rectal ulcer syndrome. Am J Gastroenterol 2006; 101(3):613–618.
81. Jarrett ME, et al. Behavioural therapy (Biofeedback) for solitary rectal ulcer syndrome improves symptoms and mucosal blood flow. Gut 2004; 53(3):368–370.
82. Choi HJ, et al. Clinical presentation and surgical outcome in patients with solitary rectal ulcer syndrome. Surg Innov 2005 12(4):307–313.
83. Felt-Bersma RJ, Cuesta MA. Rectal prolapse, rectal intussusception, rectocele, and solitary rectal ulcer syndrome. Gastroenterol Clin North Am 2001; 30(1):199–222.
84. Sitzler PJ, et al. Long-term clinical outcome of surgery for solitary rectal ulcer syndrome. Br J Surg 1998; 85(9):1246–1250.
85. Tweedie DJ, Varma JS. Long-term outcome of laparoscopic mesh rectopexy for solitary rectal ulcer syndrome. Colorectal Dis 2005; 7(2):151–155.
86. Bharucha AE, Phillips SF. Slow transit constipation. Gastroenterol Clin North Am 2001; 30(1):77–95.
87. Emmanuel AV, Kamm MA. Response to a behavioural treatment, biofeedback, in constipated patients is associated with improved gut transit and autonomic innervation. Gut 2001; 49(2):214–219.
88. Pescatori M, Spyrou M, Pulvirenti d'Urso A. A prospective evaluation of occult disorders in obstructed defecation using the "iceberg diagram." Colorectal Dis 2006; 8(9):785–789.
89. Nyam DC, et al. Long-term results of surgery for chronic constipation. Dis Colon Rectum 1997; 40(3):273–279.

13 Urogynecologic Pelvic Floor Dysfunction

Vivian C. Aguilar and G. Willy Davila

Section of Urogynecology, Department of Gynecology, Cleveland Clinic Florida, Weston, Florida, U.S.A.

INTRODUCTION

Anatomical and Functional Overlap of the Pelvic Floor

As one considers the female pelvis, it is evident that the pelvic floor functions as an integrated unit given the intimate relationship of the pelvic viscera and the coexistence of urologic, gynecologic, and gastrointestinal symptoms. It is well established that dysfunction in one organ system is often accompanied by abnormalities in another. In one study, a significant proportion of women with stress urinary incontinence had advanced pelvic organ prolapse (POP) on pelvic examination (1). Similarly, any irritative condition of one organ system may produce similar symptoms in another (2). Specialists in these systems, gynecologists, urologists, and colorectal surgeons, have traditionally addressed their area of expertise. However, lack of identification of dysfunction in an adjacent organ system may lead to serial surgeries for women. The concept of horizontal integration of pelvic floor function, rather than the traditional vertical approach, provides a comprehensive assessment of the pelvic floor with a multidisciplinary team approach (Fig. 1) (3).

NEUROMUSCULAR MECHANISMS OF URINARY CONTINENCE

In women, the important factors for continence involve anatomic support and neuronal innervation to the bladder and the urethra to maintain urethral closure. At the urethrovesical junction, increased pressure inside the urethra as compared to the bladder promotes continence and is accomplished by the internal and external urethral sphincters. Innervation of the pelvic floor is accomplished by the parasympathetic and sympathetic autonomic and peripheral somatic motor and sensory systems. The sympathetic fibers originating from spinal cord level T-11 to L-2 and their neurotransmitters enable the filling and storage capacity of the bladder through relaxation of detrusor smooth muscle, contraction of the base of the bladder, and urethral smooth muscle as well as inhibition of parasympathetic input. The parasympathetic fibers originating from spinal cord levels S-2 to S-4 and their transmitters stimulate contraction of the detrusor and relaxation of the urethral sphincter accomplishing the voiding mechanism. The somatic nerves provide innervation to the striated muscle of the external urethral sphincter and the muscles of the pelvic floor along the Pudendal nerve.

EVALUATION OF PELVIC ORGAN PROLAPSE

Evaluation tools for POP include the POP Quantification (POP-Q) system, a standardized classification and grading system approved by the International Continence Society (4). The POP-Q measures six points in the vagina and vulva in relation to their distance from the hymen, quantified in centimeters during the fullest extent of protrusion, most commonly with Valsalva or standing. Negative values represent measurements proximal to the hymen, point zero, whereas positive values signify measurements distal to the hymen. Three other landmarks are measured as well without Valsalva and quantified (Fig. 2). These points are then summated in table form and can then be used to assess the stage of prolapse. Tables 1–4 describe various identifying points in the vagina used for measurement. There are five stages of prolapse derived from the measurements obtained on split speculum examination and are described in Table 5.

The Baden–Walker half-way system is another prolapse grading system that is commonly used. This has been shown to also have reliable interobserver measurements. Prolapse is classified as cystocele, uterine or vaginal vault prolapse, rectocele, and/or enterocele individually

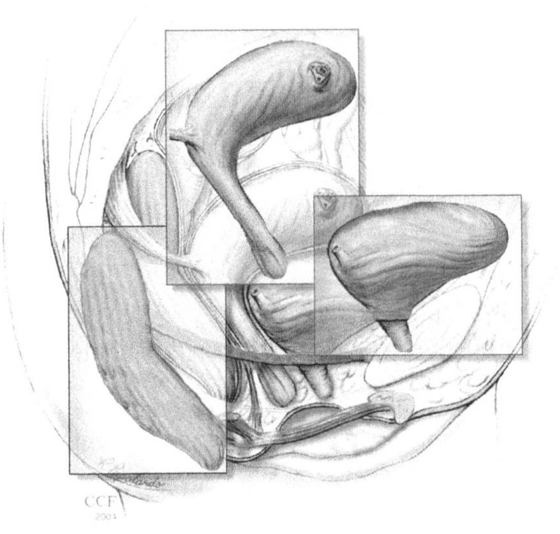

Figure 1 Horizontal integration of pelvic floor function.

and is graded in relation to its distance to the introitus. First degree describes a prolapse that is present half-way to the introitus. Second degree describes descent to the introitus. Third degree is prolapse that is present half-way beyond the introitus. Lastly, complete prolapse is that where the prolapse is completely exteriorized (5).

URINARY INCONTINENCE

Demographics

Approximately 13 million people are affected by urinary incontinence in the United States. The annual direct cost of urinary incontinence in 1995 was $16.3 billion, with 12.4 billion (76%) for women and 3.8 billion (24%) for men. These costs are twice greater for those above the age of 65 than those younger than 65 (7.6 billion vs. 3.6 billion). Routine care and management of incontinence absorbs the majority of the cost (70%), followed by nursing home care (14%), treatment (9%), complications (6%), and evaluation and diagnosis (1%) (6). The projected costs to the health-care system for the treatment of incontinence are expected to increase substantially as the population ages (7).

The International Continence Society has redefined urinary incontinence as "the complaint of any involuntary leakage of urine" to incorporate more women who may suffer from

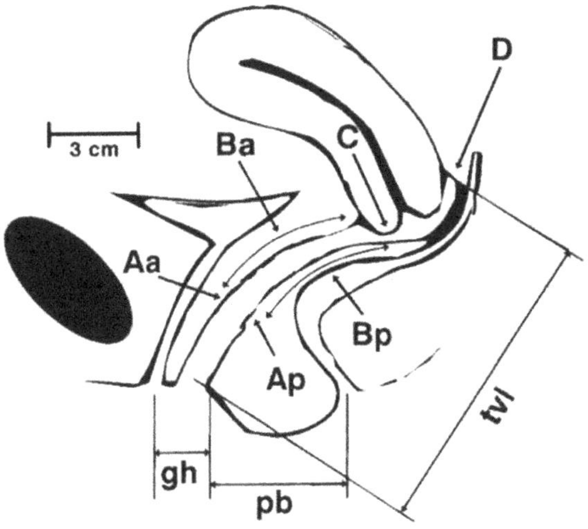

Figure 2 Pelvic organ prolapse quantification system (POP-Q).

Table 1 Points along the anterior vaginal wall: A anterior (Aa) and B anterior (Ba)

Point Aa	Located 3 cm proximal to the external urethral meatus, it is a defined point corresponding to the approximate location of the urethrovesical junction. This measurement can range from −3 cm to +3 cm depending on the degree of anterior wall descent.
Point Ba	The most distal portion of any part of the anterior vaginal wall, the anterior vaginal fornix, or anterior vaginal cuff. In the absence of any anterior vaginal wall prolapse point Ba is −3 cm.

Table 2 Points Along the Superior Vagina: C and D

Point C	Denotes the cervix when the uterus is present or the vaginal cuff following hysterectomy. Its value represents the most distal descent of the cervix or vaginal cuff with valsalva.
Point D	Represents the location of the posterior fornix in a woman who still has a cervix. It corresponds to the level of the uterosacral ligaments at their attachment to the posterior cervix. Measuring this point can differentiate between suspensory failure of the uterosacral–cardinal ligament complex from cervical elongation. Point D is omitted in the absence of the cervix.

Table 3 Points Along the Posterior Vaginal Wall: A Posterior (Ap) and B Posterior (Bp)

Point Ap	Located in the midline of the posterior vaginal wall, 3 cm proximal to the hymen. The measurement can range from −3 cm in a woman without prolapse to +3 cm with complete vaginal prolapse.
Point Bp	Corresponds to the most distal portion of any part of the posterior vaginal wall. When there is no prolapse it measures −3 cm and would have a positive value equal to the cuff measurement in a woman with complete posthysterectomy vault eversion.

Table 4 Other Landmarks

Total vaginal length (TVL)	The furthermost depth of the vagina in centimeters when point C or D is reduced to their normal position.
Genital hiatus (GH)	Measured from the middle of the external urethral meatus to the posterior midline hymen.
Perineal body (PB)	Measured from the posterior margin of the genital hiatus to the midanal opening.

Table 5 Five Stages of Prolapse

Stage 0	No prolapse is demonstrated. Points Aa, Ba, Ap, and Bp are all −3 cm and either point C or D is less than or equal to TVL −2 cm.
Stage I	The criteria for stage 0 are not met, and the most distal portion of the prolapse in greater than one cm above the level of the hymen.
Stage II	The most distal portion of the prolapse is less than or equal to 1 cm proximal or distal to the plane of the hymen (i.e., its quantitation value is greater or equal to −1 cm but less or equal to +1 cm).
Stage III	The most distal portion of the prolapse is greater than 1 cm below the plane of the hymen protrudes no further than 2 cm less than the total vaginal length in centimeters (i.e., its value is greater than 1 cm but less than TVL-2 cm).
Stage IV	Complete vaginal eversion is demonstrated. The most distal portion of the prolapse protrudes to at least TVL—2 cm (i.e., its value is greater or equal to TVL—2 cm).

incontinence without the further complication of being a "social or hygienic problem" (8). Although this increases the overall number of women who are affected, fewer than half the women with incontinence report seeking medical care for the problem (9). Johnson et al. (10) reported that individuals were more likely to seek professional help if they had to use pads for their incontinence, had large volumes of leakage with episodes, had significant impairment of their daily activities, and men were more likely to seek medical attention than women.

Types of Urinary Incontinence

There are five major types of urinary incontinence: stress urinary incontinence, detrusor overactivity, mixed incontinence, overflow incontinence, and functional incontinence.

Stress urinary incontinence is the involuntary loss of urine that occurs when intravesical pressure exceeds the maximal urethral closure pressure during activities such as coughing, laughing, sneezing, or exercising. This can be due to damage to the proximal urethra from radiation, prior surgeries, estrogen deficiency, or a congenital weakness. Stress urinary incontinence is foremost attributed to neuromuscular damage to the urethrovesical junction resulting from vaginal childbearing.

Detrusor overactivity is the involuntary loss of urine that occurs by spontaneous and uninhibited detrusor contractions. In some cases, a very strong need to urinate or "urge" can accompany these contractions and is commonly referred to as "urge incontinence". Overactive bladder (OAB) is a broader term, which encompasses the spectrum of urinary urgency, frequency, nocturia, and urge incontinence.

Mixed Incontinence is the presence of both stress incontinence and detrusor overactivity. Treatment should be aimed at the predominant type of incontinence according to the patients' complaints.

Overflow incontinence is urinary leakage associated with overdistension and overfilling of the bladder. In these cases, urine loss is described as constant or frequent dribbling. It is commonly caused by lower motor neuron disease as seen with diabetes mellitus, prior pelvic surgery with urinary outflow obstruction, or with advanced POP.

Functional incontinence can be a temporary or chronic condition occurring as a result of other cognitive, physical, or psychological impairments that interfere with proper toilet habits or the ability to reach the toilet. This type of incontinence may also occur or worsen in the setting of an underlying bladder problem.

Risk Factors for Urinary Incontinence

Urinary incontinence is two to three times more common in women than in men and this gender difference persists for all types of incontinence. As age increases, so does the prevalence of urinary incontinence. Brown et al. (11) established that there is a 30% greater prevalence for each five year increase in age. Conventionally, Caucasian women have been deemed at a higher risk for urinary incontinence than other races. Several studies have demonstrated this trend where non-Hispanic whites were 2.8 times more likely to have weekly stress incontinence than non-Hispanic blacks. In addition, Caucasian women were more likely to develop stress incontinence, whereas African-American women were more often diagnosed with detrusor overactivity (11,12).

Many women experience symptoms of urinary incontinence during their pregnancy, and these symptoms can persist following vaginal delivery from injury to the muscle and connective tissue that support the bladder neck. Estrogen deficiency and urogenital atrophy also affect the anatomic integrity of the urethra, bladder trigone, and pubococcygeal muscles which have a high affinity for estrogen receptors. Obesity and smoking also appear to have a consistent causal relationship with incontinence (13,14).

Diagnosis and Evaluation of Urinary Incontinence

History

A detailed description of the episodes of incontinence should be obtained as to the type of urinary leakage, activities resulting in loss of urine, the amount lost per episode, and sensations related to urine loss. Daytime and night-time voiding patterns and frequency should be established as well as the presence of nocturnal enuresis. Risk factors for urinary incontinence should be explored as well as reversible causes of urinary incontinence such as urinary tract infection, excessive fluid or caffeine intake, medication side effects, or uncontrolled diabetes. The patient's past medical history should identify other possible causative factors including neurological disease, pulmonary disease, diabetes, obesity, constipation or fecal impaction, or prior malignancy and treatment. The past medical history should also include a thorough obstetric history reporting gravity, parity, number of vaginal deliveries, birth weights, instrument assistance for deliveries, and episiotomy or tears. In the gynecological history, attention to prior pelvic incontinence and/or reconstructive surgeries should be noted as well as hormonal status, any gynecologic malignancy and treatments, sexual history, and complaints. Other symptoms of urinary dysfunction should be reviewed such as recurrent urinary tract infections, hematuria, hesitancy, straining to void, poor or intermittent stream, postvoid dribbling, or the sensation of incomplete emptying. Routine bowel habits should be assessed as well as the presence of any constipation, chronic diarrhea, vaginal or perineal splinting, and flatal or fecal incontinence. The patient's medication list should be reviewed with particular attention to any drugs that may contribute to incontinence or retention such as diuretics, antihypertensive agents, estrogens, anticholinergics, or psychotropic medications. As part of the social history, other lifestyle factors that may affect incontinence such as tobacco and alcohol use, fluid and caffeine intake, chronic lifting and straining, and exercise should be noted.

Physical Examination

The physical examination occurs at the initial meeting with the patient with general observation of the degree of mobility and gait, obesity, visual impairment, odor (of urine, smoke, or alcohol), and signs of neurologic disease such as tremor, facial asymmetry, or speech pattern. Common neurologic diseases that can affect bladder function include stroke, Alzheimer's disease, Parkinson's disease, and Multiple Sclerosis. Examination of the abdomen for identification of prior surgical scars, abdominal masses, or hernias should be done. In addition, one should assess the back and flanks in order to evaluate for costovertebral angle tenderness, back surgeries, or spinal deformities. The extremities should be examined for edema, chronic venous stasis and neurologic sensation, deep tendon reflexes, and motor strength.

The pelvic examination begins with the patient in lithotomy position followed by inspection of the perineal skin and external genitalia for signs of hypoestrogenism such as atrophy or agglutination of the labia. Irritation and excoriation of the perineal area as a result of chronic wetness and pad use should be noted. The neurological examination of the perineum focuses on sacral nerve innervation from segments L1 to L2 and S2 to S4. The sensory component of the nerves is tested by discrimination of light touch and pin prick stimulation over the dermatomes of the inner thigh, vulva, and perineum. The motor component is examined by testing the clitoral and anal reflexes. Gentle touch to the clitoris or the labia majora should elicit contraction of the anal sphincter.

A speculum examination is then performed to evaluate for vaginal atrophy, lesions of the cervix, or abnormal pooling of urine that may indicate the presence of a fistula. The speculum is then split into anterior and posterior halves, and using the posterior blade each compartment of the vagina is inspected individually. The anterior vaginal wall should be inspected for the presence of any masses that may represent urethral diverticulum. POP evaluation is then performed using the POP-Q system.

Following the speculum examination, a bimanual examination is performed to assess the size, shape, and the position of the uterus and the presence of masses or fibroids that may contribute to urinary symptoms such as urgency, frequency, incontinence, or obstruction. During the bimanual examination, pelvic floor muscle strength can be assessed by having the patient attempt to squeeze the examiner's fingers present in the vagina by contracting their levator ani. The strength, duration, and symmetry of the contraction should be assessed. Women who can voluntarily contract these muscles may benefit from performing pelvic floor muscle exercises, whereas women who cannot identify or contract these muscles would benefit from structured pelvic floor rehabilitation and biofeedback (15). A rectal examination is then done to evaluate baseline sphincter tone, contraction strength and symmetry, the presence of hemorrhoids, occult blood, fecal impaction, rectal prolapse, or rectal masses.

At this initial visit, an estimation of a postvoid residual should be obtained to diagnose urinary retention. This volume may be obtained by catheterization or ultrasound. If catheterized, the urine may be sent for urinalysis and culture. A voiding diary may be given to the patient to complete either before the initial evaluation or to further clarify the nature of the incontinence. The patient measures and records all liquids consumed, the number of voids and incontinence episodes, and factors associated with incontinence over a 24 to 72 hour period. Useful information can be obtained in evaluating urinary frequency, mean and largest voided volumes, and nature and severity of incontinence in order to establish a reference to assess treatment efficacy (16).

Laboratory Evaluation

All patients should have a clean-catch urinalysis to identify conditions predisposing to urinary incontinence or other medical conditions such as glycosuria, infection, bacteruria, pyuria, or proteinuria. If the urinalysis is suspicious for infection a culture should be obtained. Urine cytology may be considered in patients with persistent hematuria or risk factors for urinary tract malignancies.

Simple Cystometry and Uroflowmetry

A simple and useful urodynamic study can be performed using a transurethral catheter, a 60 cc irrigation syringe, and sterile normal saline or water at room temperature. The patient is asked to empty her bladder and obtain a clean-catch specimen that is sent for urinalysis and culture. If suggestive for infection, the patient is treated with antibiotics and returns at a later date for re-evaluation if symptoms persist. The bladder is then catheterized and a postvoid residual can be obtained.

Next, the irrigation syringe is attached to the catheter and the bladder is filled in 50 mL aliquot increments at a rate of 50–100 mL per minute. The patient is asked to discriminate the initial sensation of fluid present in the bladder, normal desire to void, strong desire to void, or maximum capacity. Normal capacity ranges from 400 to 650 mL. Maximum capacity of less than 250 mL or greater than 650 mL is abnormal and warrants further evaluation with multichannel urodynamics. During bladder filling the meniscus in the syringe should be observed for any rise indicating bladder contractions. Overflow of the fluid over the top of the syringe signifies detrusor overactivity. At capacity, provocative measures are performed that may trigger a bladder contraction such as heel bouncing, the sound of running water, or immersing hands in cool water.

Stress urinary incontinence may be demonstrated by having the patient cough while the examiner observes for leakage. If no leakage is noted, then the patient is asked to repeat the cough stress test in the standing position. If there is a delay in the interval between the cough and the demonstration of leakage or the flow of fluid is prolonged, a diagnosis of detrusor overactivity should be considered. Women who exhibit leakage of urine with a relatively empty bladder are at risk of having intrinsic sphincter deficiency which may limit success with conservative treatment measures (17).

Indications for Complex Urodynamic Evaluation

Multichannel urodynamics is indicated in women with prior incontinence surgery, excessively small or large bladder capacity, suspicion of intrinsic sphincter deficiency, unsuccessful medical or behavioral therapy for incontinence, and nondiagnostic simple cystometrics. During multichannel urodynamics, simultaneous measurements are obtained of intravesical, abdominal, and urethral pressures during cystometry. Detrusor pressure is calculated by subtraction of the abdominal and intravesical pressures. Assessment of stress and urge leakage is performed by having the patient cough, Valsalva, or perform provocative measures at different bladder capacities. Pelvic floor muscle activity is also measured by electromyography with either a patch on the perineum or needle placement.

Cystometry assesses capacity which should range from 400 to 650 mL in an adult. Bladder compliance is measured as a change in pressure with volume and is expressed as mL/cm H_2O and assesses elasticity and bladder distensibility. Compliance in a normal individual should be less than 10 mL/cm H_2O; values $\geq$20 mL/cm H_2O are considered significant. Conditions that may affect bladder compliance include tuberculosis, radiation, interstitial cystitis, and infiltrative diseases such as sarcoidosis or scleroderma.

Normal bladder sensation is assessed during filling cystometry and is subjective and variable among patients. The first sensation is the first awareness of a cold sensation or filling of the bladder. The first desire to urinate is usually between 90 and 150 mL. A strong desire to void is described as a persistent urge to void without fear of leakage whereas urgency occurs with a fear of leakage or pain. These values may range from 200 to 400 mL and complete fullness ranges from 400 to 650 mL. Delayed sensation may be due to neurologic disease and early sensation may be attributed to chronic inflammatory conditions of the bladder, detrusor overactivity, or decreased bladder compliance.

During cystometry, the presence of any involuntary bladder contraction is evaluated and may indicate neurogenic or idiopathic detrusor overactivity. Detrusor contractions may also be triggered by increases in intra-abdominal pressure with coughing, laughing, and sneezing and may mimic stress urinary incontinence. Pressure flow studies are performed by measurement of detrusor pressure and urine flow rate and provide information regarding the presence of bladder outlet obstruction.

Leak point pressures can be assessed by measurement of the detrusor contraction or abdominal pressure with cough or Valsalva resulting in urinary leakage. Valsalva leak point pressure (VLPP) measurements less than 60 cm H_2O indicate intrinsic sphincter deficiency. Urethral pressure profile is a measure of urethral resistance obtained at rest and urethral closure pressure measurements less than 20 cm H_2O are also indicative of intrinsic sphincter deficiency.

Treatment of Urinary Incontinence

Nonsurgical Therapies for Stress Incontinence

Although there are many effective surgical options for stress urinary incontinence, many patients opt not to pursue surgery or may not be good surgical candidates. Basic therapies include antibiotic therapy in the presence of infection, estrogen therapy in those with urogenital atrophy, and timed voiding for those with large capacity bladders.

Bladder Training

Bladder retraining involves patient education and timed voids with increased interval between voids while attempting to avoid incontinent episodes. A voiding diary is kept and voiding intervals are begun every hour during the first week along with observation of fluid intake and triggers. During subsequent weeks, the voiding interval is increased incrementally by 15 to 30 minutes weekly until a goal of voiding intervals of every 2.5 to 3 hours is obtained. Bladder retraining is more successful when combined with pelvic floor muscle training (PFMT), biofeedback, and drug therapy.

PFMT

PFMT involves contraction of the pelvic floor or levator ani muscles to assist in controlling urinary leakage in women with both stress and mixed incontinence. By volitional contraction of the pelvic floor, the striated muscle of the external urethral sphincter also contracts narrowing the lumen and outflow of urine. Although women are instructed to "try to stop the flow of urine" to correctly identify the pelvic floor muscles, they should not routinely perform them during voiding or an abnormal voiding pattern may develop. In addition, contraction of the pelvic floor elevates the bladder, stretches the urethra, and causes an angulation of the urethra–vesical junction further increasing the resistance to urinary flow. Furthermore, contraction of the external urethral sphincter may lead to a reflexive relaxation of the bladder detrusor mediated by activation of Pudendal afferent nerves to inhibition of parasympathetic motor neurons via spinal interneurons (18).

Pelvic Floor Physiotherapy/Biofeedback

Biofeedback and pelvic floor physiotherapy is performed by trained professionals to help patients learn to strengthen and relax their pelvic muscles in order to improve bladder function. Biofeedback uses vaginal or rectal pressure sensors and/or electromyography to accurately measure the strength and action of the pelvic floor muscles, and provides "feedback" information to the patient so that the patient can learn to better contract the muscles. Women who cannot voluntarily contract their pelvic floor muscles may benefit from biofeedback. An important part of pelvic floor biofeedback therapy and PFMT is consistent exercise of the pelvic muscles at home and along with patient education and patient commitment to the program.

Functional Electrical Stimulation

Electrical stimulation to the pelvic floor muscles and nerves is delivered by an intravaginal or a perineal surface electrode which inhibits premature and inappropriate detrusor contractions via the direct stimulation of Pudendal nerve afferents (sensory receptors or sensory nerve fibers). Which causes a reflexive contraction of the pelvic floor musculature. In this respect, therapeutic stimulation for stress incontinence requires the same afferent input as that for urge incontinence. Low-frequency stimulation (10–20 mHz) is used for OAB, medium frequency (50–100 mHz) is used for stress urinary incontinence, and higher frequency (200 mHz) is used for urinary retention.

Surgical Procedures for Stress Urinary Incontinence

The goal of surgery for stress urinary incontinence is to provide sufficient support and urethral resistance to prevent urinary leakage during increases in intra-abdominal pressure while allowing for voluntary, complete, and low-pressure bladder emptying. There are many surgical procedures for urinary incontinence; determining the appropriate procedure entails consideration of the type of stress incontinence, bladder capacity and function, severity of incontinence and the presence of other associated conditions such as vaginal prolapse, and abdominal or pelvic pathology requiring concurrent surgical correction. One of the two main approaches to surgical correction of female stress urinary incontinence is to reposition the urethra and the bladder neck in a well-supported retropubic position while creating a backboard of support to the urethra as seen in the retropubic approaches such as the Burch or the Marshall—Marchetti–Krantz procedure. The second approach is to create coaptation or compression of the urethra by augmenting the resistance provided by the intrinsic sphincter unit with or without affecting urethral and bladder neck support as in the suburethral sling or bulking procedures. Lastly, the newest approach involves dynamic midurethral support which may provide an anti-incontinence effect by reduction of urethral hypermobility or producing a dynamic kink in the urethra during increases in intra-abdominal pressure.

Burch Procedures

Retropubic colposuspension was the procedure of choice for stress urinary incontinence until the development of the minimally invasive midurethral slings. The goal of the suspension was to return the urethra to its retropubic position and provide a backboard of support to the urethrovesical junction. The advantage of this approach is the ability to address coexisting abdominal or pelvic pathology; however, the large incision, increased morbidity, and prolonged healing as well as the inability to address other POP repair concurrently have made this a less desirable choice as an incontinence procedure.

The traditional approach involves a Pfannensteil or low vertical incision, dissection and exposure of the retropubic space, and identification of the bladder, urethra, and paravaginal fascia. Permanent sutures are then placed through the paravaginal fascia at the level of the bladder neck and then the sutures are subsequently passed through the ipsilateral ileopectineal line (Cooper's ligament). The sutures are tied elevating the urethrovesical junction with care to avoid overcorrection. Cystoscopy is recommended to confirm ureteral patency and the absence of any permanent sutures within the bladder. Cure rates appear to vary over time but are reported to be greater than 80% at four years (19). Complications include voiding dysfunction (0.3%), de novo detrusor overactivity (17%), and POP (13.6%) such as enterocele, cystocele, and rectocele (20).

Retropubic Sling Procedures

The sling procedures also aim to provide a backboard of support to the urethrovesical junction as well as create some urethral compression or coaptation. Sling materials include autologous grafts, allografts, xenografts, and synthetic material. Slings are placed at the level of the urethrovesical junction and the proximal urethra and tied with minimal or no tension to avoid causing bladder outlet obstruction. Long-term studies using autologous or synthetic materials have published cure rates of 80% and improvement in over 90% of cases. Use of synthetetic materials has been associated with an increased risk of urethral or vaginal erosion (21).

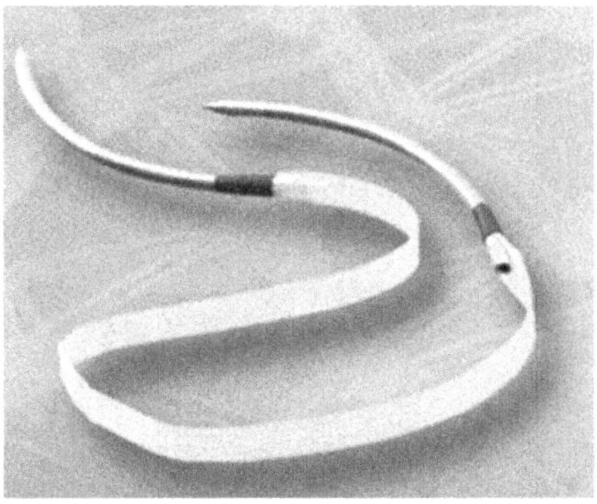

Figure 3 Tension-free vaginal tape (TVT, Ethicon Inc.).

Midurethral Sling Procedures

The Tension-free vaginal tape (TVT, Ethicon Inc., U.S.A.) (Fig. 3) was developed by Ulmsten et al. (22) in the mid 1990s. The Integral Theory proposed by Petros supposes that recreating the support of the pubo-urethral ligament and suburethral vaginal tissues by placement of a polypropylene sling at the level of the midurethra can effectively treat stress urinary incontinence (23). At five-year follow-up, Nilsson and colleagues (24) reported a subjective and objective cure rate of 84.7% and a low failure rate of 4.5%. The most common complications were bladder perforation in 6%, urinary retention in up to 4%, and de novo urgency in approximately 5% of patients. Concern arose from reports of other life-threatening complications such as bowel and vascular injuries, but these have remained rare (<1%) as reported in the MAUDE database.

The procedure may be performed under general, regional, or local anesthesia depending upon the need for other concomitant vaginal reconstructive procedures. Two small incisions are made in the skin overlying the mons pubis at the superior border of the pubic ramus, approximately 1 cm from the midline. A one to two cm. incision is made in the vaginal mucosa immediately overlying the level at the midurethra, which can be confirmed by examination of the urethrovesical junction and urethra with a Foley catheter in place. The needle with attached polypropylene tape is then passed through the vaginal incision, through the periurethral space, and immediately posterior to the pubic ramus to exit the suprapubic skin incisions. There are many variations in needle passage, either transvaginally or transabdominally. In addition, tensioning the tape has not been completely standardized with most placing it in a tension-free fashion with an intervening Hegar dilator, Kelly clamp, or other instrument. The high success rate and ease of placement as well as tolerability of the TVT procedure have gained wide acceptance and applicability.

Transobturator slings (Fig. 4) were developed in 2001 in order to avoid the risks of retropubic needle passage and still maintain the hammock support of the midurethra as described by DeLancey (25). The transobturator approach involves passage of the sling percutaneously through the obturator foramen and then through a previously made vaginal incision (26)

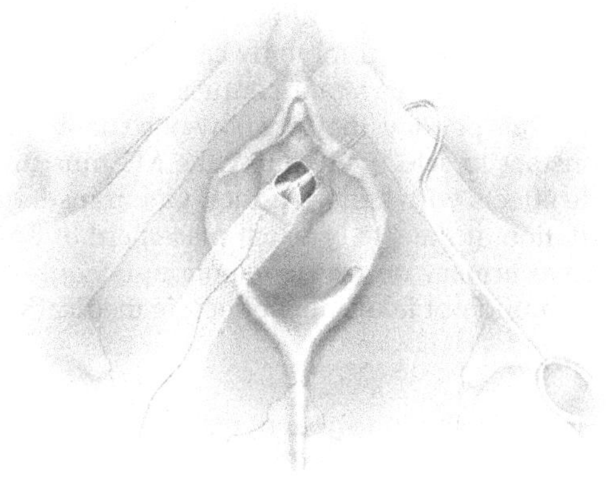

Figure 4 Transobturator sling (Monarc, AMS Inc.).

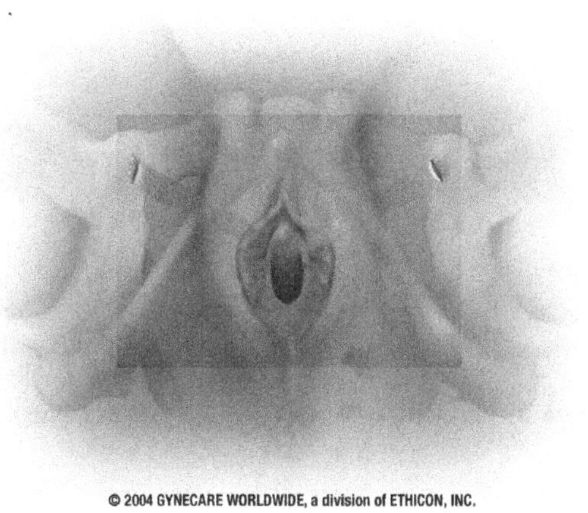

Figure 5 Final placement of transobturator sling.

(Fig. 5). In addition to reducing the risk of urinary tract injury in bypassing the retropubic space, the placement of the sling in the broad hammock position may decrease the incidence of de-novo urge symptoms. Subjective cure rates for the transobturator slings were similar to the retropubic approach in a recent metanalysis. Adverse events such as groin pain, vaginal mesh erosion, or injuries were more common in the obturator group, whereas bladder injuries and voiding difficulties were more common in the retropubic group (27). Several authors have noted that patients with impaired urethral sphincters were more likely to have recurrent stress urinary incontinence following obturator slings than those with normal urethral sphincters (28,29). Further outcome data regarding transobturator slings will become available as midurethral slings become the standard for the treatment of stress urinary incontinence.

Bulking Agents

There are many injectable agents used for the treatment of severe stress urinary incontinence including bovine glutaraldehyde cross-linked collages (GAX), carbon-coated zirconium beads, macroplastique, and autologous tissues such as fat and cartilage. Many of these options have fallen out of favor due to poor durability, migration, tissue erosion, and safety. These materials are injected either periurethrally or transurethrally to improve coaptation or resistance of the urethra at the urethrovesical junction. Although there are a few adverse outcomes attributable to bulking agents, namely transient urinary retention, UTI, and hematuria, the success rates with injectables are variable (30,31).

Treatment of Detrusor Overactivity

In addition to behavioral modification with dietary management, timed voiding, bladder retraining, and functional electrical stimulation, medical therapy is the mainstay of treatment for detrusor overactivity. Medications used for detrusor overactivity and OAB are antimuscarinics, which affect the central nervous system and muscarinic receptors in smooth muscle. They act to relax the smooth muscle of the bladder, reducing detrusor contractions and reducing urinary urgency, frequency, and urge incontinence episodes. Side effects are a result of the effect on the medication on muscarinic receptors in other parts of the body commonly causing dry mouth, and constipation, and possibly headache, dry eyes, blurred vision, confusion, and urinary retention. Initially prescribed as multidose medications per day, they are now once daily dosed in an extended release form. Newer formulations act to selectively affect the M3 muscarinic receptor in an attempt to decrease untoward side effects with better efficacy. One transdermal formulation is available with some reported irritation at the site of patch placement but minimal anticholinergic side effects. Patients who have urinary or gastric retention, uncontrolled narrow-angle glaucoma, or intending pregnancy should not take anticholinergic medication.

Hormone Therapy

A woman's bladder and urethra as well as the vagina contain estrogen, receptors since these tissues arise from the same embryologic origin. Estrogen helps maintain the strength, flexibility, and thickness of the tissues in this area by increasing the blood flow, enhancing nerve function, and maintaining tissue integrity. Theoretically, the drop in estrogen that occurs after the menopause contributes to the deterioration of the supportive tissues around the bladder and urethra, which makes these tissues weak, atrophic and may aggravate urinary incontinence.

Systemic hormone therapy is no longer prescribed specifically for urinary benefits, but vaginal estrogen may be recommended. Most experts agree that the localized effects of vaginal estrogen do not exert the same risks as systemic hormone replacement. A systematic review of the effects of estrogen therapy for the Hormones and Urogenital Therapy Committee summarized that estrogen therapies were associated with statistically significant improvements in diurnal frequency, nocturnal frequency, urgency, improved bladder capacity, and decreased the number of incontinence episodes (32).

Other Medications

Imipramine is a tricyclic antidepressant that has both anticholinergic and alpha-adrenergic effects. It relaxes the detrusor muscle of the bladder while stimulating the alpha receptors in the smooth muscles at the bladder neck to contract. It may be beneficial in the treatment of mixed, stress, and urge incontinence. One beneficial side effect of Imipramine is drowsiness; therefore it may be useful for night-time incontinence as well as to aid with insomnia. Cardiovascular side effects include irregular heartbeat, dizziness, or fainting from orthostatic hypotension, and therefore it must be used cautiously in the elderly population. Other side effects including dry mouth, blurry vision, and constipation are similar to those of other anticholinergic medications.

Desmopressin is a synthetic version of a natural body hormone, antidiuretic hormone (ADH) which decreases the production of urine. In addition, more ADH is produced at night, so the need to urinate is lower while sleeping. Desmopressin is commonly used to treat bed-wetting in children and is available as a nasal spray or pill for use before bedtime. Desmopressin may also reduce urinary incontinence in adult women. Side effects are uncommon, but there is a risk of water retention and hyponatremia in older women. Thus, serum sodium measurements and careful observation are necessary when prescribing the medication.

Sacral Nerve Neuromodulation

Sacral nerve stimulation or neuromodulation therapy is a reversible treatment for patients with urge incontinence or urinary retention, who do not respond to behavioral treatments or medication. It is indicated for the treatment of urinary urgency, frequency, urge incontinence and non-neurogenic urinary retention that has not responded to other treatment modalities. InterStim™ (Medtronic, Minneapolis, Minnesota, U.S.A.) is an implanted neurostimulation system that sends electrical pulses to the sacral nerve. Stimulation of sacral nerve may relieve the symptoms of urinary frequency, urgency, urge incontinence, and urinary retention. Prior to implantation, the effectiveness of the therapy is tested on an outpatient basis with an external temporary pacing wires and stimulatory device. The patient completes a voiding diary for a period before and after stimulation noting frequency of urination, leakage episodes, and volumes voided. If the comparison demonstrates a significant reduction of symptoms, the device is implanted. An external programming device can be used to adjust the level of stimulation and the leads being stimulated. In addition, another small hand held programming device is given to the patient to further adjust the level of stimulation, if necessary. The system can be turned off at any time. Some adverse events that have been reported include changes in bowel function, infection at the implant site, movement or malfunctioning of the lead, pain, or unpleasant stimulation at other sites.

PELVIC ORGAN PROLAPSE

Conservative Treatment for POP

Treatment options for POP include expectant management, pelvic floor or Kegel exercises, pessary placement, or surgical correction. The type of therapy selected depends upon the degree of prolapse, concomitant anatomical or functional defects, the presence of urinary incontinence, and patient preference.

Expectant Management

In women with mild or asymptomatic prolapse, close observation and follow-up may be considered with twice yearly or at annual visits. Should a patient experience any changes in symptoms

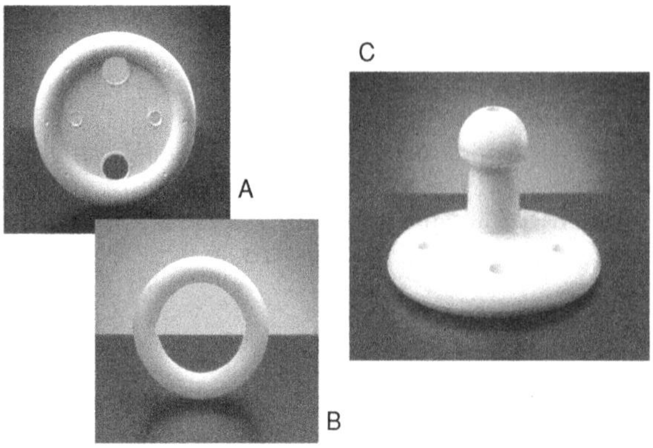

Figure 6 Pessaries for pelvic organ prolapse.

or size of the prolapse in the interim, a return examination to reassess the prolapse should be scheduled. In women who have advanced prolapse but are still asymptomatic, closer interval observation may be appropriate to reassess potential risks for infection, urinary retention, mucosal erosion, or switch to more active management (33).

Pelvic Floor Exercises

Pelvic floor muscle or Kegel exercises are intended to improve the strength of the pelvic muscles thereby increasing support to the pelvic organs. Although it is unlikely that pelvic floor exercises will correct POP, they may be beneficial for adjunctive therapy for urinary or fecal incontinence (33). Patients may be trained in performing the exercises by squeezing the examiners fingers during pelvic examination. Patients are then instructed to carry out the exercises throughout the day in several sets of 10 repetitions, holding each for approximately five seconds. If the patient cannot identify the pelvic floor muscles adequately or has significant weakness, they may benefit from working with a pelvic floor physical therapist. Although pelvic floor exercises may provide some improvement in symptoms, adherence to the regimen is key in sustaining beneficial effects.

Pessary

Conservative management with pessaries for POP is becoming more common with the increasing population of elderly patients requiring nonsurgical management of their prolapse. Pessaries can be divided into two categories: those that support or those that are space filling. Support pessaries, such as rings, act as a lever to support the pelvic organs (Fig. 6) and are recommended for early stage prolapse. Space filling pessaries, such as the gellhorn or the donut, are indicated for more advanced prolapse. Adaptations to the pessary have been made to also address urinary incontinence. Another similar device, the Colpexin ball or sphere, can be used as a prolapse support device as well as a tool for performing pelvic floor muscle exercises. When fitted properly, the patient should not feel the pessary in place, nor should it affect bladder or bowel function. In women with urogenital atrophy, the application of local estrogen is essential in preventing erosions with pessary use. Patients who are able and willing to perform pessary management may be followed at six-month intervals to guarantee fit and ensure vaginal mucosal integrity. For these patients, we recommend removing the pessary once or twice a week along with usage of vaginal estrogen. Patients who are not able to remove the pessary on their own should be seen at two- to three-month intervals to remove the pessary and inspect the vaginal mucosa. The vagina may be irrigated with antiseptic or betadine solution to prevent anerobic overgrowth and the pessary may be then replaced along with antibiotic gel or estrogen cream. It is imperative for the clinician to ensure appropriate compliance and follow-up care to prevent adverse outcomes such as vesicovaginal or rectovaginal fistula.

Surgical Treatment of POP

Repair of the Anterior Vaginal Wall

Anterior vaginal wall prolapse may result from distinct defects in different areas of anterior vaginal wall support. This may include central defects in the midline fibromuscular layer

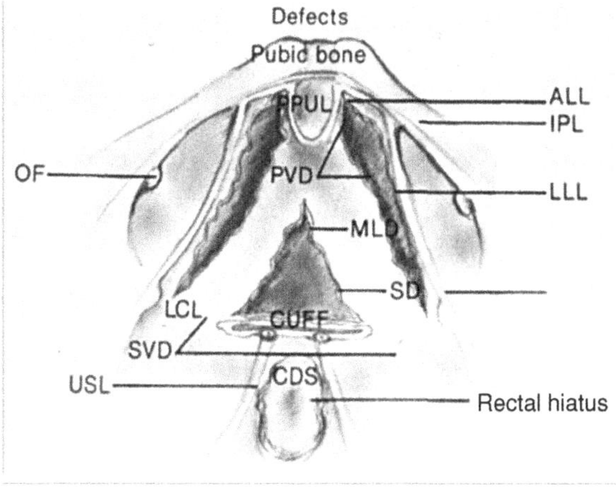

Figure 7 Defects of anterior vaginal wall support.

(central cystocele), lateral detachment of the anterior vagina to the arcus tendineous fascia pelvis (ATFP) (lateral or paravaginal defect) (Fig. 7), loss of bladder neck support, or transverse avulsion of the fibromuscular layer from the vaginal apex.

Anterior Colporrhaphy

Anterior colporrhaphy is regularly used to correct prolapse arising from a central defect. The procedure is begun using a midline vertical incision and the vaginal mucosa is separated from the underlying endopelvic fascia. Dissection is then carried out laterally to each vaginal sulcus and proximally to the vaginal apex or cervix. Once the dissection is accomplished, the endopelvic fascia is plicated in the midline, thereby repairing the central defect and elevating the bladder base. Subsequently, the fascia is reattached to the vaginal apex or cervix. Finally, excess vaginal mucosa may be trimmed and closed with 2–0 polyglycolic acid suture, and the vagina is packed for further postoperative hemostasis.

Paravaginal Defect Repair

The paravaginal defect repair is used to correct anterior vaginal wall prolapse that results from detachment of the anterior endopelvic fascia from its lateral attachment to the ATFP. The paravaginal defect repair may be carried out either through an abdominal or vaginal approach. Abdominally, this may be performed via an open laparotomy or a laparoscopic approach. Each method has the same goal of reattaching the lateral vaginal sulcus to the ATFP using bilateral nonabsorbable sutures. The initial suture is placed through the full thickness of the lateral vaginal sulcus and then through the ATFP at the level of the ischial spine. Subsequent sutures are then placed at 1 cm intervals attaching the lateral vaginal wall along the course of the ATFP to the inferior border of the pubic symphysis.

The vaginal approach to the paravaginal defect repair has undergone considerable modification with the introduction of total vaginal mesh kits.

Vaginal Vault Prolapse Repair

Surgical procedures for apical vaginal vault prolapse re-establish apical support by reconnecting the uterosacral, sacrospinous, or the anterior longitudinal ligaments to the apex of the vagina. The objective of these procedures is to maintain vaginal length, axis, and caliber as well as to re-establish the continuity of the vaginal fascial envelope.

Procedures for vaginal vault prolapse can be divided into abdominal and vaginal reconstructive approaches as well as obliterative techniques. Abdominal procedures may also be performed via laparotomy or laparoscopic approaches.

Abdominal Procedures

Abdominal Sacrocolpopexy

Abdominal sacrocolpopexy is performed by connecting the vaginal apex to the sacral promontory using a mesh bridge. The resulting suspension restores the vagina to a more physiologic

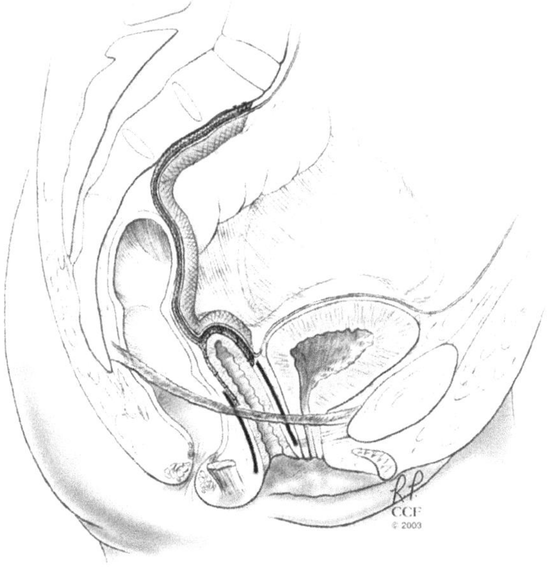

Figure 8 Abdominal sacrocolpopexy for vaginal vault prolapse.

axis than other procedures for vaginal vault prolapse (Fig. 8). Traditionally, the procedure has been performed via a transverse or vertical laparotomy incision. The laparoscopic approach for abdominal sacrocolpopexy involves considerable laparoscopic skill with a substantial learning curve. Many surgeons are utilizing robotic technology to master the laparoscopic techniques required to perform this procedure.

The procedure involves exposing the anterior longitudinal ligament of the vertebral column at the level of the sacral promontory by incising the peritoneum bordered by the right ureter and the colon. The middle sacral artery and perforating vessels are identified and care is taken to avoid injury to these structures. Once the anterior longitudinal ligament is identified and cleared of overlying adventitial and fatty tissue, a permanent suture may be placed by hand or using a bone anchoring device. Dissection is continued inferiorly along the peritoneum medial to the ureter to the level of the vaginal apex. The vaginal vault is elevated by hand or using an EEA sizer or flat retractor. The peritoneum over the vagina is dissected along the anterior and posterior vaginal walls for attachment of the Y-shaped mesh bridge. Each arm of the mesh is attached to the vagina using two to three rows of nonabsorbable sutures. The long arm of the graft is then elevated to the level of the promontory without excessive tension on the vaginal apex and attached to the sutures on the promontory. The peritoneum is then closed over the length of the mesh for prevention of bowel adhesions. Additional abdominal procedures can be performed, as indicated, such as Burch colposuspension or paravaginal repairs.

Uterosacral Ligament Suspension

Uterosacral ligament suspension of the vaginal apex can be performed as an open, laparoscopic, or vaginal procedure. The procedure involves identifying the uterosacral ligaments or their remnants and passing a nonabsorbable suture through the uterosacral ligament and attachment to the vaginal apical angles. There are several modifications of this technique which can incorporate a peritoneal culdeplasty with bilateral or unilateral attachment to each uterosacral (34). Attachment of the vaginal cuff to the uterosacral and cardinal ligament complex, as in a TeLinde suture, at the time of hysterectomy may prevent future prolapse of the vaginal vault (35).

Vaginal Procedures

Sacrospinous Ligament Fixation

Initially described in Germany and popularized by Nichols et al. (36) in the United States in the 1970s, the sacrospinous ligament fixation for suspension of the vaginal vault is the most common vaginal procedure performed for this indication. This procedure can be performed via both posterior and anterior vaginal dissection for a unilateral or bilateral attachment of the vaginal apex to the sacrospinous ligament. The sacrospinous ligament can be identified by palpation of the ischial spines and one or two nonabsorbable sutures are then placed through the ligament 1 cm medial to the ischial spine. The sutures are then passed through the fibromuscular layer of the vagina without penetrating the vaginal mucosa. With a bilateral suspension, the sutures are tied to the ligament in such a manner to maintain symmetry and a vertical axis to the vagina. Intraoperative risks of this procedure include Pudendal or inferior gluteal vessel injury with possible life-threatening hemorrhage and Pudendal or Sciatic nerve injury with gluteal pain. Postoperatively, the vagina may be at risk for anterior vaginal prolapse because of the pronounced posterior deviation of the vaginal axis with sacrospinous attachment (37).

Uterosacral Ligament Suspension

The vaginal approach to uterosacral ligament suspension was originally described by McCall in 1938 (38). The uterosacral ligament remnants are identified, grasped with Allis clamps, and sutures are then placed through the ligament and incorporated into the fibromuscular layer of the vagina as well as the vaginal epithelium, if delayed absorbable sutures are used. Unilateral or bilateral suspension sutures may be used with attachment to ipsilateral or bilateral vagina apices. Cystoscopy should then be performed to confirm ureteral patency as there is an increased risk of ureteral injury with this approach which may be as high as 11% (34).

Repair of Posterior Vaginal wall Prolapse

Posterior vaginal wall prolapse may result from distinct defects or tears in different areas of posterior vaginal wall support. This may include central defects in the midline rectovaginal septum, lateral detachment of the posterior vagina to the arcus tendineous fascia rectovaginalis, at the apical attachment of the rectovaginal fascia to the vaginal cuff resulting in an enterocele, or transverse avulsion distally from the perineal body. Symptoms of posterior vaginal wall prolapse may include vaginal bulge, pelvic pressure, obstructed defecation, and constipation. Although repair of rectoceles and enteroceles may successfully correct anatomic defects, symptoms of defecatory dysfunction and constipation may not be alleviated by surgery.

Posterior Colporrhaphy

Traditional posterior colporrhaphy is often performed with a concurrent perineorrhaphy or perineoplasty to correct a widened genital hiatus and also facilitates the restoration of the posterior deflection of the vagina in the pelvis. Allis or Kocher clamps are placed on the vaginal hymen bilaterally and then overlapped to assess a final vaginal caliber that admits two to three fingerbreadths. A third clamp is then placed in the midline on the perineum 1–2 cm below the hymen. The tissue is then infiltrated with a dilute hemostatic agent and a V-shaped incision is made on the perineum between the clamps. Excess tissue is resected and dissection is continued along the posterior vaginal wall separating the vaginal epithelium from the underlying rectovaginal septum to approximately 1 cm from the vaginal apex or above the level of the rectocele. Dissection is continued laterally to the lateral vaginal sulcus and the medial margins of the Puborectalis muscle. Plication of the rectovaginal septum is then performed with one- or zero-vicryl sutures along the length of the rectocele to the level of the hymen. Levator ani plication may be incorporated along with the rectovaginal septum, although this is associated with postoperative dyspareunia and may be omitted in sexually active women. At the hymen, a one- or zero-Vicryl suture is used to reapproximate the splayed bulbocavernosus muscle to the perineal body. Examination during and at the end of the repair should be performed to identify any vaginal narrowing or banding.

Enterocele

An enterocele is formed when the intestine protrudes through a defect in the rectovaginal or vesicovaginal pouch and an enterocystocele is a double hernia in which both the bladder and the intestines protrude. Enterocele repair may be performed by abdominal, laparoscopic, and vaginal approach, although there are little data to support the superiority of one approach over another. Traditional enterocele repair involves identification of the enterocele sac and its contents, dissection of the sac, closure with multiple circumferential permanent purse-string sutures with incorporation of the cardinal–uterosacral ligaments or their remnants, and excision of the excess sac. At the time of hysterectomy, enterocele repair may be performed in conjunction with a McCall culdeplasty and high uterosacral vault suspension. An enterocele may also be encountered at the apex of the dissection of the posterior vaginal wall during rectocele repair. This defect most likely results from transverse avulsion of the rectovaginal fascia from its cervical or vault attachment. Repair of this defect can be performed by reattachment of the superior edge of the fascia to the posterior aspect of the cervix or vault in the midline and laterally at the level of the uterosacral ligaments using permanent sutures.

SUMMARY

Urogynecologic pelvic floor dysfunction encompasses a wide array of clinical entities. These dysfunctions need to be approached systematically in an attempt to understand the true nature of the underlying problem. Once the problem has been properly identified, the options for correction may be properly presented for the patient to consider.

REFERENCES

1. Ng CS, Rackley RR, Appell RA. Incidence of concominant procedures for pelvic organ prolapse and reconstruction in women who undergo surgery for stress urinary incontinence. Urology 2001; 57(5):911–913.
2. Myers DL, Aguilar VC. Gynecolgic manifestations of interstitial cystitis. Clin Obstet Gynecol 2002; 45(1):233–241.
3. Davila GW, Ghoneim GM. Pelvic floor dysfunction: The importance of a multidisciplinary approach. Clin Colon Rectal Surg 2003; 16:3–4.
4. Bump RC, Mattiasson A, Bo K, et al. The standardization of terminology of female pelvic organ prolapse and pelvic floor dysfunction. Am J Obstet Gynecol 1996; 175:10–17.
5. Baden WF, Walker TA. Surgical Repair of Vaginal Defects. Philadelphia, PA: Lippincott, 1992:14.
6. Wilson L, Brown J, Shin G, et al. Annual direct cost of urinary incontinence. Am J Obstet Gynecol 2001; 98:398–406.
7. Wan H, Sengupta M, Valkoff V, et al. 65+ in the United States. US Census Bureau, Current Population Reports. Washington, DC: US Government Publishing Office, 2005:23–209.
8. Abrams P, Cardozo L, Fall M, et al. The standardisation of terminology of lower urinary tract function: report from the standardisation sub-committee of the International Continence Society. Am J Obstet Gynecol 2002; 187:116–126.
9. Kinchen KS, Burgio K, Diokno AC, et al. Factors associated with women's decision to seek treatment for urinary incontinence. J Womens Health 2003; 12:687–698.
10. Johnson TM, Kincade JE, Bernard SL, et al. Self-care practices used by older men and women to manage urinary incontinence. Results from the national follow-up survey of self-care and the aging. J Am Geriatr Soc 2002; 48:894–902.
11. Brown JS, Grady D, Ouslander JG, et al. Prevalence of urinary incontinence and associated risk factors in postmenopausal women. Heart & Estrogen/Progestin Replacement Study Research Group. Obstet Gynecol 1999; 94:66–70.
12. Graham CA, Mallett VA. Race as a predictor or urinary incontinence and pelvic organ prolapse. Am J Obstet Gynecol 2001; 185:116–120.
13. Mommsen S, Foldspang A. Body mass index and adult female urinary incontinences. World J Urol 1994; 12(6):319–322.
14. Bump RC, McClish DM. Cigarette smoking and pure genuine stress incontinence of urine: a comparison of risk factors and determinants between smokers and nonsmokers. Am J Ostet Gynecol 1994; 170(2):579–582.
15. Seim A, Eriksen BC, Hunskaar S. A study of female urinary incontinence in general practice. Demography, medical history, and clinical findings. Scand J Urol Nephrol 1996; 30(6):465–471.
16. Wyman JF, Choi SC, Harkins SW, et al. The urinary diary in evaluation of urinary incontinence in women: A test retest analysis. Obstet Gynecol 1998; 71:812–817.
17. Lobel RW, Sand PK. The empty supine stress test as a predictor of intrinsic urethral sphincter dysfunction. Obstet Gynecol 1996; 88:128–132.
18. Park JM, Bloom DA, McGuire EJ The guarding reflex revisited. Br J Urol 1997; 80:940–945.
19. Leach GE, Dmochowski RR, Appell RA et al. Female stress incontinence clinical guidelines panel summary report on surgical management of stress urinary incontinence. J Urol 1997; 158:875–880.
20. Colombo M, Zanetta G, Vitobello D, et al. The Burch colposuspension for women with detrusor overactivity. Br J Obstet Gynaecol 1996; 103:255–260.

21. Abrams P, Khoury S, Wein A, eds. Incontinence. 2nd ed. Plymouth, UK: Health Publications Ltd., 2002.
22. Ulmsten U. Intravaginal slingplasty (IVS): An ambulatory surgical procedure for treatment of female urinary incontinence. Scand J Urol Nephrol 1995; 29:75–82.
23. Petros PE, Ulmsten UI. An integral theory and its method for the diagnosis and management of female urinary incontinence. Scan J Urol Nephrol Suppl 1993; 153:1–93.
24. Nilsson CG, Kuuva N, Falconer C, et al. Long term results of the tension-free vaginal tape (TVT) procedure for surgical treatment of female stress urinary incontinence. Int Urogynecol J 2001; 12(suppl 2):S5–S8.
25. DeLancey JOL, Richardson AC. Anatomy of genital support. Clin Obstet Gynecol 1993; 175:311–319.
26. Delorme E. Transobturator urethral suspension: Mini-invasive procedures in the treatment of stress urinary incontinence. Prog Urol 2001; 11:1306–1313.
27. Latthe P, Foon R, Toozs-Hobson P. Transobturator and retropubic tape procedures in stress urinary incontinence: a systematic review and meta-analysis of effectiveness and complications. BJOG 2007; 114:522–531.
28. Guerette NL, Bena JF, Davila GW. Transobturator slings for stress incontinence: Using urodynamic parameters to predict outcomes. Int Urogynecol J 2008; 19(1):97–102.
29. O'Connor R, Nanigian D, Lyon M. Early outcomes of mid-urethral slings for female stress urinary incontinence stratified by Vlasalva leak point pressure. Neurourol Urodynam 2006; 25:685–688.
30. Chrouser KL, Fick F, Goel A, et al. Carbon coated zirconium beads in beta-glucan gel and bovine glutaraldehyde cross-linked collagen injections for intrinsic sphincter deficiency: Continence and satisfaction after extended follow-up. J Urol 2004; 171:1152–5.
31. Radley SC, Chapple CR, Mitsogiannis IC, et al. Transurethral implantation of macroplastique for the treatment of female stress urinary incontinence secondary to urethral sphincter deficiency. Euro Urol 2001; 39:383–389.
32. Cardozo L, Lose G, McClish D, et al. A systematic review of the effects of estrogens for symptoms suggestive of overactive bladder. Acta Obstet Gynecol Scand 2004; 83(10):892–897.
33. Weber AM, Richter HE. Pelvic organ prolapse. Obstet Gynecol 2005; 106:615–634.
34. Barber MD, Visco AG, Weidener AC, et al. Bilateral uterosacral ligament vaginal vault suspension with site specific endopelvic fascia defect repair for the treatment of pelvic organ prolapse. Am J Obstet Gynecol 2000; 183:1402–1411.
35. Rock JA, Jones HW. TeLinde's Operative Gyneocology. Philadelphia, PA: Lippincott Williams & Wilkins, 2008.
36. Nichols DH, Randalls CL. Vaginal Surgery. 3rd ed. Baltimore, MD: Williams and Wilkins, 1989:313–327.
37. Smilen SW, Saini J, Wallach SJ, et al. The risk of cystocele after sacrospinous ligament fixation. Am J Obstet Gynecol 1998; 179:1465–1472.
38. McCall ML. Posterior culdeplasty: Surgical correction of enterocele during vaginal hysterectomy: A preliminary report. Obstet Gynecol 1957; 10:595–602.

14 Anorectal Pain

Jill C. Genua
Colon and Rectal Surgeons of Southern Connecticut, Stamford, Connecticut, U.S.A.

David A. Vivas
Cleveland Clinic Florida, Weston, Florida, U.S.A.

INTRODUCTION

The chief complaint of anorectal pain is often approached with trepidation by the colorectal surgeon since the physical examination is often unremarkable with no obvious cause for this very troublesome complaint. Patients have often sought multiple prior medical opinions, or have undergone ineffective procedures. To further complicate the problem, the terms proctalgia fugax, levator syndrome, anal spasm, pelvic floor dyssynergia, and idiopathic anal pain are often used interchangeably. Therefore, the choice of an appropriate treatment is not simple. An effective approach to this chief complaint is composed of systematic evaluation, concise classification, familiarity with the available treatment options, patience, and—most importantly—realistic expectations.

EVALUATION

Various forms of anorectal pathology will present as pain. The goals of the initial evaluation are to exclude infectious, inflammatory, neoplastic, and neurologic causes, and to elicit a clear description of the idiopathic anorectal pain. The ability of a patient to describe the pain is as subjective as pain itself. A thorough history involves specific questions regarding location, character, precipitating events, triggering factors, frequency, duration, radiation, associated symptoms, and alleviating factors. Chronic medical conditions, prior surgeries (particularly pelvic and anorectal procedures), and routine medications should be identified. In females, gynecologic disorders and obstetric history should be noted. In males, a history of prostate pathology is significant. A full review of all systems should complete the history.

Physical examination includes abdominal evaluation, visual inspection, palpation, digital rectal examination, anoscopy, and proctoscopy. Palpation for points of tenderness (particularly the puborectalis and internal anal sphincter muscles) and palpation of the lymph nodes of the groin should not be overlooked. Full colonoscopy is indicated per screening guidelines or, if warranted, by history and review of systems. Evaluation to this point is often sufficient to exclude abnormalities such as hemorrhoidal disease, anal fissure, abscess/fistula, pruritis ani, dermatitis, cutaneous infections, carcinoma, and proctitis.

Coccygodynia is sometimes categorized with proctalgia or idiopathic pain. However, it should be viewed and treated as a distinct condition. Palpation, pressure, or manipulation of the coccyx elicits a distinct pain and it may be caused by tumors, trauma, avascular necrosis, or referred pain from lumbar disk prolapse (1–4).

Patients with pelvic floor prolapse warrant special consideration. Anorectal pain has been reported in 16% to 25% of these patients (5). However, this pain is often secondary to the pressure and discomfort of the prolapse rather than idiopathic anorectal pain. Thus relief of this discomfort should be considered part of the overall management of the prolapse.

If history and physical examination have not revealed a source of the pain, imaging with computed tomography (CT) scan of the abdomen and pelvis and/or magnetic resonance imaging (MRI) is the next step. The goal of imaging is to exclude pelvic masses or neurologic causes of anorectal pain. Pain is reported as one of the presenting features of presacral tumors with malignant presacral masses, with twice the likelihood of having associated pain shown in at least one study (6). Sacrococcygeal pain is the most common complaint with malignant retrorectal tumors, but rectal fullness and pressure with defecation are additional symptoms (7).

The role of endoanal ultrasound (EAUS) and physiologic testing at this step is unclear. EAUS in patients with idiopathic anal pain has revealed an abnormally thick or hypertrophied internal anal sphincter; however, treating this finding has effectively relieved the pain in only a small number of patients (8). Similarly, higher anal resting pressures have been recorded in patients with anal pain compared to a control group; however, when these pressures were reduced, the pain was not consistently relieved (9). Therefore, in the absence of concomitant pelvic floor complaints, routine EAUS and manometric testing are unlikely to affect the management of anorectal pain.

Once primary pelvic and anorectal abnormalities have been excluded, three patterns of pain exist: proctalgia fugax, levator syndrome, and pudendal neuropathy.

PROCTALGIA FUGAX, LEVATOR SYNDROME, AND PUDENTAL NEUROPATHY

Proctalgia Fugax

Proctalgia fugax is defined by recurrent episodes (lasting seconds to minutes) of sudden and severe anorectal pain; the pain disappears completely between attacks (10). Perhaps the first account describing "a peculiar and severe pain of the rectum which comes in paroxysms, generally during first sleep" was in 1841 (11), but the term "proctalgia fugax" was first used in 1935 (12). Despite the time since these first early accounts, the condition is still considered a "clinical enigma" (13). Patients describe short episodes of severe-to-excruciating pain originating in or above the anal canal. The episodes can occur without warning during the day or night. A common complaint is being disturbed from sleep by the episode of pain. The majority of patients describe a cramping, spasm-like, or stabbing pain; others describe a crushing, pricking, burning, tingling, swelling, or stretching sensation similar to an electric shock (14).

The pathophysiology of proctalgia fugax is unclear. Based on small series of patients, theories include intestinal spasm or motor abnormalities (15), spasm and tension of pelvic floor muscles (16), motor abnormalities of anal smooth muscle (17,18), hypertrophy/thickening of the internal anal sphincter (8,19,20), and vasospasm (21). However, findings in other small cohorts of patients do not consistently support these theories (9,22).

Early reports of proctalgia characterize the majority of patients as perfectionists, anxious, tense, and hypochondriacs (23). The absence of objective physical findings often tempts physicians to classify these patients as anxious or dramatic. However, a significant proportion of patients are found to be relaxed, successful, well-adjusted people with troublesome episodes of pain (24).

Levator Ani Syndrome

Levator ani syndrome is defined as chronic or recurrent rectal pain or aching, which lasts 20 minutes or longer; symptoms for a minimum of 12 weeks over one year must be present to establish this diagnosis (10). The reported discomfort is located high in the rectum with a sensation of an intrarectal object, rectal fullness, or sensation of sitting on a ball (10,25). Spasm of the levator ani muscle is believed to be responsible, and palpation of the levator ani muscle will reveal a tight painful band (25). The differences between proctalgia fugax, as described above, and levator spasm are sometimes subtle and some literature does not distinguish between the two. However, with careful interrogation, the pain can often be classified as proctalgia fugax or levator spasm. The finding of a tight band-like puborectalis muscle is consistent with levator ani syndrome, while the physical exam in proctalgia fugax patients is usually unremarkable.

Pudendal Neuropathy

There is a sufficient body of literature regarding pudendal neuropathy to distinguish it as a separate category of anorectal pain (26–32). In one series of 68 patients with proctalgia, 55 were found to have a point of tenderness corresponding to the pudendal nerve; when this specific point was palpated, it reproduced an attack of pain (28). Bicycling can produce chronic inflammation and fibrosis which entraps the pudendal nerve and precipitates this form of pain (32). Fibrosis and pudendal nerve entrapment may also be the mechanism by which radiation therapy of the prostate causes pain (33). The subtle characteristic which distinguishes pudendal neuropathy is the positional aspect: the pain increases with sitting, and is relieved by sitting on a toilet or standing (27). The only finding on physical examination may be pain with palpation at the ischial spine on digital rectal examination (26).

MANAGEMENT

The treatment of chronic rectal pain has been referred to as a "frustrating endeavor" (34). The most successful treatment algorithms involve patience and sequential trials and combination therapies. After excluding organic, treatable, and potentially dangerous conditions, the first line of therapy is reassurance and conservative measures. Bowel habits should be optimized to avoid excessive strain on the pelvic floor. Fiber supplementation may be recommended. Heat, usually in the form of warm water baths, has consistently been proven beneficial despite minimal objective data (35). Nonsteroidal anti-inflammatory mediations, if not contraindicated, and low-dose diazepam (2 mg at bedtime) can be considered as the first line medical therapy. In addition, a regimen of perineal strengthening exercises may relieve pain by inducing muscle fatigue (36,37).

When specific points of tenderness can be identified, targeted treatment is beneficial. Transanal digital massage, as part of a regimen of heat and muscle relaxants, has provided relief of symptoms of levator ani syndrome (25). Application of linearly polarized near-infrared radiation therapy to a strongly tender point has been described as a simple, safe, and effective modality (38). In cases of pudendal neuralgia, CT or ultrasound-guided nerve blocks (29,30) and surgical decompression of the nerve have been successful (26,31).

Pharmacotherapy

Several medications have been used for the treatment of anorectal pain. Some relieve muscle spasm, while others act by an unknown mechanism. Medications include oral diltiazem (80 mg twice daily) (21), oral clonidine (150 μg twice daily then one week of tapering dosage) (39), inhaled salbutamol (40), and topical nitroglycerin (8,9,41,42).

Botulinum Toxin

Injection of botulinum toxin may benefit patients by treating muscle dystonia in the anorectal area (8,9,43). In a small study, injection of 25 IU of botulinum A toxin, with supplementary 50 IU injections as needed, demonstrated high success with no morbidity (43).

Biofeedback Therapy

Biofeedback is a valuable therapy for motivated patients who have access to a dedicated and skilled biofeedback therapist (44–46). Electromyography-based biofeedback combined with techniques of muscle relaxation and cognitive-behavioral psychotherapy will help alleviate pain (44). The protocol is successful only if the patient is compliant. There is no risk of harm or worsening of symptoms with this treatment.

Electrogalvanic Stimulation

Electrogalvanic stimulation (EGS) is a therapy which delivers high-voltage, low-frequency oscillating electric current to produce sustained contraction of the levator muscle (47–52). Repeated application of the current induces muscle fatigue. The published success rates are notable, including one study which reports greater than 90% effectiveness (50). Some studies suggest this success decreases with longer follow-up time (47,52). However, EGS is considered a valuable and safe option for anorectal pain disorders (47–52).

In a short-term study of local injection therapy compared to EGS for levator ani syndrome, local injection at tender points had better results (53). In a comparison of EGS, biofeedback therapy, and steroid caudal block in 60 patients with chronic intractable rectal pain, more than half of the patients were refractory to all three therapeutic options (34). These comparison studies emphasize the need to individualize treatment. If there is an obvious area of tenderness, it should be targeted for therapy. In other cases, patient variables and characteristics may cause the patient to be refractory to multiple modalities.

Acupuncture

Acupuncture should not be regarded only for refractory cases, but should be considered as an adjunct to all steps of the treatment algorithm. Acupuncture is a therapy that has withstood the test of time, and is an option for all patients regardless of their response to conventional therapies (54). While limited in number, a variety of modern studies have reported acupuncture as effective treatment for disorders of pelvic pain (55–60).

A formal pain management program is an extremely valuable resource, particularly for those cases where the cause of the pain is likely multifactorial (61). A trained pain specialist can offer additional therapies such as differential and diagnostic pain blocks and steroid caudal blocks (62).

CONCLUSION

While some literature groups all idiopathic rectal pain into one class, the entities of coccygodynia, levator ani syndrome, proctalgia, and pudendal neuralgia should be distinguished, if possible. Classification of the pain and location of tender anatomical points are helpful for targeting therapy. The surgeon should be aware of the available options for treatment and design an algorithm tailored to the individual patient. Two important patient variables are the degree of distress caused by the pain, and their motivation to comply with treatment. Some decisions will be based on availability, such as EGS and biofeedback therapy. An effective approach to the complaint of anorectal pain is composed of a variety of factors; however, realistic expectations from both the patient and the physician are crucial.

REFERENCES

1. Ziegler DK, Batnitzky S. Coccygodynia caused by perineural cyst. Neurology 1984; 34:829–830.
2. Lourie J, Young S. Avascular necrosis of the coccyx: A cause for coccygodynia? Case report and histological findings in sixteen patients. Br J Clin Practice 1985; 39:247–248.
3. Wray C, Esom S, Hoskinson J. Coccygodynia: Etiology and treatment. J Bone Joint Surg Am 1991; 73B:335–338.
4. Postacchini F, Massobrio M. Idiopathic coccygodynia: Analysis of fifty-one operative cases and a radiographic study of the normal coccyx. J Bone Joint Surg Am 1983; 65 A:1116–1124.
5. Jelovsek JE, Barber MD, Paraiso M, et al. Functional bowel and anorectal disorders in patients with pelvic organ prolapse and incontinence. Am J Obstet Gynecol 2005; 193:2105–2111.
6. Jao SW, Beart RW Jr, Spencer RJ et al. Retrorectal tumors: Mayo Clinic experience, 1960–1979. Dis Colon Rectum 1984; 28:644–652.
7. Glasgow SC, Birnbaum EH, Lowney JK, et al. Retrorectal tumors: A diagnostic and therapeutic challenge. Dis Colon Rectum 2005; 48:1581–1587.
8. Gracia Solanas JA, Ramirez Rodriguez JM, Elia Guedea M, et al. Sequential treatment for proctalgia fugax. Mid-term follow-up. Revista Espanola de Enfermedades Digestivas 2005; 97(7):491–496.
9. Christiansen J, Bruun E, Skjoldbye B, et al. Chronic idiopathic anal pain: Analysis of ultrasonography, pathology and treatment. Dis Colon Rectum 2001; 44:661–665.
10. Whitehead WE, Wald A, Diamant NE, et al. Functional disorders of the anus and rectum [Rome II: A multinational consensus document on functional gastrointestinal disorders]. Gut 1999; 45(supp II):II-55–II-59.
11. Hall M. Severe pain in the rectum and its remedy. Lancet 1841; 1:838, 854–855.
12. Thaysen EH. Proctalgia fugax. Lancet 1935; 2:243.
13. Peery WH. Proctalgia fugax: A clinical enigma. South Med J 1988; 81:621–623.
14. De Parades V, Etienney I, Bauer P, et al. Proctalgia fugax: Demographic and clinical characteristics. What every doctor should know from a prospective study of 54 patients. Dis Colon Rectum 2007; 50:893–898.
15. Harvey RF. Colonic motility in proctalgia fugax. Lancet 1979; 2:713–714.
16. Sinaki M, Merritt JL, Stillwell GK. Tension myalgia of the pelvic floor. Mayo Clin Proc 1977; 52(11):717–722.
17. Eckardt VF, Dodt O, Kanzler G, et al. Anorectal function and morphology in patients with sporadic proctalgia fugax. Dis Colon Rectum 1996; 39:755–762.
18. Rao SSC, Hatfield RA. Paroxysmal anal hyperkinesis: A characteristic feature of proctalgia fugax. Gut 1996; 39:609–612.
19. Celik AF, Katsinelos P, Read NW, et al. Hereditary proctalgia fugax and constipation: Report of a second family. Gut 1995; 36:581–584.
20. de la Portilla F, Borrero JJ, Rafel E. Hereditary vacuolar internal anal sphincter myopathy causing proctalgia fugax and constipation: A new case contribution. Eur J Gastroenterol Hepatol 2005; 17(3):359–361.
21. Boquet J, Moore N, Lhuintre JP, et al. Diltiazem for proctalgia fugax. Lancet 1986; 1:1493.
22. Thompson WG. Proctalgia fugax in patients with the irritable bowel, peptic ulcer, or inflammatory bowel disease. Am J Gastroenterol 1984; 6:450–452.

23. Pilling LF, Swenson WM, Hill JR: The psychological aspects of proctalgia fugax. Dis Colon Rectum 1972; 8:372–374.
24. Mountifield JA. Proctalgia fugax: A cause of marital disharmony. CMAJ 1986; 134:1269–1270.
25. Grant SR, Salvati EP, Rubin RJ. Levator syndrome: An analysis of 316 cases. Dis Colon Rectum 1975; 18:161–163.
26. Ramsden CE, McDaniel MC, Harmon RL, et al. Pudendal nerve entrapment as source of intractable perineal pain. Phys Med Rehabil 2003; 82:479–484.
27. Robert R, Prat-Pradal D, Labatt JJ et al. Anatomic basis of chronic perineal pain:role of the pudendal nerve. Surg Radiol Anat 1998; 20:93–98.
28. Takano M. Proctalgia fugax:caused by pudendal neuropathy? Dis Colon Rectum 2005; 48:114–120.
29. Hough DM, Wittenberg KH, Pawling W, et al. Chronic perineal pain caused by pudendal nerve entrapment: Anatomy and CT guided perineal injection technique. Am J Roentgenol 2003; 181:561–567.
30. Kovacs P, Gruber H, Piegger J, et al. New, simple, ultrasound-guided infiltration of the pudendal nerve. Dis Colon Rectum 2001; 44:1381–1385.
31. Mauillon J, Thomas D, Leroi AM, et al. Results of pudendal nerve neurolysis transposition in twelve patients suffering from pudendal neuralgia. Dis Colon Rectum 1999; 42:186–192.
32. Ricchiuti VS, Haas CA, Seftel AD,et al. Pudendal nerve injury associated with avid bicycling. J Urol 2000; 162:2099.
33. Antolak SJ, Hough DM, Pawlina W. The chronic pelvic pain syndrome after brachytherapy for carcinoma of the prostate. J Urol 2002; 167:2525.
34. Ger GC, Wexner SD, Jorge JMN,et al. Evaluation and treatment of chronic intractable rectal pain—a frustrating endeavor. Dis Colon Rectum 1993; 36:139–145.
35. Dodi G, Bogoni F, Infantino A, et al. Hot or cold in anal pain? A study in the changes in internal anal sphincter pressure profiles. Dis Colon Rectum 1986; 29:248–251.
36. Thiele GH. Coccygodynia: Cause and treatment. Dis Colon Rectum 1963; 6:422–436.
37. Salvati EP. The levator syndrome and its variant. Gastroenterol Clin North Am 1987; 16:71–78.
38. Mibu R, Hotokezaka M, Mihara S, et al. Results of linearly polarized near-infrared irradiation therapy in patients with intractable anorectal pain. Dis Colon Rectum 2003; 46:S50–S53.
39. Swain R. Oral clonidine for proctalgia fugax. Gut 1987; 28:1039–1040.
40. Eckardt VF, Dodt O, Kanzler G, et al. Treatment of proctalgia fugax with salbutamol inhalation. Am J Gastroentrol 1996; 91:686–689.
41. Lowenstein B, Cataldo PA. Treatment of proctalgia fugax with topical nitroglycerin:report of a case. Dis Colon Rectum 1998; 41:667–668.
42. Hyman N, Cataldo P. Topical nitroglycerin for levator spasm. Dis Colon Rectum 1999; 42(3):427.
43. Sanchez Romero AM, Arroyo Sebastian A, Perez Vicente FA, et al. Treatment of proctalgia fugax with botulinum toxin: Results in 5 patients. Revista Clinica Espanola 2006; 206(3):137–140.
44. Gilliland R, Heyman JS, Altomare DF, et al. Biofeedback for intractable rectal pain: Outcome and predictors of success. Dis Colon Rectum 1997; 40:190–196.
45. Heah SM, Ho YH, Tan M, et al. Biofeedback is effective treatment for levator ani syndrome. Dis Colon Rectum 1997; 40:187–189.
46. Bassotti G, Whitehead WE. Biofeedback, relaxation training, and cognitive behaviour modification as treatments for lower functional gastrointestinal disorders. QJM 1997; 90:545–550.
47. Chiarioni G, Chistolini F, Menegotti M, et al. One year follow-up study on the effects of electrogalvanic stimulation in chronic idiopathic constipation with pelvic floor dyssynergia. Dis Colon Rectum 2004; 47:346–353.
48. Sohn N, Weinstein MA, Robbins RD. The levator syndrome and its treatment with high-voltage electrogalvanic stimulation. Am J Surg 1982; 144:580–582.
49. Oliver GC, Rubin RJ, Salvati EP, et al. Electrogalvanic stimulation in the treatment of levator syndrome. Dis Colon Rectum 1985; 28:662–663.
50. Nicosa JF, Abcarian H. Levator syndrome: A treatment that works. Dis Colon Rectum 1985; 28:406–408.
51. Billingham RP, Isler JT, Friend WG, et al. Treatment of levator syndrome using high-voltage electrogalvanic stimulation. Dis Colon Rectum 1987; 30:584–587.
52. Hull TL, Milsom JW, Church J, et al. Electrogalvanic stimulation for levator syndrome: How effective is it in the long term? Dis Colon Rectum 1993; 36:731–733.
53. Park D-H, Yoon S-G, Kim KU, et al. Comparison study between electrogalvanic stimulation and local injection therapy in levator ani syndrome. In J Colorectal Dis 2005; 20:272–276.
54. Frank LP. Acupuncture for pelvic floor dysfunction. In: Davila GW, Ghoniem GM, Wexner SD, eds. Pelvic Floor Dysfunction: A Multidisciplinary Approach. London: Springer Verlag, 2006:259–262.
55. Chang PL. Urodynamic studies in acupuncture for women with frequency, urgency and dysuria. J Urol 1988; 140:563–566.
56. Pigne A, DeGoursac C, Barrat J. Acupuncture and unstable bladder. In: Proceedings of 15th Annual Meeting of International Continence Society, London, 1985:186–187.

57. Shaoguang W. Electroacupuncture treatment for constipation due to spasmodic syndrome of the pelvic floor. J Trad Chin Med 2001; 21(3):205–206.
58. Wedenberg K, Moen B, Norling A. A prospective randomized study comparing acupuncture with physiotherapy for low-back pain in pregnancy. Acta Obstet Gynecol Scand 2000; 79:331–335.
59. Martin DC, Ling FW. Endometriosis and pain. Clin Obstet Gynecol 1999; 42:664–686.
60. Steege JF, Stout AL, Somkuti SG. Chronic pelvic pain in women: Toward an integrative model. Obstet Gynecol 1991; 3:30.
61. Gobrial W. Pain localization and control. In: Davila GW, Ghoniem GM, Wexner SD, eds. Pelvic Floor Dysfunction: A Multidisciplinary Approach. London: Springer Verlag, 2006:259–262.
62. Amaranth L, Wexner SD. Caudal epidural block in the management of proctalgia fugax. Am J Pain Manage 1994; 4:153–155.

15 Anorectal Abscess

Orit Kaidar-Person and Benjamin Person
Department of General Surgery B, Rambam Healthcare Campus, Haifa, Israel

INTRODUCTION

An abscess is an acute process in which pus is accumulated in a cavity in the tissue as a reaction to an infection or a foreign material (1). Anal fistula is a pathology that often coexists with anorectal abscess. The exact pathologic relationship is yet to be determined, but it is believed that anorectal abscess is an acute presentation of a fistula (2).

Anorectal abscess is a common surgical condition; however, the exact incidence of this disease cannot be estimated since most of the cases do not necessarily result in hospitalization, as some rupture spontaneously while others are treated in the physician's office without any official documentation. An abscess usually requires immediate surgical intervention (3). Understanding the anorectal anatomy, knowledge of the pathophysiology of anorectal abscess, identification of possible colorectal pathologies that may contribute to the presence of an abscess, and identification of potential complex cases that may require in-hospital drainage are crucial in order to achieve a satisfactory response to treatment and to avoid devastating consequences.

HISTOLOGY, ANATOMY, AND PATHOPHYSIOLOGY

The anal canal is approximately 5 cm in length; it begins a few centimeters proximal to the dentate line and ends at the anal verge.

Histology and Pathophysiology

The lining of the anal canal is a composition of various types of epithelium and glands that take part in the pathologic process of abscess formation. The proximal end of the anal canal is a transitional zone (5–20 mm above the dentate line) where the columnar epithelium of the rectum becomes a transitional epithelium. The mucosa in the transitional zone is cuboidal and is thought to be important for discrimination between gas and stool (4). This epithelium changes into stratified squamous epithelium at the mucocutaneous junction at the dentate line. Thus, proximal to the dentate line the epithelium of the anal canal is mucosa, and distal to the dentate line it is stratified nonkeratinized squamous epithelium. Anal glands lie within the intersphincteric plane at the level of the dentate line. They secrete mucus that empties into the anal crypts (into the lumen of the anal canal) through the anal ducts. The anal crypts macroscopically appear as small pits along the anal valve at the dentate line (5–8). Eisenhammer (9) and Parks' (10) cryptoglandular theory relates the formation of anorectal abscess to infection at the site of the anal glands. Similar to that theory, Whitney's (11) "cryptitis" theory closely resembles the cryptoglandular theory and differs only in terminology. These authors proposed that, as the intramuscular anal glands become infected, the ducts become obstructed by debris resulting in stasis of the glandular secretions which interferes with the body's defense mechanisms. When the ducts are obstructed, the glands cannot drain into the anal canal. It is unclear which comes first, the infection within the gland or the stasis; a disorder that causes primarily mucous retention in the crypts might result in secondary infection (9). Moreover, Parks (12) demonstrated that approximately 50% of the crypts are not connected to the anal glands, and that the ducts end blindly, usually downward into the submucosa. In two-thirds of the specimens, he noted that one or more branches of the duct enter the sphincter, and in one half, the branches cross the internal anal sphincter (IAS). The consequence of these histologic findings is that obstruction or infection of the duct itself may result in an abscess and subsequently fistula formation. Infection of the anal gland as a stage in the development of fistula-in-ano was first suggested by Chiari (13). A subsequent histopathologic report documented that up to 80% of the anal glands are submucosal, 8% extend to the IAS, 8% to the conjoined longitudinal muscle, 2% to the intersphincteric space, and 1% penetrate the external anal sphincter (EAS) (14). This might be the pathologic explanation of transphincteric fistula and the various locations of anorectal abscess.

The anal canal ends at the anal verge, which is the point where the stratified squamous epithelium becomes skin; this is marked by the presence of hair follicles and sweat glands. It also contains apocrine glands that may be associated with hidradenitis suppurativa. This disease is an inflammatory process that involves the apocrine glands which are located in different areas of the body such as the axilla, scalp, and perineum. The disease does not present prior to puberty and may well result in abscesses and fistulas in various locations, including the anorectal region (15).

Anatomy and Pathophysiology

The musculature of the anal canal forms the anal sphincter mechanism. Familiarity with these structures is essential for understanding the course of the disease, therapeutic approach, and is imperative in order to avoid devastating complications such as fecal incontinence.

The anal canal is composed of two circular muscular layers; each is formed by different types of muscle fibers and has a distinct role in the evacuation process. The inner muscle layer is composed of smooth muscle, is approximately 3 cm in length, and is a direct continuation of the inner circular muscle of the lower rectum. This layer is known as the IAS. It is widely accepted that injury of the IAS may result in incontinence (16). Alterations in the IAS may occur with age, gender, and previous injury. Some authors have reported that thickness of the IAS increases with age, most probably associated with fibrous thickening (17–19).

The external muscle layer composes the EAS, which is a skeletal muscle and is thus under voluntary control. There is a distinct anatomic plane between the IAS and the EAS occupied by longitudinal connective tissue fibers which are continuous with the outer longitudinal muscle wall of the rectum. This area is termed the intersphincteric plane, in which the anal glands lie at the level of the dentate line, and is frequently the area where the infection begins and through which it spreads (Fig. 1). The EAS is arbitrarily separated into three components: subcutaneous, superficial, and deep. The deep division of the EAS is part of the puborectalis muscle and it appears to be significant for maintaining fecal continence (20). The anatomy of the anal canal and perianal structures as defined by phased-array magnetic resonance imaging (MRI) was described by Morren and coworkers (21) and showed that the EAS was shorter in females than in males, and occupied, respectively, 30% and 38% of the length of the anal canal.

The potential anorectal spaces are the basis of a widely used classification of anorectal abscesses. This classification is crucial for proper eradication of the inflammatory process and may aid in identification of the fistulous tract (Fig. 1). These spaces include the intersphincteric, perianal, ischioanal, supralevator, and deep postanal spaces.

As mentioned earlier, the intersphincteric space lies between the IAS and the EAS and is bounded superiorly by the rectal wall. Inferiorly, the intersphincteric space continues with the perianal space. The perianal space is located superficially in the area of the anal verge. It is bounded by the ischioanal fat laterally and extends medially to the distal portion of the anal canal. The ischioanal space extends from the levator ani muscle to the perineum. Anteriorly, it is bounded by the transverse perineal muscles and posteriorly by the gluteus maximus muscle and the sacrotuberous ligament. Its lateral border is formed by the obturator internus muscle and medially it is bounded by the levator ani and the EAS. The supralevator space is bounded laterally by the pelvic wall, medially by the rectal wall, superiorly by the peritoneum, and inferiorly by the levator ani muscle. The deep postanal space is located deep to the EAS and the IAS, between the coccyx posteriorly, and lies below the levator ani and above the anococygeal ligament (2).

The infection may spread in several directions, giving rise to a variety of abscesses and fistulas (12). Infection usually begins in the intersphincteric plane. If the infection spreads downward, a perianal abscess will result; if it tracks upward, a high intersphincteric or supralevator abscess will be formed. Infection that crosses the EAS will result in an ischiorectal abscess, and upward spread across the levator might also result in a supralevator abscess. A circumferential spread that may occur in each of the above-mentioned compartments will form a horseshoe abscess. Accumulation of pus in each of these spaces will result in different presenting symptoms and will necessitate a different surgical approach. The term submucosal abscess (or submucous)

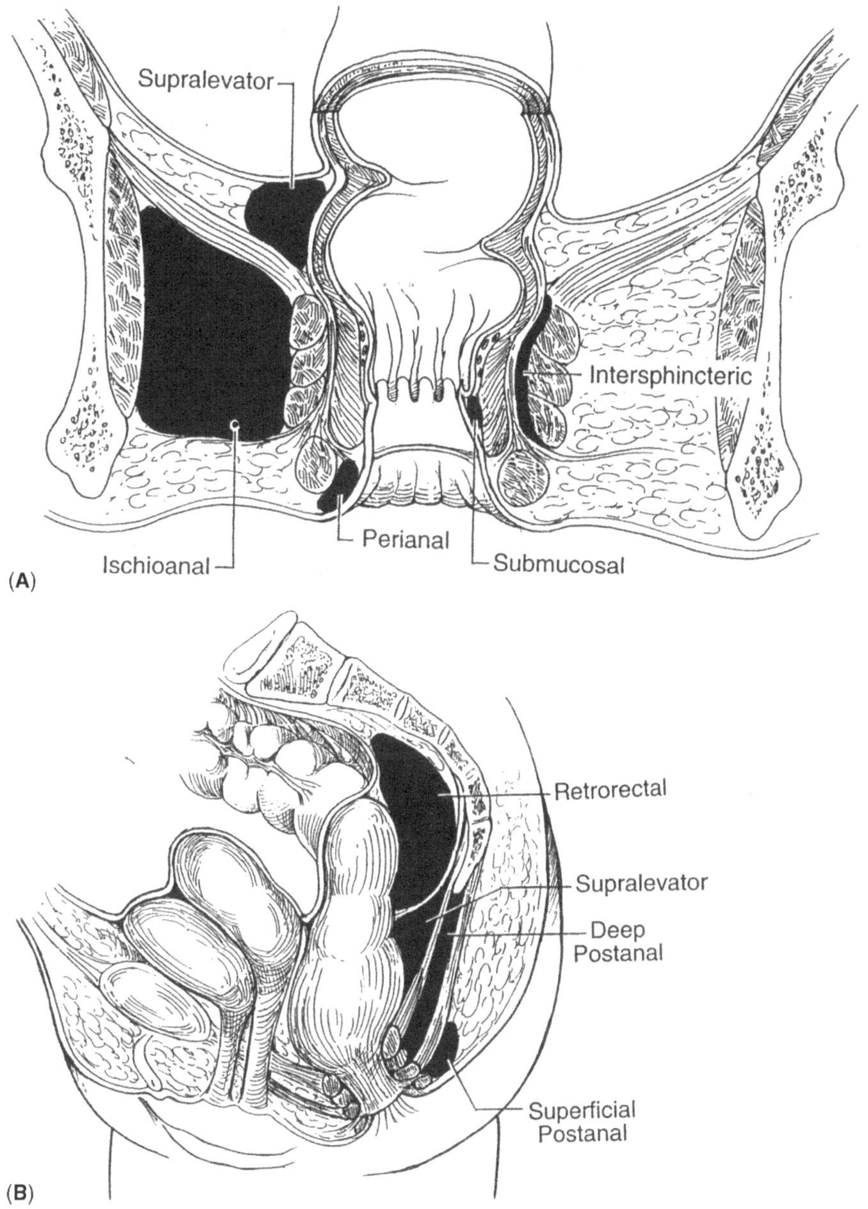

Figure 1 Anorectal spaces. **(A)** Coronal section. **(B)** Sagittal section. *Source*: From Ref. 75.

is confusing since it is unclear whether it is simply a misnomer for an intersphincteric abscess that migrated upward and protruded into the lower rectum, since it is not located in the submucosa (22,23). Some textbooks have actually diagramed a submucosal abscess at the level of the anal canal, either near the anal verge or proximal to the dentate line (2,24); however, if it does exist in this location, this is also a misnomer since the line liying below the dentate line is not mucosa but stratified nonkeratinized epithelium (25).

This classification is not absolute and many patients have more than one abscess component (anatomically); in these patients, the classification can be made for convenience according to the major component of the abscess (22). In a series of 1023 patients treated in the section of colorectal surgery at Cook County Hospital, the abscesses were classified according to the major component. Perianal abscesses were most frequently encountered and were seen in 42.7% of cases, ischiorectal and intersphincteric abscesses were almost equal in incidence at

22.8% and 21.4%, respectively. The least common abscesses were supralevator and submucous (high intersphincteric) abscess (22).

Abscesses can also be subdivided according to their circumferential location around the anal canal. Parks (12) reported that 24% were located anteriorly and 61% were located posteriorly. According to the Cook County Hospital experience, 50% of the abscesses were located in the posterior quadrant and one-third in the lateral quadrants. Only 12.1% of the abscesses were located anteriorly (22). The higher incidence of anorectal abscess in the posterior quadrant of the anorectum may be explained by the fact that many of the anal crypts and glands are located in this quadrant.

ETIOLOGY

It is estimated that approximately 90% of all anorectal abscesses are the result of cryptoglandular infection (2), although very few subsequent studies confirm or refute Eisenhammer and Parks' findings. The remainder may be a consequence of conditions such as previous colorectal or pelvic surgery, inflammatory bowel diseases, trauma, malignancy, and others (Table 1) (15,26–32).

Table 1 Predisposing Conditions and Causes of Anorectal Abscess

- Cryptoglandular origin
- Inflammatory bowel disease
  - Crohn's disease
  - Ulcerative colitis
- Infectious
- Hidradenitis suppurativa (15)
- Extension of a Pilonidal abscess
- Tuberculosis (26)[a]
  - Actinomycosis (27,28)[a]
  - Lymphogranuloma venereum (29,30)[a]
- Nontyphoidal Salmonella (31)
- Cryptococcal infection (32)
- Rectal schistosomiasis
- Amebiasis
- Trauma
  - Penetrating trauma
  - Hematoma
- Hard stool/ Diarrhea
- Foreign body (Swallowed, gastrointestinal tract, urinary tract)
- Autoerotic/erotic
- Psychiatric
- Therapeutic
- Trauma
- Surgery
  - Hemorrhoidectomy
  - Internal anal sphincterotomy
  - Episiotomy
  - Prostatectomy
  - Colorectal surgery
  - Excision of rectal endometriosis
- Anal fissure
- Malignancy
  - Carcinoma
  - Leukemia
  - Lymphoma
- Radiation
- Immune-compromised state (prior to bone marrow transplantation)
- Acquired immunodeficiency syndrome (AIDS)
- Diabetes mellitus

[a]Either as inflammatory bowel disease or manifestation of an extraintestinal disease.

MICROBIOLOGY AND ANTIBIOTICS

A few studies that evaluated the microbiology of anorectal abscesses have suggested that an acute anorectal abscess that was colonized with enteric microorganisms (such as Escherichia coli, Bacteroides, Bacillus, and Klebsiella species) rather than nonenteric bacteria (skin bacteria: coagulase-negative Staphylococci and Peptostreptococcus species) was more likely to be associated with an anal fistula. The authors recommended that when the microbiological analysis yields enteric bacteria, but no fistula has been found in the initial drainage operation, repeat examinations with various modalities (such as manual and endoanal ultrasound examinations) were mandatory to identify an occult fistula-in-ano (33,34).

Traditionally, cultures taken from an inflammation site are usually obtained for determining the appropriate antibiotic treatment; this is not the case in most anorectal abscesses. According to the guidelines established by the American Society of Colon and Rectal Surgeons (35), perianal abscesses require immediate incision and drainage and that additional antibiotics in cases of uncomplicated anorectal abscesses were not needed. These recommendations follow evidence that the addition of antibiotics to incision and drainage of cutaneous abscesses did not improve outcomes (36). These recommendations do not apply in cases of immunocompromised patients, patients with diabetes mellitus, prosthetic devices, systemic sepsis, or evidence of extensive soft-tissue cellulitis. The recommendations of the American Heart Association should be enforced, and preoperative antibiotic coverage should be given to patients with prosthetic cardiac valves, previous endocarditis, complex congenital heart disease and malformations, surgically constructed systemic pulmonary shunts or conduits, acquired valve dysfunction, hypertrophic cardiomyopathy, and mitral valve prolapse with valvular regurgitation and/or thickened leaflets (35,37).

It appears that there is a minor role for antibiotics in the primary management of anorectal abscess, except in selected cases. The treatment of anorectal abscesses should not be delayed by a course of antibiotics, and there is no indication for delaying drainage while "waiting for the abscess to mature" and fluctuance to develop. The treatment should be an immediate incision and drainage. Delay of such treatment is only justified if the patient presented to the office, and the office setting was not optimal to perform the procedure; these cases will be discussed later in this chapter. The surgeon should evaluate the extent of the infection, the clinical status of the patient and follow the recommendations of the American Heart Association for prevention of endocarditis (2,35). Special consideration should be given for individual cases such as patients with an increased risk for opportunistic infections (29,32), patients with foreign bodies (such as intrauterine device (27,28), and immigrants from endemic areas (26,28).

EPIDEMIOLOGY

As cited above, the exact incidence of anorectal abscess cannot be estimated since some rupture spontaneously, while still others are treated in the physician's office without any official documentation. Thus, it may be difficult to conduct large longitudinal studies in order to assess the incidence or prevalence of this condition. Nelson (38) suggested evaluating the incidence of anorectal abscesses from available data on anal fistulas, since fistulas are unlikely to resolve spontaneously and usually require surgical intervention. Calculating backwards from numerous studies brought to a coarse estimation of incidence of 68,000 and 96,000 cases of anal abscess in United States, and since an abscess is an acute state, the incidence usually exceeds the prevalence.

Anorectal abscesses occur nearly twice as frequently in men than in women (23,39). Other studies have also indicated a male predominance (40,41). The majority of patients are in the third or fourth decades of life (37,38,42).

SYMPTOMS AND CLINICAL EVALUATION

Symptoms depend on the site of the abscess and the extent of the infection. The classic symptoms of acute suppuration—a tender erythematous swelling—often accompany perianal abscess due to its superficial location. In this case, the inflammatory mass will be present outside

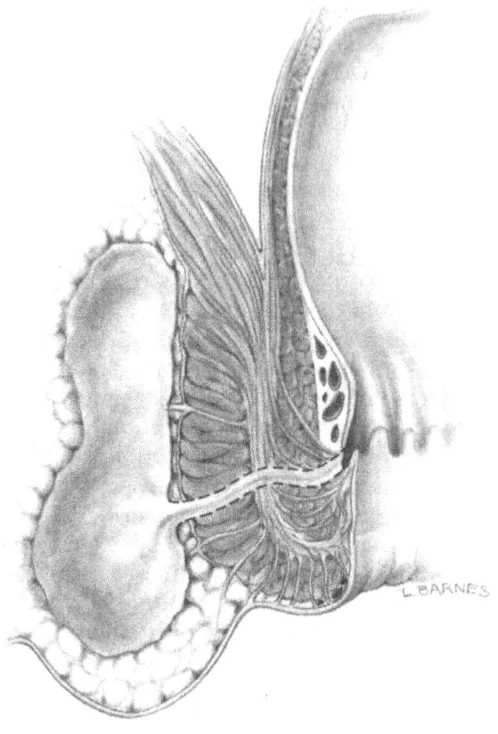

Figure 2 Ischiorectal abscess. *Source*: From Ref. 23.

the anal verge and fluctuance might not be present. In the other types of anorectal abscesses that are located deep within the pelvic tissue, a mass may not be easily evident on physical examination, or it may only be palpated or visualized during a rectal exam or anoscopy (Fig. 1) (43). If present, it may be located on the upper part of the anal canal or the lower part of the rectum. Because of the location, the patient may recount a history of prolonged symptoms (pain, fever), and is more likely to have systemic symptoms such as fever and leukocytosis compared to a superficial perianal abscess. An ischiorectal abscess, if swelling and erythema are involved, will appear medially at the buttock, lateral to the anal verge (Fig. 2). A deep postanal abscess can be associated with severe rectal discomfort, pain radiating to the sacrum, coccyx, or buttocks, and may be confused for coccydynia. An intersphincteric abscess is usually associated with severe pain and frequently requires an evaluation under anesthesia (EUA). Pain associated with an anorectal abscess is often exacerbated by or appears after evacuation.

Of the 1023 patients evaluated in the Cook County Hospital study, pain was a universal symptom and was present in all patients (22). If the abscess is associated with a fistula, the patient may complain of mucous, pus, or bloody discharge unrelated to evacuation (38). Urinary symptoms may also accompany this disease; symptoms of dysuria, retention, or inability to void may be suggestive of intersphincteric or supralevator abscess (2).

Since the majority of anorectal abscesses are resolved in the physician's office, usually during the first office visit, it is imperative to note that an anorectal abscess may be the first presentation of an anorectal cancer; moreover, patients with chronic anorectal disease are at an increased risk of developing cancer (44,45). Biopsies should be obtained if such a suspicion arises. Conditions that may be associated with anorectal pain, and should be considered in the differential diagnosis, are summarized in Table 2.

There are various diagnostic modalities that may aid in the diagnosis of an anorectal abscess including endoanal ultrasound, computerized tomography (CT), MRI, or radionucleotide white cell scanning; these modalities should not delay drainage which is both diagnostic and therapeutic, unless there is a suspicion of a coexisting pathology that may require a more complex intervention, or in cases of immunocompromised patients (38). In cases in which pain precludes a proper office examination, patients need to undergo an EUA.

Table 2 Differential Diagnosis for Anorectal Pain

Anal fissure
Anorectal abscess
Anorectal abscess with fistula
Thrombosed hemorrhoid
Proctitis (Gonococcal/ chlamydial infection)
Levator spasm
Proctalgia fugax
Sexual transmitted disease
Cancer
Foreign body
Trauma/ perianal hematoma
Perianal Crohn's disease
Ulcerative colitis
Pilonidal abscess/sinus
Bartholin's abscess
Tuberculosis
Hidradenitis suppurativa
Lymphogranuloma venereum
Solitary chronic rectal ulcer
Pruritus ani
Retrorectal cysts
Alcock's canal syndrome (entrapment of the pudendal nerve)
Testicular carcinoma
Cystitis
Prostatitis
Coccydynia
Rectal prolapse
Diverticular disease
Irritable bowel syndrome

Endoanal Ultrasound

Endoanal ultrasound can be used during the initial evaluation of the patient. Given that anorectal abscess is associated with substantial pain, patients should receive appropriate analgesia. This modality can aid in determining the location and extent of the abscess, presence of a fistula, and evaluating the integrity of the sphincter mechanism. The latter is important in patients in whom a fistulotomy is considered or if there is a history of fecal incontinence. Endoanal ultrasound may also serve for follow-up when recurrence of the abscess is suspected. The exact role of endoanal ultrasound is still controversial; Cataldo et al. (46) concluded that, in certain clinical situations, this modality can be beneficial but most cases can be managed without it, whereas Millan et al. (41) stated that endoanal ultrasound is important for accurate anatomical localization, proper drainage, and may help avoid recurrence or extrasphincteric fistula. It appears that the role of endoanal ultrasound is still evolving as ultrasound guided needle drainage of intersphincteric abscesses has been described as a treatment option (47). In cases of fistula-in-ano, injection of hydrogen peroxide through the external opening may assist with the identification of some tracts and internal openings, and enhance the appearance of the abscess on ultrasound (Fig. 3) (48).

TREATMENT

Incision and Drainage

The treatment of an anorectal abscess is prompt incision and drainage. Most patients can be treated in an outpatient setting; in selected cases, in-hospital drainage is recommended (Table 3). Antibiotic coverage should be given when indicated (2,35). Abscess drainage can be performed relatively easily; however, damage to involved or adjacent anatomical structures can cause lifelong morbidity. Moreover, approaching an anorectal abscess without examining the possibility of a potential fistula may be harmful. It is hypothesized that various types of anorectal abscesses have different incidences of fistula (Table 4) (22); this should be taken into

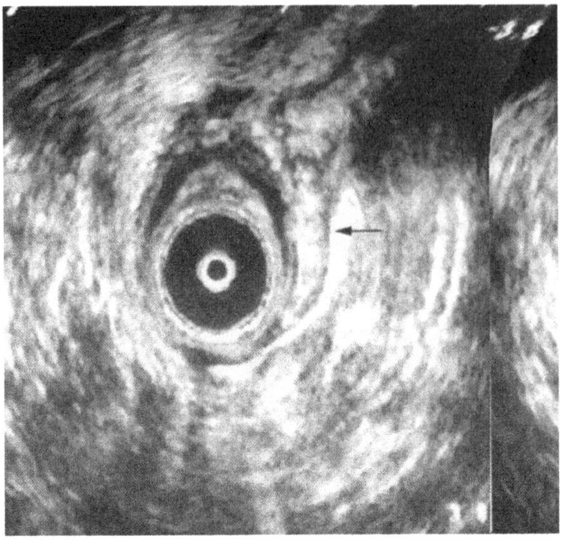

Figure 3 Ultrasound of anorectal abscess. *Source*: From Ref. 24.

account, and efforts should be made to identify the fistulous tract and internal opening, either during the primary drainage procedure or during follow-up.

A perianal abscess should be drained even when there is no fluctuance. In cases where the surgeon is uncertain, insertion of a large-bore hypodermic needle to the tenderness point may aid in the diagnosis (23). The procedure can be easily performed in the office under local anesthesia (2). The patient should be placed in a prone jackknife or left lateral position; the area should be prepped with an antiseptic solution and the most painful spot should be determined and subsequently infiltrated with 0.5% lidocaine with 1:200,000 of epinephrine. To prevent premature closure of the incision which may result in poor drainage and/or recurrence, the surgeon should create a cruciform or elliptical incision and trim its edges. Insertion of a drainage catheter or placement of a seton in case an internal opening is identified may also aid in promoting drainage (35,49). There is no need for packing of the cavity (2).

The technique of drainage of an uncomplicated ischiorectal abscess is similar to that of a perianal abscess. Ischiorectal abscesses are somewhat more challenging to treat because some are unapparent, have a high incidence of concomitant fistula, or are part of a more complex abscess such as a horseshoe abscess; thus, the patient should be properly evaluated prior to treatment. The site of the incision should be as close to the anal verge as possible (the medial side of the abscess), to allow for a smaller incision if a subsequent fistulotomy is indicated, and reduce the complexity of a subsequent fistula (2,23). After creating a cruciform or elliptical incision, the cavity can be irrigated with saline or an antiseptic solution. Although the abscess might be large, it is unnecessary to create a large incision; the incision should be located correctly to allow proper drainage, and premature closure should be prevented. A drain or seton can also be placed to promote drainage.

It is important to try and evaluate the patient during the primary procedure in order to locate an internal opening of a fistula, since up to 25% of the abscesses are associated with a

Table 3 Indications for In-Hospital Drainage

Need of general, spinal, or caudal anesthetic
Complex infection
Sepsis
Extensive cellulitis
Diabetes mellitus
Immune-compromised patient
Large abscess requiring vigorous irrigations
Indication for intravenous antibiotics
Intersphincteric abscess, horseshoe abscess, supralevator abscess, large ischiorectal abscess

Table 4 Incidence of Fistula in Different Types of Anorectal Abscesses According to the Cook County Hospital Experience

Type of abscess	*n*	Abscesses with fistula (%)
Perianal	437	34.5
Ischiorectal	233	25.3
Intersphincteric	219	47.4
Supralevator	75	42.6
High intersphincteric	59	15.2

Source: From Ref. 22.

fistula (Table 4) (22). Compressing the abscess before drainage while passing an anoscope might cause the pus to show through the internal opening and aid in its identification. Identifying an internal opening is an indication for a subsequent definitive treatment. This maneuver will cause severe pain for the patient, thus adequate anesthesia should be provided.

Drainage of a large ischiorectal, horseshoe, and/or deep postanal abscess is more complex and should generally not be performed in the outpatient setting. It requires regional or general anesthesia, while the patient is in the prone jackknife or left lateral position (2).

Patients will often have an external opening of a fistula and a preoperative diagnosis of a horseshoe fistula can be made by physical examination in up to 48% of cases; other diagnostic modalities that may aid in the diagnosis include contrast fistulography, ultrasound, and/or MRI (50). The surgical approach should be a midline incision made posteriorly between the coccyx and the anus (2,23,50–52). The incision should divide the superficial part of the EAS and extend to the lower half of the IAS to decompress the abscess. A counter-incision, one on either side, can be made over the ischioanal fossa to allow drainage of the anterior portion of the abscess (Hanley procedure) (Fig. 4) (2,51,52).

An intersphincteric abscess can be subdivided into high and low, according to the upward or downward extension of the pus (10). Parks and Thomson (9) found that in 55% of cases, the abscesses were associated with a bulge in the wall of the anal canal, 45% had an opening into the lumen of the anal canal, and an anal fistula was found in up to 25% of patients. In their study, none of the cases was associated with an external opening, and an opening into the lumen of the anal canal did not always indicate the presence of a fistula (9). Ramanujam et al. (22) described an incidence of fistula in up to 47.4% and 15.2% in patients with intersphincteric and high intersphincteric abscess, respectively. A protrusion of the abscess into the lumen of the anal canal or the lower rectum will aid in the diagnosis; however when there is doubt, the surgeon can introduce a needle into the intersphincteric plane while the patient is under anesthesia. The presence of pus will confirm the diagnosis. Treatment is usually performed under a general, caudal, or spinal anesthetic, in the proper setting (Table 3). The surgical approach is through the anus, by inserting an anal retractor and dividing the IAS along the length of the abscess, trimming the edges of the wound without primary closure to allow proper drainage.

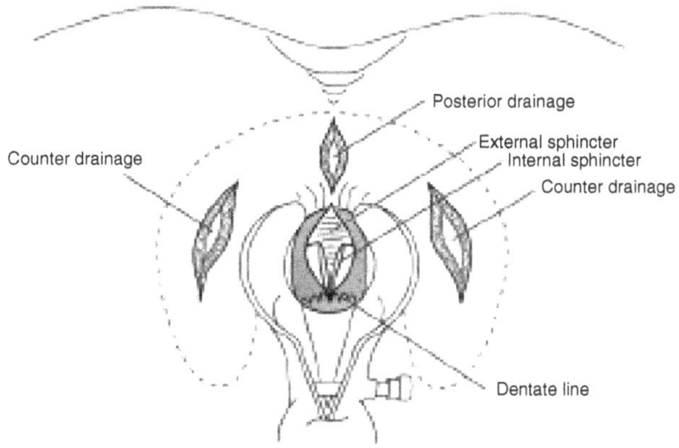

Figure 4 Drainage of horseshoe abscess. *Source*: From Ref. 2.

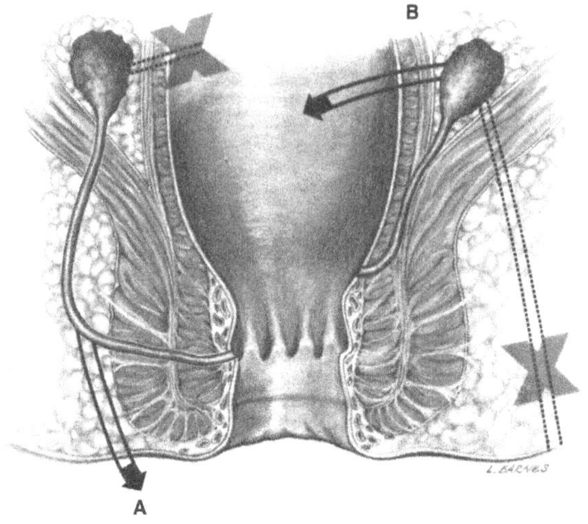

Figure 5 Suprasphincteric fistula. *Source*: From Ref. 23.

Supralevator abscesses are relatively uncommon, although in one series their incidence was up to 9.1% (40). In that series, the abscess was associated with leukocytosis, perianal pain, and/or fever in more than 70% of the cases. Gluteal pain was found in 24% of the cases and 20% of the patients were diabetic (39). Prior to treatment, the surgeon should determine the origin of the abscess: an underling pelvic inflammatory process, or an extension of another anorectal abscess such as an intersphincteric or ischioanal abscess (2). Drainage of the abscess should be performed according to its origin; incorrect drainage may result in a fistula formation. If the abscess has an intersphincteric origin or is related to pelvic sepsis, the abscess should be drained as an intersphincteric abscess at the level of the rectum, by incising the lower rectum at the appropriate level and dividing the upper part of the IAS. In this case, it is important to avoid external drainage as this can result in a subsequent suprasphincteric fistula (Fig. 5). If the abscess originates in the ischioanal fossa, it should be drained through the perianal skin (external drainage) and the incision should be as medial as possible. Intrarectal drainage in this case might result in a transphincteric fistula (Fig. 5). Packing should generally be avoided as this is usually very painful for the patient and precludes proper drainage.

Primary Closure

Primary closure of the skin after draining an anorectal abscess is not considered a common practice or standard of care. A few studies have evaluated traditional incision and drainage compared with primary closure (53–55) In one study, patients were randomized into both unroofing and packing, or into incision, curettage, and primary suture with systemic antibiotic treatment (53); patients with fistulas were excluded. The authors concluded that curettage and primary closure with systemic antibiotic treatment was significantly superior, without increased risk of recurrence or of subsequent fistula. A major flaw of this study was the relatively short follow-up of less than one year. Another randomized study (54,55) included patients with fistula, and primary fistulotomy was conducted at the time of the primary procedure if indicated. The initial report (54) suggested that primary closure resulted in lower rates of recurrence; a later publication from the same institution with a longer follow-up indicated that recurrence of abscess tended to be more frequent after skin closure (55). The healing time after skin closure was significantly shorter; thus the authors concluded that primary closure was the more attractive treatment option.

Catheter Drainage

A retrospective study from the Cleveland Clinic Foundation (56) included patients who were treated by placement of a 10–16 French soft latex mushroom catheter into the abscess cavity; antibiotics were not administered. No sutures or irrigations were used during the procedure, and the drains were removed after an average of 12 days. Four patients were diabetic and eight had a history of inflammatory bowel disease. Nine patients were treated previously for anorectal abscesses. A mean follow-up of 30 months was available for 31 patients. The authors concluded that catheter drainage of ischiorectal abscess in selected cases resulted in healing with low morbidity and significant cost savings.

This procedure can be easily performed in the office with local anesthesia while the patient is placed in a prone jackknife or left lateral position; a stab incision is made as medial as possible, thereby allowing the pus to drain. The size and length of the catheter should be determined by the size of the abscess cavity. A 10 to 16 French soft latex mushroom catheter is inserted into the abscess cavity over a probe. The shape of the catheter should hold it inside the cavity, obviating the need for a suture. The end of the catheter should be shortened to allow 2 to 3 cm to exit the skin, in order to avoid the possibility of the catheter falling into the abscess cavity. A small bandage is then applied over the catheter (2,56). In a study by Beck et al. (56), the drains were removed after an average of 12 days; the duration of the drain should be individualized according to clinical findings and progress, including the size of the original abscess, degree of granulation tissue, and amount of drainage.

Synchronous Treatment for Fistula

An anal fistula may be seen at the time of the primary drainage procedure. Whether a definitive procedure should be performed for fistula at the time of abscess drainage is still under debate. There is no doubt that the decision of performing a synchronous fistulotomy should be made according to the clinical scenario. A rigid attempt to identify and treat a fistula may result in a false passage and an unnecessary procedure. An internal opening cannot be identified in up to 66% of patients, and thus not all abscesses are associated with fistula (22,57). There are a few randomized controlled studies and subsequent meta-analyses that have addressed this issue. These studies differ in the time of randomization (prior to or after surgical exploration), the type of procedure performed for the fistula (fisulectomy vs. fistulotomy), timing of the fistulotomy, and type of abscess, bringing into question the value of the subsequent meta-analyses (39,58–64). A meta-analysis that included five trials with a total of 405 patients concluded that sphincter-cutting procedures for anorectal abscesses resulted in a 83% reduction in recurrence rate; however, there was a tendency, albeit not statistically significant, for a higher risk of fecal incontinence to gas and soiling when a primary sphincter-cutting procedure was performed ($p = 0.140$). The authors concluded that there was no conclusive evidence as to whether simple incision and drainage or sphincter-cutting procedure was better in the treatment of anorectal abscess fistula (63).

Current recommendations published in the ASCRS Textbook of Colon and Rectal Surgery (2) state that if the internal opening of a low transsphincteric fistula was readily apparent during the primary drainage procedure, it was feasible to perform a primary fistulotomy. Exceptions to this recommendation include patients with Crohn's disease or AIDS, elderly patients, those with a high transsphincteric fistula, and women with anterior fistulas and episiotomy scars. The treatment options for anal fistulas are further discussed in a separate chapter in this text.

Postoperative Care

Warm sitz baths, noncodeine analgesics, and stool bulk forming agents are recommended. Follow-up visits should be scheduled by clinical judgment; patients with an intersphincteric or supralevator fistula, large abscess, diabetes mellitus, or other significant comorbidities should be followed up within one or two weeks from the initial procedure. Other patients can be evaluated two to four weeks postoperatively. Patients who underwent a catheter drainage procedure should be evaluated within 7 to 10 days after the procedure. If the drainage has stopped and the cavity is closed around the catheter, the catheter could be carefully removed. If drainage is still required, the catheter can be left in situ or replaced with a smaller size catheter (2).

During the follow-up visits, attempts should be made to identify an external opening of a fistula if the clinical state of the patient allows. Proctosigmoidoscopy and anoscopy should also be performed at that time.

COMPLICATIONS

Recurrence

A prospective study of recurrent anorectal abscesses was carried out to elucidate the causes of recurrence. In 32% of the patients, the original diagnosis was incorrect and the patients actually had hidradenitis suppurativa which was excised. In 68% of the patients, the cause of recurrence was due to inappropriate prior treatment including fistulous abscesses requiring fistulotomy, large abscesses associated with fistula, and abscesses without associated fistula but missed adjacent components (such as ischiorectal, supralevator, postanal abscesses). The authors concluded that all patients with recurrent abscesses must be examined meticulously under anesthesia to identify associated fistulas or missed components, or to exclude hidradenitis suppurativa (15). Undiagnosed fistula is presumed to be associated with persistent infection. Failure to allow for complete drainage will also result in recurrence; this may be the result of inappropriate technique and premature closure of the wound. Recurrence is also more likely to occur in patients with a past history of abscess drainage (15,59,64). A few studies have indicated that, after incision and drainage, ischioanal and intersphincteric abscesses were associated with higher recurrence rates of fistulas and/or abscesses (59,64).

Recurrence is also likely to occur in cases in which the primary cause of the abscess and/or infection was not properly addressed; thus underlying conditions such as hidradenitis suppurativa and Crohn's disease should be considered (Table 1).

Incontinence

Prior to any anorectal procedure, the patient should be questioned about fecal incontinence. Anorectal physiological testing (such as a manometry) and endorectal ultrasound are desirable if the patient has a history of soiling and incontinence; although most patients do not require physiologic testing, this may influence which surgical treatment option is preferable. Undoubtedly, incision and drainage are the definitive treatment for an acute abscess, but primary fistulotomy should also be reconsidered in case the patient has baseline fecal incontinence.

Fecal incontinence, in any given case, can be the result of the surgical technique or poor wound care. A surgical technique that involves excessive division of the EAS while performing a primary fistulotomy or inadvertent division of the EAS while draining a perianal or deep post anal abscess may result in incontinence. As mentioned above, the puborectalis muscle has a role in maintaining continence; inappropriate division of this skeletal muscle while draining a supralevator abscess might also cause incontinence (20,65).

Although many surgeons advocate treating the fistula during the primary procedure of abscess drainage, a synchronous procedure usually has a tendency for a higher incidence of fecal incontinence (39,59,63).

Necrotizing Infection

Anorectal abscess can spread to adjacent tissues and lead to necrotizing a soft-tissue infection that involves the skin, subcutaneous fat, fascia, and muscles subsequently leading to gangrene, septicemia, and even mortality. This condition is sometimes termed Fournier's gangrene or Fournier's disease, which is a bacterial infection involving the skin, genitals, and perineum. It is often a mixed infection of anaerobic gram-negative Bacteroides with a mixed flora of Pseudomonas, E. coli, Proteus, and fungi (66). Factors contributing to the development of this condition are delay in diagnosis, inadequate and inappropriate treatment, the offending microorganism, and concomitant diseases such as diabetes mellitus, chronic renal failure, tuberculosis, AIDS, and other immunocompromised states. Factors associated with a satisfactory outcome are repeated examinations under anesthesia by a specialist, prompt and definitive surgical treatment (including drainage and radical debriedment), systemic antibiotics, nutritional and fluid support (hyperalimentation, hydration, and restoration of electrolyte balance), monitoring concomitant diseases, and, in some cases, a diverting stoma (66–69).

SPECIAL CONSIDERATIONS

Hematological Disorders

Acute anorectal infections such as abscesses and fistulas are often encountered in patients with acute and chronic hematological malignancies. The treatment strategy in these patients is controversial and should be in consideration with the patient's neutrophil counts. The trend of the neutrophil count during the infection process is an important factor affecting the perianal lesion, symptoms and clinical presentation, the choice of treatment, and prognosis. Neutropenic patients frequently present with nonfluctuating poorly defined indurations, fever, and pain. A period of normal white count during the infection usually leads to well-defined fluctuant lesions; when the clinical picture is better defined, patients usually undergo operative treatment (70,71). Reported mortality rates in patients with acute leukemia are as high as 45 to 78% (72), thus these patients should always be treated in a hospital setting. Evidence suggests that there is a correlation between the number of circulating granulocytes and the incidence of anorectal infections. In one study, the incidence of perianal infections was found to be 7.3% in patients with acute leukemia and only 0.92% of patients with chronic leukemia (70). In another trial, the most important prognostic indicator of outcome was the number of days of neutropenia during the infectious episode (71). The controversy regarding the clinical and operative management of these patients is due to the belief that septicemia may develop secondary both to diagnostic and therapeutic instrumentation, and in immunocompromised patients this may lead to a grave prognosis (72). Yet another study reviewed 39 years of experience including 54 patients with leukemia and acute rectal pathology (73); of these, 25 had perirectal abscesses and/or fistulas. Other pathologies included prolapsed or thrombosed hemorrhoids, anal fissures, and perianal excoriations. The authors reported that in 4 of the 54 cases, the clinical course clearly implied that the rectal digital examination or instrumentation may have caused the bacteremia; however, 13 of 54 patients had positive blood cultures for gram-negative organisms at some point during the course of the disease. The current approach when evaluating immunocompromised patients with suspected anorectal pathology should be a cautious one. Avoiding digital rectal examinations, suppositories, or enemas is recommended (2). Sitz baths and appropriate antibiotics form the core of therapy in these patients. Cautious surgical drainage should be offered when indicated; indications for operative treatment in these patients are obvious fluctuation, evidence of soft-tissue infection, or persistent sepsis in spite of appropriate antibiotic treatment (2).

REFERENCES

1. Concise Oxford American Dictionary. New York: Oxford University Press, 2006:3.
2. Vasilevsky CA, Gordon PH. Benign Anorectal: Abscess and Fistula. In: Wolff BG, Fleshman JW, Beck DE, Pemberton JH, Wexner SD, eds. The ASCRS Textbook of Colon and Rectal Surgery. New York: Springer, 2007:192–213.
3. Fielding MA, Berry AR. Management of perianal sepsis in a district general hospital. J R Coll Surg Edinb 1992; 37(4):232–234.
4. Rickard MJ. Anal abscesses and fistulas. ANZ J Surg 2005; 75(1–2):64–72.
5. Kaiser AM, Ortega AE. Anorectal anatomy. Surg Clin North Am 2002; 82(6): 1125–1138.
6. Dujoyny N, Quiros RM, Saclarides TJ. Anorectal anatomy and embryology. Surg Oncol Clin N Am 2004; 13(2):277–293.
7. Wendell-Smith CP. Anorectal nomenclature: fundamental terminology. Dis Colon Rectum 2000; 43(10):1349–1358.
8. Thompson-Fawcett MW, Warren BF, Mortensen NJ. A new look at the anal transitional zone with reference to restorative proctocolectomy and the columnar cuff. Br J Surg 1998; 85(11):1517–1521.
9. Parks AG, Thomson JP. Intersphincteric abscess. Br Med J 1973; 2(5865):537–539.
10. Eisenhammer S. The internal anal sphincter and the anorectal abscess. Surg Gynecol Obstet 1956; 103(4):501–506.
11. Whitney ET. Review of Gastroenterology. Gastroenterology 1948; 15:451.
12. Parks AG. Pathogenesis and treatment of fistula-in-ano. Br Med J 1961; 1:463.
13. Chiari H. Medizinische Jahrbücher 1878; 8:419.
14. Seow-Choen F, Ho JMS. Histoanatomy of anal glands. Dis Colon Rectum 1994; 37(12):1215–1218.
15. Chrabot CM, Prasad ML, Abcarian H. Recurrent anorectal abscesses. Dis Colon Rectum 1983; 26(2):105–108
16. Lund JN, Scholefield JH. Aetiology and treatment of anal fissure. Br J Surg 1996; 83(10):1335–1344.
17. Burnett SJ, Bartram CI. Endosonographic variations in the normal internal anal sphincter. Int J Colorectal Dis 1991; 6(1):2–4.
18. Nielsen MB, Pedersen JF. Changes in the anal sphincter with age. An endosonographic study. Acta Radiol 1996; 37(3 Pt 1):357–361.
19. Frudinger A, Halligan S, Bartram CI, et al. Female anal sphincter: age-related differences in asymptomatic volunteers with high-frequency endoanal US. Radiology 2002; 224(2):417–423.
20. Liu J, Guaderrama N, Nager CW, et al. Functional correlates of anal canal anatomy: puborectalis muscle and anal canal pressure. Am J Gastroenterol 2006; 101(5):1092–1097.
21. Morren GL, Beets-Tan RG, van Engelshoven JM. Anatomy of the anal canal and perianal structures as defined by phased-array magnetic resonance imaging. Br J Surg 2001; 88(11):1506–1512.

22. Ramanujam PS, Prasad ML, Abcarian H, et al. Perianal abscesses and fistulas. A study of 1023 patients. Dis Colon Rectum 1984; 27(9):593–597
23. Corman ML. Anorectal Abscess. In: Corman ML, ed. Colon and Rectal Surgery. 5th ed. Philadelphia: Williams and Wilkins, 2005:285.
24. Yebara SM, Salum MR, Cutait R. Fistulas-in-ano and abscesses. In: Wexner SD, Stollman N, eds. Diseases of the Colon. New York: Informa Healthcare, 2007:707–721.
25. Wexner SD. Personal communication. March 2007.
26. Lee YJ, Yang SK, Byeon JS, et al. Analysis of colonoscopic findings in the differential diagnosis between intestinal tuberculosis and Crohn's disease. Endoscopy 2006; 38(6):592–597.
27. Aldamiz-Echebarria San Sebastian M, Vesga Carasa JC, Aspiazu Alonso-Urquijo A, et al. An ischiorectal abscess due to Actinomyces. Rev Clin Esp 1992; 190(5): 258–260.
28. Lee IJ, Ha HK, Park CM, et al. Abdominopelvic actinomycosis involving the gastrointestinal tract: CT features. Radiology 2001; 220(1):76–80.
29. Mostafavi H, O'Donnell KF, Chong FK. Supralevator abscess due to chronic rectal lymphogranuloma venereum. Am J Gastroenterol 1990; 85(5):602–606.
30. Mindel A. Lymphogranuloma venereum of the rectum in a homosexual man. Case report. Br J Vener Dis 1983; 59(3):196–197.
31. Galanakis E, Bitsori M, Maraki S, et al. Invasive non-typhoidal salmonellosis in immunocompetent infants and children. Int J Infect Dis 2007; 11(1):36–39.
32. Calck M, Motte S, Rickaert F, et al. Cryptococcal anal ulceration in a patient with AIDS. Am J Gastroenterol 1988; 83(11):1306–1308.
33. Toyonaga T, Matsushima M, Tanaka Y, et al. Microbiological analysis and endoanal ultrasonography for diagnosis of anal fistula in acute anorectal sepsis. Int J Colorectal Dis 2007; 22(2):209–213.
34. Lunniss PJ, Phillips RK. Surgical assessment of acute anorectal sepsis is a better predictor of fistula than microbiological analysis. Br J Surg 1994; 81(3):368–369.
35. Whiteford MH, Kilkenny J III, Hayman N, et al. The Standards Practice Task Force. The American Society of Colon and Rectal Surgeons. Practice parameters for the treatment of perianal abscess and fistula-in-ano (revised). Dis Colon Rectum 2005; 48(7):1337–1342.
36. Llera JL, Levy RC. Treatment of cutaneous abscess: a double-blind clinical study. Ann Emerg Med 1985; 14(1):15–19.
37. Dajani AS, Taubert KA, Wilson W, et al. Prevention of bacterial endocarditis: recommendations by the American Heart Association. Clin Infect Dis 1997; 25(6):1448–1458.
38. Nelson R. Anorectal abscess fistula: what do we know? Surg Clin North Am 2002; 82(6):1139–1151.
39. Prasad ML, Read DR, Abcarian H. Supralevator abscess: diagnosis and treatment. Dis Colon Rectum 1981; 24(6):456–461
40. Oliver I, Lacueva FJ, Perez Vicente F, et al. Randomized clinical trial comparing simple drainage of anorectal abscess with and without fistula track treatment. Int J Colorectal Dis 2003; 18(2):107–110.
41. Millan M, Garcia-Granero E, Esclapez P, et al. Management of intersphincteric abscesses. Colorectal Dis 2006; 8(9):777–780.
42. Waku M, Napolitano L, Clementini E, et al. Risk of cancer onset in sub-Saharan Africans affected with chronic gastrointestinal parasitic diseases. Int J Immunopathol Pharmacol 2005; 18(3):503–511.
43. Hughes F, Mehta S. Anorectal sepsis. Hosp Med 2002; 63(3):166–169.
44. Nelson RL, Prasad L, Abcarian H. Anal carcinoma presenting as perirectal abscess or fistula. Arch Surg 1985; 120:632–635.
45. Avill R. The management of carcinoma of the rectum presenting as an ischiorectal abscess. Br J Surg 1984; 71:665.
46. Cataldo PA, Senagore A, Luchtefeld MA. Intrarectal ultrasound in the evaluation of perirectal abscesses. Dis Colon Rectum 1993; 36(6):554–558.
47. Epstein, Giordano P. Endoanal ultrasound-guided needle drainage of intersphincteric abscess. Tech Coloproctol 2005; 9(1):67–69.
48. Buchanan GN, Bartram CI, Williams AB, et al. Value of hydrogen peroxide enhancement of three-dimensional endoanal ultrasound in fistula-in-ano. Dis Colon Rectum 2005; 48(1):141–147.
49. Isbister WH. A simple method for the management of anorectal abscess. Aust N Z J Surg 1987; 57(10):771–774.
50. Inceoglu R, Gencosmanoglu R. Fistulotomy and drainage of deep postanal space abscess in the treatment of posterior horseshoe fistula. BMC Surg 2003; 26:3,10.
51. Hanley PH. Conservative surgical correction of horseshoe abscess and fistula. Dis Colon Rectum 1965; 8(5):364–368.
52. Hanley PH, Ray JE, Pennington EE, et al. Fistula-in-ano: a ten-year follow-up study of horseshoe-abscess fistula-in-ano. Dis Colon Rectum 1976; 19(6):507–515.
53. Leaper DJ, Page RE, Rosenberg IL, et al. A controlled study comparing the conventional treatment of idiopathic anorectal abscess with that of incision, curettage and primary suture under systemic antibiotic cover. Dis Colon Rectum 1976; 19(1):46–50.

54. Christensen K, Kronborg O, Olsen H. Primary suture, with or without a clindamycin cover, in the treatment of anorectal abscesses. Ugeskr Laeger 1983; 21, 145(8):576–578.
55. Kronborg O, Olsen H. Incision and drainage v. incision, curettage and suture under antibiotic cover in anorectal abscess. A randomized study with 3-year follow-up. Acta Chir Scand 1984; 150(8):689–692.
56. Beck DE, Fazio VW, Lavery IC, et al. Catheter drainage of ischiorectal abscesses. South Med J 1988; 81(4):444–446.
57. Read DR, Abcarian H. A prospective survey of 474 patients with anorectal abscess. Dis Colon Rectum 1979; 22(8):566–568.
58. Hebjorn M, Olsen O, Haakansson T, Andersen B. A randomized trial of fistulotomy in perianal abscess. Scand J Gastroenterol 1987; 22(2):174–176.
59. Schouten WR, van Vroonhoven TJ. Treatment of anorectal abscess with or without primary fistulectomy. Results of a prospective randomized trial. Dis Colon Rectum 1991; 34(1):60–63.
60. Ho YH, Tan M, Chui CH, et al. Randomized controlled trial of primary fistulotomy with drainage alone for perianal abscesses. Dis Colon Rectum 1997; 40(12):1435–1438.
61. Tang CL, Chew SP, Seow-Choen F. Prospective randomized trial of drainage alone vs. drainage and fistulotomy for acute perianal abscesses with proven internal opening. Dis Colon Rectum 1996; 39(12):1415–1417.
62. Knoefel WT, Hosch SB, Hoyer B, et al. The initial approach to anorectal abscesses: fistulotomy is safe and reduces the chance of recurrences. Dig Surg 2000; 17(3):274–278.
63. Quah HM, Tang CL, Eu KW, et al. Meta-analysis of randomized clinical trials comparing drainage alone vs primary sphincter-cutting procedures for anorectal abscess-fistula. Int J Colorectal Dis 2006; 21(6):602–609.
64. Holzheimer RG, Siebeck M. Treatment procedures for anal fistulous cryptoglandular abscess—how to get the best results. Eur J Med Res 2006; 11(12):501–515.
65. Seow-Choen F, Nicholls RJ. Anal fistula. Br J Surg 1992; 79(3):197–205.
66. Lichtenstein D, Stavorovsky M, Irge D. Fournier's gangrene complicating perinal abscess: report of two cases. Dis Colon Rectum 1978; 21(5):377–379.
67. Bode WE, Ramos R, Page CP. Invasive necrotizing infection secondary to anorectal abscess. Dis Colon Rectum 1982; 25(5):416–419.
68. Huber P Jr, Kissack AS, Simonton CT. Necrotizing soft-tissue infection from rectal abscess. Dis Colon Rectum 1983; 26(8):507–511.
69. Adinolfi MF, Voros DC, Moustoukas NM, et al. Severe systemic sepsis resulting from neglected perineal infections. South Med J 1983; 76(6):746–749.
70. Buyukasik Y, Ozcebe OI, Sayinalp N, et al. Perianal infections in patients with leukemia: importance of the course of neutrophil count. Dis Colon Rectum 1998; 41(1):81–85.
71. Glenn J, Cotton D, Wesley R, et al. Anorectal infections in patients with malignant diseases. Rev Infect Dis 1988; 10(1):42–52.
72. Barnes SG, Sattler FR, Ballard JO. Perirectal infections in acute leukemia. Improved survival after incision and debridement. Ann Intern Med 1984; 100(4): 515–518.
73. Boddie AW Jr, Bines SD. Management of acute rectal problems in leukemic patients. J Surg Oncol 1986; 33(1):53–56.
74. Vasilevsky CA, Gordon PH. The incidence of recurrent abscesses or fistula-in-ano following anorectal suppuration. Dis Colon Rectum 1984; 27(2):126–130.
75. Vasilevsky CA. Anorectal abscess and fistula-in-ano. In: Beck D, ed. Handbook of Colorectal surgery,. 2 nd ed. New York: Informa Health Care, 2003:345.

16 Fistula-in-Ano

Rodrigo Ambar Pinto and Cesar Omar Reategui Sanchez
Department of Colorectal Surgery, Cleveland Clinic Florida, Weston, Florida, U.S.A.

Mari A. Madsen
Department of Colon and Rectal Surgery, Cedars Sinai Medical Center, Los Angeles, California, U.S.A.

INTRODUCTION

A fistula is an abnormal connection between two epithelial lined surfaces. The term fistula derived from the Latin meaning "of reed, pipe, or flute." An anal fistula is a tract which usually communicates an infected anal gland to a secondary opening in perianal skin, which is often lined with granulation tissue.

ETIOLOGY

Cryptoglandular disease is responsible for 90% of fistula-in-ano. Anorectal abscesses, presented in the preceding chapter, represent the acute presentation of cryptoglandular disease, while fistulae are the chronic evolution of the same process. An abscess will always have preceded a fistula, although at the time of presentation it may have been so long ago that the patient cannot recall. Other less common causes of fistulae are Crohn's disease, trauma, anal fissures, carcinoma, radiation therapy, tuberculosis, and chlamydial infections. A complete listing of the differential diagnosis for fistula-in-ano is listed in Table 1.

INCIDENCE

In the United States, the incidence of abscess is 68,000 to 96,000 per year. Of these, 26% to 37% will persist as fistulae, resulting in 20,000 to 25,000 new cases of fistula per year. Table 2 reviews the incidence of fistula formation corresponding to the presenting abscess type. The gender ratio is 2:1 (male:female) (2).

CLASSIFICATION

The classification system for fistula-in-ano has undergone numerous revisions to arrive at the current Parks classification system, which is predominantly used today (Table 3) (3). Prior to development of the Parks system, multiple classification systems often resulted in confusion and difficulty comparing results in the literature. At that time, the most used system had been developed by Milligan and Morgan in 1934 (4). While Parks relates fistulous tracts to the internal and external anal sphincter muscle, the Milligan–Morgan system related the fistula tracts to the anorectal ring.

From a purely practical standpoint, fistulae are frequently classified as either *simple* or *complex*. Simple fistulae are considered to be intersphincteric or low transsphincteric (<30% sphincter compromise). Fistulotomy is the best treatment for this kind of fistula, and is not expected to put a patient's continence at risk. Complex fistulae involve more than 30% of the sphincter and usually are transsphincteric, suprasphincteric, or extrasphincteric. Special consideration is given to anterior fistulae in women, the presence of multiple tracts, recurrent fistula, preexisting incontinence, local irradiation, and Crohn's disease, thereby classifying these groups as complex fistulae as well (5). It is specifically for these patients that alternative treatments to fistulotomy have been developed.

Table 1 Differential Diagnosis of Fistula-in-ano

Nonspecific 90%
Cryptoglandular
Specific 10%
Trauma
Foreign body
Obstetric
Hemorrhoidectomy
Radiation therapy
Inflammatory bowel disease
Crohn's disease
Cancer
Adenocarcinoma of the rectum
Squamous cell carcinoma of the anus
Lymphoma
Infectious
Tuberculosis
Actinomycosis
Lymphgranuloma venereum
Abdominal
Diverticulitis
Pelvic inflammatory disease
Appendicitis
Extra-anal sources
Presacral cyst
Bartholin's cyst
Pilonidal disease
Hidradenitis suppurativa

Parks divided fistulae into four types depending on the relationship with the anal sphincters:

Intersphincteric is the chronic phase of a perianal abscess. The tract is located within the intersphincteric space [Fig. 1 (B) and (C)].

Transsphincteric results from an ischiorectal abscess. The tract passes through the internal and external sphincters to the ischiorectal fossa [Fig. 1 (D)]. The level at which the fistula passes through the sphincter muscles determines whether it is considered low or high. This has further implications on the risk of incontinence with fistulotomy and therefore another management option should be selected for high fistulae.

Suprasphincteric is the result of a supralevator abscess. The tract is located above the puborectalis and curves downward lateral to the external anal sphincter in the ischiorectal space to the perineal skin [Fig. 1 (E)]. Suprasphincteric fistulae can also be the result of an intra-abdominal process, such as Crohn's disease. In these cases, management is most appropriately directed toward treatment of the intra-abdominal process.

Extrasphincteric is the least common type of fistula. The tract originates from the dentate line, and passes above the levators before reversing to pass back through them to the perineal skin via the ischiorectal space [Fig. 1 (F, G)].

Table 2 Incidence of Fistula by Type of Anorectal Abscess

Type	Number of abscesses	Fistula formation	% Fistulization
Perianal	437	151	34.5
Ischiorectal	233	59	25.3
Intersphincteric	219	104	47.4
Supralevator	75	32	42.6
Submucous	59	9	15.2

Ramanujam diseases of the colon and rectum 1984 (1).

Table 3 Classification of Anal Fistulae

Types of fistula	Subclassification	Primary tract	Frequency (%)	Other possible tracts
Intersphincteric	Simple low tract High blind tract High tract with rectal opening Rectal opening without perineal opening Extrarectal extension Secondary to pelvic disease	Via internal sphincter to the intersphincteric space and to the perineum	70	High blind tract, high opening into the rectum, no opening, or pelvic extension
Transsphincteric	Uncomplicated High blind tract	Low via internal and external sphincters into the ischiorectal fossa	23	High tract with perineal opening; high blind tract
Suprasphincteric	Uncomplicated High blind tract	Via intersphincteric space, superiorly above puborectalis muscle through ischiorectal fossa to perineal skin	5	High blind tract
Extrasphincteric	Secondary to anal fistula, trauma, anorectal disease, pelvic inflammation	From the rectum above the elevators and through the elevators to perineal skin	2	–

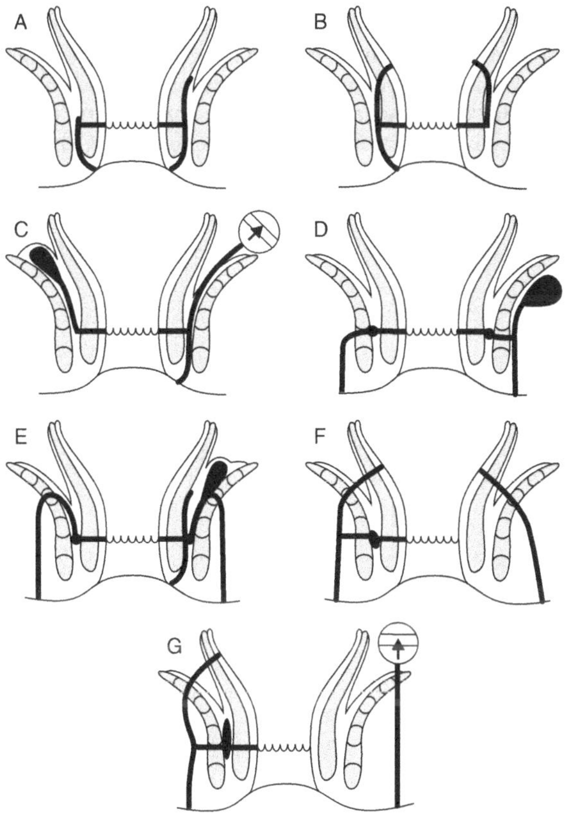

Figure 1 Fistula-in-ano classification. A superficial fistula tracks below both the internal anal sphincter and the external anal sphincter complexes. (**A**) An intersphincteric fistula tracks between the internal anal sphincter and the external anal sphincter in the intersphincteric space. (**B**) An intersphincteric fistula tracks that ascend through supralevator space (**C**) A transsphincteric fistula leaves the intersphincteric space and penetrates the ischiorectal space before tracking down to the skin (**D**) An extrasphincteric fistula tracks outside the external anal sphincter and penetrates the levator muscle into the rectum. (**E**) An extrasphincteric fistula tracks outside the external anal sphincter that can have a secondary tract in intersphincteric space. (**F**) An extrasphincteric fistula tracks outside the external anal sphincter that can have a secondary tract in intersphincteric space or penetrate supralevator space (**G**). *Source*: From Ref. 3.

EVALUATION

Symptoms

A patient with a fistula-in-ano will often have a history of an abscess that was either drained spontaneously or surgically. It is not unusual for the patient to have suffered with the fistula for years before seeking attention for it. There can be intermittent or continuous discharge. If it is intermittent, the patient may have increased pain and pressure prior to recurrent drainage, which gives relief. Other symptoms include bleeding, soreness, pruritusm, or perianal dermatitis. The patient's history and physical examination are the basis of the evaluation.

Physical Examination

Inspection

The external or secondary opening can be seen as an elevation of granulation tissue discharging pus. This may be elicited on the digital rectal examination. Scar from earlier procedures may be appreciated as well as chronic skin changes such as thickened and redness from persistent drainage. Occasionally, the secondary opening is more subtle or difficult to detect against a background of perianal inflammation. Under these circumstances, gentle palpation of the surrounding skin can exude a small amount of pus, thereby identifying the external opening.

Palpation

Digital rectal examination may reveal an indurated cord-like structure beneath the skin in the direction of the internal opening. Inability to palpate the fistula tract implies a deeper course and therefore higher transsphincteric fistula. Internal openings may be felt as indurated nodules or pits that correspond to enlarged papilla, leading to a thickened tract.

Anoscopy

This examination allows visualization of the dentate line for possible identification of internal openings before surgery, as well as identification of other pathology such as Crohn's disease or carcinoma.

In 1900, Goodsall and Miles (6) published their findings on the course of anorectal fistulae. Their conclusion is now widely known as Goodsall's rule, which states that secondary openings located posteriorly to the coronal line are associated with tracts that curve to the posterior midline before entering the anal canal. Secondary openings anterior to the coronal line track straight toward the internal opening of the anal canal. This observation has held up with one modification from Ciroco and Reilly (7), who noted that Goodsall's rule holds true within 3 cm from the anal verge (Fig. 2).

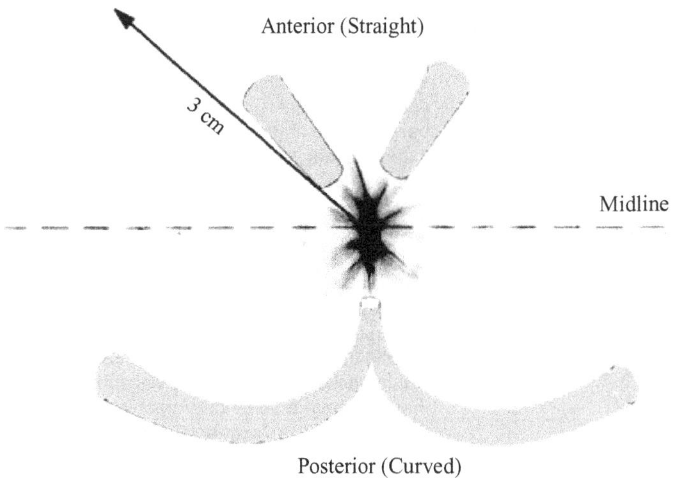

Figure 2 Goodsall's rule.

Radiological Evaluation

Radiology has a limited role in the evaluation of anal fistulae. Most cases can be diagnosed and treated only based on clinical examination. Radiological examinations are useful in atypical cases or after recurrences.

Fistulography

Fistulography involves cannulation of the external opening with injection of water soluble contrast and a small fitting tube. It may be useful for evaluation of recurrent or complex fistulae. However, its use has been generally discouraged because of risk of septicemia in a small amount of patients and poor visualization of anatomic landmarks. This study has been substituted by other diagnostic modalities (8,9).

CT Scan

CT scan has a minor role in the assessment of anal fistulae. The main use of CT scan is to distinguish an abscess requiring drainage from perirectal cellulites. It is done with intravenous and rectal contrast. It may be useful if MRI is not available or contraindicated (10).

Endoanal Ultrasound

Anal ultrasound, as described by Bartram, was revolutionary in the assessment of anal sepsis (8). The role of ultrasound is to identify the fistula tract in relation to the internal and external sphincters, as well as to determine if the fistula is simple or complex and define the location of the primary opening.

Cataldo et al. (11) found that anal ultrasound was best used for evaluation of complex and recurrent abscesses. That said, the presence of scar or other artifact could limit anatomic definition by ultrasound. It may also have limitations in the evaluation of superficial, extrasphincteric, secondary, and supralevator tracts. Anal ultrasound is optimally used in cases of intersphincteric or transsphincteric fistula tracts. Despite this, others have described anal ultrasound to have almost 100% accuracy in the detection of abscesses and differentiate simple from complex anal sepsis (12–14).

The injection of hydrogen peroxide into the fistula opening during ultrasound improves identification of fistulae and their internal openings by making them hyper instead of hypoechoic. The addition of hydrogen peroxide increased the detection of fistulous tracts by 24% and the detection of internal openings by 28% (12–15).

The advent of 3-D ultrasound with volume acquisition and multiplanar imaging of the anal canal improved the accuracy of ultrasound techniques to over 80%, when compared to endocoil MRI (9). It has been proven useful for evaluation of the extent of the fistulous tract and its relation to sphincter muscles, the position of the internal opening in relation to the anal margin, and secondary tracts or cavities. In addition, the use of hydrogen peroxide yielded an additional benefit. The only two limitations with this method are the limited field of 2 cm from the anal probe and the poor distinction of supralevator and high infralevator sepsis (13).

Magnetic Resonance Image

The main role of magnetic resonance imaging (MRI) is in evaluating patients with complex, recurrent fistulae and those with anatomic distortion from earlier surgery. The technique is based on endoanal coil, body coil, and phase array coil. The major advantage is a multiplanar visualization of the sphincter muscles and differentiation of supralevator from infralevator injuries. MRI can also demonstrate the course of the primary tract as well as secondary extensions (9). In addition, it has the ability to differentiate the tract from granulation tissue and sphincter muscles (16).

MRI does have some limitations; neural and vascular structures as well as chemical artifacts filled with fluid could lead to erroneous identification of a fistula tract (17). However, accurate classification of fistulae with MRI is possible in 89% of patients compared to 61% using 2-D anal ultrasound. Although MRI seems superior to endoanal ultrasound in the assessment of fistula-in-ano, anal ultrasound tends to be more useful than MRI because it is more widely available, can be performed quickly in the office setting, and is less expensive (18). MRI is therefore best reserved for cases where ultrasound has already failed to identify the fistula and internal opening.

Anal Manometry

Anal manometry has a role in recurrent and complex fistulae in which preoperative resting and squeezing pressures may guide the extent and type of treatment (19).

TREATMENT

Multiple techniques have been proposed over the centuries for the treatment of fistula. Injection of 3% or 4% silver nitrate solution along the length of the fistula was popularized in the late 18th century. Similar procedures were described such as injection of a bismuth paste by Pennington, and the use of a quinine and urethane solution advocated by Blond in 1940. Destruction of the fistula tract with a carbon dioxide laser was proposed in the 1980s by Slutski (20). The fact that there are multiple procedures currently employed by surgeons for the treatment of fistula-in-ano, coupled with the greater number of procedures that are no longer en vogue, speaks to the delicate balance between curing the fistula, preventing recurrence, and preserving sphincter function.

Surgery is the basis of treatment of anorectal fistulae. It has been proposed that if a fistula is asymptomatic by the patients' estimation, inaction is an appropriate measure; however, it is important to recall that over time, the estimated risk of developing a carcinoma is 0.1% (21).

The first step of treatment is identification of the internal opening. This can present a challenge because it may be closed. Keeping Goodsall's rule in mind, the typical steps taken to identify the fistula tract and the internal opening include (1) gentle passage of a fistula probe, taking care not to create a false passage; (2) injection of dye into fistula tract using hydrogen peroxide, methylene blue, or milk to identify appearance at the internal opening; (3) follow the granulation tissue; and (4) pull on the fistula tract to identify dimpling at internal opening; this is most effective for anteriorly located, straight tracts.

Fistulotomy

Fistulotomy is a procedure that was first described in the 14th century by John Arderne (20). It consists of the gentle passage of a probe from the external to the internal opening, after its identification. The sphincter muscle is palpated. If the amount of muscle is deemed to be insufficient as to cause incontinence, the fistulous tract is opened along its length. The base of the tract will be covered with granulation tissue. The presence of granulation tissue confirms correct identification of the fistulous tract, as opposed to having created a false passage. The granulation tissue can be removed with a curette or gauze to reveal the fibrous fistula tract underneath, which should be investigated to identify any secondary, or daughter, tracts of the main fistula which could complicate healing. Removal of immediately adjacent skin and subcutaneous fat ensures against premature closure of the wound. Alternatively, marsupialization with approximation of the skin edges to the opened fistula tract is also effective.

Seton

Setons were first described by Hippocrates. The term is derived from the Latin word *seta*, meaning bristle (20). Generally, they are used in more complex situations such as a high transsphincteric fistula or complex fistulous disease. If the tract is at a higher level crossing the sphincter muscles, a seton can be a good option to use independently or in combination with the laying open technique (Figs. 3 and 4). The material used for setons is always nonabsorbable. There are two different ways of using setons, as described later.

Cutting Seton

The cutting seton was promoted by Hanley (22). The technique consists of division of the lower half of the internal anal sphincter, isolation of the fibers of the external anal sphincter, and passage of a nonabsorbable suture, usually silk, around the remaining external anal sphincter. Silk is often used because it promotes fibrosis while the seton is gradually tightened over an eight-week period, and slowly divides the sphincter muscle. This allows healing and fibrosis proximally, thereby preventing separation of the muscle ends as they are divided. A cutting seton allows for the conversion of a high transsphincteric fistula to a low transsphincteric fistula, either to lay open the remaining fistula or to allow passage of the seton all the way through.

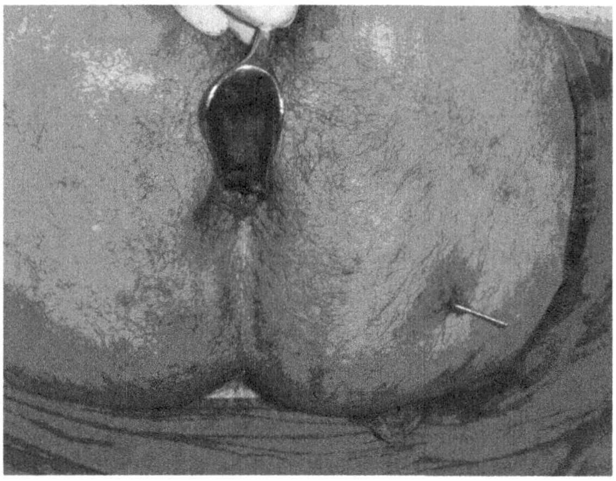

Figure 3 Combined seton in a lay open technique (identification of fistula tract with probe).

Table 4 illustrates the results of the use of cutting setons for anal fistulae, with low recurrence rates and variable grades of incontinence.

Draining Seton

A seton may also be used as a drain, which is left loosely in the fistula tract to provide prolonged drainage without dividing sphincter muscles. Materials such as silicone are used to minimize reaction and facilitate drainage, as well as to allow drainage and closure of any secondary tracts. It has a specific use for patients with Crohn's fistulae, complex AIDS, and those patients who are debilitated (30). The aims of loose setons are (1) long-term drainage of the fistula in patients too infirm to undergo more invasive procedures or risk of recurrent sepsis, and (2) to allow healing of secondary tracts in preparation for a second stage operation.

Immunodeficient patients with neutropenia, hematologic malignancy, organ transplant, and complex AIDS may be best served with drainage alone. These patients are susceptible to poor healing, and are at risk for uncontrolled local or systemic sepsis if a more aggressive repair is attempted, thus antibiotic coverage is a must. Intervention in these patients should be tailored on a case-by-case basis; however, it is good to remember that conservative management with Sitz baths, long-term antibiotics, and a draining seton may be the safest and most viable option.

Advancement Flaps

Endorectal Advancement Flaps

Endorectal advancement flaps were first described by Noble 1902, specifically for the treatment of rectovaginal fistulae (30). This treatment modality consists of removal and patching of the internal opening with a muscular–mucosal flap of rectal wall. The first requirement for this

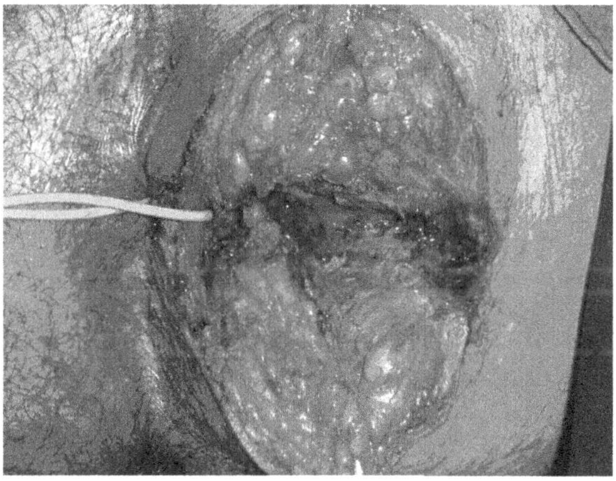

Figure 4 Combined seton and lay open technique.

Table 4 Results of Cutting Seton for Anal Fistula

Author	Time to cut through (wk)	Recurrence (%)	Minor incontinence (%)	Major incontinence (%)
Joy & Williams (23)	20	6	50	20
Durgan (24)	–	0	20	0
Theerapol (25)	9	2	–	0
Zbar (26)	14	11	6	0
Hamel (27)	–	0	0	0
Pescatori (28)	–	–	6	12
Mentes (29)	<3	5	20	0

Williams colorectal disease 2007 (30).

procedure is that the patient must have a mature single fistula tract with no active extensions and no uncontrolled sepsis. Frequently, a draining seton has been in place for six weeks to ensure these conditions prior to scheduling the rectal advancement flap.

Advantages of this technique include a reduction in duration of healing, reduced associated discomfort, lack of deformity to the anal canal, and little potential additional damage to the sphincter muscles since no muscle is divided. This technique should be considered for patients with complex fistulous disease, as described earlier. It may also be used to close rectovaginal and rectourethral fistulae.

The procedure requires a full mechanical and antibiotic bowel preparation. Generally, the procedure is done with the patient in the prone jackknife position, although occasionally for a posterior internal opening, a lithotomy position may be preferred. Under regional or general anesthetic, after insertion of a Foley catheter, the fistula tract is identified with a probe and the internal opening is either cored out or curetted. Following that, a broad-based, muscular–mucosal flap is raised, such that the flap base should be twice the width of the apex. The flap should be sufficiently mobilized so that it can easily be advanced 1 cm below the level of internal opening. The remaining internal opening is then sutured closed with an absorbable suture so it is watertight. Finally, the flap is brought down over the previous internal opening so that it is covered without tension. The flap is then secured in place with absorbable material. Longer tracts should be drained with a de Pezzer catheter to prevent recurrence of sepsis, which can lead to flap failure (Fig. 5).

Traditionally, in the immediate postoperative period, patients were placed on a clear liquid diet and antidiarrheals—a so-called medical colostomy; however, randomized clinical trials comparing with early oral intake showed no difference in morbidity or sepsis, but increased cramps, nausea, and discomfort. Therefore, most practitioners have abandoned the practice of postoperative bowel confinement. The main cause of flap failure is inadequate blood supply that can be accessed by observation of color or capillary refill by gentle pressure to the perineal skin (30).

Relative contraindications to the transanal rectal advancement flap procedure are shown in Table 5. Transanal rectal advancement flaps are generally safe, but not all patients are appropriate candidates for this treatment modality. Table 6 reviews the results of the endorectal advancement flap. Initially, the reported success of the procedure was in the range of 80%; however, more recent data suggests the effectiveness is in the range of 60% to 70%. Functional results are good with minimal or no disturbance of continence.

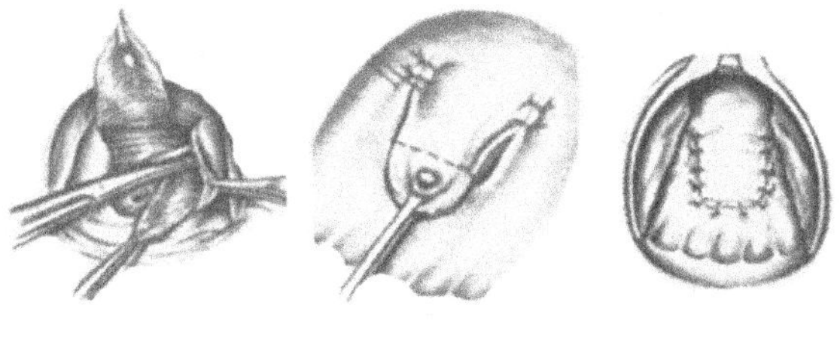

Figure 5 Endorectal advancement flap technique. *Source*: From Vasilevsky CA. Fistula in ano. Wexener SD and Beck DE, eds. *Fundamentals of Anorectal Surgery, Second Edition.*

Table 5 Contraindications for Transanal Rectal Advancement Flap

Presence of proctitis, especially in patients with Crohn's disease
Undrained sepsis and/or persisting secondary tracks
Severe perianal scarring from previous fistula surgery
Rectovaginal fistula with a diameter >3 cm
Malignant or radiation-related fistula
Fistula of <4-wk duration
Stricture of the anorectum
Severe sphincter defect

Island Flap Anoplasty

Dermal island advancement flap anocutaneous advancement flap was first introduced for the treatment of anal strictures and ectropion. Its use in the treatment of fistulae started in the past decade, basically to avoid incontinence and mucosal ectropion after mucosal flap advancement. This procedure has been reported for transsphincteric fistulae with or without suprasphincteric extension and for complex or recurrent cases. There are good results in terms of healing, postoperative complications, pain, and incontinence. Most published series include a reduced number of patients. Larger patient numbers are reported in a meta-analysis and appear to support the long-term efficacy of this technique (Table 7).

Fibrin Glue

Fibrin glue as a treatment of anal fistulae was first introduced in the early eighties (42,43). It is an activated mixture of solution containing fibrinogen, factor XIII, fibronectin, and aprotinin (44). When applied to the fistula tract, the fibrin clot seals the tract and stimulates migration, proliferation, and activation of fibroblasts.

The reported success rate was approximately 50% of patients, followed over a variable period of time. After licensing of commercial fibrin glues in 1999, usage greatly increased. More recent, series in the literature have revealed more disappointing results over a longer period of follow-up so that the use of fibrin glue is now uncommon (Table 8).

Preoperative preparation is similar to that of the endorectal advancement flap. Shorter fistula tracts are preferable for this modality. Secondary tracts and undrained infection will predictably lead to failure. The operative technique involves identification and curettage of the internal and external openings. Fibrin glue is injected into the fistula, thus filling the entire tract. Ideally, a bead of glue can be seen extruding from both the internal and external openings (Figs. 6–8). The main advantage of fibrin glue is that it avoids the risk of incontinence and can be performed on an outpatient basis with minimal morbidity. In the event of failure, the technique may be repeated several times; however, the possibility of using a different technique is not eliminated.

Anal Fistula Plug

This fistula plug made from lyophilized porcine intestinal collagen is designed to occlude the fistula tract from the internal to the external opening. The plug provides a scaffold for the ingrowth of native tissue. Advantages of this technique are the mechanical stable configuration,

Table 6 Results of Endorectal Advancement Flap

Author	Number	Crohn's (%)	F/U[a]	Healing (%)	Recurrence (%)	Incontinence (%)
Ozuner (31)	101	47	31	94	29	NS
Miller (32)	25	0	14	80	0	0
Ortiz (33)	103	0	12	93	7	8
Makowiec (34)	32	100	19.5	89	30	3
Sonoda (35)	99	44	17	64	36	NS
Lewis (36)	8	75	2–24	75	25	12.5

[a]Median follow-up in months (range).
Abbreviation: NS, not stated.

Table 7 Results of Island Flap Anoplasty

Author	Number	Crohn's (%)	Follow-up[a]	Healing (%)	Recurrence (%)	Incontinence (%)
Jun (37)	40	0	17	95	2.5	0
Amin (38)	18	0	19	83	11	0
Del Pino (39)	11	27	1–10	72	28	NS
Nelson (40)	65	NS	NS	NS	20	NS
Hossack (41)	16	NS	NS	98	1.7	0

[a]Median follow-up in months (range).
Abbreviation: NS, not stated.

minimal foreign body reaction, and infection resistance (Figs. 9 and 10). Champagne et al. (62) reported an 83% closure rate with a median follow-up of 12 months. However, more recently, other authors have not enjoyed the same success rates with less than 50% closure rates in longer follow-up (63–66).

SUMMARY

Fistula-in-ano represents the chronic phase of cryptoglandular disease. Diagnosis on the basis of history and physical examination is generally straightforward, although the possibility of other pathologies, such as Crohn's disease, should be kept in mind. Unless complex or recurrent disease is anticipated, examination under anesthesia with the possibility of definitive management is an appropriate first step once the diagnosis has been made. Accordingly, radiologic studies such as ultrasound or MRI should be reserved for cases of complex or recurrent disease.

Selection of the appropriate operative management mandates a thorough understanding of both the regional anatomy and the pathophysiology. Successful treatment of the fistula and preservation of continence can be a daunting process which may require repeated attempts. As a result, it is important to be well versed in the multiple treatment modalities currently available and to stay abreast of new developing technologies in the battle of this, at times, challenging disease. Figure 11 shows a suggested algorithm for the management of fistula-in-ano.

Table 8 Fibrin Glue Success Rates

Author (year)	*n*	Etiology	Success rate (%)	Follow-up (mo)
Hjortrup (1991) (45)	23	CG	75	4
Abel (1993) (46)	10	CG, RVF, HIV, CD	60	3–12
Venkatesh (1999) (47)	30	CG, RVF, HIV, CD	60	9–57
Aitola (1999) (48)	10	CG	0	6
Ramirez (2000) (49)	9	CG	50	–
Cintron (2000) (50)	79	CG, RVF, HIV, CD	61	12
Patrlj (2000) (51)	69	CG	74	18–36
El-Shobaky (2000) (52)	30	–	87	–
Salim (2001) (53)	6	–	100	3
Lindsey (2002) (54)	19	CG, CD	63	3
Chan (2002) (55)	10	–	60	–
Sentovich (2003) (56)	48	CG, CD	69	6–46
Zmora (2003) (57)	24	CG, CD	33	1–36
Buchanan (2003) (58)	22	CG	14	14
Loungnarath (2004) (59)	39	CG, CD	31	26
Vitton (2005) (60)	14	CD	14	23
Singer (2005) (61)	75	CG, HIV, CD	35	27

Abbreviations: N, number; CG, crypto-glandular disease; RVF, rectovaginal fistula; CD, Crohn's disease.
Source: Singer, M. *Surg Clin N Am* 2006.

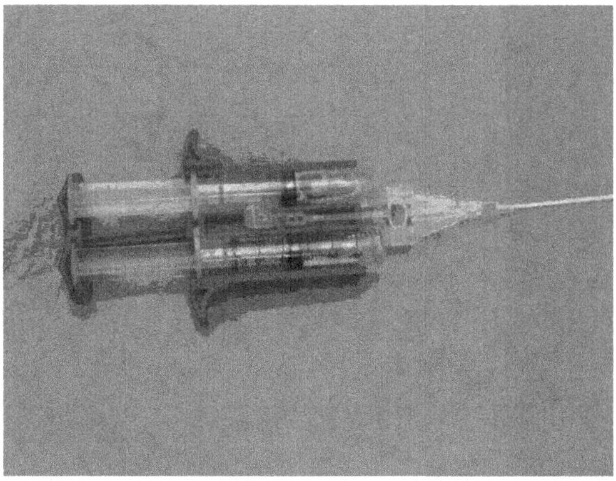

Figure 6 Fibrin glue syringe.

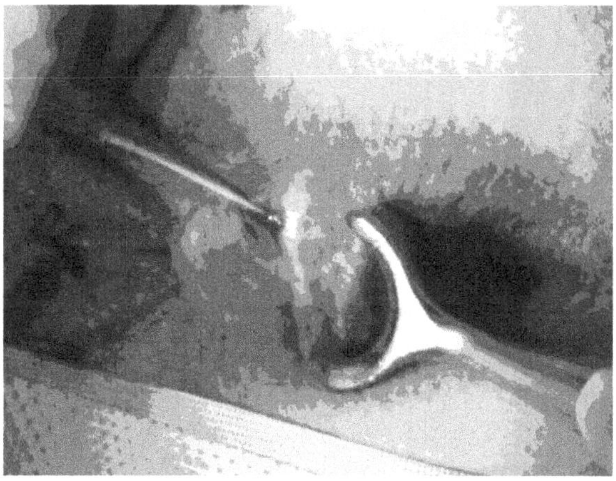

Figure 7 Placement of fibrin glue.

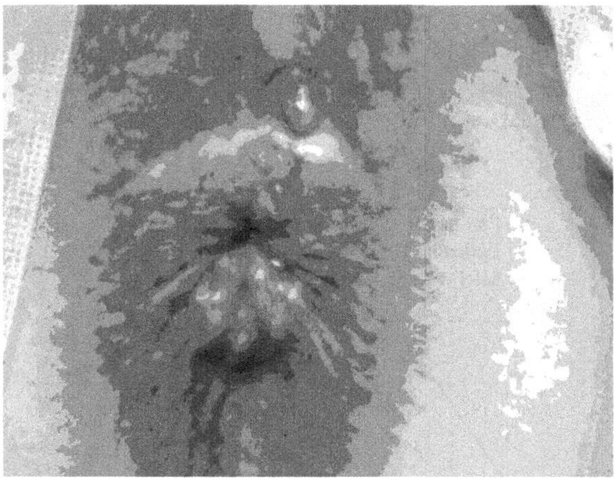

Figure 8 Post fibrin glue placement.

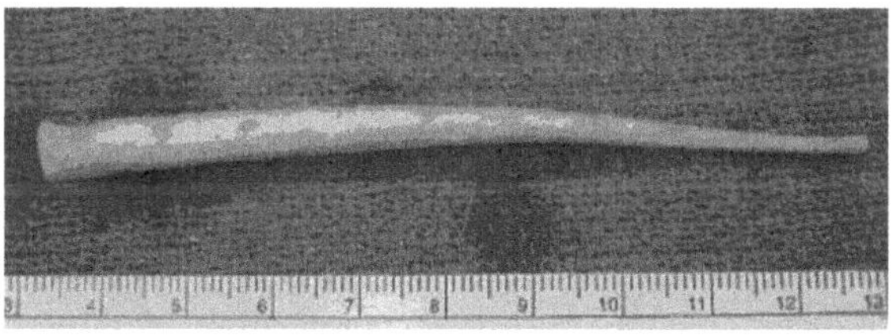

Figure 9 Collagen plug.

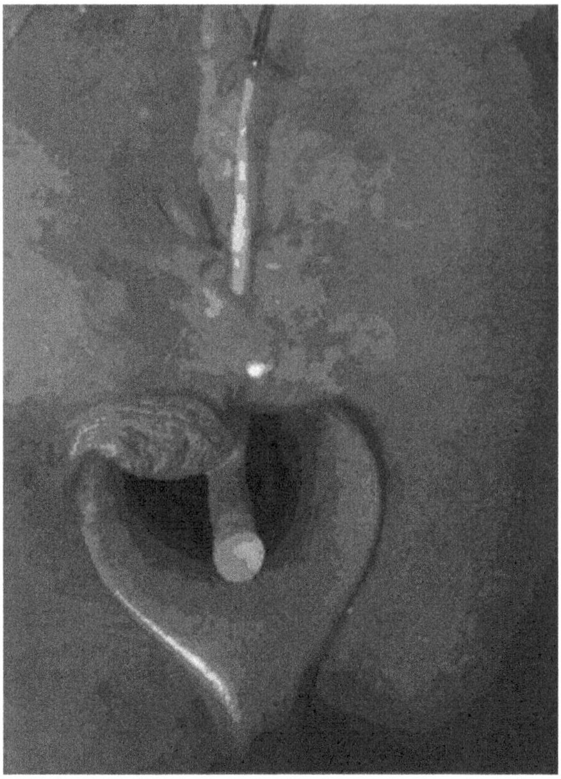

Figure 10 Placement of collagen plug.

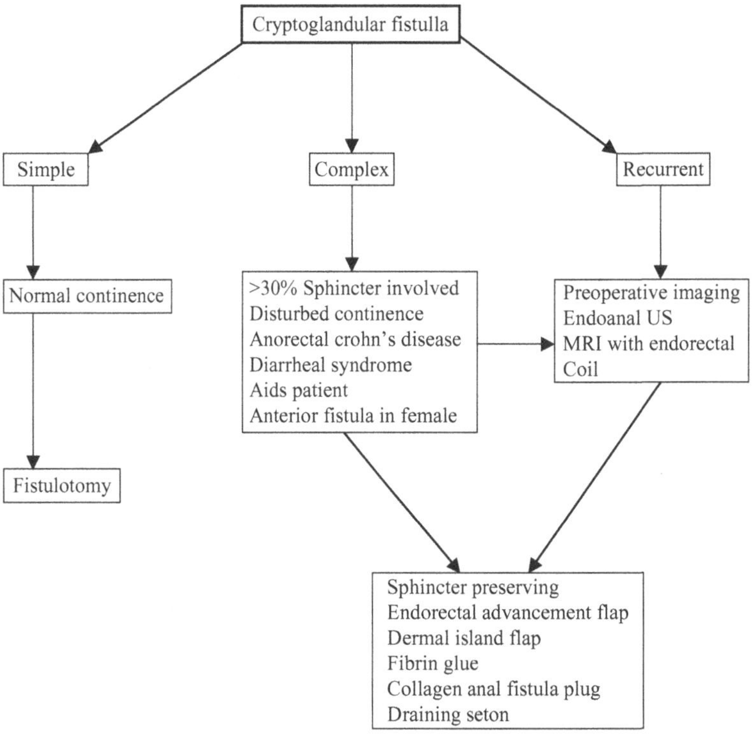

Figure 11 Cryptoglandular fistula management algorithm.

REFERENCES

1. Ramanujam PS, Prasad ML, Abcarian H, et al. Perianal abscesses and fistulae. A study of 1023 patients. Dis Colon Rectum 1984; 27:593–597.
2. Sainio P, Husa A. A prospective manometric study of the effect of anal fistula surgery on anorectal function. Acta Chir Scand 1985; 151:279–288.
3. Parks AG, Gordon PH, Hardcastle JD. A classification of fistula-in-ano. Br J Surg 1976; 63:1–12.
4. Milligan ETC, Morgan CN. Surgical anatomy of the anal canal with special reference to anorectal fistulae. Lancet 1934; 2:1213–1217.
5. Thompson HR. The orthodox conception of fistula-in-ano and its treatment. Proc Roy Soc Med 1962; 55:754–756.
6. Goodsall DH, Miles WE. Anorectal fistula. Dis Colon Rectum 1982; 25:262–278.
7. Cirocco WC, Reilly JC. Challenging the predictive accuracy of Goodsall's rule for anal fistulae. Dis Colon Rectum 1992; 35:537–542.
8. Bartram C, Buchanan G. Imaging anal fistula. Radiol Clin North Am 2003; 41:443–457.
9. Barker PG, Lunniss PJ, Armstrong P, et al. Magnetic resonance imaging of fistula in ano: Technique, interpretation and accuracy. Clin Radiol 1994; 49:7–13.
10. Wolff BG, Fleshman JW, Beck DE, et al. The ASCRS Textbook of Colon and Rectal Surgery. 1st ed. Springer: London, 2006:192–214.
11. Cataldo PA, Senagore A, Luchtefeld MA. Intrarectal ultrasound in the evaluation of perirectal abscesses. Dis Colon Rectum 1993; 36:554–558.
12. Law PJ, Talbot RW, Bartram CI, et al. Anal endosonography in the evaluation of perianal sepsis and fistula in ano. Br J Surg 1989; 76:752–755.
13. Regadas SMM, Regadas FSP. Two and Three-Dimensional Ultrasonography in Abscess and Fistula. Imaging Atlas of the Pelvic Floor and Anorectal Diseases. London: Springer, 2008.
14. Sudol-Szopinska I, Gesla J, Jakubowski W, et al. Reliability of endosonography in evaluation of anal fistulae and abscesses. Acta Radiol 2002; 43:599–602.
15. Sudol-Szopinska I, Szczepkowski M, Panorska AK, et al. Comparison of contrast-enhanced with non-contrast endosonography in the diagnostics of anal fistulae. Eur Radiol 2004; 14:2236–2241.
16. Halligan S. Imaging fistula-in-ano. Clin Radiol 1998; 53:85–95.
17. Myhr GE, Myrvold HE, Nilsen G, et al. Perianal fistulae: Use of MR imaging for diagnosis. Radiology 1994; 191:545–549.
18. Lunniss PJ, Barker PG, Sultan AH, et al. Magnetic resonance imaging of fistula-in-ano. Dis Colon Rectum 1994; 37:708–718.
19. Saino P, Husa A. A prospective manometric study of defective anal fistula surgery on anorectal function. Acta Chir Scand 1985; 151:279–288.
20. Lockhart-Mummery JP. Discussion on fistula-in-ano. Proc Roy Soc Med 1929; 22:1331.
21. McAnnaly AK, Dockerty MB. Carcinoma developing in chronic draining cutaneous sinuses and fistulae. Surg Gynecol Obstet. 1949; 88(1):87–96.
22. Hanley PH. Anorectal abscess fistula. Surg Clin North Am. 1978; 58:487–503.
23. Joy HA, Williams JG. The outcome of surgery for complex anal fistulae. Colorectal Dis 2002; 4:254–261.
24. Durgan V, Perek A, Kapan M, et al. Partial fistulotomy and modified cutting seton procedure in the treatment of high extrasphincteric perianal fistulae. Dig Surg 2002; 19:56–58.
25. Theerapol A, So BY, Ngoi SS. Routine use of setons for the treatment of anal fistulae. Singapore Med J 2002; 43:305–307.
26. Zbar AP, Ramesh J, Beer-Gabel M, et al. Conventional cutting vs. internal anal sphincter-preserving seton for high trans-sphincteric fistula: A prospective randomized manometric and clinical trial. Tech Coloproctol 2003; 7:89–94.
27. Hamel CT, Marti WR, Oertli D. Simplified placement and management of cutting setons in the treatment of trans-sphincteric anal fistula: Technical note. Int J Colorectal Dis 2004; 19:354–356.
28. Pescatori M, Ayabaca S, Caputo D. Can anal manometry predict anal incontinence after fistulectomy in males? Colorectal Dis 2004; 6:97–102.
29. Mentes BB, Oktemer S, Tezcaner T, et al. Elastic one-stage cutting seton for the treatment of high anal fistulae: preliminary results. Tech Coloproctol 2004; 8:159–162.
30. Wiliams JG, Farrands PA, Williams AB, et al. The treatment of anal fistula: ACPGBI Position Statement. Color Dis 2007; 9(suppl 4):18–50.
31. Ozuner G, Hull TL, Cartmill J, et al. Long-term analysis of the use of transanal rectal advancement flaps for complicated anorectal/vaginal fistulae. Dis Colon Rectum 1996; 39:10–14.
32. Miller GV, Finan PJ. Flap advancement and core fistulectomy for complex rectal fistula. Br J Surg 1998; 85:108–110.
33. Ortiz H, Marzo J. Endorectal flap advancement repair and fistulectomy for high trans-sphincteric and suprasphincteric fistulae. Br J Surg 2000; 87:1680–1683.
34. Makowiec F, Jehle EC, Becker HD, et al. Clinical course after transanal advancement flap repair of perianal fistula in patients with Crohn's disease. Br J Surg 1995; 82:603–606.

35. Sonoda T, Hull T, Piedmonte MR, et al. Outcomes of primary repair of anorectal and rectovaginal fistulae using the endorectal advancement flap. Dis Colon Rectum 2002; 45:1622–1628.
36. Lewis P, Bartolo DC. Treatment of trans-sphincteric fistulae by full thickness anorectal advancement flaps. Br J Surg 1990; 77:1187–1189.
37. Jun SH, Choi GS. Anocutaneous advancement flap closure of high anal fistulae. Br J Surg 1999; 86:490–492.
38. Amin SN, Tierney GM, Lund JN, et al. V-Y advancemen flap for treatment of fistula-in-ano. Dis Colon Rectum 2003; 46:540–543.
39. Del Pino A, Nelson RL, Pearl RK, et al. Island flap anoplasty for treatment of transsphincteric fistula-in-ano. Dis Colon Rectum 1996; 39:224–226.
40. Nelson RL, Cintron J, Abcarian H. Dermal island-flap anoplasty for transsphincteric fistula-in-ano: Assessment of treatment failures. Dis Colon Rectum 2000; 43:681–684.
41. Hossack T, Solomon MJ, Young JM. Ano-cutaneous flap repair for complex and recurrent supra-sphincteric anal fistula. Colorectal Dis 2005; 7(2):187–192.
42. Hedelin H, Nilson AE, TegerNilsson A-C, et al. Fibrin occlusion of fistulae postoperatively. Surg Gynecol Obstet 1982; 154:366–368.
43. Kikegaard P, Madsen P. Perineal sinus after removal of the rectum. Occlusion with fibrin adhesive. Am J Surg 1983; 145:791–794.
44. Atrah HI. Fibrin glue (Editorial). Br Med J 1994; 308:933–934.
45. Hjortrup A, Moesgaard F, Kjaergard J. Fibrin adhesive in the treatment of perineal fistulae. Dis Colon Rectum 1991; 34:752–754.
46. Abel ME, Chiu YSY, Russell TR, et al. Autologous fibrin glue in the treatment of rectovaginal and complex fistulae. Dis Colon Rectum 1993; 36(5):447–449.
47. Venkatesh KS, Ramanujam P. Fibrin glue application in the treatment of recurrent anorectal fistulae. Dis Colon Rectum 1999; 42:1136–1139.
48. Aitola P, Hiltunen KM, Matikainen M. Fibrin glue in perianal fistulae—a pilot study. Ann Chir Gynaecol 1999; 88:136–138.
49. Ramirez RT, Hicks TC, Beck DE. Use of tisseel fibrin sealant for complex fistulae using conscious sedation. Dis Colon Rectum 2000; 43:A1–A62.
50. Cintron JR, Park JJ, Orsay CP, et al. Repair of fistuale-inano using fibrin adhesive. Long-term follow up. Dis Colon Rectum 2000; 43:944–950.
51. Patrlj L, Kocman B, Martinac M, et al. Fibrin glue-antibiotic mixture in the treatment of anal fistulae: Experience with 69 cases. Dig Surg 2000; 17:77–80.
52. El-Shobaky M, Khafagy W, El-Awady S. Autologous fibrin glue in the treatment of complex cryptoglandular fistula in ano. Colorectal Dis 2000; 2(Suppl):17.
53. Salim AS, Ahmed T. KTP-laser and fibrin glue for treatment of fistulae in ano. Saudi Med J 2001; 22:1022–1024.
54. Lindsey I, Smilgin-Humphreys MM, Cunningham C, et al. A randomized, controlled trial of fibrin glue vs. conventional treatment for anal fistula. Br J Surg 2002; 45:1608–1615.
55. Chan KM, Lau CW, Lai KK, et al. Preliminary results of using a commercial fibrin sealant in the treatment of fistula-in-ano. J R Coll Surg Edinb 2002; 47:407–410.
56. Sentovich SM. Fibrin glue for anal fistulae. Long term results. Dis Colon Rectum 2003; 46:498–502.
57. Zmora O, Mizrahi N, Rotholtz N, et al. Fibrin glue sealing in the treatment of perineal fistulae. Dis Colon Rectum 2003; 46:584–589.
58. Buchanan GN, Bartram CI, Phillips RK, et al. The efficacy of fibrin sealant in the management of complex anal fistula: A prospective trial. Dis Colon Rectum 2003; 46:1167–1174.
59. Loungnarath R, Dietz DW, Mutch MG, et al. Fibrin glue treatment of complex anal fistulae has low success rate. Dis Colon Rectum 2004; 47:432–436.
60. Vitton V, Gasmi M, Barthet M, et al. Long term healing of Crohn's anal fistulae with fibrin glue injection. Aliment Pharmacol Ther 2005; 21(12):1453–1457.
61. Singer M, Cintron J, Nelson R, et al. Treatment of fistulae in- ano with fibrin sealant in combination with intra-adhesive antibiotics and/or surgical closure of the internal fistula opening. Dis Colon Rectum 2005; 48:799–808.
62. Champagne BJ, O'Connor LM, Ferguson M, et al. Efficacy of anal fistula plug in closure of cryptoglandular fistulae: Long-term follow-up. Dis Colon Rectum 2006; 49:1817–1821.
63. Lawes DA, Efron JE, Abbas M, et al. Early experience with the bioabsorbable anal fistula plug. World J Surg 2008; 32(6):1157–1159.
64. Ky AJ, Sylla P, Steinhagen R, et al. Collagen fistula plug for the treatment of anal fistulas. Dis Colon Rectum 2008 51:838–843.
65. Schwandner O, Stadler F, Dietl O, et al. Initial experience on efficacy in closure of cryptoglandular and Crohn's transsphincteric fistulae by the use of the anal fistula plug. Int J Colorectal Dis 2008; 23(3):319–324.
66. Safar B, Jobanputra S, Cera S, et al. Anal Fistula Plug: Initial Experience and Outcomes. Oral presentation. St.Louis, MO: American Society of Colon and Rectal Surgeons Annual meeting, 2007.

17 Pilonidal Disease

Jorge A. Lagares-Garcia and Matthew Vrees
R.I. Colorectal Clinic, LLC, Pawtucket, Rhode Island, U.S.A.

EPIDEMIOLOGY

Pilonidal disease is a complicated process of the subcutaneous tissue and skin. The etiology remains a debate, and theories include both an acquired disease process versus congenital cause. In the acquired theory of development, it is postulated that one either gets hair implantation in the sacral region, or there is rupture of a hair follicle leading to a foreign body reaction. Supportive evidence for this theory is that the disease is most common in hirsute males, and a similar disease process occurs in the fingers of barbers. The congenital theories include medullary canal remnants, dermal inclusion cysts, or vestigial sex glands. The onset of disease typically ranges from the early teenage years to the 30s but certainly can be seen in older populations. The classic acute clinical presentation is pain and swelling located over the upper portion of the gluteal area, typically in the midline. When the patient does not seek early medical advice, the process may progress to erythema or possibly a fluctuant mass. Not uncommonly, the patient will have purulent drainage from open sinuses which temporarily relieves the clinical symptoms. In chronic cases, the disease usually causes persistent drainage of bloody and purulent fluid and intermittent flares or abscess formation from occluded sinuses. If left untreated, the disease spectrum may range from a simple noninfected pilonidal sinus (Fig. 1) to a complex soft tissue infection with multiple tracts (Fig. 2) originating just over the postsacral fascia and progressing in all directions. Although infections in this area are almost always secondary to pilonidal disease, other potential etiologies include hidradenitis suppurativa and cryptoglandular disease with a long fistula tract. The latter must be ruled out prior to definitive therapy since the surgical management of this process is considerably different.

William Mayo originally described a pilonidal cyst and associated abscess in the medical literature (1), but the disease was more popularized as "jeep's disease" when the occurrence in World War II caused nearly 80,000 admissions and an average hospital stay of 55 days following surgical intervention (2,3).

It is postulated that vacuum forces and negative pressure in the natal clefts cause rupture of hair follicles with penetration of hair and other debris leading to obstruction and infection (4). Sondena et al. (5) reported that 15% of patients will have only aerobes, 29% only anaerobes, and 10% will have both aerobes and anaerobes. Nearly 44% of patients will have no growth from operative cultures.

ACUTE PRESENTATION

Pilonidal Abscess

In the acute setting, the treatment is no different than any other abscess. Adequate drainage can usually be performed in the office or, at most, in an outpatient setting. Successful outpatient treatment involves having a cooperative patient which is predicated by adequate information given to the patient. In the prone position, the buttocks are spread with the use of wide tape. Any hair in the area is shaved and then cleansed with either an alcohol-based solution or betadine. The site is then anesthetized using a mixture of 1% lidocaine and 0.5% marcaine with epinephrine. Once adequate anesthesia is accomplished, a 15 blade is used to excise a 1 cm area of skin overlying the abscess. A hemostat is then used to open the cavity, along with any loculated areas. Evacuation of hair or any other foreign body facilitates healing and closure. By excising a small amount of skin to prevent rapid closure, one can avoid the need for packing which is both painful and quite costly. A simple sterile dressing is adequate. Wide excision of the affected area in the acute setting is generally not recommended. Antibiotic coverage is unnecessary

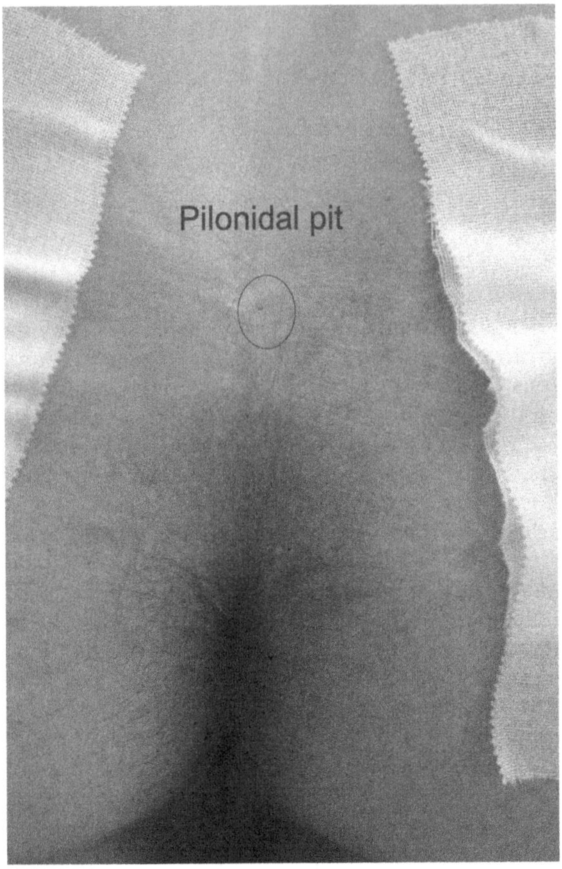

Figure 1 A simple pilonidal pit.

unless significant cellulitis is present or the patient is immunocompromised. Standard practice consists of routine follow-up in the office every other week or on an as-needed basis until the area has completely healed. It is also recommended that the patient have somebody shave the area weekly to avoid the theoretical problem of hair entering the wound Other maneuvers to keep the area clean during the healing process are wound irrigation with a handheld shower head which is preferable but not always possible. Standard Sitz baths will suffice in most cases.

CHRONIC PRESENTATION

Draining Pilonidal Sinus

The ideal surgical therapy for chronic pilonidal disease is one that is technically easy to perform, associated with a short recovery, minimal pain, and a low recurrence rate. To date, multiple options have been described.

In 1994, simple treatment by strip shaving a 5 cm circumferential area in the gluteal cleft was described by Armstrong and Barcia (6). In a study heavily criticized of its methodology, they demonstrated an advantage using this technique in comparison to surgeries such as midline excision with/without marsupialization, primary total or partial closure, packing, rotational flaps, Z-plasty, and skin grafting.

This treatment is always recommended as the initial conservative therapy in patients with localized disease and no inflammation.

Other conservative treatments have been reported recently including the use of laser hair removal. Schulze et al. (7) reported no recurrences in 19 patients using laser epilation in addition to surgical therapy. This low recurrence rate was duplicated in a small series of 14 patients by Odili and Gault (8). Although these series include small numbers of patients, this may be an

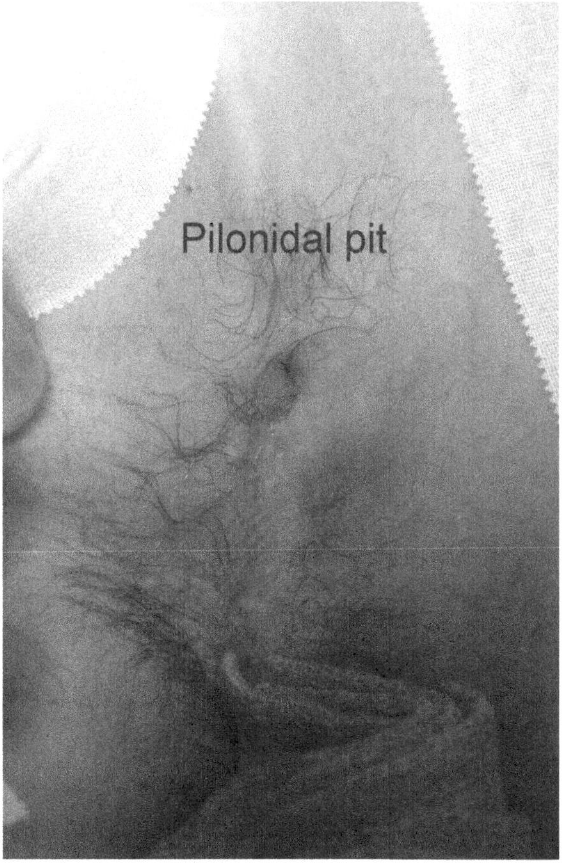

Figure 2 Complex multiple pilonidal sinuses.

acceptable nonsurgical technique that can be implemented prior to extensive resection, with or without complex flap reconstruction.

Sinus Excision

Prior to sinus excision, the patient prepares with a Fleet® enema® (Fleet phosphosoda, Lynchburg, Virgin Islands, U.S.A.) preparation to allow for an adequate rectal examination. If simple excision is to be performed, it is recommend that MAC anesthesia be implemented, thus avoiding an endotracheal tube. The patient is placed in the prone jackknife position, and the buttocks are retracted exposing the cleft. The patient is sedated using propofol and fentanyl, unless there are patient-specific contraindications to these medications. Shaving and sterile preparation as well as draping of the area are performed. Injection of methylene blue using an angiocatheter (Fig. 3) aids in localization of the tract and will also demonstrate possible communications with other sinuses. Routine local anesthetic is infiltrated (50% mixture of 1% lidocaine and 0.5% marcaine), and the sinus is excised with at least 1 cm in diameter of surrounding normal skin (Figs. 4 and 5) (9). The wound is left open and packed with gauze after cleansing with sterile saline (Fig. 6). This therapy, studied retrospectively in 62 patients, yielded a 1.6% recurrence rate with a median follow-up of 12 months. Furthermore, it was associated with a 54% high satisfaction rate and 79% of the patients would recommend this therapy to other patients.

Primary Excision and Closure by Granulation

The drawback to this technique is the lengthy time to recover and the daily dressing changes, which are both inconvenient and unpleasant. In a survey sent to 103 patients, Menzel et al. (10) reported an average length of time to return to work of four weeks. A recurrence rate of 12% was noted with a follow-up ranging from 12 to 47 months.

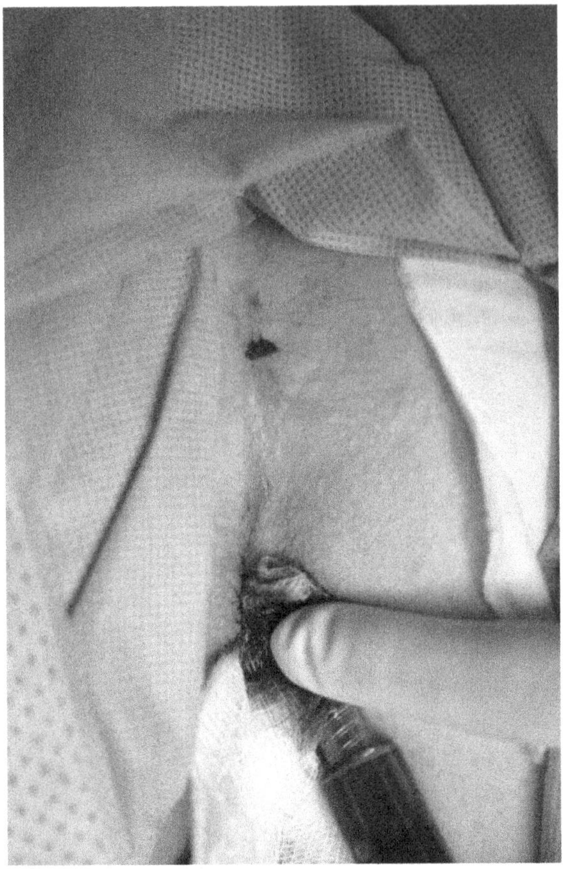

Figure 3 Injection of methylene blue to identify tracts.

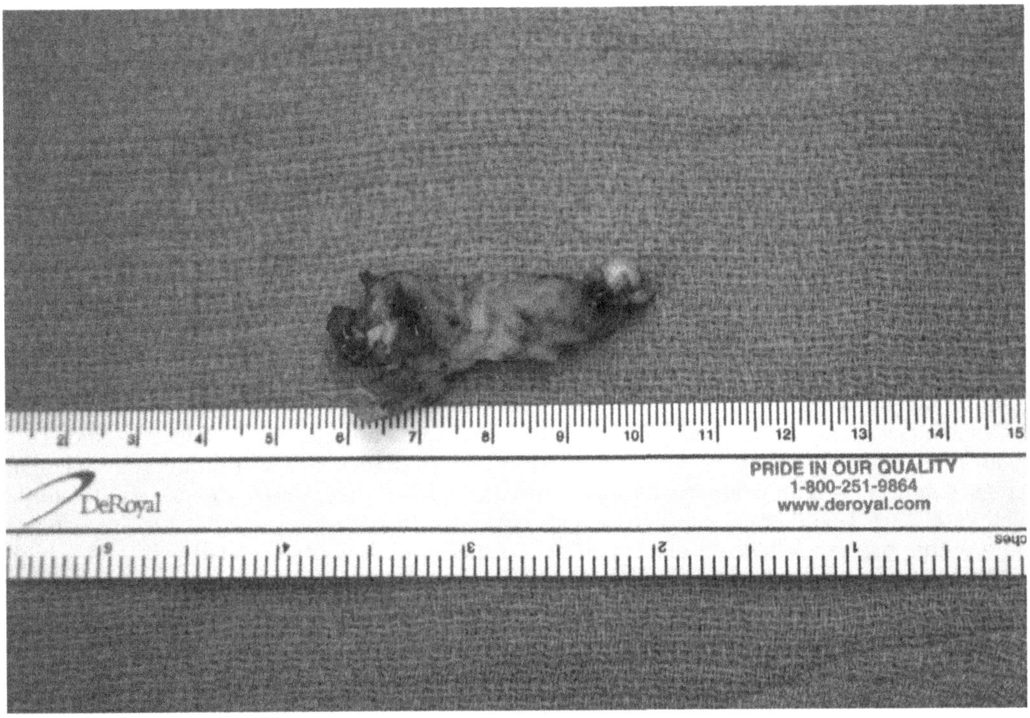

Figure 4 Pilonidal sinus specimen.

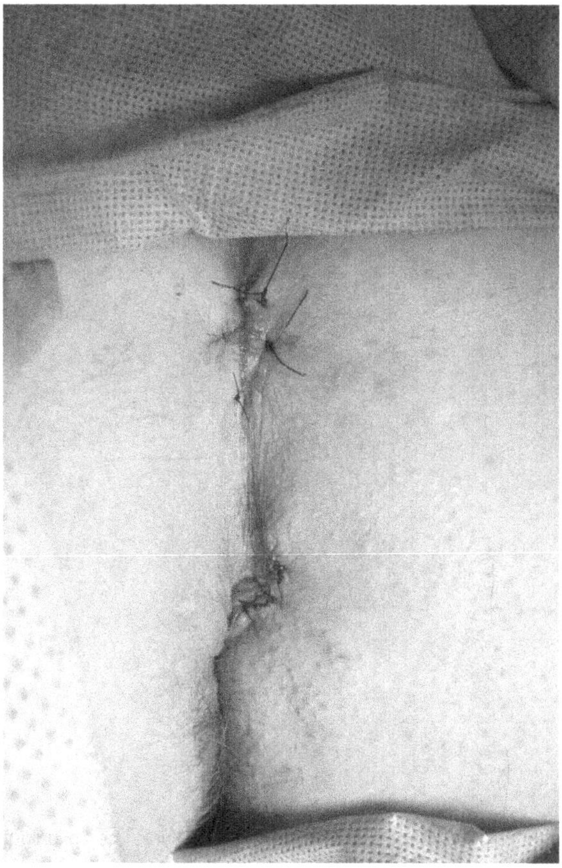

Figure 5 Primary closure of pilonidal sinus.

Other techniques of primary excision have been described using radiofrequency to shorten the recovery time, time off from work, mean analgesic requirement, and time to complete healing (11). In a comparative study between open and primary closure of the midline, Perruchoud et al. (12) reported a similar recurrence rate of 6% with fewer postoperative visits required and a shorter time to return to work, favoring primary closure. More recently, case reports have been published in regards to the VAC system, promoting more rapid wound healing. Reports in both the adult and pediatric literature cite success in all patients and conclude a benefit to this therapy. Although many patients do not tolerate the VAC system as well as wounds in other areas due to the location, it remains a viable option in patients with difficult wound healing.

Limberg Flap Repair

A primary rhomboid sinus excision and fasciocutaneous flap (Limberg flap) has been described as a closure technique for chronic pilonidal disease. Considering the origin of the disease, the use of a flap eradicates the gluteal cleft with less hairy areas used for the reconstruction as well as theoretically less postoperative perspiration (Figs. 7 and 8) (13).

Kapan et al. (13) reported a 10 year series with an average follow-up of 69 (range 9–120) months using this technique in 85 patients. A total of three recurrences (3.5%) were noted, all occurring between 24 and 30 months after the original surgery. Complications from the surgery included edema (1.2%), wound infection (1.2%), and wound hematoma under the flap (2.3%). These complications all resolved and there was no report of any ischemic loss of tissue to the area. The average length of hospital stay was 5.3 days and return to daily activities occurred three weeks postoperatively.

Daphan et al. (14) reported a larger series of 147 patients with a shorter follow-up of 13 (range 1–40) months. The recurrence rate was 4.8%. Local complications included seroma formation (2%) and wound dehiscence (4.1%). Patients remained in the hospital for an average of 5.9 days and full return to daily activities occurred on an average of 18.8 days.

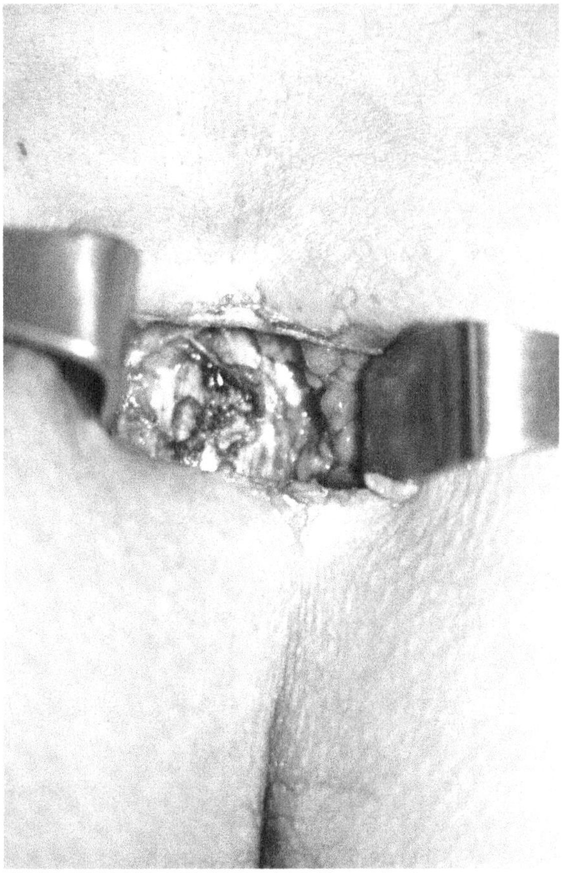

Figure 6 Secondary closure of pilonidal excision.

Karydakis Flap Technique

Originally described in 1973, the use of this asymmetrical flap technique has reported recurrence as low as 1% (15–17). The original description involves an asymmetric midline incision causing flattening and lateralization of the natal cleft (Fig. 9) (15). The use of drainage after the excision and reconstruction is controversial. In order to determine the role of drainage, a total of 50 patients were evaluated following a Karydakis flap. The mean hospital length of stay was 2.5 days in each group. Comparison between the two groups revealed a statistically significant decrease in fluid collection in the group without a suction drain (8% vs. 32%, respectively). There was no long-term follow-up reported in this study.

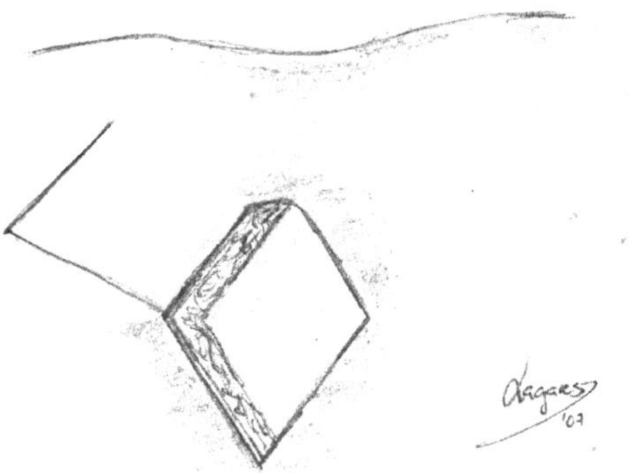

Figure 7 Limberg flap: Flap drawing for coverage.

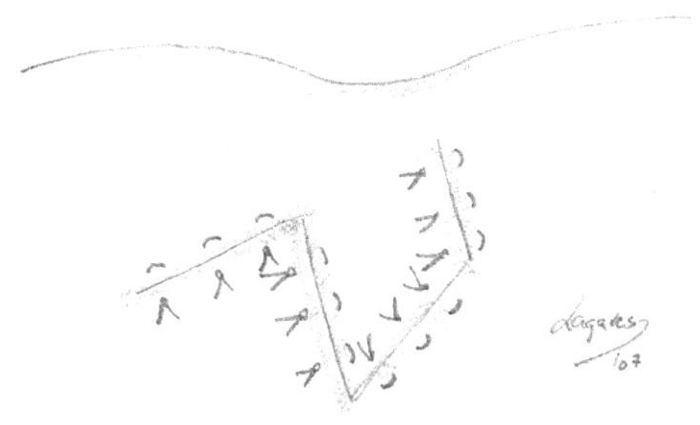

Figure 8 Limberg flap: Closure with the flap.

In another study assessing the role of Karydakis flap, Keshava et al. (18) studied a total of 70 patients with an average follow-up of 36 (range 1–79) months. The endpoints of this retrospective study were superficial and complete wound breakdown (38% and 8.4%, respectively) with a recurrence rate of 4.2%. A smaller study with 28 patients reported no recurrence at a median follow-up of 3 years (19). A modification of the flap with subcutaneous fistulectomy in 14 patients yielded one seroma postoperatively, with no closure failures and no recurrence at a median follow-up of 16.2 (range 4–36) months (20).

Comparison between Karydakis flap and wide midline excision has revealed a lower recurrence rate (0% vs. 11%, respectively) with similar early complication rates in the less common pediatric population (21).

Gluteus Maximus Myocutaneous Flap

A complex rotational flap using the gluteus maximus has been described to cover large areas in the sacrum when complex tracts or malignant degeneration require such aggressive wide local excisions (22).

MALIGNANT DEGENERATION

Chronic sinuses and long standing neglect of surgical care for nonhealing wounds may potentially cause a rare malignant degeneration of a pilonidal sinus. De Bree et al. (23) reviewed the current literature in regard to malignancy associated with chronic pilonidal disease. Although a rare entity, unusual nonhealing wounds should be suspect and warrant biopsy. The vast majority of these malignancies (92%) were squamous cell carcinoma followed by basal cell and adenocarcinoma in 5% and 3%, respectively. The mean age of presentation was 52 years and the duration of symptoms averaged 22 years; 12% had lymph node involvement at the time of presentation. Treatments described for this type of malignancy include surgery alone, concomitant chemotherapy and radiation therapy, or a combination of surgery with neoadjuvant or adjuvant chemotherapy and radiation therapy. The mean follow-up was 28 months with local recurrence rates, regional lymph node recurrence, and a distant metastasis rate of 31%, 4%, and 15%, respectively. Cancer-related deaths were 20% at a mean follow-up of 30 months.

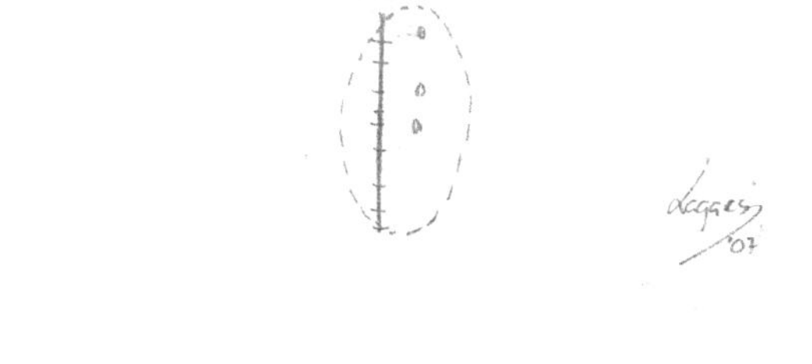

Figure 9 Karydakis flap: Incision on the left and subcutaneous dissection underneath.

If surgery is undertaken, the ability to maintain tumor-free margins may require the role of multiple specialists and should be well planned in advance with individualized therapeutic strategies.

FOLLOW-UP AND SURVEILLANCE

Routinely, the follow-up of patients depends on the procedure performed. A visit is scheduled within the first two weeks postoperatively and, depending on the status of the wound, closer or more spaced follow-up visits are then scheduled.

On average, patients will require between two to three months when wounds are left open and then four weeks when primary closure is done. Routine skin hygiene includes direct hand-held shower application and, once the wound is closed, shaving or depilation is recommended.

REFERENCES

1. Mayo OH. Observations on Injuries and Diseases of the Rectum. London: Burgess and Hill, 1833:45–46.
2. Casberg MA. Infected pilonidal cyst and sinuses. Bull US Army Med Dept 1949; 9:493–496.
3. Bascom J, Bascom T. Failed pilonidal surgery: new paradigm and new operations leading to cures. Arch Surg 2002; 137:1146–1150.
4. Hull TL, WU J. Pilonidal disease. Surg Clinc North Am 2002; 82:1169–1185.
5. Sondenan K, Nesvik I, Andersen E, et al. Bacteriology and complications of chronic pilonidal sinus treated with excision and primary closure. Int J Colorect Dis 1995; 10:161–166.
6. Armstrong JH, Barcia PJ. Pilonidal sinus disease: the conservative approach. Arch Surg 1994; 129(9):914–917.
7. Schulze SM, Patel N, Hertzog D, et al. Treatment of pilonidal disease with laser epilation. Am Surg 2006; 72(6):534–537.
8. Odili J, Gault D. Laser depilation of the natal cleft- an aidto healing the pilonidal sinus. Ann R Coll Surg Engl 2002; 84(1):29–32.
9. Kement M, Oncel M, Kurt N. Sinus excision for the treatment of limited chronic pilonidal disase: results after a medium-term follow up. Dis Colon Rectum 2006; 49: 1758–1762.
10. Menzel T, Dörner A, Cramer J. Excision and open wound treatment of pilonidal sinus. Rate of recurrence and duration of work incapacity. Dtsch Med Wochenschr 1997; 122(47):1447–1451.
11. Gupta PJ. Comparative study between radiofrequency sinus excision and open excision in sacrococygeal pilonidal sinus disease. Dig Surg 2005; 22(6):459–463.
12. Perruchoud C, Viulleumier H, Givel JC. The treatment of pilonidal disease of the sacrococcygeal region by the method of limited excision and open wound healing. Swiss Surg 2002; 54(1):27–31.
13. Kapan M, Kapan S, Pekmezci S, et al. Sacrococcygeal pilonidal sinus disease with Limberg flap repair. Tech Coloproctol 2002; 6:27–32.
14. Daphan C, Tekelioglu MH, Sayilgan C. Limberg flap repair for pilonidal sinus disease. Dis Colon Rectum 2004; 47:233–237.
15. Karydakis GE. New approach to the problem of pilonidal sinus. Lancet 1973; 2:1414–1415.
16. Karydakis GE. Easy and successful treatment of pilonidal sinus after explanation of its causative processes. ANZ J Surg 1992; 62:385–389.
17. Peterson S, Koch R, Stelzner S, et al. Primary closure techniques in chronic pilonidal sinus. Dis Colon Rectum 2002; 45:1458–1467.
18. Keshava A, Young CJ, Rickard MJ, et al. Karydakis flap repair for sacrococcygeal pilonidal sinus disease: how important is technique. ANZ J Surg 2007; 77(3):181–183.
19. Anyanwu AC, Hossain S, Williams A, et al. Karydakis operation for sacrococcygeal pilonidal sinus disease: experience in a district general hospital. Ann R Coll Surg Engl 1998; 80(3):197–199.
20. Kulacoglu H, Dener C, Tumer H, et al. total subcutaneous fistulectomy combined with karydakis flap for sacrococcygeal pilonidal disease with secondary perianal opening. Colorectal Dis 2006; 8(2):120–123.
21. Morden P, Drongowski RA, Geiger JD, et al. Comparison of Karydakis versus midline excision for treatment of pilonidal sinus disease. Pediatr Surg Int 2005; 21(10):793–796.
22. Perez-Gurri JA, Temple WJ, Ketcham AS. Gluteus maximus myocutaneous flap for the treatment of recalcitrant pilonidal disease. Dis Colon Rectum 1984; 27:262–264.
23. De Bree E, Zoetmulder FAN, Christodoulakis M, et al. Treatment of malignancy arising in pilonidal disease. Ann Surg Oncol 2001; 8(1):60–64.

18 Perianal Crohn's Disease

Marat Khaikin and Oded Zmora

Department of Surgery and Transplantation, Sheba Medical Center, Sackler School of Medicine, Tel Aviv, Israel

INTRODUCTION

Crohn's disease is a chronic relapsing inflammatory bowel disease, with skip areas of transmural involvement. Although the etiology remains unknown, the current concept is that some unknown offending factors, which may be environmental, dietary, infectious, intraluminal flora, or others, lead to inappropriate stimulation of the epithelial mucosal immune system in genetically susceptible individuals (1). This excessive response causes an exaggerated inflammatory process and tissue damage, with gastrointestinal and extraintestinal manifestations.

Crohn's disease can affect any part of the gastrointestinal tract from the mouth to anus, but most commonly involves the terminal ileum and the right colon. The classic age distribution at diagnosis is bimodal with a main peak in the second decade of life, and the second in the fifth decade (2). There is a slight female gender predominance, and the disease is more common in Caucasians and in the Jewish population (3,4).

Perianal Crohn's disease is the involvement of the perineal area in the inflammatory process. It may primarily be present at the perianal region in 5% to 25% of patients and can be associated with active disease in the proximal gastrointestinal tract or colon in about one third to half of the patients, respectively (5).

CLINICAL PRESENTATION

Perianal Crohn's disease most commonly presents as perineal abscesses and fistulas, including rectovaginal fistulas. However, it may also present with anal fissures, anal ulcers, and edematous skin tags. Patients may also experience fecal incontinence as well as anal stenosis. The activity of the perianal disease usually parallels intestinal flare-up, presenting with diarrhea, fever, intermittent abdominal pain, fatigue, weight loss, and anorexia. However, up to 25% of the patients may predominantly suffer from anal symptoms with quiescent abdominal disease (6). In some cases, perianal disease may be the initial presenting symptom of Crohn's disease, preceding the abdominal symptoms, thereby leading to the diagnosis of Crohn's disease.

Crohn's disease is a chronic disease, and curative intent of any therapy is currently not realistic. The main goal of both medical and surgical therapies is to improve and protect quality of life. Perianal disease is frequently associated with significant disability and morbidity, affecting daily activity and severely jeopardizing quality of life. Correct diagnosis of the perianal conditions and sound use of the various medical and surgical treatment options are paramount in the treatment of these patients.

PHYSICAL FINDINGS OF CROHN'S DISEASE

Skin Tags

In patients with perianal Crohn's disease, skin tags are usually edematous, large, cyanotic, and occasionally painful. They often arise from a healed anal ulcer or fissure and, if large, can cause perianal hygiene problems. Perianal skin involvement may also present as skin ulcers and maceration with poor prolonged healing.

Anal Fissures

Anal fissures in patients with Crohn's disease are usually eccentric, multiple, and painless in contrast to single, midline, and very painful conventional fissures (7). They may be associated

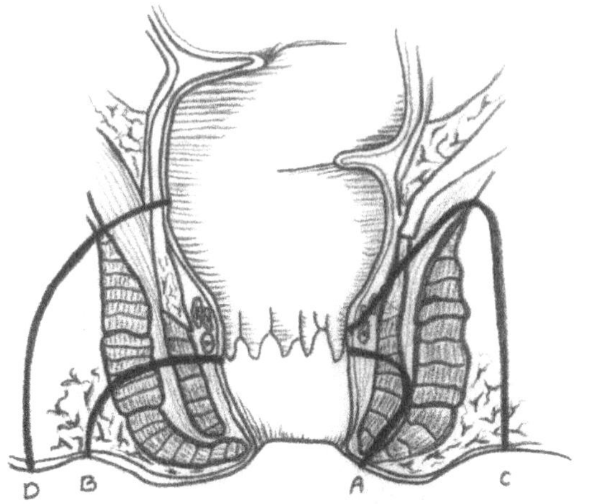

Figure 1 Park's classification of perianal fistulas. (A) intersphincteric fistula, (B) low trans-sphincteric fistula, (C) high trans-sphincteric fistula, (D) supra-sphincteric fistula.

with large skin tags and heal spontaneously in more than 80% of the patients (8). Perianal abscess should be strongly suspected in patients with severe pain or fever.

Anal Ulcers

Anal ulcers appear in consequence of anorectal inflammation and may present with rectal bleeding and pain. They may lead to anal stenosis, perianal abscess, or fistula.

Anal Stenosis and Anorectal Stricture

Anal stenosis and anorectal stricture may arise as a complication of ongoing active inflammatory anorectal disease, recurrent perianal abscesses and fistulas, or repeated perianal operations.

Perianal Abscesses and Fistulas

Perianal abscesses and fistulas are the most common suppurative manifestations of perianal Crohn's disease and are frequently multiple, complex, and recurrent. The etiology of perianal Crohn's abscesses and fistulas may be the result of infected anal glands in the intersphincteric space (Park's cryptoglandular theory), or they may arise from the transmural penetration of deep anal ulcers into the perirectal tissue (9,10). The presence of perianal pain, fever, tenderness, and induration with or without fluctuation and purulent discharge requires examination under anesthesia (EUA) to exclude the presence of perianal abscess.

Several anorectal spaces may become infected in perianal Crohn's disease and result in abscesses and fistulas. These include perianal, intersphincteric, supralevator, and deep postanal spaces. Park describes five classification of perianal fistulas with respect to the external anal sphincter: superficial, intersphincteric, transsphincteric, suprasphincteric, and extrasphincteric (Fig. 1) (11). These fistulas are also classified as either simple (low) or complex (high). A simple fistula is superficial, intersphincteric, or low transsphincteric, has a single external opening, without fluctuation or pain, and is not associated with rectovaginal fistula, active rectal inflammation, or anorectal stricture. A complex fistula is high transsphincteric, suprasphincteric, or extrasphincteric, and encompasses a significant portion of the external anal sphincter. High fistulas and those associated with active proctocolitis, multiple external openings, abscess, rectovaginal fistula, and anorectal stenosis makes surgical treatment more difficult, with higher risk of complications and lower success rate.

Rectovaginal Fistulas

Rectovaginal fistulas may occur in 3% to 10% of women with Crohn's disease (12). The etiology is similar to other Crohn's perianal fistulas, with most originating from deep anterior anorectal ulcers penetrating into the vagina. They may be low or high, but usually occur in the midportion of the rectovaginal septum.

Most women with rectovaginal fistulas present with anorectal pain, intermittent vaginal discharge of pus, or passage of gas through the vagina. It may be associated with perianal abscess or fistula, active proctitis, or anorectal stricture. These fistulas are challenging to treat and have high recurrence rates after surgical repair. Rectovaginal fistulas have also been frequently reported in patients who were diagnosed with Crohn's disease after restorative proctocolectomy for presumably ulcerative colitis, and may originate at the level of the ileoanal anastomosis.

Symptomatic Fecal Incontinence

Fecal incontinence may occur in up to 39% of patients with long-standing complicated perianal Crohn's disease (13). The incontinence may be related to severe inflammation of the anorectum resulting in chronic fibrosis and loss of compliance and reservoir function, and may be the end result of multiple aggressive fistulotomies and other surgical interventions. In female patients, obstetric trauma may also contribute to fecal incontinence. A thorough history, physical examination, and additional imaging modalities help to correctly detect the cause of incontinence in these patients.

Carcinoma

A long duration of perianal disease and the presence of chronic nonhealing perianal fistulas may theoretically increase the risk for anorectal malignancy. The risk for squamous-cell carcinoma of the anus does not appear to be increased in patients with perianal Crohn's disease; however, should anal carcinoma develop the anorectal inflammation may delay diagnosis (14). Because of this risk, a biopsy of long-standing nonhealing lesions should be considered.

DIAGNOSIS

The diagnosis of perianal Crohn's disease in patients with a known history of Crohn's disease presenting with anorectal complaints is obvious. However, Crohn's disease should also be suspected in patients with multiple and complex perianal abscesses and fistulas, nontraumatic rectovaginal fistulas, recurrent nonhealing eccentric fissures, and persistent perineal wounds.

In the presence of known or suspected perianal Crohn's disease, diagnostic efforts are frequently focused to define the type, location, and nature of perianal involvement.

History and Physical Examination

A thorough history and physical examination is often sufficient for a diagnosis of most perianal lesions, and specialized imaging studies are not routinely required. Patients should be questioned as to the exact presentation of current symptoms, past events, abdominal symptoms, medications, and continence. Physical examination should include careful inspection of the perianal area for any sign of undrained abscess as well as any external opening of perianal fistulas. The fistula can frequently be gently probed in the office, delineating its relation to the sphincter mechanism. However, if associated with severe pain, probing should be withheld. A digital anorectal examination may reveal tenderness or fluctulance, anorectal masses, and deformities, and should also include an assessment of anal pressures. In severe cases, digital rectal examination may be limited because of significant anal pain and tenderness. Anoscopy, if possible, may show purulent discharge, internal openings of perianal fistulas, and suggest the presence or absence of mucosal inflammation of the anal canal.

Examination Under Anesthesia

In any case of suspected perineal sepsis not adequately drained, EUA should be promptly performed without delay. Deep perianal abscesses and other anorectal manifestations of Crohn's disease may not be clinically apparent on external examination, and in some cases rectal examination may be limited because of pain and tenderness. Any patients with perineal Crohn's disease with sepsis, perianal tenderness, or discharge should be considered for EUA. This outpatient procedure consists of inspection, probing of the fistula tracts, along with concomitant surgical incision, and drainage of any perianal infection. One must also consider deep placement of seton drains in order to prevent recurring episodes of perianal sepsis.

Imaging and Diagnostic Modalities

Imaging and other diagnostic modalities, such as endoscopy, ultrasound, contrast studies, computerized tomography (CT), and pelvic magnetic resonance imaging (MRI) can help in the

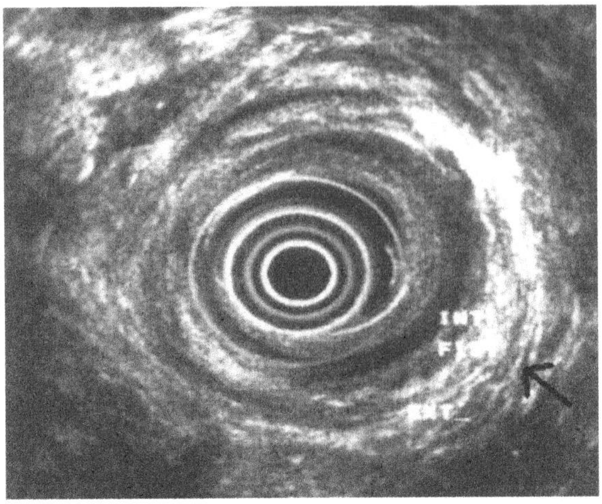

Figure 2 Trans-rectal ultrasound showing perianal fistula. Arrow shows hyper-echoic enhancement after injection of H_2O_2.

diagnosis and classification of perianal Crohn's disease (15–17). These techniques may assist in the localization of undrained abscesses not evident on physical examination, and are helpful in delineating the number and location of perianal fistulas, their secondary tracts, as well as associated collections. In addition, one may gain insight as to the relationship of the fistula tract to the sphincter mechanism. Careful attention to these parameters is essential in selecting the correct treatment option for each patient.

Transanal Endoscopic Ultrasound

Transanal endoscopic ultrasound (EUS) is a circular ultrasound in which the probe is inserted into the anal canal and rectum. As the probe is in proximity to the pathology, it is very sensitive for the detection of abscesses and fistulas (Fig. 2) (18). The correct reading of this examination is user dependent; therefore, diagnostic accuracy ranges from 56% to 100%. The accuracy of EUS in the detection of perianal fistulas may be enhanced by the use of hydrogen peroxide, and EUS findings may change the surgical management in 10% to 15% of cases (19). In patients in whom severe anal tenderness precludes digital rectal exam, transanal EUS without anesthesia is usually impossible. However, this may be brought into the operating room and used as part of the EUS.

Static Transperineal Ultrasound

Static transperineal ultrasound is a new modality for the assessment of the perianal region (20,21). In this examination the ultrasound transducer is applied on the perineal skin (Fig. 3). The procedure is less invasive than conventional anorectal EUS, and may also be informative in cases with severe anal pain and tenderness. Preliminary results are encouraging, but future

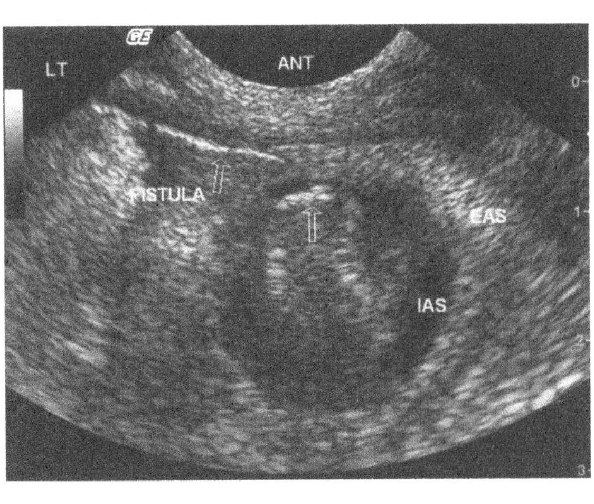

Figure 3 Trans-perineal ultrasound of perianal fistula. (Courtesy of Mark Bear Gabel, MD, Sheba Medical Center, Israel.)

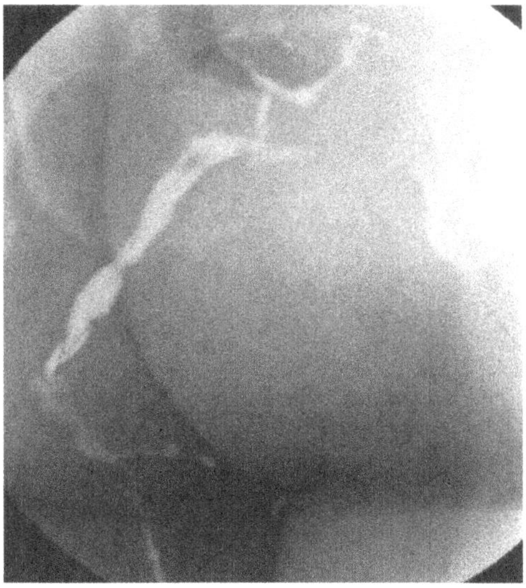

Figure 4 Water-soluble contrast fistulography.

experience is needed to determine the role of this modality in the evaluation of perianal Crohn's disease.

Endoscopy

Endoscopy is essential for the identification of active proctitis and colitis, biopsy of any suspicious lesion of the anal canal and rectum, and may help to locate internal openings of perianal fistulas draining to the lower rectum.

Gastrograffin or Barium Enema and Conventional Fistulography

Gastrograffin or barium enema and conventional fistulography are helpful in the localization of fistulas and associated collections or secondary tracts, but cannot define their relationship to the sphincter mechanism (Fig. 4) (22,23). A Gastrograffin enema and vaginography may be useful in detecting rectovaginal fistula, and methylene blue or betadine infused into the rectum with a tampon in the vagina, or rectal insufflation with air while the vagina is filled with saline may further support the diagnosis.

Pelvic CT

Pelvic CT may be informative for perianal abscesses not seen on physical examination and confirm the extent of perirectal sepsis and proctocolitis; however, this modality is not accurate for perianal fistulas and is not routinely used for this purpose.

Pelvic MRI

Pelvic MRI with phased array or endoanal coils has proven accurate in classifying perianal Crohn's fistulas (Fig. 5) (24,25). The diagnostic accuracy of this test is at least similar to EUS and EUA. The main limit for its widespread use is the high cost and limited availability of an appropriately equipped anal MRI.

A prospective study from the Mayo Clinic showed that pelvic MRI, rectal EUS, and EUA are all reasonably accurate methods of classifying perianal Crohn's disease. They suggested that the optimal approach to patients with Crohn's disease suspected of having a perianal fistula or abscess may be the combination of any two of these three methods (26).

Anorectal Manometry

Anorectal manometry measures the anorectal pressures at rest and squeeze, rectal sensitivity, and compliance. This test may be helpful in addition to physical assessment of anal continence, both in cases of impaired continence, and before surgical procedures which may potentially affect the anal sphincter.

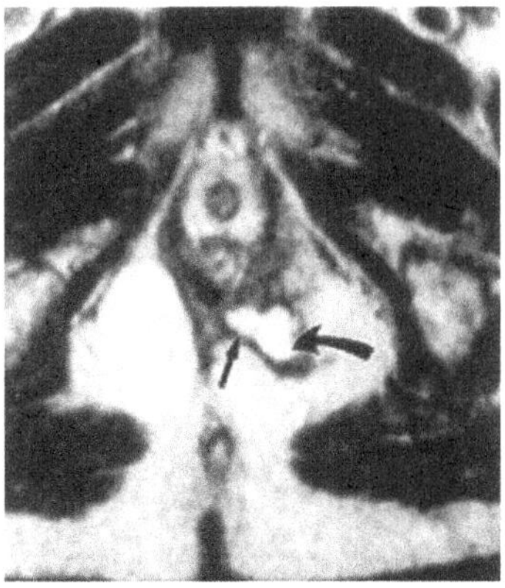

Figure 5 Pelvic MRI of perianal fistula. Arrows point to an associated cavity. (Courtesy of Marian Amitai, MD, Sheba Medical Center, Israel.)

MEDICAL AND SURGICAL MANAGEMENT

A multidisciplinary approach between the patient, surgeon, gastroenterologist, radiologist, pathologist, nutritionist, and other specialists makes the successful treatment of perianal Crohn's disease possible. The acute and long-term management of such patients depends on knowledge of type and location of the lesions and sites involved, diagnostic modalities, perianal anatomy, the severity of the patient's symptoms, and the medical and surgical options. Moreover, the general condition of the patient and proximal intestinal tract should also be evaluated and treated, if necessary. Several studies have suggested that if perianal manifestations persist in the presence of proximal luminal disease, resection of the inflammed bowel may improve perianal disease; however, practical use of this principle is still controversial (27,28).

Patients with perianal Crohn's disease experience significant morbidity and are at risk for incontinence either directly through the destructive inflammatory process or as a result of inadvertent damage during aggressive surgery. The primary management of such patients combines medical and surgical treatment aiming to improve quality of life and alleviate suffering. A comprehensive multidisciplinary approach is paramount, as either one alone is frequently not efficacious.

Medical Treatment

Prior to selection of medical treatment, thorough identification of the site of the fistula tracts, exclusion of perirectal abscess, and evaluation for the presence of active proctocolitis are advised. Current medical therapy includes antibiotics, immunomodulating antimetabolites such as azathioprine and 6-mercaptopurine (6-MP), infliximab, and occasionally cyclosporine, and tacrolimus. Corticosteroids are usually not beneficial in the therapy of perianal Crohn's disease and may retard wound healing and exacerbate abscess formation (29). Aminosalicylates are also ineffective in healing of fistulas. However, treatment of active rectal inflammation with topical corticosteroids or mesalamine may improve anal symptoms.

Antibiotic Therapy

There are no controlled trials showing that antibiotics are effective in the treatment of Crohn's perianal fistulas (1). Currently, metronidazole at doses from 750 to 1500 mg/day and/or ciprofloxacin 1000 mg/day are the main agents used for up to three–four months. Response rates may reach 80%, but long-term therapy is required to prevent exacerbation. Adverse events of metronidazole such as paresthesias, which may persist after drug discontinuation, nausea, glossitis, metallic taste, and a distal peripheral sensory neuropathy may limit its long-term use.

Antimetabolites

Antimetabolites such as azathioprine and 6-MP are widely used in the current clinical practice. A meta-analysis of controlled trials and uncontrolled case series showed that in the fistula healed after four months of therapy in 54% of patients and the fistula may be healed in most of the patients after nine months of treatment; however, recurrence is common after discontinuation in 95% of patients (30). Azathioprine at doses of 2 to 3 mg/kg/day and 6-MP at a dose of

1.5 mg/kg/day are effective for the treatment of perianal Crohn's disease; adverse reactions may include leukopenia, pancreatitis, drug-induced hepatitis, infection, and allergy.

Cyclosporine A

Uncontrolled case series have suggested that using intravenous cyclosporine at a dose of 4 mg/kg/day for seven days leads to an improvement in 83% of patients, but with high exacerbation rates after conversion to oral therapy (31). Severe side effects such as renal insufficiency, hypertension, infection, hepatotoxicity, paresthesias, and seizure are associated with cyclosporine, and its use is not routinely indicated for perianal Crohn's disease.

Infliximab

Infliximab is a mouse–human chimeric monoclonal antibody against tumor necrosis factor. Controlled trials have shown that infliximab at a dose of 5 mg/kg administered as a three dose induction regimen at zero, two, and six weeks is effective in at least a 50% decrease in purulent discharge of the fistula (8,32). Maintenance therapy with infliximab 5 mg/kg every eight weeks prolongs the time to loss of response, and is required in many patients for long-term symptom control (1). Adverse events of this therapy may include infusion reactions, drug-induced lupus, and infections such as pneumonia, tuberculosis, aspergillosis, histoplasmosis, and coccydioidomycosis. However, the treatment is generally well tolerated and effective, and is widely used in patients unresponsive to antibiotics and antimetabolites. The gradual development of antichimeric antibodies against infliximab frequently requires upscaling the dose, and may eventually lead to loss of the drug's effectiveness.

Tacrolimus

One small placebo-controlled trial showed that tacrolimus at a dose of 0.2 mg/kg/day for 10 weeks reduced the number of draining fistulas without complete closure (29). The major toxicity of this treatment was renal impairment. Thus, although currently not routinely used, tacrolimus may be a potential therapeutic agent in patients unresponsive to azathioprine, 6-MP, or infliximab (32).

Surgical Treatment

The surgical management of perianal Crohn's disease does not cure the disease, but offers effective palliation. Therefore, the goal of surgical treatment is to improve quality of life, based on careful patient selection, and is reserved for patients who develop perianal complications of the disease or are unresponsive to aggressive medical therapy. Crohn's disease tends to progress despite surgical therapy, and most patients will require at least one operation during their lifetime (33).

Surgical treatments of perianal Crohn's disease may be divided into two general categories: urgent and elective treatment. Urgent surgical care is mainly aimed at controlling perineal sepsis by adequate incision and drainage, while elective treatment addresses perianal fistulas and anal strictures. Similar to abdominal surgery for Crohn's disease, the perineal procedure should be effective enough to control sepsis or alleviate discomfort, while it should be somewhat limited and nonaggressive to avoid sphincter damage and preserve sphincter function. A larger surgery is not necessarily a better one, and as has been addressed by Sir Alexander-Williams in 1974, "Fecal incontinence is the result of aggressive surgeons and not progressive disease" (34).

Collaboration on surgical intervention with the gastroenterologist, radiologist, pathologist, nutritionist, and other specialists takes on particular importance in the success of therapy, especially when active proximal luminal disease exists. These patients are often immunocompromised, malnourished, and dehydrated. They often have diarrhea, which causes dehydration and electrolyte imbalances. One should address the patient's nutritional status and adrenocortical function prior to surgical intervention. Active proximal luminal inflammation should be appropriately treated with the goal of reducing stool liquidity that irritates the perianal area.

Urgent or Emergent Surgery

Urgent or emergent surgery for control of perineal sepsis and abscesses includes EUA for diagnosing the source of sepsis and drainage of simple or deep abscesses without fistulotomy of an associated fistula. Operative procedures may be performed under general, regional, or

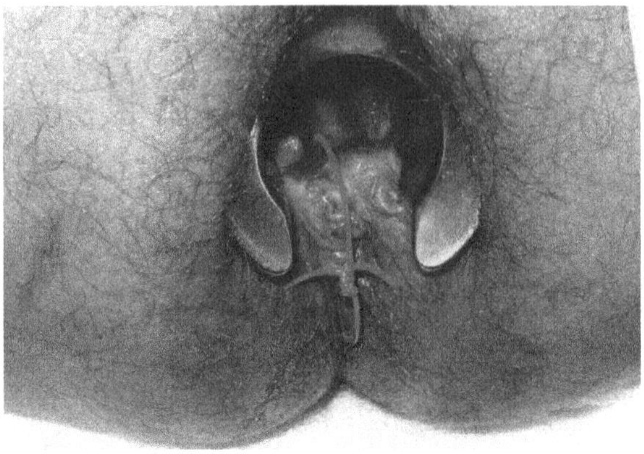

Figure 6 Noncutting seton.

local anesthesia with intravenous sedation as appropriate. For the drainage of perianal abscess, a small semicircular stab wound is made over the medial aspect of the overlying skin close to the anal verge. If a fistula cannot be identified, a 12- to 16-Fr mushroom catheter may be inserted into the abscess cavity. If a fistula tract is identified, a noncutting seton (nonabsorbable suture or vessel loop) is often placed through the fistula tract with the two ends tied loosely together (Fig. 6). The seton drain ensures continuous drainage leading to the resolution of the perianal sepsis.

Elective Surgery

Elective surgical treatment for perianal Crohn's disease may include procedures for nonfistulous complications such as dilatation of anorectal strictures and lateral sphincterotomy in selected patients with anal fissure. Most commonly, however, patients with perianal Crohn's disease will require surgical treatment in an attempt to repair perianal and rectovaginal fistulas that are unresponsive to medical therapy. This may include fistulotomy, fibrin glue injection, transanal endorectal flap advancement, and gracilis muscle interposition. Occasionally, temporary diverting colostomy or ileostomy is required to control symptoms. In severe cases resistant both to medical and surgical therapy, proctectomy or proctocolectomy may be required (35,36).

Nonfistulous Conditions

Typical Crohn's edematous and painful skin tags arise from a healed anal ulcer or fissure, and their excision is not recommended because of poor wound healing and the risk of perianal sepsis. Biopsy is recommended in cases where malignancy may be suspected (37). Soft and painless skin tags that cause hygiene problems can be safely excised.

Treatment of hemorrhoids in patients with Crohn's disease should be noninvasive. If symptomatic prolapse or bleeding hemorrhoids persist in the absence of active anorectal disease, rubber band ligation may be effective. Hemorrhoidectomy is usually not advised in these patients because of a high rate of nonhealing wounds, anal stenosis, and perianal septic complications.

Crohn's fissures are usually painless and heal spontaneously in more than 80% of the patients (15). Painful fissures should raise suspicion for intersphincteric abscess, and should lead to prompt EUA with drainage of abscess, if found. In most cases, internal sphincterotomy may be performed to allow adequate drainage without jeopardizing continence. If painful fissure persists without local abscess on EUA, medical management and observation are preferred. Invasive procedures such as botulinium toxin injection or lateral internal sphincterotomy should be reserved for patients with fissures resulting from diarrhea owing to bowel disease, without perianal activity and who have failed all conservative treatments.

Anorectal strictures may arise as a result of chronic inflammation, abscesses, fistulas, anal ulcers, and multiple anorectal surgical procedures (38). Asymptomatic strictures do not require surgery. Symptomatic anorectal strictures with difficult defecation or tenesmus may be treated with single or repeated digital dilatations, usually after medical therapy of active proctocolitis. In persistent severe cases, fecal diversion or proctectomy may be appropriate.

The possibility of cancer should always be considered in chronic nonhealing fistulas, ulcers, fissures, diverted rectums, and areas of chronic perianal inflammation. In these cases,

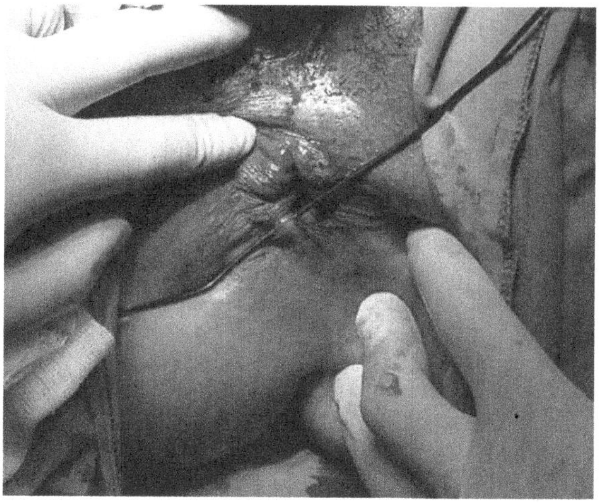

Figure 7 Lay open fistulotomy of a superficial fistula.

biopsies should be promptly obtained and, if positive, standard oncologic principles should be applied.

Treatment of Fistulas

Treatment of fistulas in patients with perianal Crohn's disease is challenging because of poor wound healing and the risk of secondary incontinence. Selection of the most appropriate surgical approach depends largely on the type of fistula, past attempts at repair, severity of symptoms, and current continence status.

Limited Fistulotomy

A limited fistulotomy can be safely performed for simple (low) fistulas not including any significant portion of the external anal sphincter, without active proctitis with well-controlled proximal luminal disease, and in patients with adequate continence. The fistula tract should be identified, probed throughout its length, and intraoperatively assessed prior to the decision to proceed with fistulotomy. The internal opening may be identified using a probe inserted through the external opening. When unsuccessful, injection of hydrogen peroxide through the external opening with visualization of "bubbles" in the anus and rectum may be helpful (39). Retrograde probing from the suspected crypt at the dentate line toward the external opening may occasionally facilitate passage of the probe. Following adequate assessment, the fistula is laid open using electrocautery, and the fistula tract is curetted (Fig. 7).

Rectovaginal fistulas in patients with perianal Crohn's disease should not be treated with fistulotomy, even with low fistulas, due to the risk of fecal incontinence. In women, the anterior portion of the anal sphincter mechanism is shorter and weaker than the posterior aspect as there is no puborectalis muscle at the anterior anal sphincter, and therefore division of the sphincter mechanism in these cases may lead to a significant impairment in continence (40).

Complex (high) fistulas require nonaggressive surgical procedures to avoid destruction of the sphincter mechanism. A noncutting seton is most commonly used which provides drainage of the fistula tract and reduces formation of perianal abscesses (41,42). The seton drain may be left in place for a long duration until the inflammation is quiescent. Premature removal of the seton increases the incidence of recurrent perianal sepsis.

Endorectal Advancement Flap

Endorectal advancement flap (EAF) is a surgical technique aimed at repairing perineal fistulas with preservation of the anal sphincter function. This procedure can be performed only when no active proctitis is evident, and may be especially helpful in the anterior location and in rectovaginal fistulas in women (43,44). The patient is placed in the prone jackknife or lithotomy position, depending on the fistula location and the surgeon's preference. The anal canal and fistula tract are examined using an operative anoscope. A broad-based, U-shaped incision is made using cautery, and a flap of lower rectum including mucosa, submucosa, and a superficial part of the muscular layer is raised (45). Several surgeons inject saline or local anesthetic solution

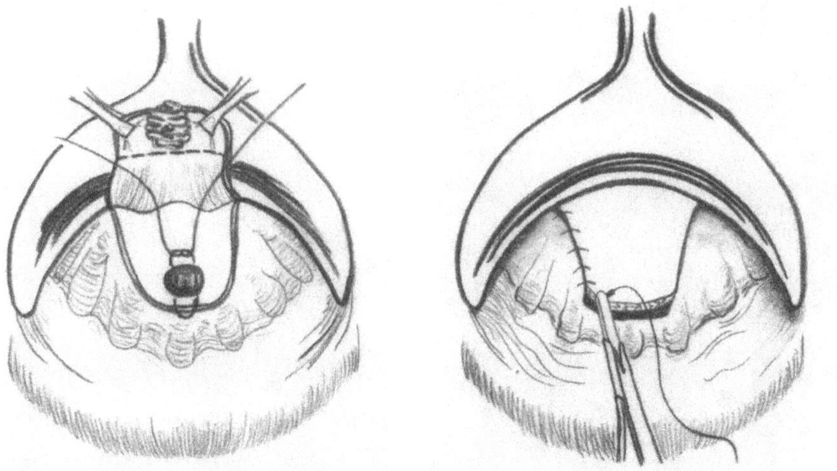

(A) (B)

Figure 8 Endorectal advancement flap.

with or without adrenaline to provide easier dissection and better hemostasis. The base of the flap should be approximately 3 cm cephaled to the internal opening and twice as wide as the apex, to ensure adequate blood supply. Following mobilization, the internal opening under the flap is closed using 3–0 Vicryl or PDS sutures, and the apex, which includes the mucosal defect, is excised. The flap is pulled down to cover the internal opening, and sutured in place using interrupted absorbable sutures. The external tract is curetted and enlarged for adequate drainage (Fig. 8). A mushroom-tip catheter may be useful to ensure drainage until complete healing of the internal opening is evident.

The reported success rate of EAF in patients with Crohn's perianal fistulas ranges between 25% and 100%, while the success using EAF for rectovaginal fistulas ranges from 50% to 100% (8,43,46–48).

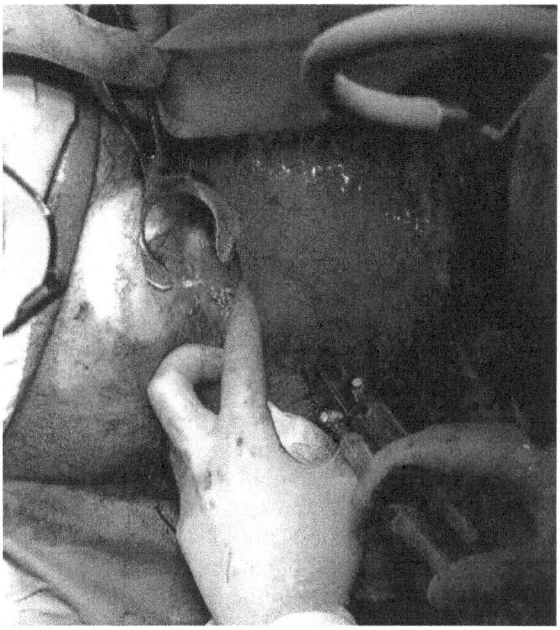

Figure 9 Instillation of fibrin glue.

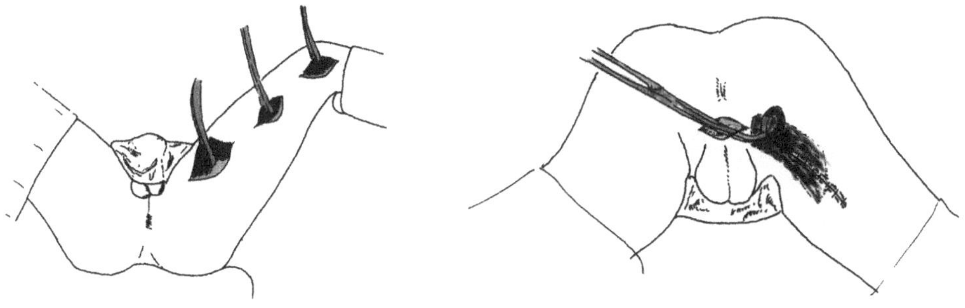

(A) (B)

Figure 10 Gracilis muscle transposition: (**A**) thigh incisions and (**B**) perianal incision and muscle transposition. *Source*: From Zmora O et al. Gracilis muscle transposition for iatrogenic rectourethral fistulas. Ann Surg 2003; 237(4):483–487.

Fibrin Glue

Installation of fibrin glue is a technically simple procedure for the treatment of perianal fistulas, associated with low risk and early return to normal activity. Fibrin glue is a blood product which uses the activation of thrombin to form a fibrin clot, mechanically sealing the fistula tract. The clot promotes tissue healing processes while being gradually absorbed by fibrinolysis.

The fistula tract is probed throughout its length and then cleasned using a fine Volkmann's currete or brushed with a pipe cleaner. A flexible catheter tip attached to a double armed syringe is inserted through the external opening and advanced toward the internal opening. The glue is injected while slowly withdrawing the catheter, until glue is seen sealing both openings (Fig. 9).

Published series with the use of fibrin glue for perianal fistulas of mixed etiologies suggest success rates of approximately 30% to 70%. There are currently no series addressing the use of the glue specifically for perianal Crohn's disease, but subgroup analysis of series with mixed types of fistulas suggest that the cause of fistula does not significantly affect success rate (49).

Fistula Plug

The anal fistula plug may also be used to treat perianal fistulas associated with Crohn's disease. The clear advantage in using this technique is that it is simple to perform and avoids cutting of sphincter muscle. The early studies of the Surgisis (Cook Surgical) anal fistula plug invented by Armstrong reported an overall success rate of 82% (50). However, he excluded patients with Crohn's disease. He later reported on 20 consecutive patients with perianal Crohn's disease who underwent anal fistula plug placement. A total of 36 fistula tracts were identified in those 20 patients. At his final follow up, he noted that all fistula tracts were closed in 16 of the 20 patients for an overall success rate of 80%. In total, 30/36 (83%) of the individual fistula tracts were closed at follow up. Armstrong notes best success in patients with one fistula tract initially (51). Other studies have shown success using the anal fistula plug in patients with Crohn's disease with an overall success rate of 85% reported by Schwandner et al. (52).

Gracilis Muscle Transposition

Gracilis muscle transposition is a major procedure used for the repair of perineal fistulas in patients with severe symptoms who have failed simpler procedures, and is especially helpful in the treatment of persistent rectovaginal and rectourethral fistulas. The gracilis muscle at the medial aspect of the thigh is detached from its attachments near the knee, and dissected free through three small thigh incisions (Fig. 10). Care should be taken to protect the neurovascular bundle supplying the muscle near its origin. The plain between the rectum and the vagina is then dissected to divide the fistula tract, and the rectal opening is repaired. The gracilis muscle is rotated and sutured to interpose between the rectum and the vagina. The success rate with the use of this procedure for Crohn's rectal vagina fistulas is approximately 70% (53).

Ileostomy and Colostomy (Temporary Diversion)

Extensive perianal fistulas associated with active proctitis, severe recurrent perirectal sepsis or rectovaginal fistulas, in which perineal procedures are unsuccessful, may require creation of a temporary diverting ileostomy or colostomy. Fecal diversion alleviates the symptoms associated with the perianal disease. Diversion may also allow healing and closure of perineal fistulas, and avoids the risk of persistent nonhealing perineal wounds frequently associated with proctectomy (6,54). However, in selected patients with severe uncontrolled perineal sepsis and active proctitis despite aggressive medical and surgical treatment, proctectomy may ultimately be required to improve quality of life.

REFERENCES

1. Podolsky DK. Inflammatory bowel disease. N Engl J Med 2002; 347:417–429.
2. Knutson D, Greenberg G, Cronau H. Management of Crohn's disease-a practical approach. Am Fam Physician 2003; 68:707–714.
3. Loftus EV, Sandborn WJ. Epidemiology of inflammatory bowel disease. Gastroenterol Clin N Am 2002; 31:1–20.
4. Yamada T, Alpers DH, et al., eds. Inflammatory bowel disease. Textbook of Gastroenterology. 3d ed. Philadelphia: Lippincott Williams & Wilkins, 1999: 1776–1778.
5. Rankin GB, Watts D, Melnyk CS, et al. National Cooperative Crohn's Disease Study: extraintestinal manifestations and perianal complications. Gastroenterology 1979; 77:914–920.
6. McClane SJ, Rombeau JL. Anorectal Crohn's disease. Surg Clin North Am 2001; 81:169–183.
7. Metcalf AM. Anal fissure. Surg Clin North Am 2002; 82:1291–1297.
8. Sandborn WJ, Fazio VW, Feagan BG, et al. AGA technical review on perianal Crohn's disease. Gastroenterology 2003; 125:1508–1530.
9. Allan A, Keighley MR. Management of perianal Crohn's disease. World J Surg 1988; 12:198.
10. Fuhrman GM, Larach SW. Experience with perirectal fistulas in patients with Crohn's disease. Dis Colon Rectum 1989; 32:847.
11. Parks AG, Gordon PH, Hardcastle JD. A classification of fistula-in-ano. Br J Surg 1976; 63:1–12.
12. Hull T, Fazio VW. Rectovaginal fistula in Crohn's disease. In: Phillips RK, Lunniss PJ, eds. Anal Fistula: Surgical Evaluation and Management. London: Chapman and Hall, 1996:143.
13. Felt-Bersma R, Poen AC, Cuesta MA, et al. Anal lesions and anorectal function in perianal Crohn's disease. Gastroenterology 1999; 116:714.
14. Buchman AL, Ament ME, Doty J. Development of squamous cell carcinoma in chronic perineal sinus and wounds in Crohn's disease. Am J Gastroenterol 1991; 86:1829.
15. Tio TL, Mulder CJ, Wijers OB, et al. Endosonography of peri-anal and peri-colorectal fistula and/or abscess in Crohn's disease. Gastro Endosc 1990; 36:331–336.
16. Schratter-Sehn AU, Lochs H, Vogelsang H, et al. Endoscopic ultrasonography versuscomputed tomography in the differential diagnosis of perianorectal complications in Crohn's disease. Endoscopy 1993; 25:582–586.
17. Berliner L, Redmond P, Purow E, et al. Computed tomography in Crohn's disease. Am J Gastroenterol 1982; 77:548–553.
18. Orsoni P, Barthet M, Portier F, et al. Prospective comparison of endosonography, magnetic resonance imaging and surgical findings in anorectal fistula and abscess complicating Crohn's disease. Br J Surg 1999; 86:360–364.
19. Sloots CE, Felt-Bersma RJ, Poen AC, et al. Assessment and classification of fistula-in-ano in patients with Crohn's disease by hydrogen peroxide enhanced transanal ultrasound. Int J Colorectal Dis 2001; 16:292–297.
20. Kkeinubing H Jr, Jannini JF, Malafaia O, et al. Transperineal ultrasonography: new method to image the anorectal region. Dis Colon Rectum 2000; 43:1572–1574.
21. Rubens DJ, Strang JG, Bogineni-Misra S, et al. Transperineal sonography of the rectum: anatomy and pathology revealed by sonography compared with CT and MR imaging. AJR AM J Roentgenol 1998; 170:637–642.
22. Kuijpers HC, Schulpen T. Fistulography for fistula-in-ano. Is it useful? Dis Colon Rectum 1985; 28:103–104.
23. Weisman RI, Orsay CP, Pearl RK, et al. The role of fistulography in fistula-in-ano. Dis Colon Rectum 1991; 34:181–184.
24. Zbar AP, Kmiot WA. Anorectal investigation. In: Phillips RKS, ed. Colorectal surgery: a companion to specialist surgical practice. London: WB Saunders, 1998:1–32.
25. Zbar AP. Magnetic resonance imaging and the coloproctologist. Tech Coloproctol 2001; 5:1–7.
26. Schwartz DA, Wiersema MJ, Dudiak KM, et al. A comparison of endoscopic ultrasound, magnetic resonance imaging, and exam under anesthesia for evaluation of Crohn's perianal fistulas. Gastroenterology 2001; 121:1064–1072.
27. Heuman R, Bolin T, Sjodahl R, et al. The incidence and course of perianal complications and arthralgia after intestinal resection with restoration of continuity for Crohn's disease. Br J Surg 1981; 68:528.

28. Orkin BA, Telander RL. The effect of intra-abdominal resection or fecal diversion on perianal Crohn's disease in pediatric Crohn's disease. J Pediatr Surg 1985; 20:343.
29. Stein RB, Lichtenstein GR. Medical therapy for Crohn's disease. Surg Clin North Am 2001; 81:71–101.
30. Pearson DC, May GR, Fick GH, et al. Azathioprine and 6-mercaptopurine in Crohn's disease. A meta-analysis. Ann Intern Med 1995; 123:132–142.
31. Gurundu SR, Griffel LH, Gialanella RJ, et al. Cyclosporine therapy in inflammatory bowel disease: short-term and long-term results. J Clin Gastroenterol 1999; 29:151–154.
32. Egan LJ, Sandborn WJ. Advances in the treatment of Crohn's disease. Gastroenterology 2004; 126:1574–1581.
33. Shorb PE. Surgical therapy for Crohn's disease. Gastroenterol Clin North Am 1989; 18:111–128.
34. Alexander-Williams J. Fistulae-in-ano: management of Crohn's fistula. Dis Colon Rectum 1976; 19:518.
35. Nelson R. Anorectal abscess fistula: what do we know? Surg Clin North Am 2002; 82:1139–1151.
36. Schwartz DA, Pemberton JH, Sandborn WJ. Diagnosis and treatment of perianal fistulas in Crohn disease. Ann Intern Med 2001; 135:906–918.
37. Keighley MR, Allan RN. Current status and influence of operation on perianal Crohn's disease. Int J Colorectal Dis 1986; 1:104–107.
38. Linares L, Moreira LF, Andrews H, et al. Natural history and treatment of anorectal strictures complicating Crohn's disease. Br J Surg 1988; 75:653.
39. Rosen L. Anorectal abscess-fistulae. Surg Clin North Am 1994; 74:1293—1308.
40. Saclarides TJ. Rectovaginal fistula. Surg Clin North Am 2002; 82:1261–1272.
41. Larson DW, Pemberton JH. Current concepts and controversies in surgery for IBD. Gastroenterology 2004; 126:1611–1619.
42. Williams JG, MacLeod CA, Rothenberger DA, et al. Seton treatment of high anal fistulae. Br J Surg 1991; 78:1159–1161.
43. American Gastroenterological Association Medical Position Statement: perianal Crohn's disease. Gastroenterology 2003; 125:1503–1507.
44. Kodner IJ, Mazor A, Shemesh EI, et al. Endorectal advancement flap repair of rectovaginal and other complicated anorectal fistulas. Surgery 1993; 114:682–690.
45. Joo JS, Weiss EG, Nogueras JJ, et al. Endorectal advancement flap in perianal Crohn's disease. Am Surg 1998; 64:147–150.
46. O'Leary DP, Durdey P, Milroy CE. Definitive repair of anovaginal fistula in Crohn's disease. Ann R Coll Surg Engl 1998; 80:250.
47. Fry RD, Kodner IJ. Management of anal and perineal Crohn's disease. Infect Surg 1989; 8:209.
48. Hull TL, Fazio VW. Surgical approaches to low anovaginal fistula in Crohn's disease. Am J Surg 1977; 173:95.
49. Zmora O, Mizrahi N, Rotholtz N, et al. Fibrin glue sealing in the treatment of perineal fistulas. Dis Colon Rectum 2003; 46(5):584–589.
50. Johnson EK, Gaw JU, Armstrong DN. Efficacy of anal fistula plug vs. fibrin glue in closure of anorectal fistulas. Dis Colon Rectum 2006; 49(3):371–376.
51. Champagne BJ, O'Connor LM, Ferguson M, et al. Efficacy of anal fistula plug in closure of cryptoglandular fistulas: long-term follow-up. Dis Colon Rectum 2006; 49(12):1817–1821.
52. Schwandner O, Stadler F, Dietl O, et al. Initial experience on efficacy in closure of cryptoglandular and Crohn's transsphincteric fistulas by the use of the anal fistula plug. Int J Colorectal Dis 2008; 23(3):319–324.
53. Rius J, Nessim A, Nogueras JJ, et al. Gracilis transposition in complicated perianal fistula and unhealed perineal wounds in Crohn's disease. Eur J Surg 2000; 166(3):218–222.
54. Schraut WH. The surgical management of Crohn's disease. Gastroenterol Clin N Am 2002; 31:255–263.
55. Present DH, Rutgeerts P, Targan S, et al. Infliximab for the treatment of fistulas in patients with Crohn's disease. N Engl J Med 1999; 340:1398–1405.

19 Pruritis Ani

Eliad Karin and Shmuel Avital
Department of Surgery A, Sourasky Medical Center, Tel Aviv, Israel

INTRODUCTION

Pruritus ani is a common condition afflicting up to 5% of the population and characterized by an unpleasant, severely irritating, and sometimes burning sensation of the perianal region (1). In the majority of patients, pruritis ani is a primary (idiopathic) condition with no apparent pathological cause. The idiopathic condition varies in its incidence from 25% to 95%, according to different series (2,3). Conversely, secondary pruritis ani may result from a large number of medical disorders including dermatological, proctological, and systemic diseases.

In secondary pruritus ani, a specific medical disorder is generally responsible for causing the perianal irritation. This may be a specific skin process, local infection, anal soiling from anorectal diseases such as fistulas or fissures, or a systemic disease affecting the perianal area. Assessing and treating the specific medical disorder will frequently solve a secondary pruritis ani. In idiopatic pruritus ani, the causative mechanism is unclear. There are two major contributing factors that may initiate or aggravate this process: perianal wetness and patients' excess fixation and attention to the perianal region.

Irritation of the perianal area is mediated by sensory nerve endings of unmyelinated C-fibers. There are some peripheral mediators that also play a role in the mediation of this sensation including histamine, serotonin, prostaglandins, endogenous opioids, and neuropeptides (4). Histamine, which is the main mediator, has been shown to activate central motor areas which are linked to the action of scratching, thereby supporting the observed itch–scratch–itch behavior that may aggravate any pruritus condition regardless of its etiology (5).

PRIMARY (IDIOPATHIC) PRURITIS ANI

Any condition that creates moisture in the perianal area may lead to primary pruritus ani. Common factors may include loose stools, fecal seepage, and the use of local creams. Most often, an initial sensation of pruritus becomes exacerbated by excess attention to the this area with vigorous perianal hygiene using irritating soaps, creams, or ointments that leads to repeated scratching with further damage and maceration of the skin and increased local inflammation and symptoms (6).

Patients with idiopathic pruritus ani have abnormal transient internal sphincter relaxation and an abnormally profound decrease in the anal canal pressure during rectal distention, as well as early incontinence on saline continence tests, implying that intermittent seepage from the anal canal may be a causative factor (7–10). A decrease in resting anal canal pressure with coffee (caffeine) intake has also been reported, which may explain the documented exacerbation of symptoms after ingestion of caffeine (11). Other food types associated with pruritus ani include spices, citrus fruits, tea, chocolate, and tomatoes (7,8).

Fecal contamination may also play a role in the development of perianal pruritus. Feces containing some potential allergens, bacteria, and endopeptidases of bacterial origin can cause itching and inflammation (12–14). In addition, there is some evidence to support an association between pruritus ani of long duration and the presence of anal, rectal, or colon cancer, although the causative relation is not well understood (15).

SECONDARY PRURITIS ANI

Pruritis ani may be secondary to dermatological disorders that may afflict this area. Contact dermatitis can be caused by applied "therapies" such as topical anesthetics, lanolin, Neosporin, or even overuse of topical steroids. Other conditions such as psoriasis, lichen planus, seborrhea, and hormonal deficiency in menopausal women are rather uncommon, but are specific causes of pruritus ani (6).

Infection with pinworms (*Enterobius Vermicularis*) is the most common cause of pruritis ani in children, and is characterized by intense nocturnal itching caused by migration of the worms to the anus to lay their eggs, during the night. Diagnosis is made by identification of the pinworms' eggs under a microscope from a swab taken from a cellophane tape that was attached to the child's perianal skin in the early morning. Other anal warts and dermatoses such as lichen sclerosis or atrophicus will also cause perianal irritation.

Lichen sclerosus is a lymphocyte mediated inflammatory condition, which has a predilection for the anogenital epithelium. The etiology is unknown, although there is a definite association with autoimmune disorders. The majority of cases occur in adults, usually postmenopausal women. In addition, a significant number of prepubertal children develop lichen sclerosus. Management is mainly medical, using ultra-potent topical corticosteroid. There is no indication for surgical excision of lichen sclerosus unless malignancy, intraepithelial neoplasia, or problematic scarring has developed. In fact, lichen sclerosus is a disease process that has the potential for scarring and surgery may actually exacerbate the disorder and cause additional scaring. However, surgery is indicated for some of the postinflammatory sequelae or if squamous cell carcinoma develops, although this is rare (16).

Lichen simplex chronicus or idiopathic essential pruritus is a chronic pruritc condition of unknown etiology. There are generally no signs of skin disease apart from lichenification and excoriation; the skin markings are increased and the skin is mildly scaly and leathery. Lichen simplex chronicus encompasses the term "chronic pruritus ani" (17). In older patients, pruritis may be a presenting symptom for anal tumors including Bowen's and Paget's disease (which are tumors in situ) and invasive anal cancer (6).

Common proctological disorders such as fissures, fistulas, and prolapsed rectal mucosa or hemorrhoids may cause pruritus, as well as systemic medical disorders such as diabetes. Secondary causes of pruritis ani are listed in Table 1 and are classified into dermatologic, proctologic, and systemic causes.

EVALUATION

An important part of the evaluation for prurits ani is a diagnostic workup, in order to differentiate primary from secondary pruritis. Evaluation is carried out with a detailed history, physical examination, and laboratory and imaging studies, as necessary.

Specific aspects that should be addressed in history taking are the time of onset of symptoms and their duration, stool consistency and association of symptoms with bowel movements, stool leakage, sensation of seepage or moisture around the anus, scratching of the perianal area, and any overuse of soaps or other cleansing agents in this area.

Physical examination should include a thorough examination of the peri-anal skin, a digital rectal examination with emphasis on anal sphincter tone, palpation of polyps or tumors, anoscopy, and rectoscopy. Based on the patient's history and age, a colonoscopy for investigation of inflammatory bowel disease or colorectal polyps and carcinomas may be warranted.

Evaluating patients based on acute versus chronic symptoms is very helpful. Acute anal pruritis is often secondary to acute dermatological or anorectal disorders. Considering the dermatological etiologies, one should examine the perianal skin for signs of bright red erythema, weeping, and significant skin irritation, which are signs of acute eczematous dermatitis or allergic contact dermatitis, inflammatory plaques or folliculitis, satellite lesions of extensive candidiasis, and signs of borrows and scabetic nodules as part of scabies infestation. In children or young adults, pinworms might be diagnosed during the examination, explaining the anal irritation as well as perianal cellulites due to beta-hemolytic infection. Erosions and vesicles caused by herpes simplex virus and condyloma accuminatum from human papilloma virus are also occasionally noted.

In addition, anorectal disorders such as anal fissure, perianal fistula, external thrombosed hemorrhoids, prolapsed internal hemorrhoids, and findings consistent with fecal soiling on the perianal skin or underwear should be evaluated in searching for etiology.

Table 1 Etiologic Factors in Anal Pruritis

1. Idiopathic anal pruritis
2. Secondary anal puruitis
   a. Dermatologic causes
      1. Psoriasis
      2. Contact dermatitis
      3. Lichen planus
      4. Lichen sclerosus
      5. Seborrhea
      6. Post menopausal
      7. Fungal or bacterial infections–candida, dermatophyte, group A and group B streptococcus and staphylococcus aureus.
      8. Scabies
      9. Herpes simplex
      10. Hidradenitis
      11. Paget's disease
      12. Bowen's disease
   b. Proctologic conditions
      1. Anal fissure
      2. Fistula in ano
      3. Rectal mucosal prolapse and prolapsed hemorrhoids
      4. fecal incontinence
      5. condyloma
      6. Inflammatory bowel disease
      7. Proctitis
      8. Cloacogenic carcinoma
      9. Villous adenoma of rectum
      10. Pinworms–Enterobius vermicularis
   c. Systemic disorders
      1. Diabetes mellitus
      2. Lymphoma
      3. uremia
      4. Psychogenic factors.

Chronic anal pruritis is often less explosive and has a history of gradual onset. Once the potential causes of acute anal pruritis are considered and either treated or discarded, the quest for chronic etiology begins. These may include the papulosquamous disorders, primary inflammatory disorders of the anoderm or anal canal, malignancies, mechanical causes, and psychogenic factors. Papulosquamous disorders such as seborrheic dermatitis, psoriasis, and atopic dermatitis rarely present with perianal lesions alone.

The perianal area is a common site for the inflammatory dermatoses lichen sclerosus and lichen planus. The fragile atrophic skin secondary to lichen sclerosus is easily irritated and can be pruritic.

Malignancies of the perianal area are often slow growing and can cause low-grade pruritis. Bowen's disease (anal squamous cell carcinoma in situ) and Paget's disease (anal adenocarcinoma in situ) may mimic dermatitis with erythematous plaques and variable scaling. Any apparent dermatoses not responding to treatment should be further investigated by biopsy.

There is often no evidence of discrete pathology, and the appearance of the perianal skin may vary. Examination may reveal either normal skin or lichenification and excoriation. These findings may be classified using the Washington Hospital Center criteria (18) as:

Stage 1—skin is erythematous and inflamed; Stage 2—white lichenified skin; Stage 3—lichenified skin with coarse ridges of skin and ulceration. In these cases, the pruritis is considered idiopathic, and treatment should be aimed at alleviation of symptoms.

TREATMENT

Potential causative disorders of pruritis ani found following the initial evaluation should be appropriately treated and then followed up for resolution of symptoms. Any suspicious skin or anal canal lesions should be biopsied. Following treatment and resolution of the potential causes, patients with idiopathic pruritis ani or nonresolving pruritis should be counseled regarding appropriate anal hygiene and reassured that this is a benign condition.

The patient is often unwittingly creating or worsening the problem, since most patients with anal discomfort tend to overclean the perianal region with harsh soaps and frequent scrubbing. In many cases, all that is required is to treat the underlying conditions causing the anorectal discomfort, and break the vicious cycle.

The initial recommended treatment algorithm is to identify and resolve any underlying conditions such as hemorrhoids, fissures, or dermatologic conditions, as well as regulating bowel habits with a high fiber diet, fiber supplements, and increase in fluid intake. Patients should be instructed to maintain perianal hygiene by gently washing and completely drying the perianal area after defecation. In addition, soaps, medicated wipes, or ointments and creams that may irritate the perianal area should be discontinued. An additional measure to help absorb moisture is to dust cornstarch on the perianal area to keep it dry and clean (6). Hydrocortisone cream (1%) can be applied sparingly two to three times daily for a short period of time (7–14 days), and it may be effective for nonfungal types of pruritis ani. However, the role of local steroids in pruritis ani is limited. In a study by Oztas et al. (19), there were no differences noted between treatments with local steroids versus the use of perianal cleanser in patients with pruritis ani; both were found to be equally effective in approximately 90% of patients. Treatment for long periods with local steroids should be avoided since they can cause atrophy, bacterial and fungal infections, allergic contact dermatitis, telangiectasia, purpura, and scar formation (19).

Antihistamines (17) are sometimes indicated; however, their use is empiric since there are no controlled studies for treatment of pruritis ani.

The initial treatment approach described above is beneficial for the majority of patients with pruritis ani. However, in some cases, refractory to this first-line care, further treatment is required. Intractable idiopathic pruritis ani may become a socially embarrassing condition for the patient and a therapeutic challenge for the physician. Although the proportion of these intractable cases is relatively small, the actual numbers may be considerable owing to the high incidence of anal pruritis (8,15). Diverse treatment modalities have been proposed for this resistant form of pruritis ani, including intradermal alcohol injection, ultraviolet phototherapy, cryotherapy, radiotherapy, or even surgical therapy to denervate or remove the affected skin (16,17). Unfortunately, none of these often invasive and expensive approaches has gained widespread acceptance.

Available treatments options that are easy to administer and that have been deemed beneficial include:

Topical Capasaicin

Capasaicin is a natural alkaloid derived from plants of the Solanaceae family. Topical capasaicin is known to be safe and effective to alleviate the pain and itching. Evidence suggests that capasaicin exercises an active depressant effect in the synthesis, storage, transport, and release of substance P. Capasaicin probably elicits its effect on C fiber sensory affert neurons which contain substance P by activating capasaicin (vanilooid) receptor. Capasaicin functions to activate and then, at higher doses and longer times, desensitize this class of neurons.

In a randomized double blind placebo-controlled study on the treatment of idiopathic pruritis ani with capasaicin cream (0.006%) applied to the anal area three times daily for four weeks, capasaicin was found to be effective in 70% of patients who experienced relief during treatment. The beneficial effect of capasaicin was immediate or within three days in most patients. Side effects included local burning sensation and one patient developed urticaria. Long-term follow up (10–20 months) revealed that most patients remained more or less asymptomatic on a regimen of a once-daily application of capasaicin; some patients were completely asymptomatic and did not require further treatment (20).

Intradermal Methylene Blue Injection

Eusebio and coworkers (21) first described the method of intradermal methylene blue injection for pruritis in 1990. Subsequently, in 1997 Farouk and Lee (22) reported six patients who were treated with this method. In 2004, Mentes et al. (23) reported the results of 30 patients with

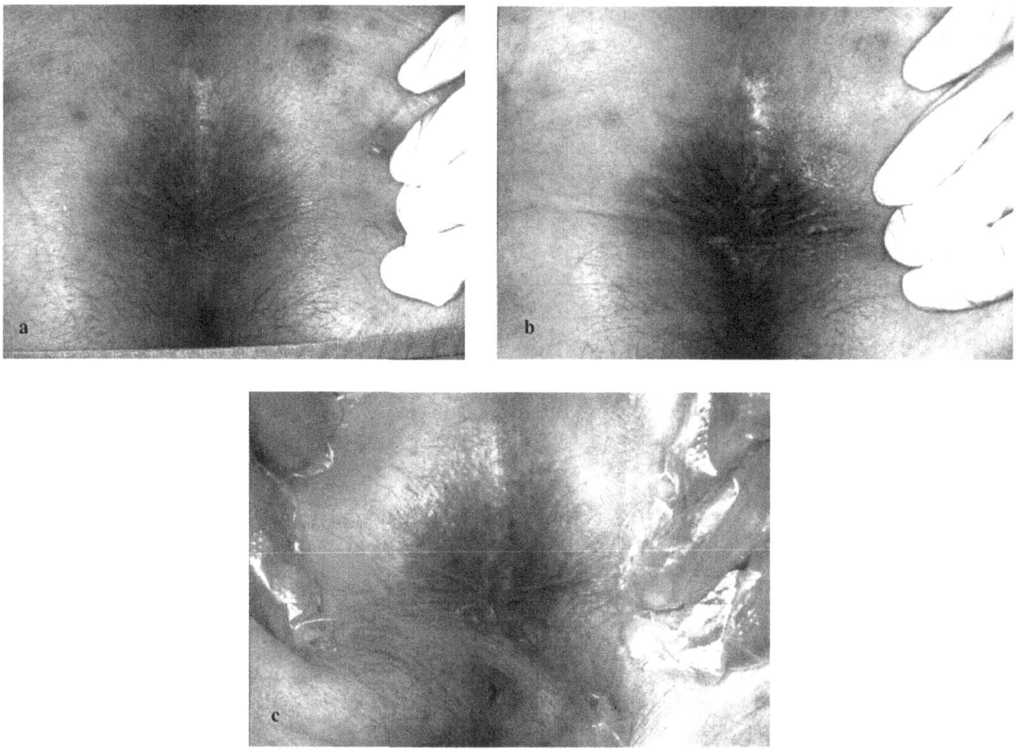

Figure 1 Iidiopathic intractable pruritus ani. a: Typical skin breakdown, maceration, and lichenification. b: Appearance immediately after methylene blue injection. c: Symptomatic healing following methylene blue injection was generally accompanied by disappearance of perianal excoriation and lichenification. *Source: From Ref. 23.*

intractable pruritis ani treated by intradermal methylene blue and concluded that this is a fast, safe, easy, and efficient method of treating intractable idiopathic pruritis ani (Fig. 1).

Methylene blue probably acts by ablation of the sensory nerve endings in the perianal skin, which appears to reduce the sensation of itch, resulting in a decreased desire to scratch. This then allows disruption of the vicious cycle of itch–scratch into which these patients inevitably become trapped.

In a study by Botterill and Sagar (24), patients with chronic idiopathic intractable pruritis ani were treated by intradermal injection of a 20 mL mixture containing 15 mL of 1% lidocaine, 5 mL of methylene blue, as well as 100 mg of hydrocortisone. As a result, 64% of patients were symptom free after the first injection, while 72% became asymptomatic after the second injection. The overall success rate was 88%. There were no cases of permanent discoloration. One potential transient side effect is mild fecal seepage (4%), but this resolved after two days (24).

SUMMARY

Pruritis ani is a common proctological condition and should be evaluated initially with history taking and physical examination. It is helpful to categories pruritus ani as acute or chronic, and it is most important to differentiate between primary and secondary pruritis ani. Primary idiopathic pruritis ani will usually respond to local measures that will keep the perianal area dry, although some of the cases may be intractable and those patients should be treated with special measures discussed in this chapter.

REFERENCES

1. Mazier WP. Hemorrhoids fissures and pruritus ani. Surg Clin North Am 1994; 74:1277–1292.
2. Bernardi RS, Chen HP. Perianal extramammary Paget's disease. Surg Gynecol Obstet 1988; 167:359.
3. Wexner SD, Daily TH. Pruritus Ani: Diagnosis and management. Curr Concepts Skin Dis 1986; 7:5–9.

4. Etter L, Myers SA. Pruritus in systemic disease: Mechanism and management. Dermatol Clin 2002; 20:249–272.
5. Hasieh J, Hagermark O, Stable-Backdahl M, et al. Urge to scratch represented in the human cerebral cortex during itch. J Neurophys 1994; 72:3004–3008.
6. Billingham RP, Isler JT, Kimmins MH, et al. The diagnosis and management of common anorectal disorders. Curr Probl Surg 2004; 41(7):586–645.
7. Braun Falco O, Plewig G, Wolff HH, et al. Dermatologic proctology. In: Braun Falco O, Plewig G, Wolf HH, et al, eds. Dermatology. 2nd ed. Berlin: Springer, 2000:1693–1700.
8. Aucoin EJ. Pruritus ani. Postgrad Med 1987; 82:76–80.
9. Farouk R, Duthie GS, Pryde A, et al. Abnormal transient internal sphincter relaxation in idiopathic pruritus ani: Physiologic evidence from ambulatory monitoring. Br J Surg 1994; 81:603–606.
10. Allan A, Ambrose NS, Silverman S, et al. Physiological study of pruritus ani. Br J Surg 1987; 74:576–579.
11. Smith LE, Henrichs D, McCullah RD. Prospective studies on the etiology and treatment of pruritus ani. Dis Colon Rectum 1982; 25:358–363.
12. Ive FA. The umbilical, perianal and genital regions. In: Champion RH, Burtan JL, Burns DA, et al., eds. Textbook of Dermatology. 6th ed. Oxford: Blackwell Science, 1998:3163–3238.
13. Kocsard E. Pruritus ani. A symptom of fecal contamination. Cutis 1981; 27:518.
14. Silverman SH, Youngs DJ, Allan A, et al. The fecal microflora in pruritus ani. Dis Colon Rectum 1989; 32:466–468.
15. Daniel GI, Longo WE, Vernava AM. Pruritus ani: Causes and concerns. Dis Colon Rectum 1994; 37:670–674.
16. Neill SM, Ridley CM. Management of anogenital lichen sclerosus. Clin Exper Dermatol 2001; 26:637–643.
17. Weichert GE. An approach to the treatment of anogenital pruritus. Dermatol Ther 2004; 17:129–133.
18. Smith LE. Perianal dermatologic disease. In: Gordon P, Nivatvongs S, eds. Principles and Practice of Surgery for the Colon, Rectum and Anus. St. Louis: Quality Medical Publishing, 999:303–21.
19. Oztas MO, Oztas P, Onder M. Idiopathic perianal pruritus: Washing compared with topical corticosteroids. Postgrad Med J 2004; 80:295–297.
20. Lysly J, Sistiery-Ittah M, Israelit Y, et al. Topical capasaicin—a novel and effective treatment for idiopathic intractable pruritus ani: A randomized, placebo controlled, crossover study. Gut 2003; 52:1323–1326.
21. Eusebio EB, Graham J, Mody N. Treatment of intractable pruritus ani. Dis Colon Rectum 1990; 33:770–772.
22. Farouk R, Lee PWR. Intradermal methylene blue injection for the treatment of intractable idiopathic pruritus ani. Br J Surg 1997; 84:670.
23. Mentes BB, Akin M, Leventoglu S, et al. Intradermal methylene blue injection for the treatment of intractable idiopathic pruritus ani: Results of 30 cases. Technique Coloproctol 2004 8(1):11–14.
24. Sagar PM, Botterill ID. Intradermal methylene blue, hydrocortisone and lidocaine for chronic intractable pruritis ani. Colorectal Dis 2002; 4(2):144–146.

20 Viral Sexually Transmitted Diseases

Peter M. Kaye
Department of Surgery, St. Luke's/Roosevelt Hospital Center, New York, New York, U.S.A.

Mitchell Bernstein
Columbia University College of Physicians and Surgeons, and St. Luke's/Roosevelt Hospital Center, New York, New York, U.S.A.

INTRODUCTION

Sexually transmitted diseases (STDs) remain a common public health problem with the prevalence of some STDs such as lymphogranuloma venereum and syphilis on the rise. The anorectum is particularly susceptible to STDs. The anorectal mucosa is easily disrupted during anoreceptive intercourse allowing for the easy transmission of pathogens. In addition, multiple organisms are often present in patients with anorectal STDs and determining which pathogens are causing symptoms may be challenging.

Diagnosis and management of patients with anorectal STDs begin with a thorough history. It is important to understand that symptoms may differ depending on the location most affected in the anorectum. Due to the abundant network of sensory nerve endings in the anal canal, infections here can manifest with severe pain and tenesmus. Alternatively, infections above the dentate line often result in a proctitis that manifests as blood or mucus discharge, rectal pain, and tenesmus. A simple but thorough anorectal examination is usually all that is required for diagnosis. Good lighting (i.e., headlight, spotlight, or lighted scopes), an anoscope, and a proctoscope are requirements for a thorough physical examination. Having the patient in the prone jackknife position yields the best results; however, lateral decubitus is also adequate.

Careful inspection of the perineum and perianal region is first performed to identify any ulcers, lesions, or condyloma. Palpation around the perianal area may elicit pus, blood, or mucus discharge from the anus. Digital rectal examination followed by anoscopy and proctoscopy is subsequently performed. If such an examination proves too painful for the patient, an examination under anesthesia is best performed.

Viruses are some of the most common STDs that directly affect the colon, rectum, and anus. Although the manifestations of these diseases can be seen independently, it is difficult to discuss viral STDs without mentioning human immunodeficiency virus (HIV) and acquired immunodeficiency syndrome (AIDS), with which other viral STDs are usually intimately associated.

HIV is an RNA lentivirus from the retrovirus family that is transmitted through sexual contact. It replicates via a reverse transcriptase and incorporates its cDNA into the host genome of CD4+ T-lymphocytes. Natural progression of the disease causes destruction of the CD4+ T-lymphocytes to the point where the body is unable to restore its numbers, resulting in an immunocompromised state that enables opportunistic infection and AIDS-related malignancies to prosper. The introduction of highly active antiretroviral therapy (HAART) has resulted in a decreased incidence of opportunistic infections and AIDS-related malignancy, a decrease in HIV-related death, and an increase in the life expectancy of HIV patients (1).

Anorectal disease is the most common reason for surgical referrals in the HIV-positive population (2). As with HIV-negative patients, pain, itching, and bleeding are the most common complaints (3). The most common pathology seen in these patients is condyloma, caused by the human papilloma virus (HPV) and perianal ulcerations (3,4). Ulcerations are typically caused by herpes simplex virus (HSV); however, cytomegalovirus (CMV) can also cause ulcers of the anorectum. However, in severely immunocompromised patients, a causative organism cannot be isolated and such ulcers have been classified as idiopathic AIDS-related ulcers. These ulcers have a characteristic appearance that distinguishes them from other ulcers. They are usually located in the posterior midline of the anus, often extend distal to the dentate line and can be quite erosive (3,5). With worsening immunosuppression and progression to AIDS, these ulcers can be the cause of perianal sepsis and fecal incontinence.

Despite the success of HAART in the HIV population, the prevalence and distribution of anorectal pathology have not changed (1). Because of the affect anorectal disease has on quality of life, the possibility of complications such as perianal sepsis and malignant potential, knowledge of viral STDs, and their management are essential for the colorectal surgeon.

HERPES SIMPLEX VIRUS

HSV is a large enveloped DNA virus noted for its ability to cause a latent infection. Of the two types of HSV, Type II is responsible for 90% of anogenital herpes (6). The virus is spread via oral–genital, genital–genital, and anal–genital intercourse, where it gains access to the body via breaks in the epithelium. The incubation period for the virus is 4 to 21 days as the virus replicates locally in the skin or the mucosa at the initial site of infection. The HSV then migrates along the sensory neuron, becoming latent in the sensory ganglion cells until it is reactivated. Upon reactivation, the virus migrates peripherally down the neuron and again replicates in the skin (3,7).

Anal herpes usually presents as small painful vesicles with surrounding erythema. These ulcers can coalesce to form large ulcers that can extend from the perianal skin into the anal canal and just beyond to the distal rectum. Ulcers that persist for greater than one month are considered an AIDS-specific condition (7). The initial infection is often accompanied by systemic symptoms such as fever, chill, and malaise. Patients describe exquisite anorectal pain exacerbated by anoreceptive intercourse and defecation, mucopurulent discharge, and tenesmus. The pain with defecation may be such that patients will avoid defecating causing a psychogenic constipation that can lead to fecal impaction (6). Due to sacral nerve root involvement, some patients may complain of parasthesias or pain radiating down the posterior thighs, impotence, dypareunia, painful urination, and urinary retention (3).

Patients who present to the office with the above-mentioned symptoms should be evaluated with anoscopy and/or proctoscopy. However, an examination under anesthesia may be necessary if pain precludes an adequate examination and a diagnosis cannot be made by history and identification of characteristic vesicles in the perianal tissues; tissue cultures and biopsies can be obtained. Giemsa staining should reveal multi-nucleated giant cells, and intranuclear inclusion bodies.

HSV infection, regardless of where it is located anatomically, is not curable. Antiviral agents that are on the market are used to shorten the clinical course and decrease the severity of the infection (6). Acyclovir, valacyclovir, and famciclovir are guanosine analogs that are monophosphorylated by the viral enzyme thymidine kinase, and di- and tri-phosphorylated by the host cell resulting in a nucleotide analog that competes with dGTP as a substrate for viral DNA polymerase. When incorporated into the viral DNA, acyclovir triphosphate causes premature DNA-chain termination. Valacyclovir and famcilovir have the advantage of twice daily dosing, as opposed to acyclovir which is administered anywhere from three to five times daily. Patients with severe immunosuppression, such as CD4+ T lymphocyte count less than 200 cells/mm^3, should be placed on suppressive antiviral therapy as these patients will have frequent and prolonged recurrence (3,7).

A small percentage of the population, who are afflicted with HSV, are infected with mutant strains which are thymidine kinase deficient and are thus resistant to the guanosine analog antiviral drugs. These patients have been found to respond well to Foscarnet, which is a pyrophosphate derivative that inhibits viral DNA and RNA polymerases, thereby terminating chain elongation (3,8).

Along with antiviral medications, patients should be encouraged to use Sitz baths, analgesics, and stool softeners to help control their symptoms through the acute phase of infection (3,6).

HUMAN PAPILLOMAVIRUS

Human papillomavirus (HPV) is a double-stranded DNA virus that infects the basal keratinocytes of the epithelium where it replicates and integrates its DNA into the host genome, causing an overexpression of viral genes E6 and E7. The protein products of E6 and E7 are responsible for disabling tumor suppressor genes p53 and pRB, respectively, which results in uncontrolled cell growth and malignant transformation.

As many as 80 subtypes of HPV have been identified, with some having greater oncogenic potential than others. The role of HPV in genital warts, cervical intraepithelial neoplasia (CIN), and cervical cancer has been extensively studied. Subtypes 6, 11, 42, 43, and 44 are more commonly associated with condyloma and have a low oncogenic risk. Subtypes 16, 18, 31, 33, 35, 39, 45, 51, 52, 56, and 58 are more often related to more severe dysplasia, the precursor to squamous cell carcinoma (9). Data regarding the relationship of HPV to CIN and cervical cancer justified the establishment of the cervical cancer screening protocol that is used today.

HPV has gained a lot of attention in the field of colorectal surgery. In addition to being the causative agent responsible for condyloma accuminata (anal warts), it has been associated with anal intraepithelial neoplasia (AIN), a possible precursor to squamous cell carcinoma of the anus. Questions remain as to the significance of HPV in association with AIN and its possible progression to squamous cell carcinoma of the anus. Studies have been performed in an attempt to identify the patient population at risk of contracting HPV and developing anal squamous cell carcinoma, and potentially identify a population that would benefit from routine screening (3,10).

The population with the highest infection rate appears to be that of the HIV-positive homosexual male (10). When compared in cross-sectional studies, the HIV-positive homosexual male has a statistically significantly greater infection rate than that of the HIV-negative homosexual male (93% vs. 61% in one study, and 61% vs. 17% in another) (10,11). Palefsky et al. (10) and Breese et al. (11) demonstrated that the HIV-positive patients were typically infected with multiple subtypes of HPV, which often tend to have a higher oncogenic potential and that CD4+ T cell levels are inversely proportional to the number of subtypes and their oncogenic potential. In addition, with increased immunosuppression, high risk subtypes of HPV 31, 33, and 35, and exclusive of subtype 16, were consistently present (11).

Data such as these might suggest that HIV-positive homosexual males are the targeted population who would benefit from screening; however, it is apparent that other groups of patients still have a significant risk. In Palefsky's study (10), 61% of the HIV-negative patients were infected, which is a statistically significant segment of the study sample. Among this population, the detection of HPV was associated with anoreceptive intercourse. Although anoreceptive intercourse is considered a major risk factor for HPV transmission, it is not a prerequisite for HPV infection and AIN. Renal transplant patients and intravenous drug users have also been identified as populations at risk for HPV and AIN (12). Due to the difficulty in identifying the populations at risk for progression from AIN to squamous cell carcinoma of the anus, a protocol for screening for HPV and AIN has yet to be devised and widely accepted.

Patients with HPV infection typically present with complaints of the characteristic "cauliflower-like" exophytic, hyperkeratotic, perianal lesions. Often, the lesions cause no discomfort. It is not unusual, however, for patients to seek medical attention because they have symptoms such as pruritus ani, bleeding, or a mucopurulent discharge. Condyloma is the most common problem encountered by the colorectal surgeon in HIV-positive patients (2,4). The perianal region should be inspected followed by anoscopy or proctoscopy to identify the presence of internal lesions. When the lesions are small or flat, identification may be aided with the application of acetic acid. This causes the lesions to turn white in contrast to the surrounding pink mucosa. Biopsies can be obtained and, in the case of benign condyloma, the specimen will demonstrate hyperkeratosis, papillomatosis, and poikilocytosis. Characteristic dysplastic changes will be demonstrated in the case of AIN.

Treatment for condyloma is mainly office based. Since HPV is not curable, treatment focuses on cytodestruction of the lesions by any number of methods. Podophyllin is a resin extracted from the podophyllum plant whose active ingredient is podophyllotoxin, which is an antimitotic agent that causes tissue necrosis. The resin is applied to the wart and left to dry for four to six hours, and is then washed off. This is done once per week for four to six consecutive weeks by a physician. Podophyllin has demonstrated a clearance rate of 30% to 60% with a recurrence rate of 30% to 60%. The use of podophyllin is limited secondary to local and systemic toxicity. Podophyllotoxin has been isolated and approved for home treatment. It is less toxic and has a higher clinical clearance rate after application twice per day for three consecutive days. It has similar recurrence rates to podophyllin (13,14).

Bichloroacetic acid and trichloroacetic acid are topical agents that cause chemical coagulation of wart proteins. Although these agents have not been extensively studied, they have been associated with significant recurrence rates. Several weeks of a once-weekly application by a physician must be done carefully to avoid damaging surrounding normal tissue (13).

Cryotherapy, involving the application of liquid nitrogen, has also been used in the destruction of anal warts. Because of associated pain, local anesthesia using EMLA cream and/or lidocaine injection should be administered. Cryotherapy has a clearance rate ranging from 50% to 70%, but recurrence rates can reach 70% at six-month follow-up. Cryotherapy is recommended for limited disease (13).

Due to the high recurrence rate associated with topical treatments, surgical cytodestruction with electrocautery is the preferred treatment modality at our institution. The procedure can be done in the office using either local anesthesia with or without conscious sedation. Acetic acid is first applied to illuminate less obvious lesions. Suspicious lesions are excised and sent to pathology, and the remaining lesions are fulgurated producing a white coagulum that is the equivalent of a superficial second-degree burn. Larger lesions can be excised using scissors. Care should be taken to prevent deep burns that can cause scarring and, potentially, anal stenosis. Clearance can be as high as 100% with recurrence rates ranging from 5% to 25% (3,13).

An effective adjunct to surgical cytodestruction is the application of Imiquimod, which has poorly understood immunomodulator properties, but it stimulates the release of cytokines, including interferon; these possess antiproliferative and antiviral properties. Imiquimod therapy alone has a high recurrence rate; however, it is thought to complement the efficacy of surgical intervention for warts. Further randomized trials need to be performed to evaluate its clearance and recurrence rates when combined with surgery (13).

The persistence of HPV infection and the risk of malignancy have prompted development of HPV-directed vaccines capable of destroying infected cells and preventing new infection; these vaccines are currently undergoing clinical trials. Two of these vaccines specifically target HPV-16 because it is the most commonly found subtype associated with dysplasia and carcinoma. In addition, there is often cross reactivity between HPV-16 and other subtypes. The vaccines are composed of a mutant E7 protein that has been found to induce both a cell-mediated and humoral immune response. Both vaccines have demonstrated regression and, in some cases, eradication of anal lesions. Unfortunately, the trials that were performed included a very small number of patients (15,16). More powerful prospective randomized trials need to be completed to truly demonstrate the efficacy of these vaccines.

CYTOMEGALOVIRUS

CMV is a DNA virus that is the largest member of the herpes viridae family. Similar to the other herpes viruses, CMV goes into a latent phase after causing mild mononucleosis-like symptoms upon initial infection. Reactivation commonly occurs with immunosuppression.

CMV, which is a sexually transmitted virion, may also be transmitted via saliva, placental transfer, breastfeeding, blood transfusion, solid-organ transplantation, and hematopoietic stem-cell transplantation. Serologic studies reveal a prevalence of seropositivity of 40% to 80% in industrialized nations, as high as 94% in homosexual males, and close to 100% in patients with AIDS (17–19).

In patients with AIDS, the predominant colorectal manifestation of CMV infection is CMV ileocolitis, although CMV lesions may be present throughout the gastrointestinal tract. The patient typically presents with intractable diarrhea, sometimes with hematochezia or melena, fever, and weight loss. Diagnosis is confirmed via endoscopic biopsy. Colonoscopy can reveal ulcers that are either small and shallow or deep, vast, coalesced, and sometimes covered in a yellowish membrane. Biopsies of the ulcer should be obtained as the differential diagnosis based on the appearance of the ulcer includes ulcerative colitis and pseudomembranous colitis (7). Biopsies should be submitted for histopathologic evaluation that may reveal the characteristic basophilic intranuclear and intracytoplasmic inclusion bodies. Viral cultures should also be sent for immunohistochemistry for detection of viral antigens and PCR amplification for detection of viral DNA (7,17).

Bleeding and perforation of ulcers in ileocolitis are emergent problems encountered by the colorectal surgeon; both are usually multi-focal. The bleeding is typically massive and the perforation is severe, with significant fecal contamination. Because of their multi-focality, the appropriate operation is usually a subtotal colectomy with end ileostomy. A primary anastomosis should not be attempted since the patient's poor immunologic state will not promote healing (7).

Although uncommon, there have been case reports describing perianal CMV ulcers. Clinically, these ulcers resemble those caused by HSV. Theories regarding the mechanism of CMV-related perianal ulceration include disruption of the perianal skin secondary to prior HSV infection and sexual trauma, fecal shedding, and spread of infection from contiguous sites along the gastrointestinal tract. The ulcers typically appear when the CD4+ T-lymphocyte count is less than 50 cells/mm (2,18). Owing to the fact that several organisms are often isolated from these perianal ulcers and that CMV is ubiquitous in AIDS patients, it is uncertain whether CMV causes the primary infection, a super infection, or is simply colonizing the wound.

Treatment of CMV includes ganciclovir. Sitz baths and analgesics will control symptoms caused by the anal ulcers (18).

SUMMARY

Knowledge of viral STD presentation and the associated risk factors for transmission is essential in a modern colorectal practice. In a well-equipped office, viral STDs can be diagnosed and effectively treated in an out-patient setting. Conscientious follow-up by the patient, as well as an interdisciplinary approach to the disease by the practitioners, is necessary to optimize clinical outcome.

REFERENCES

1. Gonzalez-Ruiz C, Heartfield W, Briggs B. Anorectal pathology in HIV/AIDS-infected patients has not been impacted by highly active antiretroviral therapy. Dis Colon Rectum 2004; 47:1483–1486.
2. Barrett WL, Callahan TD, Orkin BA. Perianal manifestations of human immunodeficiency virus infection: Eexperience with 260 patients. Dis Colon Rectum 1998; 41:606–612.
3. Brar HS, Gottesman L, Surawicz C. Anorectal pathology in AIDS. Gastrointest Endosc Clin North Am 1998; 8:913–931.
4. Yuhan R, Orsay C, DelPino A. Anorectal Disease in HIV-infected patients. Dis Colon Rectum 1998; 41:1367–1370.
5. Modesto VL, Gottesman L. Surgical debridement and intralesional steroid injection in the treatment of idiopathic AIDS-related anal ulcerations. Am J Surg 1997; 174:439–441.
6. Wexner SD. Sexually transmitted diseases of the colon, rectum, and anus: The challenge of the nineties. Dis Colon Rectum 1990;33:1048–1062.
7. Pare AA, Gottesman L. Anorectal diseases. Gastroenterol Clin North Am 1997; 26:367–378.
8. Safrin S. Treatment of acyclovir-resistant herpes simplex virus infection in patients with AIDS.J Acquir Immune Defic Syndr Hum Retrovirol 1992; 5:S5.
9. Abbasakoor F, Boulos PB. Anal intraepithelial neoplasia. Br J Surg 2005; 92:277–290.
10. Palefsky JM, Holly EA, Ralston ML, et al. Prevalence and risk factors for human papillomavirus onfection of the anal canal in human immunodeficiency virus (HIV)-positive and HIV-negative homosexual men. J Infect Dis 1998; 177:361–367.
11. Breese PL, Judson FN, Penley KA, et al. Anal human papillomavirus infection among homosexual and bisexual men: Prevalence of type-specific infection and association with human immunodeficiency virus. Sex Transm Dis 1995; 22:7–14.
12. Piketty C, Darragh TM, Da Costa M, et al. High prevalence of anal papillomavirus infection and anal cancer precursors among HIV-infected persons in the absence of anal intercourse. Ann Intern Med 2003; 138:453–459.
13. Rivera A, Tyring SK. Therapy of cutaneous human papillomavirus infections. Dermatol Ther 2004; 17:441–448.
14. Von Krogh G, Longstaff E. Podophyllin office therapy against conyloma should be abandoned. Sex Transm Infect 2001; 77:409–412.
15. Goldstone S, Palefsky J, Winnett M. Activity of HspE7, a novel immunotherapy in patients with anogenital warts. Dis Colon Rectum 2002; 45:502–507.

16. Hallez S, Simon P, Maudoux F, et al. Phase I/II trial of immunogenicity of a human papillomavirus (HPV) type 16 E7 protein-based vaccine in women with oncogenic HPV-positive cervical intraepithelial neoplasia. Cancer Immunol Immunother 2004; 53:642–650.
17. Gandhi MK, Khanna R. Human cytomegalovirus: Clinical aspects, immune regulation, and emerging treatments. Lancet Infect Dis 2004; 4: 725–738.
18. Nico MMS, Cymbalista NC, Hurtado YCP,et al. Perianal cytomegalovirus ulcer in a HIV infected patient: Case report and review of literature. J Dermatol 2000; 27:99–105.
19. Puy-Montbrun T, Ganansia R, Lemarchand N, et al. Anal ulcerations due to cytomegalovirus in patients with AIDS. Dis Colon Rectum 1990; 30:1041–1043.

21 Bacterial Sexually Transmitted Diseases

David E. Beck
Department of Colon and Rectal Surgery, Ochsner Clinic Foundation, New Orleans, Louisiana, U.S.A.

Johnny B. Green
Kitsap Colorectal Surgery, Bremerton, Washington, U.S.A.

INTRODUCTION

Sexually transmitted diseases (STDs) are a major health concern in the United States. Over 15 million STDs present annually, with over 25 etiologic organisms (1–3). Infection with multiple organisms is common and symptoms of genital infection overlap with symptoms from infection of the distal anal canal, anoderm, and perianal skin (2). These symptoms often lead the patient to seek a colorectal specialist who should have an understanding of these diseases.

Anorectal STDs are most often acquired through anal intercourse. However, contiguous spread from genital infection or transmission through oral–anal contact is also possible (3). Some organisms, usually considered enteric pathogens, can also be transmitted through direct or indirect oral fecal contact (4–7).

The frequency of homosexual and ano-erotic intercourse is not well documented. It is estimated that 2% of the male population in the United States regularly practices anoreceptive intercourse. Anorectal transmission of STDs may actually occur more frequently in females since 5% to 10% engage in unprotected anal intercourse (3).

After a significant decrease in the incidence of bacterial STDs following the onset of HIV, there has been a resurgence of gonorrhea and syphilis since 1996. This coincides with the availability of highly active antiretroviral therapy (HAART). Studies have shown that the increases are predominately among men who engage in sexual intercourse with men and coincide with an increase in high-risk sexual behavior. This may represent "safer sex" burnout, or an attitude that HIV is not as dangerous now that there is treatment (8–11).

Control of bacterial STDs is important because the presence of a bacterial infection in either partner increases the transmission rate of concomitant viral infections. Bacterial lesions in the patient with a viral infection increases viral shedding and sexual fluids. Lesions in a seronegative patient increase the risk of transmission through breaks in the epithelial barrier, as well as increasing the local presence of target cells (10–12). Bacterial anorectal and genital infections are transmitted through contact of infected secretions with breaks in the epithelial barriers in the dermis or genital, anorectal, or pharyngeal mucosa. Transmission is only prevented by condoms if the condom prevents contact. Lesions that are not covered by the condom or only covered during part of the sexual experience remain infective.

Identification of the causative organism of a bacterial STDs is made more difficult due to the lack of specific symptoms, the frequent presence of multiple organisms (both bacterial and viral), and, until recently, the lack of rapid diagnostic tests. This chapter will focus on the common bacterial STDs, their diagnosis, and treatment (Table 1).

CHLAMYDIA

Chlamydia remains the most common STD in the United States, with over 3 million infections reported per year (1). Many immunotypes have been identified, with serovars D–K responsible for most STD cases in the United States. Serovars L1–L3 cause lymphogranuloma venereum, which is much less common in developed countries (1). Most women and a large portion of men have asymptomatic chlamydia infections. Positive anorectal cultures were found in 4% to 8% of asymptomatic men and 5% to 21% of asymptomatic women. While most male patients are thought to have anorectal chlamydia as a result of anoreceptive intercourse, contiguous spread from genital infection is thought to be common in women. Non-LGV chlamydia proctitis is

Table 1 Common Bacterial Sexually Transmitted Diseases

Organism	Symptoms	Anoscopy and proctoscopy	Laboratory test	Treatment
Chlamydia	Tenesmus	Friable, often ulcerated rectal mucosa ± rectal mass	Serological antibody titre: biopsy for culture	Doxycycline 100 mg PO BID or erythromycin 500 mg PO QID for 7 days, azithromycin 1 g PO single dose
Gonorrhea	Rectal discharge	Proctitis, mucopurulent discharge	Thayer–Mayer culture of discharge	Ceftriaxone 125 mg IM single dose plus doxycycline 100 mg PO BID for 7 days
Chancroid Haemophiluys ducrei	Anal pain	Anorectal abscesses and ulcers	Culture	PO QID for 21 days Erythromycin 500 mg mg PO QID for 7 days, ciprofloxin 500 mg PO BID for 3 days, single dose ceftriaxone 250 mg IM, single dose azithromycin 1 g PO
Syphilis	Rectal pain	Painful anal ulcer	Dark-field exam of fresh scrapings	Benzathine penicillin 2.4 million units IM
Granuloma inguinale	Perianal mass	Hard, shiny peri-anal masses	Biopsy of mass	Doxycycline 100 mg PO BID, bactrim DS one tab PO BID, ciprofloxin 750 mg PO BID, erythromycin 500 mg PO QID for 21 days
Campylobacter jejuni	Diarrhea, cramps bloating	Erythema, edema grayish-white ulcerations of rectal mucosa	Culture stool using selective media	Erythromycin 500 mg PO QID for 7 days
Shigella	Diarrhea, cramps	Diarrhea, cramps	Culture stool	Azithromycin 500 mg daily for 3 days

Provider should check reference material for current indicated medication. BID-Twice daily; IM, intramuscularly; PO, per os; QID, Four times daily; DS, Double strength.

typically very mild with superficial small sores and mucosal edema with mild-to-moderate mucopurulunt discharge. Lymphogranuloma venereum causes more severe pain with perianal, anal, and perineal ulcerations. Abscesses with fistula and stricturing can occur. After several weeks adenopathy may develop in perirectal, inguinal, and femoral lymph nodes (13,14).

Diagnosis by culture is difficult due to handling requirements and has a high false negative rate. Urethral and cervical infections may now be diagnosed more rapidly and more accurately through nucleic acid amplification testing using cervix or urethral swabs or first void urine samples (15,16). Direct fluorescent antibody (DFA) testing has been done for anorectal and pharyngeal specimens, but local laboratories must do independent validation. Anorectal DFA testing is particularly technically challenging due to bacterial contamination and fecal debris (16).

Current recommended treatment regimens include azithromycin, 1 g orally as a one-time dose or doxycycline 100 mg twice daily for seven days. Partners should also be screened for gonorrhea. Lymphogranuloma venereum patients should be treated with doxycycline 100 mg twice daily or erythromycin 500 mg four times daily for three weeks (17).

NEISSERIA GONORRHEA

The gonorrhea infection rate declined steadily throughout United States until the mid-1990s then increased to approximately 650,000 cases per year. Females aged 15 to 19 years and males aged

20 to 24 years are most commonly affected. The infection rate is nearly 30 times higher among young African-Americans than among Caucasians. Gonorrhea affects mucous membranes and is frequently asymptomatic in the urethra, cervix, rectum, or pharynx (1,18–21). Up to 50% of males and nearly 95% of females are asymptomatic. The incubation period is typically three to five days. Anorectal infection typically causes a mucopurulunt discharge, which can be observed passing from the anal crypts during anoscopy (22,23). Pruritis and mild tenderness are also typical but bloody discharge is less common. Anoscopy or proctoscopy reveals a nonspecific proctitis. Disseminated infection may also cause arthritis, skin lesions, myocarditis, endocarditis, and meningitis (25).

Diagnosis by culture is difficult due to culture requirement and has a high false negative rate. Thayer–Martin or chocolate agar plates are required (22–24,26–29). Recent availability of nucleic acid amplification tests has increased diagnostic accuracy. The major drawback is that antimicrobial sensitivity cannot be tested. As with chlamydia testing, local laboratory validation is required for nonculture tests of anorectal or pharyngeal specimens (26–29).

Penicillinase-producing gonorrhea species are now quite common; therefore penicillin is no longer recommended for this infection. Intramuscular ceftriaxone, 125 mg as a one-time dose remains effective. Resistant strains to quinolones have become common in Asia, and are increasing in frequency in Hawaii and California, particularly among men who have sexual intercourse with men. Quinolones are no longer recommended to treat gonorrhea in men who have sex with men. Patients should also be treated for chlamydia as up to 40% of patients have dual infection. Disseminated infection requires intravenous therapy until 24 to 48 hours after signs of infection have improved, then oral treatment should be continued for one week (17,24,29).

CHANCROID

Chancroid is caused by the bacterium Haemophilus ducreyi. It is only transmitted by sexual contact, although autoinoculation into other body areas has been shown in patients with genital ulcers. It is endemic in many developing countries, but has only been seen in focal outbreaks in the United States in recent years (30–33). Studies have shown that the early papule stage affects men and women equally, but men progress to the pustule stage much more frequently (36). Uncircumcised men are three to four times more likely to have *H. ducreyi* infection. Ulcers are more commonly single and painful in men. Women with ulcers have an average of 4.5 around the introitus, but generally do not complain of pain (34). The "chancroid triad" of a moderate-to-severely painful ulcer with an undermined ulcer edge having a purulent dirty gray base is only present in less than half of men. Painful unilateral inguinal adenitis is present in up to 40%. Enlarged nodes may suppurate. Previously, aspiration of the suppurative adenitis has been recommended over incision and drainage but, more recently, drainage has proven to be superior with more rapid healing. Untreated disease leads to prolonged genital ulcers with incomplete healing.

Genital ulceration with *H. ducreyi* has been shown to increase the transmission of HIV by 10 to 100 times (31). The presence of HIV reduces the response and cure rate by 30%. All patients with genital ulcers should be tested for HIV. Culture of *H. ducreyi* is difficult, and PCR is now the recommended method of diagnosis (38).

To date, all strains are sensitive to third generation cephalosporins (17,39). Single dose regimens such as 250 mg ceftriaxone intramuscularly are recommended. Cefotaxime, ceftizoxine, and ceftazidine are also effective. Azithromycin and erythromycin are effective orally. Azithromycin has the advantage that only a 1 g oral dose is required, although this causes emesis in 6% of patients. Erythromycin requires 250 mg orally for seven days. Cipromyacin at 250 mg bid is also effective. Many strains have developed resistance to sulphonomides, tetracycline, kanamycin, chloramphenicol, and ampicillin; therefore these should not be used for chancroid.

SYPHILIS

Syphilis has been called "the great imitator" due to the lack of unique features and variable presentation. Classically, syphilis presents as one or more genital papules 14 days to 21 days after exposure. The papule gradually ulcerates, leaving a 1 to 2 cm indurated lesion with a clear base, called a chancre. Genital ulcers are typically painless and are clinically indistinguishable from ulcers caused by chancroid or lymphogranuloma venereum, and these infections may coexist. There may be a modest increase in lymph nodes and any body part may be affected (40,41). Anorectal lesions are more commonly painful (42–44). Antibody testing such as RPR may be negative early in the infection. Chancres typically heal in six weeks to eight weeks. Secondary syphilis usually occurs in 4 to 10 weeks after the appearance of the ulcers. A macular rash on the trunk and extremities, typically on the palms and soles of the feet, is the primary finding; vesicles are rare. Mucosal ulcers may also be present. Secondary symptoms such as malaise, sore throat, headache, weight loss, low-grade fever, muscle aches, or pruritis may also be present. Lymph node enlargement may be present. Large raised gray or whitish lesions—called condyloma lata—may develop in warm most regions such as the axilla, groin, or perineum and are full of spirochete organisms. Central nervous symptoms such as iritis, uveitis, or synovitis may also be present. The rash usually resolves over 3 to 12 weeks, as do other secondary symptoms. Antibody testing at the time of secondary symptoms is usually positive. Latent syphilis is described as greater than one year from infection. At this time there may not be cutaneous signs or symptoms. Antibody testing such as RPR is positive. The presence of a positive RPR test without a history of primary chancre or rash suggests a latent neurosyphilis. This can only be excluded by cerebrospinal fluid testing. Alternatively, treatment for neurosyphilis may be administered. Some studies suggest that HIV-positive patients may progress to neurosyphilis more rapidly than HIV-negative patients.

Diagnosis can be made by dark field examination of the exudates from a chancre, proctitis, or condyloma lata. Treponema may also be found in the skin of secondary lesions, but the skin must first be abraded and saline applied; false negatives are common (41). More often, however, the diagnosis is made by serologic testing. The RPR test is usually positive by the time the diagnosis is entertained, but may be at low levels (<1:16). Tests that measure antibody to T. pallidum surface proteins (TPHA or MHA-TP) will be positive approximately 90% of the time during the initial evaluation for STD. The MHA-TP remains positive for life and cannot be used in future for diagnosis or to follow disease activity, but remains useful to rule out the diagnosis. RPR returns to negative over the course of one to two years in most patients, if the organism has been eradicated. Persistent positive RPR should suggest retreatment. A positive RPR test after documented negative test indicates reinfection.

To date, no resistance to penicillin has been noted in syphilis (17,45,46). Treatment for primary and secondary syphilis remains 2.4 million units of density in penicillin, intramuscularly, in patients who are not allergic to penicillin. Antibody testing should be repeated every six months until negative, usually in one to two years. In some patients, the VDRL test will remain positive throughout their lifetime. Penicillin-allergic patients may be treated with ceftriaxone intravenously every other day for 10 days (five doses). Alternatively, erythromycin or tetracycline, 500 mg four times daily for 30 days, is also effective. Azithromycin has been used in Russia with good results, but this has not been validated elsewhere. Latent neurosyphilis in HIV negative patients should be treated with 2.4 million units of sustained penicillin weekly, for two doses. A spinal tap should be considered or a third dose given. Failure is more common in HIV-positive patients. This has led some authors to recommend alternative regimens such as 1.2 million units of procaine penicillin daily for 10 to 15 days, or ceftriaxone 1 g daily for 10 to 15 days. However, both of these regimens have also had occasional failures. Erythromycin and tetracycline cannot be used in neurosyphilis as they do not reach the spinal fluid. Pregnant patients may be treated the same as nonpregnant patients. A reaction to treatment, called the Jarish–Herxheimer reaction will occur in one third to two thirds of patients, manifested by fever, chills, rash, arthralgia, and headache. This reaction is actually due to released endotoxin with the death of the treponema pallidum organisms. The reaction usually occurs four to six hours after treatment and resolves in 24 hours. Aspirin or ibuprofen is usually effective, as is reassurance. In some patients it may be difficult to differentiate this reaction from a penicillin allergy.

GRANULOMA INGUINALE (DONOVANOSIS)

Granuloma inguinale or donovanosis is due to the gram-negative bacterium calymmatobacterium granulomatis. The disease is rare in the United States, but is endemic in areas of South

Africa, India, New Guinea, and aboriginal Australia (47,48). The incidence of HIV infection has been noted to rise rapidly in areas with endemic donovanosis, illustrating the increased HIV transmission in the presence of genital ulcerative disease. Four types of donovanosis are described: (1) ulcerogranulomatous is the most common type with nontender single or multiple beefy red friable ulcers, (2) hypertrophic or verrucous ulcerated lesions with a raised irregular border and possibly a dry base, (3) necrotic deep foul-smelling ulcers with tissue destruction; this type may be confused with squamous cell cancer, and (4) sclerotic or cicatricial ulcers causing extensive fibrosis and scar tissue.

The natural history of donovanosis is not well documented due to the focal endemic distribution of the disease and due to the fact that most patients are in lower socio-economic classes with poor availability of medical care. The incubation period has been described as 17 to 360 days, but in some studies lesions appeared on an average of 50 days after inoculation. Genital ulceration is present in 90% of cases and the inguinal area is involved in 10%. In men, the lesions are usually on the prepuce, coronal sulcus, frenum, and glans penis. The labia majora and fourchette are most often involved in women. Extragenital lesions have been described in the anus, lip, gums, cheek, palate, pharynx, neck, nose, larynx, and chest. Extragenital lesions are most often seen in patients who also have primary genital disease; lymphadenitis is uncommon. Disseminated donovanosis has been described with spread to the liver and bone, usually associated with pregnancy or severe cervical lesions. Anal stenosis has been described with the sclerotic type.

Diagnosis has been difficult due to rigorous culture requirements. Polymerase chain reaction testing has been developed but is not widely available. The diagnostic donovan bodies can be found in tissue from the ulcer. Tissue may be obtained by curettage or biopsy then prepared with a crush technique between two slides. Leischmann or Giemsa stains will demonstrate dense inflammation with donovan in monocytes. Papanicolaou smear has also shown donovan bodies.

Treatment must be prolonged for at least three weeks. The most cost-effective regimen is azithromycin 1 g once weekly for three weeks. Doxycycline 100 mg twice daily, Ciprofloxacin 750 mg twice daily, erythromycin 500 mg four times daily, and trimethoprim/sulfamethoxazole 800/160 twice daily, all for three weeks have also been proven effective. If tissue destruction or fibrosis is extensive, reparative surgery may be required after healing is complete.

ENTERIC PATHOGENS (SHIGELLA, CAMPYLOBACTER)

Shigella and campylobacter are usually recognized as enteric pathogens causing acute diarrheal illness. They are usually acquired by ingestion of contaminated food or water. However, they can be transmitted by sexual practices that include direct or indirect oral anal contact (49–51). Symptoms include abdominal pain and watery or bloody diarrhea. Campylobacter tends to be more severe and may be confused with appendicitis or inflammatory bowel disease. Campylobacter may also be associated with systemic symptoms of cellulitis or pneumonia, especially in immunocompromised patients. Sigmoidoscopy will demonstrate nonspecific proctocolitis, but the diagnosis is made by stool cultures on selective media. Treatment is usually supportive but severe cases or cases with cellulitis, pneumonia, or immune suppression can be treated with azithromycin 500 mg daily for three days or erythromycin 500 mg four times daily for one week.

REFERENCES

1. Centers for Disease Control and Prevention. Tracking the hidden epidemics. Trends in STDs in the United States. April 2001; 1–26.
2. Centers for Disease Control and Prevention. Trends in Reportable Sexually Transmitted Diseases in the United States 2003—National Data on Chlamydia, Gonorrhea and Syphillis, 2003.
3. Halperin DT. Heterosexual anal intercourse: prevelance, cultural factors, and HIV infection and other health risks, Part 1. AIDS Patient Care STDs 1999; 13: 717–730.
4. Rompalo AM. Diagnosis and treatment of sexually acquired proctitis and proctocolitis: an update. Clin Infect Dis 1999; 28(suppl 1):S84–90.
5. Sorvillo FJ, Lieb LE, Waterman SH. Incidence of camplobacteriosis among patients with AIDS in Los Angeles County. J Acquir Immune Def Syndr 1991; 4:598–602.

6. Allos BM, Blaser MJ. Campylobacter jejuni and the expanding spectrum of related infections. Clin Infect Dis 1994; 20:1092.
7. Tee W, Mijch A. Campylobacter jejuni bacteremia in human immodeficiency virus (HIV)-infected and non-HIV-infected patients: comparison of clinical features and review. Clin Infect Dis 1998; 26:91–96.
8. Centers for Disease Control and Prevention. Resurgent bacterial sexually transmitted disease among men who have sex with men-Kind County, Washington, 1997–1999. Morb Mortal Wkly Rep 1999; 48:773–777.
9. Centers for Disease Control and Prevention. STD Surveillance 2003, Special Focus Profiles, Men Who Have Sex With Men, 2003, 1–5.
10. Klausner JD, Kent CK. HIV and sexually transmitted diseases-Latest views on synergy, treatment and screening. Postgrad Med 2004; 115:3, 79–84.
11. Taylor MT. The increasing importance of sexually transmitted diseases in HIV-infected persons. Perspective 2003; 11:169–172.
12. Kozlowski PA, Neutra MR. The role of mucosal immunity in prevention of HIV transmissions. Curr Mol Med 2003; 3:217–228.
13. Schacter J, Stephens R. Infections caused by chlamydia trachomatis. In: Morse SA, Ballard RC, Holmes KK, Moreland AA, eds. Atlas of Sexually Transmitted Diseases and AIDS. Edinburgh: Mosby, 2003: 73–96.
14. Geisler WM, Whittington WLH, Suchland RJ, et al. Epidemiology of anorectal chlamydial and gonoccal infections among men having sex with men in Seattle-using serovar and auxotype strain typing. Sex Transm Dis 2002; 29:189–195.
15. Golden MR, Astet SG, Galvan R, et al. Pilot study of COBAS pcr and ligase chain reaction for detection of rectal infections due to *Chlamydia trachomatis*. J Clin Micro 2003; 41:2174–2175.
16. Rompalo AM, Suchland RJ. Rapid Diagnosis of chlamydia trachomatis rectal infection by direct immunofluroescence staining. J Infect Dis 1987; 155:1075.
17. Centers for Disease Control and Prevention. Sexually transmitted diseases treatment guidelines 2002. Morb Mortal Wkly Rep 2002; 51(RR-6):1–77.
18. Hook III EW, Handsfield HH. Gonococcal infection in the adult. In: Holmes KK, Sparling PR, Mardh PA, et al., eds. Sexually transmitted diseases. New York: McGraw-Hill, 1999:451–466.
19. Centers for Disease Control and Prevention. Sexually transmitted disease surveillance 2002 supplement. Gonococcal Isolate Surveillance Project Annual Report. Atlanta, Georgia: U.S. Department of Health and Human Services, October, 2003.
20. Cates W. Estimates of the incidence and prevalence of sexually transmitted diseases in the United States. Sex Trans Dis 1999; 26(suppl):S2–S7.
21. Rietmeijer CA, Patnaik JL, Judson FN, et al. Increases in gonorrhea and sexual risk behaviors among men who have sex with men: A 12-year trend analysis at the Denver Metro Health Clinic. Sex Transm Dis 2003; 30:562–567.
22. Rompalo AM. Diagnosis and treatment of sexually acquired proctitis and proctocolitis: An update. Clin Infect Dis 1999; 28(suppl 1):S84–S90.
23. Klein EJ, Fisher LS, Chow AW, et al. Anorectal gonococcal infection. Ann Intern Med 1977; 86:340–346.
24. National Network of STD-HIV Prevention Training Centers. Gonorrhea. June 2004.
25. Mehrany K, Kist JM, O'Connor WJ, et al. Disseminated gonococcemia. Int J Dermatol 2003; 42:208–209.
26. Young H, Manavi K, McMillan A. Evaluation of ligase chain reaction for the non-cultural detection of rectal and pharyngeal gonorrhea in men who have sex with men. Sex Transm Infect 2003; 79:484–486.
27. Stary A, Ching SF, Teodorowicz L, et al. Comparison of ligase chain reaction and culture for detection of Neisseria gonorrhoeae in genital and extragenital specimens. J Clin Microbiol 1997; 35:239–242.
28. Deheragoda P. Diagnosis of rectal gonorrhea by blind anorectal swabs compared to direct vision swabs taken via a proctoscope. Br J Venereal Dis 1977; 53:311–313.
29. Farley TA Cohen DA, Wu SY, et al. The value of screening for sexually transmitted diseases in an HIV clinic. J Acquir Immune Defic Syndr 2003; 33:642–648.
30. McGee ZA, Grewal NG. The CDC's STD Treatment Guidelines Need a New Paradigm. Sex Transm Dis 2002; 29:674–677.
31. Ronald AR, Albritton W. Chancroid and Haemophilus ducreyi. In: Holmes KK, Mardh P-A, Lemon SM, Stamm WE, Piot PP, Wasserheit JN, eds. Sexually Transmitted Diseases. New York: McGraw-Hill, 1999:515–520.
32. Trees DL, Morse SA. Chancroid and Haemophilus ducreyi: An Update. Clin Microbiol Rev; 8(3):357–375.
33. Al-Tawfiq JA, Spinola SM. Haemophilus ducreyi: clinical diagnosis and pathogenesis. Curr Opin Infec Dis 2002; 15:43–47.
34. Spinola SM, Bauer ME, Munson RS. Immunopathogenesis of *Haemophilus ducrei* infection (Chancroid). Inf Immun 2002; 70:1667–1676.
35. DiCarlo RP, Martin DH. The clinical diagnosis of genital ulcer disease in men. Clin Infect Dis 1997; 25:292–298.

36. Bong CTH, Harezlak J, Katz BP, et al. Men are more susceptible than women to pustule formation in the experimental model of haemophilus ducreyi infection. Sex Transm Dis 2002; 29:114–118.
37. Bong CTH, Bauer ME, Spinola SM. Haemophilus ducreyi: clinical features, epidemiology and prospects for disease control. Microbes Infect 2002; 4:1141–1148.
38. Orle KA, Gates CA, Martin DH, et al. Simultaneous PCR detection of Haemophilus ducreyi, Treponema pallidum, and herpes simplex virus types 1 and 2 from genital ulcers. J Clin Micro 1996; 34:49–54.
39. Schmid GP. Treatment of Chancroid, 1997. Clin Infect Dis 1999; 28(suppl 1): S14-S20.
40. Centers for Disease Control and Prevention. Primary and secondary syphilis – United States 2002. Morb Mortal Wkly Rep 2003; 52:1117–1120.
41. Cox D, Liu H, Moreland A, et al. Syphilis. In: Morse SA, Ballard RC, Holmes KK, et al., eds. Atlas of Sexually Transmitted Diseases and AIDS. Edinburgh:Mosby, 2003:23–51.
42. Center for Disease Control and Prevention. Primary and secondary syphilis among men who have sex with men-New York City. Morb Mortal Wkly Rep 2001; 51:853–856.
43. D'Souza G, Lee JH, Paffel JM. Outbreak of syphilis among men who have sex with men in Houston, Texas. Sex Transm Dis 2003; 30:872–873.
44. Goligher JC. Sexually transmitted diseases. In: Diseases of the Anus, Rectum and Colon. 5th ed. London: Bailleire Tindall, 1985:1033–1045.
45. Augenbraun MH. Treatment of Syphilis 2001: Nonpregnant adults. Clin Infect Dis 2002; 35(suppl 2):S187–S190.
46. Centers for Disease Control and Prevention. The National Plan to Eliminate Syphilis from the United States. Atlanta, Georgia: U.S. Department of Health and Human Services. 1999:1–84. Available at http://www.cdc.gov/stopsyphilis/plan.pdf.
47. O'Farrell N. Donovanosis. Sex Transm Infect 2002; 78:452–457.
48. Jamkhedkar PP, Hira SK, Shroff HJ, et al. Clinico-epidemiologic features of granuloma inguinale in the era of acquired immune deficiency syndrome. Sex Transm Dis 1998; 25:196–200.
49. Centers for Disease Control and Prevention. HIV infection as a risk factor for shigellosis. Emerg Infect Dis 1999; 5:820–823.
50. Dritz SK, Back AF. Shigella enteritis venereally transmitted. N Eng J Med 1974; 291:1194.
51. Gaudio PA, Sethabutr O, Echeverria P, et al. Utility of a polymerase chain reaction diagnostic system in a study of the epidemiology of shigellosis among dysentery patients, family contacts, and well controls living in a shigellosis-endemic area. J Infect Dis 1997; 176:1013–1018.

22 Anal Intraepithelial Neoplasia

Patrick Colquhoun
Department of Surgery, University of Western Ontario, London, Ontario, Canada

INTRODUCTION

Anal intraepithelial neoplasia (AIN) is a histologic diagnosis characterized by malignant transformation of the anal canal (Fig. 1) without invasion below the basement membrane. Other terms used to describe this phenomenon include dysplasia and carcinoma in situ of the anal canal.

Confusion exists in the literature between AIN and Bowen's disease, with many authors suggesting the two diseases are "synonymous" (1–3). Although the two problems have many common attributes, they are two clearly distinct clinical entities. Similar to AIN, Bowen's disease is a form of intraepithelial squamous neoplasia (4). However, AIN cannot be clinically diagnosed. The diagnosis by definition requires histopathology. Bowen's disease differs in its consistent clinical presentation. It is characterized by a well-demarcated erythematous plaque with an irregular border and surface crusting with or without ulceration (4). It has been reported as a manifestation at numerous sites throughout the body, most commonly the trunk and lower extremities, least commonly the palms of the hands and soles of the feet (4). AIN is limited to the anal canal. Bowen's disease has a characteristic epidemiology most commonly afflicting males over the age of 60 (4). AIN affects individuals who have multiple sexual partners and a prior exposure to a sexually transmitted diseases; it also has a very strong correlation with the human papilloma virus and a high prevalence in the immunosuppressed, especially individuals with human immunodeficiency virus (HIV)/acquired immune deficiency syndrome (AIDS) (10–12). As in AIN, Bowen's disease is associated with invasive squamous cell carcinoma (SCC) (4). The degree of cellular atypia found in cases of Bowen's disease has not been associated with risk of transformation to SCC. The situation in AIN is clearly different. There appears to be a difference in the natural progression of high-grade AIN and low-grade AIN to invasive anal carcinoma. Analogous to the literature's approach to SCC, where a clear distinction between SCC of the anal canal and SCC of the skin has been made, AIN is distinct from Bowen's disease and the two should not be viewed as synonymous. The discussion of intraepithelial neoplasia within this chapter will be limited to AIN. Any references to SCC refer to SCC of the anal canal.

AIN was first described by Fenger et al. in 1986 (5). Although previous authors had made mention of "in situ carcinoma," Fenger was the first to attempt to demonstrate correlation between the degree of neoplasia and the risk of transformation to SCC, using the same criteria used to describe cervical intraepithelial neoplasia (CIN).

CIN was first described by Richart (6) based on the frequent observation of dysplasia/in situ carcinoma adjacent to SCC in resected specimens of the cervix. Clinicians speculated that invasive carcinoma likely evolved from an in situ cancer and hypothesized that identification and eradication of the in situ form might prevent SCC of the cervix. Cervical cancer was hypothesized to be "the end stage of a continuum of progressively more atypical changes in which one stage merges with the next" (7). Atypical cells were thought to occupy the lower third of the epithelium (CIN I), evolving to the lower third to two thirds (CIN II), and to involvement of the entire membrane (CIN III), leading to malignant transformation (SCC) (Fig. 2) (7). This hypothesis was substantiated by studies that demonstrated the risk of progression to SCC appeared to correlate well with the CIN stage (8). Validation of the concept of CIN is best demonstrated by the dramatic decrease in the incidence of cervical cancer through screening and eradication of CIN (8,9).

The similarities shared between cervical and AIN are undeniable. The cervix and anus share the same cloacogenic origin. They both represent regions where transition occurs from squamous to columnar epithelium. Histology of cervical and anal cancer is virtually identical. Invasive carcinoma is often seen in the face of intraepithelial carcinoma. Epidemiology is also very similar (10–12).

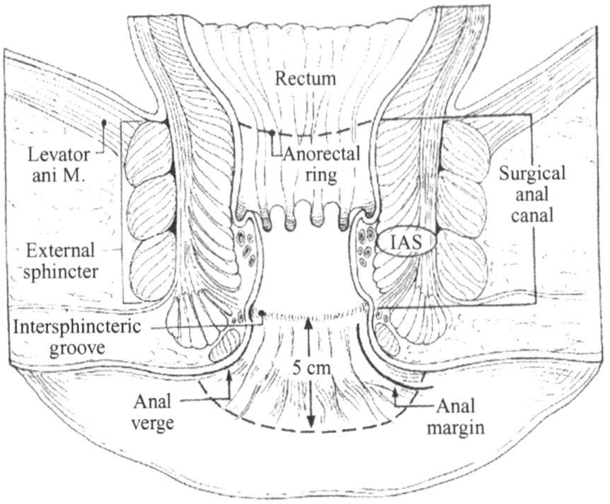

Figure 1 Anatomy of the anal canal and margin. *Source*: From Ref. 39.

These similarities have led to the hypothesis that the tumorigenesis clearly documented in cervical cancer will be observed in SCC of the anal canal. Since Fenger's publication in 1986 (5), the literature has demonstrated an association between AIN and anal SCC (13). An increased incidence of anal SCC has also been witnessed (14,15). This observation appears to be due to a rise in carcinoma witnessed in those individuals suffering with HIV (16). Current data suggest that SCC of the anus in homosexual males may be as common as cervical cancer in heterosexual women (10). The increase in SCC has been mirrored in AIN. Based on these observations there has been speculation that identification and eradication of AIN will lead to the same results as screening and intervention for CIN. It must be emphasized, however, that

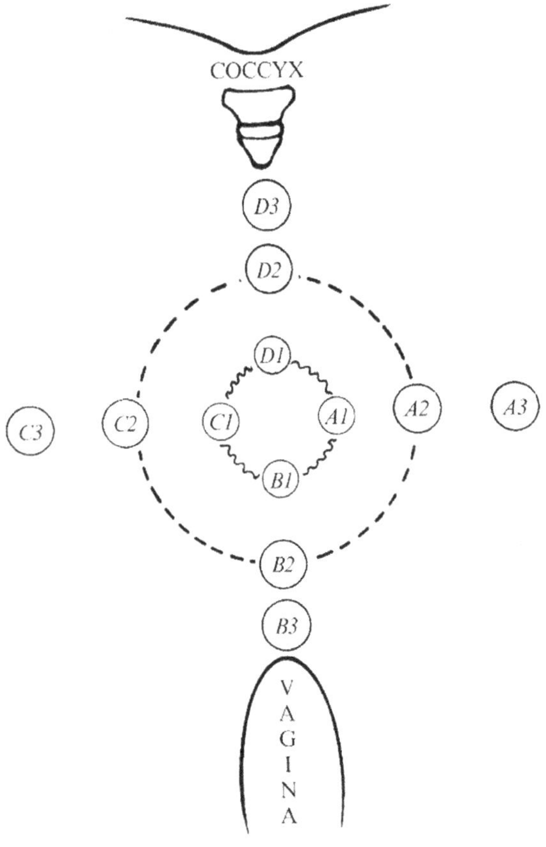

Figure 2 Schematic diagram detailing approach to mapping biopsies performed to document extent and location of intraepithelial neoplasia. **A1–D1,** biopsies at dentate line; **A2–D2,** biopsies at anal verge; and **A3–D3,** biopsies at anal margin. *Source*: From Ref. 39.

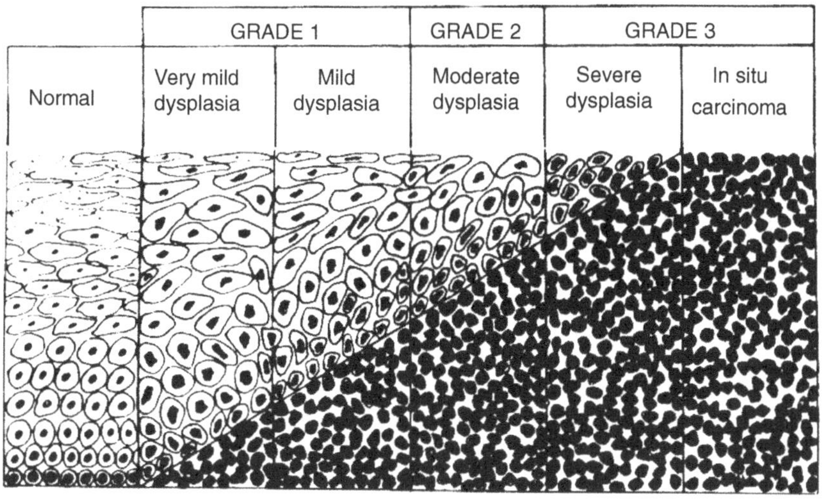

Figure 3 Schematic representation of intraepithelial neoplasia grades from 1 to 3. Each grade possesses a progressive increase in the number of undifferentiated malignant cells and a decrease in superficial cell differentiation paralleling increasing severity of intraepithelial neoplasia. *Source*: From Ref. 7.

the natural progression of AIN is still unknown and no publications to date have demonstrated direct transformation of AIN into SCC.

A recent examination of pathologists' interpretation of AIN has also called the current grading system into question. Colquhoun et al. (17) demonstrated significant inconsistency in the histologic interpretation of AIN (Fig. 3). This inconsistency was witnessed both internally (pathologist had a Kappa score of 0.64 when comparing initial interpretation to a second reading of the histology) and externally (Kappa scores varied 0.38–0.7). These results suggest the understanding of the natural progression of AIN may be limited by the grading system in use. It also suggests that interventions based on this grading system may also result in variable results.

These inconsistencies have led to confusion regarding the management of AIN in the literature. Recommendations have ranged from simple observation, anal cytology to aggressive eradication. There are no formalized practice guidelines for AIN.

CLINICAL APPROACH TO AIN

It must be acknowledged that a radical increase in anal SCC has been witnessed (14,15). This appears to be in patients who practice anoreceptive intercourse especially those who suffer with HIV (16). It is therefore imperative that physicians be vigilant about examining the anus for evidence of SCC in individuals from these populations who possess palpable anal lesions, rectal bleeding, or anal pain. At the very least, such individuals should undergo a digital rectal examination and detailed anoscopy with a plan to biopsy detectable lesions.

For asymptomatic patients, while there may be a logical argument that can be made for some form of screening for anal SCC especially in the HIV and homosexual populations, it must be acknowledged that AIN does not meet the acknowledged criteria to justify screening to prevent anal cancer (Table 1). There is a lack of understanding of the natural progression of AIN and no study has demonstrated that intervention of AIN prevents anal cancer. Currently, there are no observations reported describing the results of simple clinical surveillance of the anal canal in this population. This may be because it has been assumed that the stage of disease

Table 1 Criteria for Justification of Cancer Screening

Cancer must be an important public health problem causing significant cancer-related morbidity and mortality
Natural history must be understood and amenable to intervention
Screening modalities must be proven safe, acceptable, and cost-effective
Interventions available to prevent a given cancer must be proven safe, acceptable, and cost-effective

witnessed in the symptomatic population with anal cancer will be witnessed in the surveyed asymptomatic patients. Literature does not exist to justify surveillance for anal cancer even in high risk populations. For the time being, screening for AIN and interventions should be viewed as experimental and should only be performed within the context of research protocols.

For incidental dysplasia identified on biopsy, the management is based on the histologic interpretation. Although Fenger argued for a three-stage system for AIN (5), more recent literature suggests a two-stage system (high-grade vs. low-grade AIN) may be more practical (17).

Low-grade AIN appears to be much more common than the incidence of SCC of the anus (12). As a result, it appears that progression of low-grade AIN to invasive carcinoma is not absolute and the incidence of transformation is rare. Regression has also been observed in this situation (12). Surawicz et al. (12) have suggested that low-grade AIN may merely represent histologic response to the human papilloma virus. The incidence of subclinical invasive SCC of the anus is low (18).

Patients with low-grade AIN should be thoroughly examined for other areas of SCC that occur in this population (genital areas including penis, vulva, vagina, and cervix). Inguinal lymph node basins should be checked for clinical evidence of metastasis. Any identifiable clinical lesions should be biopsied. Results of eradication are extremely variable. Treatments are morbid. No literature has demonstrated that eradication prevents malignant transformation or survival of anal cancer. Recurrence rates appear high, most likely due to continued exposure to risk factors, inability to eradicate HPV, and persistent immunosuppression. These individuals should be counseled that they may be at heightened risk of anal cancer. Surveillance by physical and digital rectal examination and anoscopy should be instituted. The frequency of surveillance has not been studied in detail; however, an annual examination appears to be acceptable.

High-grade AIN appears to be a more worrisome lesion; it has been suggested that AIN may be a marker of subclinical invasive carcinoma (18). Risk of malignant transformation appears to be higher. Eradication of high-grade AIN has been attempted with a number of modalities, all of which have had variable results. There has been no demonstrated improvement in the literature of survival based on aggressive interventions of high-grade AIN.

Similar to patients with low-grade AIN, those with high-grade AIN should be examined for SCC in the other areas of the perineum that occur in this population. Inguinal lymph node basins should be checked for clinical evidence of metastasis. Any identifiable clinical lesions should be biopsied or excised. If anoscopy is hampered by patient intolerance, examination under anesthesia should be considered to insure complete evaluation of the anal canal.

Interventions for high-grade AIN have been reported in the literature. Surgery has been associated with significant morbidity and recurrence rates (18,19). Some benefit has been demonstrated in the identification and eradication of subclinical invasive carcinoma (18); however, no reports have stated that this translated into improved survival. Extensive resections have necessitated ostomy formation (20) and, consequently, patients with premalignant lesions who are trying to avoid ostomy formation for invasive SCC through chemoradiotherapy are being diverted.

Less invasive interventions have been reported including topical 5-fluorouracil, imiquimod, and photodynamic therapy. Topical 5-fluorouracil has been used in the treatment of Bowen's disease (21) and perianal intraepithelial adenocarcinoma (22). Variable success has been reported for anal condylomata. Graham et al. (23) treated patients with "anal Bowen's disease" involving more than 50% of the circumference of the perianal skin with topical 5-fluorouracil (23). The treatment was applied to the effected area once daily for a period of 16 weeks and appeared to be well tolerated. Temporary cessation of treatment occurred in one patient for four to seven day intervals due to pain and inflammation. At one year, all eight patients treated with topical 5- fluorouracil were disease free.

Imiquimod (*Aldara*) is an immune modifier which stimulates inflammatory mediators that are thought to have antitumor and antiviral activity. Case series have been published demonstrating a positive effect on intraepithelial neoplasia of the penis (24) and vagina (25). Kreuter et al. (26) reported a preliminary study of 10 patients with AIN who tolerated the treatments well and demonstrated regression of disease. However, long-term data are still pending.

Case reports using photodynamic therapy suggest the potential utility of this modality in the treatment of AIN. Treatments involve exposure to a photosensitizer which localizes to neoplastic tissue and is cytotoxic when exposed to specific bands of light. It has been used in

Table 2 Anal Pap Smear Technique

Moisten Dacron swab with saline or tap water
Insert swab into distal rectum at least 2 cm from anal verge
Rotate swab while withdrawing through the anal canal
Smear swab onto glass slide and fix with spray fixative or immersion in alcohol within 10 seconds of withdrawl
Stain fixed smear by routine Pap method for cytologic presentation

Source: Adapted from Ref. 34.

in situ forms of cancer, specifically Paget's and Bowen's disease (27,28). Case reports of its use in AIN suggest that it may be an effective future treatment (29,30).

To date, the medical literature has not resolved the issue of the most effective treatment of high-grade AIN nor has it determined the risk of malignant transformation. Patients should be informed that they have microscopic evidence of superficial cancer cells without clinical evidence of a cancer. They should also be aware that there is no evidence in the medical literature to show that any of the interventions mentioned above are curative. Simple observation of the area via clinical surveillance every three to six months by digital rectal examination and anoscopy is reasonable. However, in exchange for avoiding short-term morbidity, patients must be willing to accept the possibility that they may develop an overt malignancy during surveillance.

If patients desire intervention in an attempt to avoid transformation, any of the above options are reasonable. Patients should be examined under anesthesia and have mapping biopsy performed to determine the extent of the disease (Table 2). Any areas involving less than 50% of the circumference of the anus can be considered for surgical excision, under general anesthesia, to eradicate the area and detect subclinical cancer. In such cases, a 5 mm margin should be attained.

In patients whose lesions involve multiple areas or in whom the distribution involves more than 50%, topical treatments (Aldara or 5-fluororacil) or photodynamic therapy can be considered to reduce the morbidity associated with surgery for such lesions.

A great deal of literature has recently discussed the merits of anal cytology for the early detection and intervention of AIN (31–33). Palefsky's group at the University of California, San Francisco has published extensively on this subject. Currently they are in the process of detailed screening of non-HIV infected males practicing anoreceptive intercourse, HIV infected males, and females with CD4+ T–lymphocyte counts below 500 cells per mm^3, HIV infected and non-HIV infected individuals with CIN (34). Such individuals are subjected to anal Pap smear (Table 2) every 6 to 12 months. Results have been variable (34) with more recent publications suggesting acceptable sensitivity and specificity for detection of dysplasia, but an inability to accurately differentiate grades of dysplasia (36,37). Histopathology is still endorsed as the gold standard for the diagnosis and differentiation of grades of AIN. In order to facilitate histopathology, high-resolution anoscopy (colposcopy of the anus) has been hypothesized as a useful tool in those with positive anal pap smears (38). Time will tell if such strategies will allow for the development of adequate surveillance programs for high risk individuals and those patients who have incidental identification of AIN (asymptomatic individuals with AIN). For the time being, anal Pap smear and high-resolution anoscopy should be viewed as experimental and their use should be limited to research protocols.

REFERENCES

1. Cleary RK, Scalendbrand JD, Fowler JJ, et al. Perianal Bowen's Disease and anal intraepitheilial neoplasia. Dis Colon Rectum 1999; 42:945–951.
2. Brown SR, Skinner P, Tidy J, et al. Outcome after surgical resection for high-grade anal intraepithelial neoplasia (Bowen's Disease). Br J Surg 1999; 86:1063–1066.
3. Marchesa P, Fazio VW, Soledad O, et al. Perianal Bowen's disease: a clinicopathologic study of 47 patients. Dis Colon Rectum 1997; 40:1286–1293.
4. Cox NH, Morton CA. Guidelines for management of Bowen's disease. Br J Dermatol 1999; 141:633–641.
5. Fenger C, Thue Neilsen V. Intraepithelial neoplasia in the anal canal. Acta Path Microbial Immunol Scand 1986; 94A:343–349.

6. Richart RM. Cervical intraepithelial neoplasia. A review. Pathology Annual 1973. New York: Appelton-Centrury-Crofts, 1973; 8:301–328.
7. Cortran RS, Kumar V, Robbins SL. Robbins Pathologic Basis of Disease. 4th ed. Toronto: WB Saunders, 1989.
8. Cox JT. Management of precursor lesions of cervical carcinoma: history, host defense, and a survey of modalities. Obs Gyne Clin 2002; 29(4):843–868.
9. Waggoner SE. Cervical cancer. Lancet 2003; 361:2217–2225.
10. Palefsky JM. Anal squamous intraepithelial lesions in human immunodeficiency virus positive men and women. Semin Oncol 2000; 27:471–479.
11. Palefsky JM. Anal squamous intraepithelial lesions: relation to HIV and human papillomavirus infection. JAIDS 1999; 21:S42–45.
12. Surawicz CM, Kiviat NB. Rational approach to anal intraepithelial neoplasia Semin Colon Rect Surg 1998; 9(2):99–106.
13. Scholefield JH, Ogunbiyi A, Smith JHF, et al. Treatment of anal intraepithelial neoplasia. Br J Surg 1994; 81:1238–1240.
14. Johnson LG, Madeleine MM, Newcomer LM, et al. Anal cancer incidence and survival: The surveillance, epidemiology, and end results experience, 1973–2000. Cancer 2004; 101(2):281–288.
15. Welton ML. The etiology and epidemiology of anal cancer. Surg Oncol Clin North Am 2004; 13(2):263–275.
16. Klencke BJ, Palefsky JM. Anal cancer: And HIV associated cancer. Hematol Oncol Clin North Am 2003; 17:859–887.
17. Colquhoun P, Nogueras JJ, Dipasquale B, et al. Interobserver and intraobserver bias exists in the interpretation of anal dysplasia. Dis Colon Rectum 2003; 46(10):1332–1336.
18. Scholefield JH, Ogunbiyi OA, Smith JH, et al. Treatment of anal intraepithelial neoplasia. Br J Surg 1994; 81:1238–1240.
19. Chang GJ, Berry JM, Jay N, et al. Surgical treatment of high-grade anal squamous intraepithelial lesions: A prospective study. Dis Colon Rectum 2002; 45(4):453–458.
20. Thomas SS, Chenoy R, Fielding JW, et al. Vulvoperineal reconstruction after excision of anogenital multifocal intraepithelial neoplasia ("MIN"). Br J Plast Surg 1996; 49(8):539–546.
21. Cox NH, Eedy DJ, Morton CA. Guidelines for management of Bowen's disease. British Association of Dermatologists. Br J Dermatol 1999; 141(4):633–641.
22. Haberman HF, Goodall J, Llewellyn M. Extramammary Paget's disease. Can Med Assoc J 1978; 118:161–162.
23. Graham BD, Jetmore AB, Foote JE, et al. Topical 5-fluorouracil in the management of extensive anal Bowen's disease: a preferred approach. Dis Colon Rectum 2005; 48:444–450.
24. Orengo I, Rosen T, Guill CK. Treatment of squamous cell carcinoma in situ of the penis with 5% imiquimod cream: a case report. J Am Acad Dermatol 2002; 47(4 suppl):S225–S228.
25. Diakomanolis E, Haidopoulos D, Stefanidis K. Treatment of high-grade vaginal intraepithelial neoplasia with imiquimod cream. N Engl J Med 2002; 347(5):374.
26. Kreuter A, Hochdorfer B, Stucker M, et al. Treatment of anal intraepithelial neoplasia in patients with acquired HIV with imiquimod 5% cream. J Am Acad Dermatol 2004; 50(6):980–981.
27. Petrelli NJ, Cebollero JA, Rodriguez-Bigas M, et al. Photodynamic therapy in the management of neoplasms of the perianal skin. Arch Surg 1992; 127(12):1436–1438.
28. Runfola MA, Weber TK, Rodriguez-Bigas M, et al. Photodynamic therapy for residual neoplasms of the perianal skin. Dis Colon Rectum 2000; 43(4):499–502.
29. Webber J, Fromm D. Photodynamic therapy for carcinoma in situ of the anus. Arch Surg 2004; 39(3):259–261.
30. Scholefield JH. Treatment of grade III anal intraepithelial neoplasia with photodynamic therapy: report of a case. Dis Colon Rectum 2003; 46(11):1555–1559.
31. Klencke BJ, Palefsky JM. Anal cancer: an HIV-associated cancer. Hematol Oncol Clin North Am 2003; 17(3):859–872.
32. Palefsky JM. Anal squamous intraepithelial lesions in human immunodeficiency virus-positive men and women. Semin Oncol 2000; 27(4):471–479.
33. Goldie SJ, Kuntz KM, Weinstein MC. Cost-effectiveness of screening for anal squamous intraepithelial lesions and anal cancer in human immunodeficiency virus-negative homosexual and bisexual men. Am J Med 2000; 108(8):634–641.
34. Northfelt DW, Swift PS, Palefsky JM. Anal neoplasia. Pathogenesis, diagnosis, and management. Hematol Oncol Clin North Am 1996; 10(5):1177–1187.
35. Panther LA, Wagner K, Proper J, et al. High resolution anoscopy findings for men who have sex with men: inaccuracy of anal cytology as a predictor of histologic high-grade anal intraepithelial neoplasia and the impact of HIV serostatus. Clin Infect Dis 2004; 38(10):1490–1492.
36. Friedlander MA, Steir E, Lin O. Anorectal cytology as a screening tool for anal squamous lesions: cytologic, anoscopic, and histologic correlation. Cancer 2004; 102(1):19–26.

37. Fox PA, Seet JE, Stebbing J, et al. The value of anal cytology and human papillomavirus typing in the detection of anal intraepithelial neoplasia: a review of cases from an anoscopy clinic. Sex Transm Infect 2005; 81(2):142–146.
38. Jay N, Barry JM, Hogeboom CJ. Colposcopic appearance of anal squamous intraepithelial lesions: relationship to histopathology. Dis Colon Rectum 1997; 40(8):919–928.
39. Wexner SD, Beck DE, eds. Fundamentals of Anorectal Surgery. 2nd ed. London: W.B. Saunders, 1996.

23 Wound Management

Hao Wang, Badma Bashankaev, and Helen Marquez
Department of Colorectal Surgery, Cleveland Clinic Florida, Weston, Florida, U.S.A.

INTRODUCTION

The majority of colorectal operations begin and end with the incision; thus wound complications are still the highest among all complications. They decrease the patient's quality of life and increase medical and financial expenses, resulting in increased morbidity and rarely postoperative mortality. Surgeons maintain a constant effort to improve postoperative results, and comprehensive knowledge of wound management is of great importance in that process. This chapter will focus on wound management in the outpatient colorectal setting, including the basics of the wound healing process, factors associated with wound healing, wound types, principles of wound care, wound dressings, various management options, and specific colorectal conditions.

WOUND HEALING PROCESS

Wound closure types include primary, secondary, and tertiary repair, according to the intent to close the wound. Primary or first-intention closures are wounds that are immediately sealed, such as the direct closure at the end of a surgical procedure. Secondary closure indicates that there is no direct closure at the end of a surgical procedure. In general, the presence of fecal peritonitis restricts the primary closure, which would result in increased infection rates and would compromise patient outcomes. The wound (usually the skin and the subcutaneous tissue) is left open to prevent infection and close spontaneously. Tertiary closure is also used for the contaminated wound, but the difference to secondary closure is that another surgical intervention is required to close the wound (1).

Wound healing has been one of the most frequently discussed subjects in the medical literature and one of the most complex and delicate pathological processes of our bodies. Wound healing includes three phases: the inflammatory phase, the proliferative phase, and the maturational phase. The inflammatory phase is the immediate response after the surgical injury; it includes hemostasis and inflammation during the first four to six days. The first phase represents the attempt to limit the damage by stopping the bleeding, sealing the surface of the wound, secreting the cytokines and growth factors, and activating migration of the cells. The proliferative phase usually begins four days after the injury and lasts for several weeks. This stage is characterized by the formation of granulation tissue, which consists of a capillary bed, fibroblasts, collagen, and fibronectin. The last maturational phase begins about eight days after the injury and last for one year or longer. This phase is the period of scar contraction with collagen deposition and remodeling (1,2). Approximately 20% of normal tensile strength is measured at three weeks after surgery, and it will reach 70% to 80% after one year (3).

Due to inflammation in the first phase, more exudate is produced by the wound. The wound is examined and the dressings changed daily during the first three days. At this time, absorbent dressings are recommended. By the third day, the exudate is decreased and clear serous or serosanguinous, which means that the wound is transfering from the inflammatory phase to the proliferative phase. Since there is less exudates, there is no need for frequent dressing changes during this phase. The granulation tissue can be palpated from seven to nine days after the operation, and is known as the healing ridge, which indicates good wound healing and the beginning of the maturational phrase. If there is persistent exudate after three days, the wound healing process may be delayed; therefore attention should be paid to risk factors which should be identified and corrected to prevent infection or other complications.

Wounds left open because of infection or secondary or tertiary closure undergo a different healing process. The inflammation phase lasts until the infection is under control, necrotic tissue is removed, and risk factors are corrected. More exudate is produced during this phase and thus must be drained. The proliferative phase is longer because more granulation tissue is needed to fill a larger space as a result of a larger defect in the open wound. Occasionally, the wound develops into a nonhealing chronic wound, which is quite different from the acute wound from a biological and chemical environment perspective. Researchers found the fibroblast senescence (4,5) and the abnormal levels of proteinases (6), growth factors, and cytokines (7) in the chronic wound. However, these changes are the consequence of delayed healing and not the cause of nonhealing surgical wounds. The first key point is to perform wound bed preparation, which is the topical treatment for forcing the chronic wound to resume the characteristics of an acute wound (8). The other key point is to check the case history carefully and correct the possible risk factors that may prevent adequate healing.

FACTORS IMPEDING WOUND HEALING

The factors impeding wound healing are divided into two main groups: personal factors and surgical factors (Table 1). The personal factors can be subdivided into (1) the systemic factors related to the entire body and (2) the local factors, associated with the wound directly. Risk factors may also be divided into three groups: (1) preoperative, (2) operative, and (3) postoperative (2,9–12).

Often a patient is seen with multiple coexisting risk factors, and that combination increases the postoperative morbidity rate. For example, diabetic patients commonly suffer from impaired nutrition and anemia. Tissue hypoalbuminemia due to impaired local circulation causes locally prohibited chemotaxis and disabled movement capacity of inflammatory cells. As a result, diabetic wounds are predisposed to develop infection. The malnutrition and hypoproteinemia are coexisting in surgical patients with malignancies. These patients sometimes undergo chemotherapy or radiotherapy, which is also negatively influencing the future wound healing.

There is evidence in the literature that shows systemic factors are of great importance, not only to wound healing but also to patient outcome. Monitoring of the vital signs, controlling serum glucose and albumin levels, electrolyte balance, oxygen saturation, and adequate

Table 1 Factors Impeding Wound Healing

Category	Factors
	Advanced age
	Obesity
	Anemia
	Hypoxia
Systemic	Malignancy
	Jaundice
	Smoking
Personal	Underlying disease: diabetes, severe systemic diseases
	Malnutrition: deficiencies of vitamins, hypoalbuminemia
	Immunosuppression: steroids, chemotherapy
	Ischemia
Local	Infection
	Debris or necrotic tissue
	Local radiotherapy
	Major operation
	Long operation time and incision
	Intraoperative contamination
	Intraoperative hypotension
	Inadequate hemostasis
Surgical	Too much tension
	Broken or loose suture
	Foreign body
	Ostomy next to the wound
	Increased abdominal pressure

nutrition are mandatory for high-risk patients at all stages of the perioperative period, including anesthetic management.

Surgical factors that are important include meticulous techniques, adequate hemostasis, and maintaining a sterile field. Recently, research has indicated that various suture materials also make a difference. However, one meta-analysis indicated there are no differences between absorbable sutures and nonabsorbable sutures in the management of traumatic lacerations and surgical wounds as far as cosmetic outcomes and complications are concerned (12). In many practices, the midline incision is closed using two #1 double-stranded PDS-2 sutures (or #1 Vircryl suture) from each end of the incision, with both sutures meeting in the middle and the knots buried below the fascia. The skin is often closed with clips after the subcutaneous layers are irrigated and verified for meticulous hemostasis. One may avoid application of the electric coagulation, or curette the edge of the subcutaneous tissue in order to remove those damaged by electric coagulation for obese patients. For high-risk patients, retention sutures are suggested. This closure method has a good outcome because the wound is closed in bulk and no foreign body (suture knot) is left in the subcutaneous layers.

WOUND MANAGEMENT PRINCIPLES

Wound care in the colorectal ambulatory setting primarily deals with wounds with minor complications, and sometimes chronic wounds. Wounds with serious complications usually require additional surgical operations, and may even require consultation with the plastic surgeon.

There are several common principles for wound management: removal of necrotic tissue and foreign bodies, eliminating dead space, drainage of exudates, prevention from and control of infection, keeping the wound moist, and protection of the wound and the skin around the wound. All of these principles are equally important in wound management. Based on these principles, the **TIME** acronym is accepted as the principle for the wound bed preparation for the chronic wound: **T**issue, nonviable or deficit; **I**nfection or inflammation; **M**oisture imbalance; **E**dge of wound, advancing or undermined. The edge of wound is recognized as an important factor for chronic wound healing (8,13).

Historically, it was believed that the dry environment promotes wound healing, since the exudate would increase infection and it needs to be drained. In 1962, Winter (14), in a study in pigs, reported that the moist environment is better for healing and increases the rate of epithelization of superficial skin wounds. Currently, it is widely accepted that moisture is optimal for wound healing because of multiple physiological activities, including cell maneuvering, growth, function, and proliferation, all of which are facilitated in a moist environment (15). However, it is not easy to keep a wound moist due to the duel processes of wound evaporation and hydration. Therefore, it is necessary to maintain the moisture balance to evaluate wounds and choose an appropriate dressing. Dead space implies a space or cavity, which is apt to accumulate exudates. Although this promotes a moist environment, this may predispose to infection. In order to prevent this from causing infection, it has been suggested to fill the dead space with a dressing and keep the outlet large enough to drain the exudate and facilitate packing.

WOUND DRESSINGS

Wound dressing materials are one of the fastest developing fields in medical industry. Various new products are introduced every year providing different choices for surgeons and nurses involved in wound care, therefore helping to improve patient clinical outcomes. The modern dressings are devised to overcome local risk factors and promote wound healing. It is important to know the characteristics of different types of dressings and choose the optimal one for a specific wound. Wound dressings are divided into various groups which are shown in Table 2 (2,15–18).

Some dressings are composed of multiple components such as hydrofiber plus silver (Aquacel-AG), which can absorb exudate and simultaneously inhibit bacteria growth. This has gained extensive application in the management of the infectious wound. The dressing

Table 2 Types and Properties of Wound Dressings

Dressings type	Typical example	Properties
Absorb	Polyurethane Foam dressings Hydrofiber Ca-alginates	The absorbent dressing used to absorb exudate while maintaining a moist wound environment, they are used for wounds with moderate to large amounts of exudate thus preventing a wet and infectious medium. The alginates and hydrofibers can absorb 15 to 20 times their weight of fluid and are suitable for moderate to large exuding wounds.
Hydrate	Normal saline Hydrogel	The hydrating dressing can donate water to the wound and help keep a moist environment, used for wounds without or with minimal exudate.
Debride	0.25% Dakins Enzyme	Debride dressings can exliminate necrostic tissue as one method of nonsurgical debridement.
Antiseptic and Antibacterial	Silver dressings 0.25% Dakins 0.25% Acetic acid Cadexomer iodine	The silver dressings are used very extensively. Antibacterials are used to decrease wound bioburden
Biologicals	Enzyme Collagen Acellular dermal matrix	The biological dressings can provide biological factors, for example, collagen to the wound bed to enhance healing, or the enzyme to remove or liquefy necrotic tissue as one method of nonsurgical debridement.
Occlusive	Hydrocolloid Transparent films	The occlusive dressing is used to protect and separate the wound from outside contamination. Autolytic debridement is facilitated with this dressing
Negative pressure	Vacuum assisted Wound closure	Negative pressure dressings are used for removing drainage from wounds and encouraging granulation, especially for the wound with a high-output enterocutaneous fistula and abdominal wall defect.
Healing supplements	Arnica, Bromelain, Vitamin K cream	The nutritional supplement from dressings is under research, but hasn't gained extensive application.
Chinese traditional dressings	Multiple herb component	Debridement of necrotic tissue and promotion of granulation tissue growth

combination of alginate and collagen (Fibracol Plus) can drain the exudate and provide structural support to the wound.

The Vacuum Assisted Wound Closure system (VAC)—or VAC dressings—is an important development in this field. This system includes several items: foam, drape, pad, canisters, and pump. After the black granular foam dressing is cut to fit the wound, the thin and adhesive film drape is used to cover the foam and keep the entire wound completely sealed. A round 1.5 cm diameter hole is then cut out of the drape. A pad is attached to the hole and connected to the pump. The foam dressing has reticulated pores to help evenly distribute negative pressure to the entire wound. The VAC system has multiple roles: it removes the exudates and infectious material, reduces edema, promotes granulation, and provides an airtight wound. This may be an effective device for difficult and complicated wounds.

WOUND ASSESSMENT AND MANAGEMENT OPTIONS

Wound assessment is the initial step in wound management. This includes three steps: (1) inquiry, (2) inspection, and (3) palpation. Upon initial evaluation, the patient's history (medical and surgical) and symptoms need to be reviewed. The wound is then carefully examined and the entire incision exposed. The location, size, and depth of the wound need to be recorded, together with the description of the wound bed. The type, color, smell, and amount of the exudates must also be assessed. Palpation of the wound and inspection of the surrounding skin (color, tenderness, edema, and induration) should also be assessed. One should look for any signs of inflammation, soft tissue cellulites, and possible wound abscess. The clinical assessment

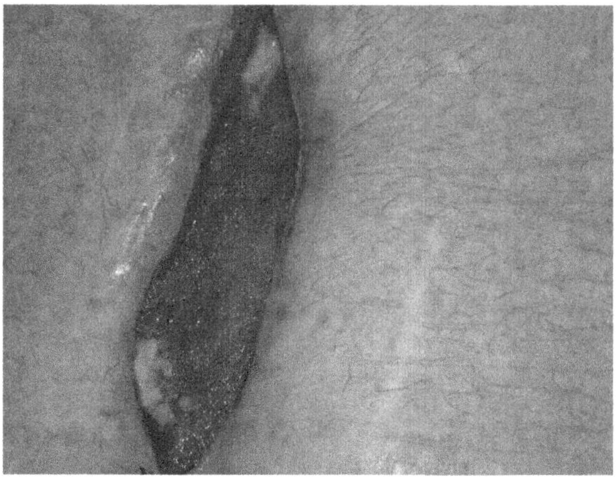

Figure 1 Clean granulating wound.

of the wound may be supplemented by tissue culture and biopsy. In some difficult situations, repeated observations must be carried out over the next few hours or in next few days to identify the trend of the particular wound. At the same time, patients are educated about the wound and instructed on how to change the dressing by themselves or with the assistance of the home health-care staff. Finally, wound reassessment and adjustment are required during the follow-up period.

WOUND DESCRIPTIONS

Clean Granulating Wound

The clean granulating wound has healthy granulation tissue which is red and firm; this indicates that the wound is in the proliferative phase and is healing well (Fig. 1). This is usually seen after the necrotic tissue is removed and the infection is under control. It is not difficult to care for this kind of wound, but the surgeon needs to adhere to two principal aspects: (1) eliminating the dead space and encouraging healing from the bottom to the top; (2) keeping a moist environment. Hydrocolloid dressings are suggested for shallow wounds with little exudates, while the alginates or foam dressings can be applied to deeper wounds with significant exudate.

An exception to this basic rule is wounds related to Crohn's disease; these patients present with loose nongranular tissue (Fig. 2) which is not healthy granulating tissue. This tissue is semitransparent light red in color and soft, which is often different from the healthy granulation tissue. This impaired repair phenomenon is not clearly defined, but this tissue should be removed by silver nitrate (Fig. 3) or debridement (normal saline wet to dry gauze, enzymes, conservative sharp) to promote healthy granulation tissue.

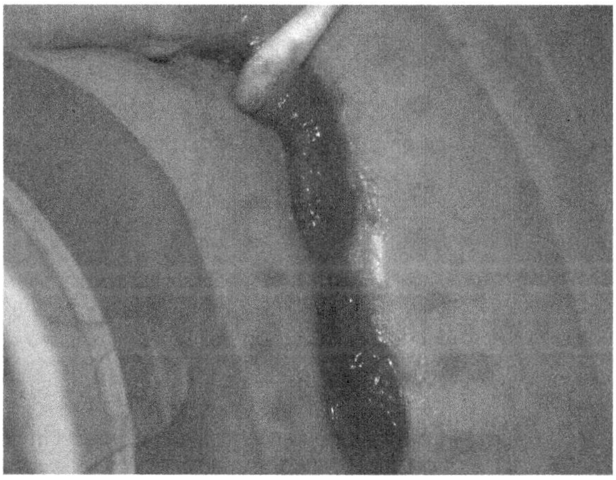

Figure 2 Loose nongranular tissue.

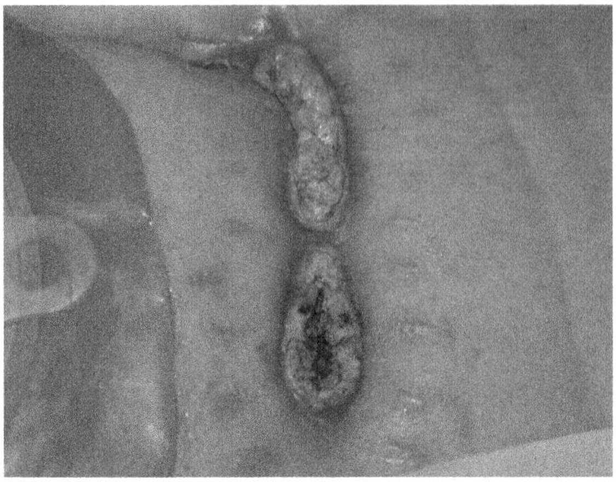

Figure 3 Loose nongranular tissue treated by silver nitrate.

Infected Wound

Postoperative wound infections are a major cause of morbidity, especially in patients undergoing colorectal surgery where the colon is opened and the wounds are exposed to a variety of bacteria in very high numbers. Konishi et al. (19) reported that the incidence of incisional infection is higher in rectal surgery than in colon surgery. Risk factors for developing incisional infection in colon surgery are patients undergoing a stoma closure and a lack of oral antibiotics, while in patients undergoing rectal surgery, preoperative steroids, preoperative radiation, and ostomy creation are risk factors. Wound infection rates are higher for patients with a stoma creation (19,20). Stoma creation is common in colorectal surgery on either a temporary or permanent basis. It is important to separate the contaminated stomal contents from the wound and to change the dressings frequently in patients with a stoma (Fig. 4). Preoperative administration of antibiotics, meticulous hemostasis to prevent wound hematomas, prevention of stool spillage, and eliminating accumulation of exudates (Fig. 5) are very important in reducing the rate of wound infections.

Infection usually involves the skin or subcutaneous tissue around the incision with symptoms or signs of infection such as pain, tenderness, localized swelling, redness, or heat (21,22). The most important principle in managing the infected wound is the complete drainage of pus. The incision should be left open and if the wound is deep, it should be packed with normal saline-moistened gauze or an antibacterial dressing. Application of silver absorptive dressings (Aquacel Ag) would help the tissue repair process and address bacterial loads. Antibiotics are not necessary in most cases, but should be considered for severe infection and surrounding cellulitis. The choice of antibiotics will depend on the culture report and clinical experience.

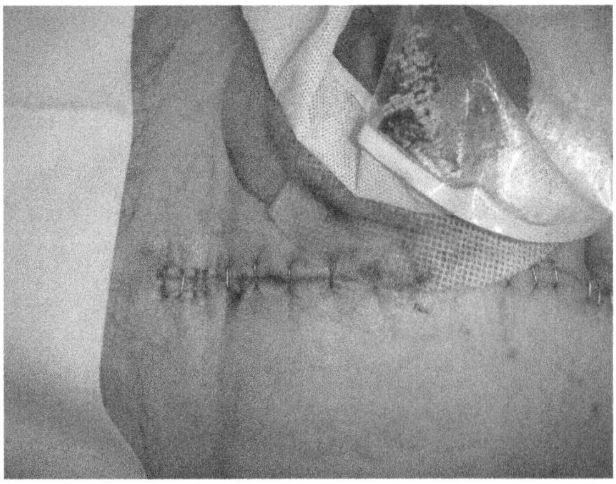

Figure 4 Wound contamination by stool from leaking ostomy bag.

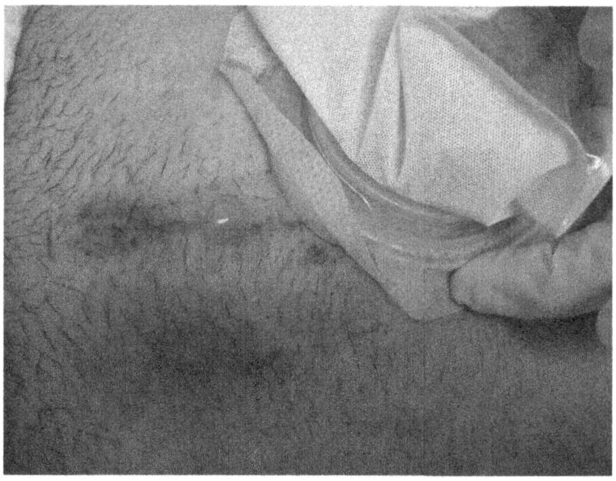

Figure 5 Wound infection next to ostomy.

Necrotic Wound

The tissue will develop necrosis because of ischemia (Fig. 6) and infection. Furthermore, the nonviable tissue is a good medium for bacterial growth. This may cause pain, infection, and delayed wound healing. It is important to remove necrotic tissue from the wound, either by surgical debridement or by nonsurgical methods. Nonsurgical debridement of necrotic tissue can be performed in different ways; autolytic, biological, chemical, and mechanical methods have all been used (23).

Surgical methods (sharp debridement), either in the operation room or in the office, can remove not only the nonviable tissue, but also the ischemic, unhealthy tissue, thick fibrotic wall, and redundant skin edges. A scalpel, curette, or scissors can be used. Debridement is quick and effective and can be used for all kinds of necrotic tissue, especially for abundant necrotic tissue or tough tissue such as fascia. Local or general anesthesia may be required and the procedure requires an experienced surgeon to avoid serious complications such as intestinal fistula from the dehisced abdominal wound.

Among nonsurgical methods, the autolytic debridement by phagocytic cells and proteolytic enzymes is a natural part of wound healing. This process is accelerated in the moist environment and inhibited by infection.

The chemical/antiseptic method was been used for many years. For example, Dakin's solution, developed during World War I, contains sodium hydrochloride and boric acid which can dissolve dead cells. However, Dakin's solution has simultaneous harmful effects on healthy tissue and is less often used as a result. Dakins is considered safe to granulation tissue in lower concentrations (0.25%); however, the skin adjacent to the wound should be protected with a skin sealant or Vaseline.

Mechanical debridement is commonly used and may vary from normal saline forceful irrigation and normal saline wet to dry gauze. In order to remove necrotic tissue via mechanical

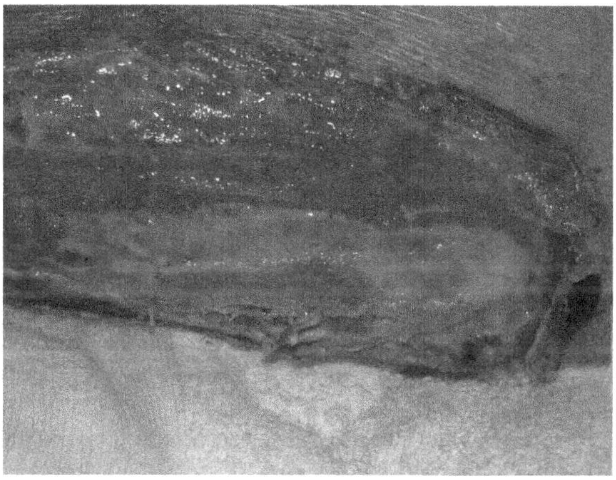

Figure 6 Necrotic tissue.

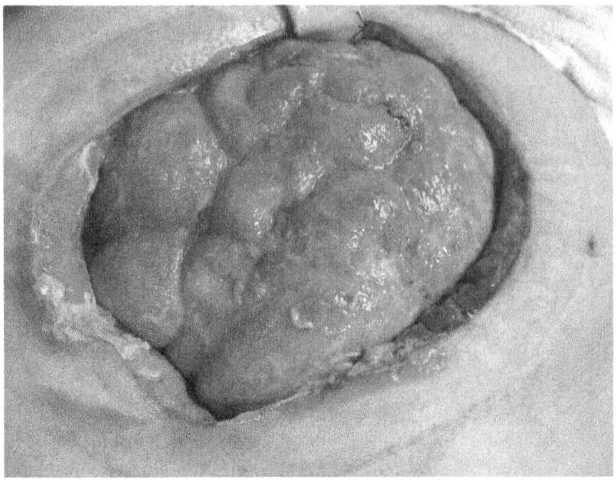

Figure 7 The open wound exposed bowel.

forces, a new development has been described. Granick et al. (24) reported the clinical outcome of a new device, Versajet Hydrosurgery, which removes the necrotic and adjacent tissue by force of the high velocity stream of sterile saline. Forty patients who had waterjet debridement were retrospectively compared with 22 patients with similar wounds who underwent operative surgical debridement. The waterjet group had significantly fewer procedures, which resulted in less expense. This new device has benefits in certain patients; however, a prospective study needs to be conducted.

Dehisced Wound

Fascial dehiscence (or full-thickness dehiscence) of the abdominal incision is a serious complication following colorectal surgery (Figs. 7 and 8). It usually occurs about one week after the initial surgery, although it is possible to occur even on the first day after surgery. Multiple factors may contribute to this type of wound, including most of the factors mentioned in Table 1. Surgical technique is one of the most important among them. Applying retention sutures and the use of an abdominal binder may help to prevent this complication in high-risk cases. Typical symptoms include acute incisional pain and a popping sensation following a violent cough or difficult defecation, which cause increased abdominal pressure. Physical examination may show the characteristic pink serous drainage from the incision if the skin is intact or the small intestine herniation if gross evisceration occurs.

The open abdomen may be complicated by serious electrolyte abnormalities, disabled intestinal function, intestinal fistula, and fatal abdominal infection. Therefore, it is best to reclose the incision with retention sutures as soon as possible. For those patients who cannot withstand this surgery, such as those suffering from critical wound infection or are in poor general health, conservative treatment provides another option. In this situation, the main objective of wound management is not only to promote wound healing, but also to separate and protect the

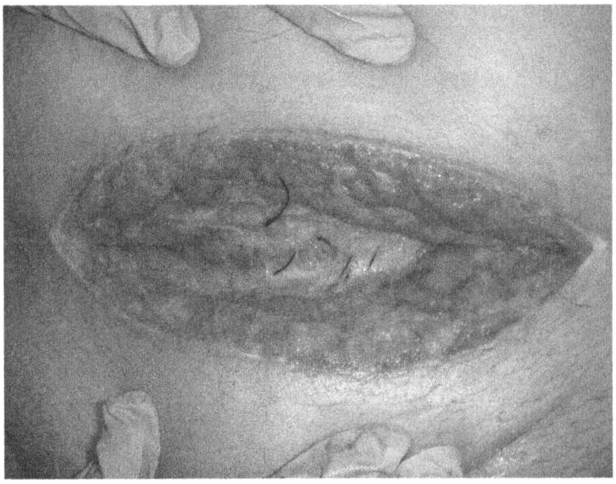

Figure 8 Fascial dehiscence because of broken suture.

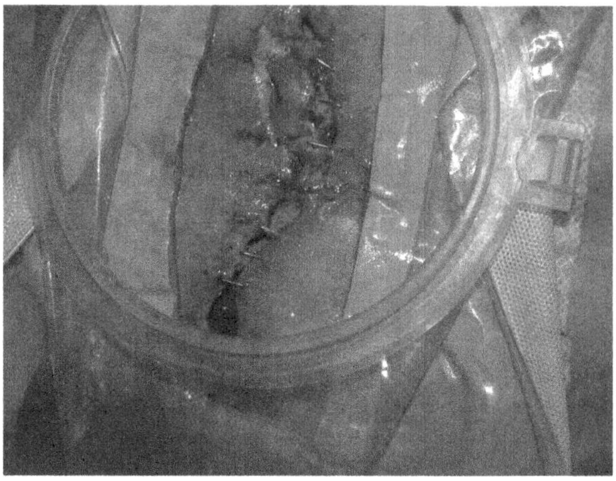

Figure 9 Traditional TX Wound Manager Pouch.

abdominal cavity from external contamination. A variety of dressings mentioned above could be used to meet this objective (Figs. 9 and 10) (2). The VAC dressings are routinely used in these situations, which have many advantages over the traditional saline-soaked gauze dressings. There are several key points that need to be considered for the VAC dressing: (1) the wound must be adequately debrided, (2) all necrotic tissue must be removed along with old suture material, (3) a nonadhesive dressing should be used to separate the bowel from the VAC dressing, and (4) no signs of abdominal sepsis may be present.

Heller et al. (25) reported VAC therapy for 21 patients suffering from wound dehiscence; 13 of these patients had fascial dehiscence. Stable cutaneous coverage was ultimately achieved in all patients by skin grafting (nine patients), local abdominal skin advancement flap (six patients), or secondary intention healing (six patients). During the follow-up period of more than six months, no patients required reassessment for wound healing problems and no patients developed reopening of the wound. Rao's group (26) treated 29 patients suffering from open wounds with a VAC dressing, six of whom developed a small bowel fistula. Four of these patients died, all from multi-organ failure. This study raises concerns that a high incidence of intestinal leakage is a result of VAC therapy and suggests that this may be ideal therapy for patients with a bowel anastomosis or enterotomy repairs. Petroleum-based gauze and low negative pressure (125 mm Hg) are the keys to preventing new fistulae from developing in the dehisced abdominal wound. In the ambulatory setting, most patients will use the Freedom VAC, which is a smaller portable unit.

After the infection is controlled or the general health status is improved, tertiary wound closure or skin grafting is considered. At this time, the implantation of biological dressings (acellular dermal matrix; ADM) (Fig. 11) or Vicryl mesh is practical. There have been reports that show good outcomes even in contaminated wounds. Schuster et al. reported on the application of ADM for 18 patients with contaminated abdominal wall defects (27). Primary closure was

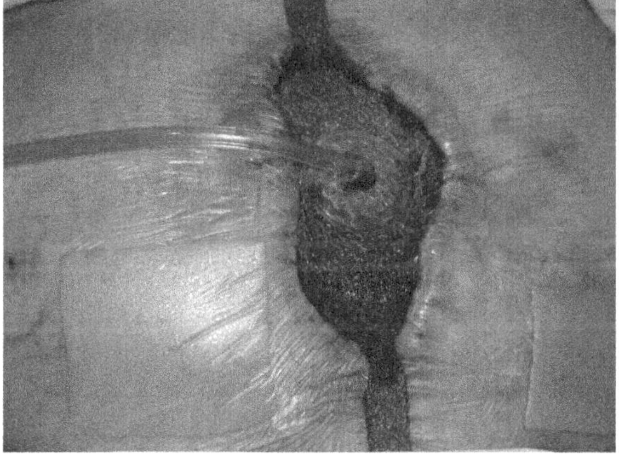

Figure 10 VAC for dehisced wound.

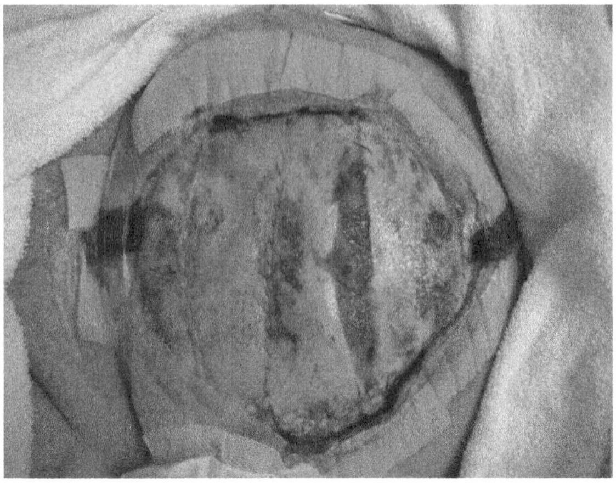

Figure 11 The implantation of Alloderm (acellular dermal matrix).

performed on 12 patients while six were left with open wounds. During the average follow-up period of 9.1 months, patients who did not have primary closure had a higher recurrence rate (5/6 vs. 4/12). Patton et al. placed ADM for 67 patients with complex and contaminated abdominal wound (28). The mean follow-up period was 10.6 months; 16 patients developed a wound infection, two required removal of the ADM, and 12 developed a recurrent hernia. This type of material provides an opportunity for high-risk patients, but the long-term outcome is still questionable.

Foreign Body

The common foreign body seen in the surgical wound is suture material (Fig. 12) followed by artificial implants. In colorectal surgery, the most common artificial implants are synthetic mesh, artificial bowel sphincter, anal fistula plugs, and stimulator devices for sacral nerve stimulation. In the unhealed and chronic wound, the suture knot (Fig. 13) can induce infection and should be removed. Meticulous adherence to aseptic technique is the key to preventing infectious complications of the artificial implant. In cases of infection, the implant should be removed from the wound.

SPECIFIC CONSIDERATIONS

Wound with Enterocutaneous Fistula

Historically this problem posed a challenge and resulted in a high mortality. The alkaline enzymatic pancreatic and bilious secretions from the small bowel erode the wound itself and the surrounding skin, which leads to difficult to manage wound infection (Fig. 14).

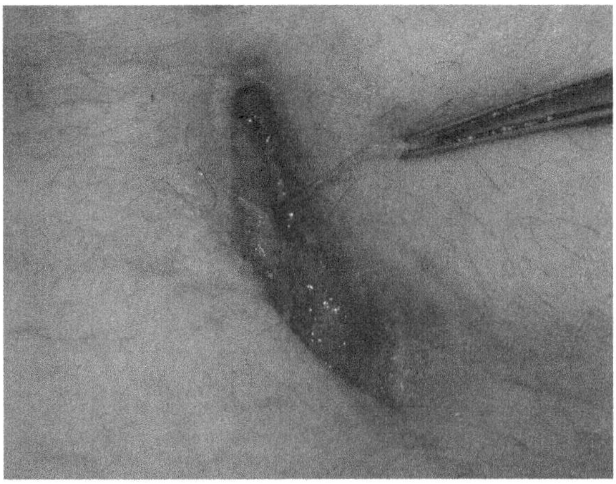

Figure 12 #12 PDS Suture.

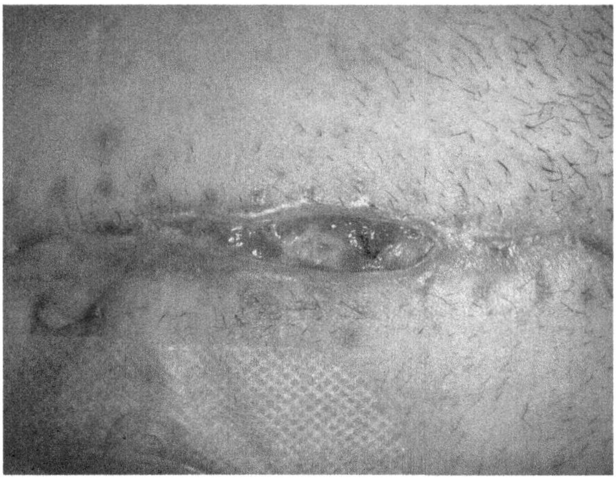

Figure 13 Suture knot.

Currently, the use of VAC dressings (Fig. 15(A–E)) and total parenteral nutrition has improved outcomes of fistula wound management. Many institutions use a VAC treatment including the placement of a single layer of petroleum-based gauze or equivalent (cellulose, Versafoam, nonadherents) in order to separate the bowel from the foam (Fig. 16). Small fistulas can contact the granular foam directly, but the nonadherent dressing and Versafoam are needed to protect the mucosa of the fistula and the pseudostoma (Fig. 17).

With VAC treatment, fistula sometimes closes and the wounds often granulose. A larg wound may be left for skin grafting. Sometimes the fistula develops into a pseudostoma and will need reoperation after the systemic and local conditions are improved. A new method was introduced to close a high-output enterocutaneous fistula and an associated abdominal wall defect (29). The serratus muscle or a composite free latissimus dorsi-serratus flap and a musculocutaneous latissimus dorsi flap have been used to close the fistula and the large abdominal defect respectively. The VAC system has been placed between the two flaps, resembling a sandwich. The fistula of a 73-year-old patient closed successfully after seven months of failed treatment. The authors believe this "sandwich" design provides an extraperitoneal approach with tension-free closure of the fistula and the abdominal wall.

Perineal Wound

The perineal wound is another challenge to colorectal surgeons because it is prone to contamination and gross infection (Fig. 18). Perineals wounds are created after all types of anal surgery such as hemorrhoidectomy, fistula surgery, implantation of artificial bowel sphincter, transanal resection of tumors, and abdominoperineal resections (APRs). One option to manage the perineal wound is to control the bowel movement, either by medically incuding constipation or by surgically diverting the fecal stream. Another option is to leave the wound open for drainage. The patients are instructed to wash the open wounds daily and after defecation.

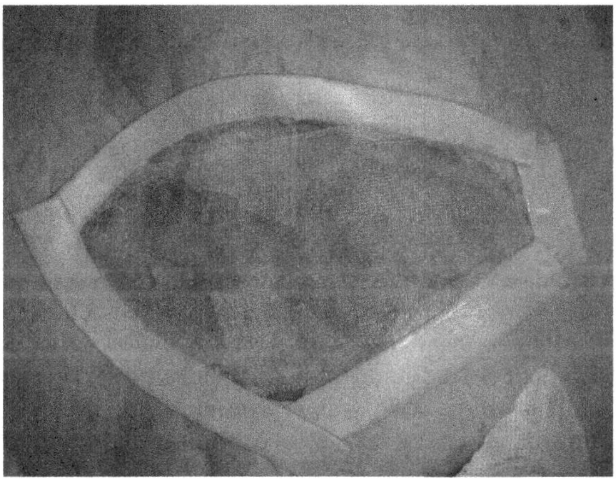

Figure 14 Wound with fistula and full-thickness abdominal wall defect.

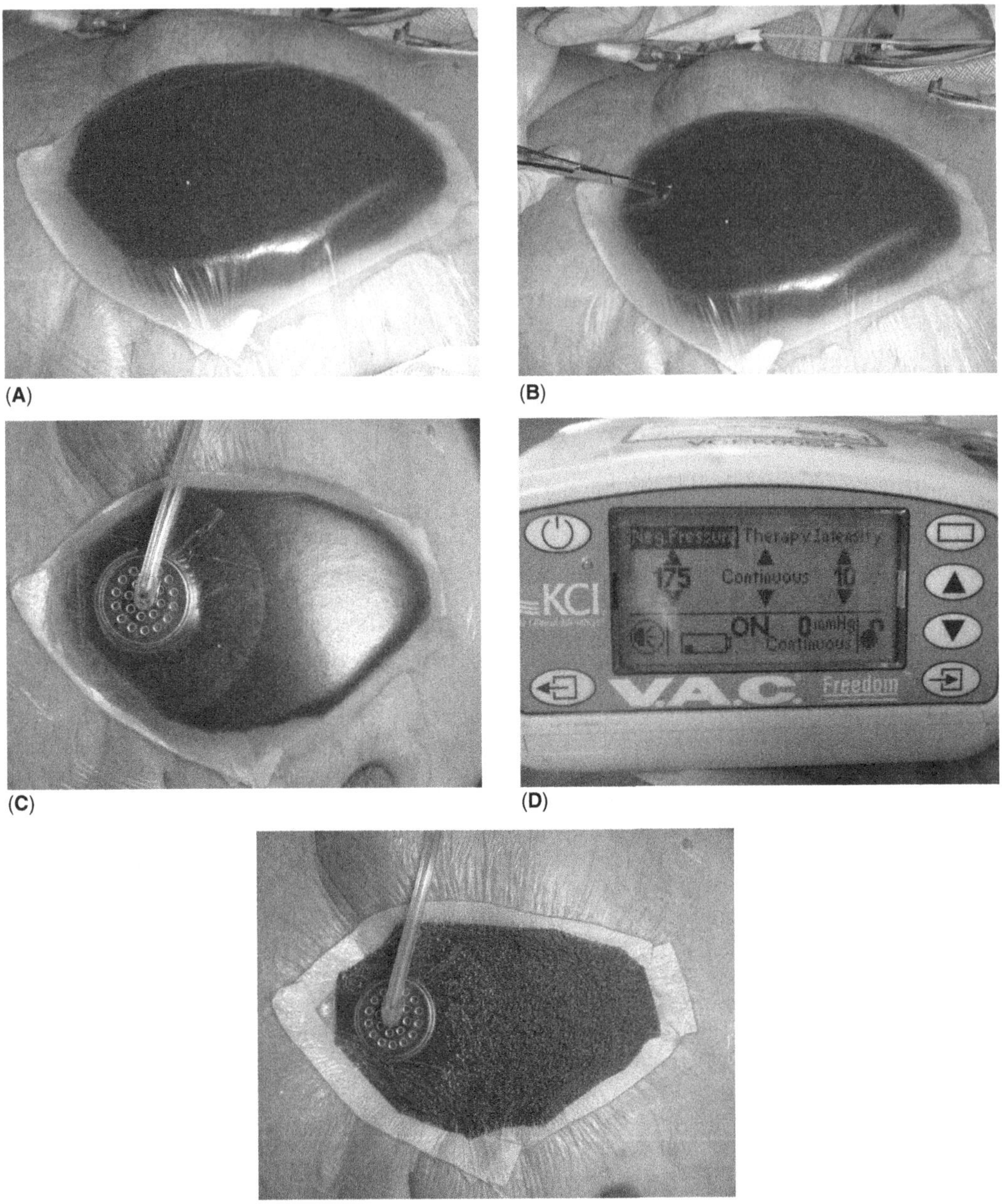

Figure 15 (**A**) VAC drape used to cover foam dressing and surrounding skin with an airtight seal. (**B**) Cutting a hole in the drape with a diameter of 1.5 cm just above the fistula for maximum suction. (**C**) VAC trac-pad and collection tube connected to canister on pump. (**D**) Freedom VAC system with a negative pressure of 175 mm Hg used for home care of the wound. (**E**) VAC foam after negative pressure initiated (air suctioned).

Another unique situation is the perineal wound after APR. Although multiple methods have been reported to decrease the rate of septic perineal wound complications after APR (30), the unhealed perineal wound remains a major problem, especially for patients with risk factors. The dead space created by removing large amounts of tissue, the bony pelvis resulting in drainage accumulation and infection, the difficulties associated with dressing these wounds, and changing the dressings, combined with the effects of chemotherapy and radiation, all make this a very difficult wound to treat. Often risk factors for impaired perineal wound healing include distant metastases, excessive alcohol consumption, and smoking (31). Hyman has defined the

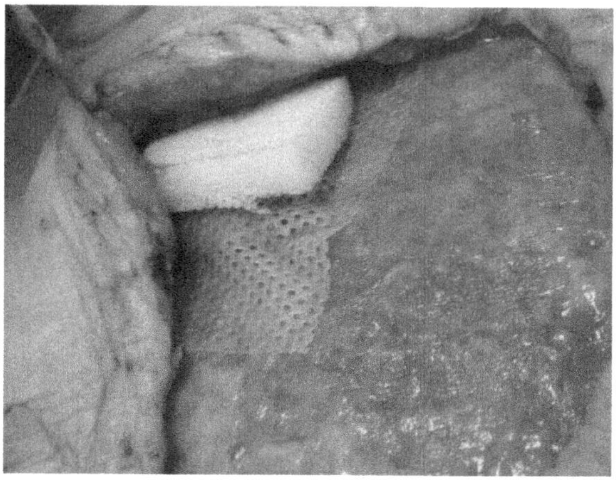

Figure 16 Nonadherent dressing and Versafoam to protect the pseudostoma.

unhealed perineal wound as that wound that is unhealed six months after operation (32). A wound with superficial sinuses could be successfully treated by curettage which can be repeated several times to ensure that healing occurs from the bottom up, while the large open may require a two-step procedure for closure and healing. This process may include complete debridement of the fibrotic rind followed by placement of healthy, well-vascularized tissue such as the gracilis muscle (32).

Laparoscopic Wound

It is now widely accepted that there are fewer wound-related complications after laparoscopic surgery than after open surgery. Yamamoto et al. (33) showed stoma creation and intraoperative hypotension to be significant risk factors for wound infection specific to elective laparoscopic surgery for colorectal carcinoma. The laparoscopic patients required less hospital readmissions and reoperations, which resulted in fewer hospital costs. Dobson et al. (34) compared 603 consecutive laparoscopic colorectal procedures with 2246 consecutive open colorectal surgery. They identified wound infection in 5.8% ($n = 25$) of the laparoscopic group and 4.8% ($n = 65$) of the open group. Only one of the laparoscopic patients required hospital readmission but none required reoperation, while in the open surgery group 52% (34/65) required hospital readmission and 12% (8/65) required reoperation. In addition, patients in the open surgery group had far greater expenses related to wound dressing changes and VAC application.

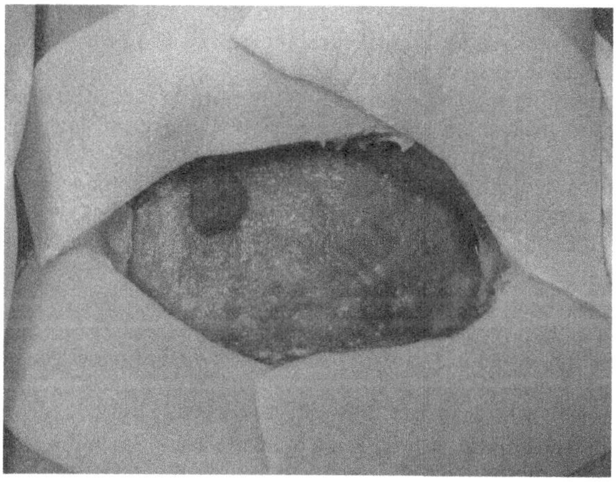

Figure 17 Pseudostomas may need surgical closure.

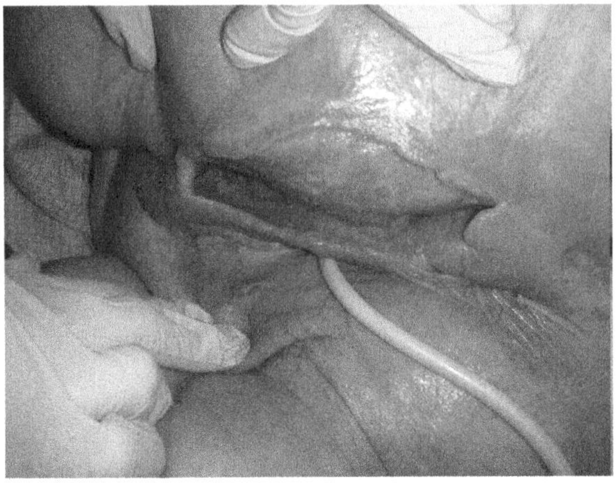

Figure 18 Perineal wound.

SUMMARY

In the wound management practice, multiple risk factors that impede the healing of wounds should be identified and corrected. The specific characteristics of the wound should then be assessed in detail in order to choose optimal management and dressings based on the wound healing principles, as outlined. In addition, other clinical considerations should be assessed. In this way, wound healing can be accelerated and good clinical outcomes obtained.

REFERENCES

1. Phillips LG, Leong M. Wound Healing. In : Townsend CMJ, ed. Sabiston Textbook of Surgery. St. Louis: Elsevier, 2004.
2. Hahler B. Surgical wound dehiscence. Medsurg Nurs 2006; 15(5):296–300.
3. Jones V, Bale S, Harding K. Acute and chronic wounds. In: Baranoski S, Ayello EA, eds. Wound Care Essentials: Practice Principles. Philadelphia: Lippincott-Williams and Wilkins, 2004:61–78.
4. Henderson EA. The potential effect of fibroblast senescence on wound healing and the chronic wound environment. J Wound Care 2006; 15(7):315–318.
5. Mendez MV. Fibroblasts cultured from distal lower extremities in patients with venous reflux display cellular characteristics of senescence. J Vasc Surg 1998; 28(6):1040–1050.
6. Pirila E. Collagenase-2 (MMP-8) and matrilysin-2 (MMP-26) expression in human wounds of different etiologies. Wound Repair Regen 2007; 15(1):47–57.
7. Trengove NJ, Bielefeldt-Ohmann H, Stacey MC. Mitogenic activity and cytokine levels in non-healing and healing chronic leg ulcers. Wound Repair Regen 2000; 8(1):13–25.
8. Schultz GS. Wound bed preparation: a systematic approach to wound management. Wound Repair Regen 2003; 11(suppl1):S1–S28.
9. Adams SB Jr, Sabesan VJ, Easley ME. Wound healing agents. Foot Ankle Clin 2006; 11(4):745–751.
10. Pompeo M. Misconceptions about Protein Requirements for Wound Healing: Results of a Prospective Study. Ostomy Wound Manage 2007; 53(8):30–44.
11. Chadwick MA. Short course preoperative radiotherapy is the single most important risk factor for perineal wound complications after abdominoperineal excision of the rectum. Colorectal Dis 2006; 8(9):756–761.
12. Al-Abdullah TA, Plint C, Fergusson D. Absorbable versus nonabsorbable sutures in the management of traumatic lacerations and surgical wounds: a meta-analysis. Pediatr Emerg Care 2007; 23(5):339–344.
13. Carville K. Which dressing should I use? It all depends on the 'TIMEING'. Aust Fam Physician 2006; 35(7):486–489.
14. Winter GD. Formation of the scab and the rate of epithelization of superficial wounds in the skin of the young domestic pig. Nature 1962; 193:293–294.
15. Brett DW. A review of moisture-control dressings in wound care. J Wound Ostomy Continence Nurs 2006; 33(6 suppl):S3–S8.
16. Jones V, Grey JE, Harding KG. Wound dressings. Br Med J 2006; 332(7544): 777–780.
17. Hess C, Dressings. In : Kowalak J, ed. Clinical Guide: Wound Care. Philadelphia: Springhouse, 2002:140–442.
18. Driver VR. Silver dressings in clinical practice. Ostomy Wound Manage 2004; 50(9 A suppl):11 S–15 S.

19. Konishi T. Elective colon and rectal surgery differ in risk factors for wound infection: results of prospective surveillance. Ann Surg 2006; 244(5):758–763.
20. Tang R. Risk factors for surgical site infection after elective resection of the colon and rectum: a single-center prospective study of 2,809 consecutive patients. Ann Surg 2001; 234(2):181–189.
21. Moore Z, Cowman S. Effective wound management: identifying criteria for infection. Nurs Stand 2007; 21(24):68,70,72.
22. Horan TC. CDC definitions of nosocomial surgical site infections,1992: a modification of CDC definitions of surgical wound infections. Am J Infect Control 1992; 20(5):271–274.
23. Falabella AF. Debridement and wound bed preparation. Dermatol Ther 2006; 19(6):317–325.
24. Granick MS. Efficacy and cost-effectiveness of a high-powered parallel waterjet for wound debridement. Wound Repair Regen 2006; 14(4):394–397.
25. Heller L, Levin SL, Butler CE. Management of abdominal wound dehiscence using vacuum assisted closure in patients with compromised healing. Am J Surg 2006; 191(2):165–172.
26. Rao M. The use of vacuum-assisted closure of abdominal wounds: a word of caution. Colorectal Dis 2007; 9(3):266–268.
27. Schuster Rl. The use of acellular dermal matrix for contaminated abdominal wall defects: wound status predicts success. Am J Surg 2006; 192(5):594–597.
28. Patton JH Jr, Berry S, Kralovich KA. Use of human acellular dermal matrix in complex and contaminated abdominal wall reconstructions. Am J Surg 2007; 193(3):360–363.
29. de Weerd L. The sandwich design: a new method to close a high-output enterocutaneous fistula and an associated abdominal wall defect. Ann Plast Surg 2007; 58(5):580–583.
30. Meyer L. Perineal wound closure after abdomino-perineal excision of the rectum. Tech Coloproctol 2004; 8(suppl 1):S230–S234.
31. Artioukh DY, Smith RA, Gokul K. Risk factors for impaired healing of the perineal wound after abdominoperineal resection of rectum for carcinoma. Colorectal Dis 2007; 9(4):362–367.
32. Hyman NH. Unhealed perineal wound. In: Fazio VW, Church JM, Delaney CP, eds. Current Therapy in Colon and Rectal Surgery. Philadelphia: Mosby, 2005, 241–243.
33. Yamamoto S, Fujita S, Akasu T, et al. Wound infection after elective laparoscopic surgery for colorectal carcinoma. Surg Endosc 2007; 21(12):2248–2252.
34. Dobson MW. Minimal wounds, minimal wound infections: laparoscopic surgery decreases morbidity of surgical site infections and decreases the cost of wound care. Dis Colon Rectum 2007; 50(5):722.

24 Ostomy Management

Mary Lou Boyer
Department of Colorectal Surgery, Cleveland Clinic Florida, Weston, Florida, U.S.A.

INTRODUCTION

A number of diagnoses may result in determining that a patient will undergo surgery requiring an ostomy. However, the specific diagnosis impacts what type of ostomy will be created, whether the ileostomy or colostomy will be temporary or permanent, where it will be located and even the patient's acceptance, and how he or she copes with the outcome. Informing the patient and family members of what procedure is to be performed and scheduling testing and other pre-op appointments can be a daunting task with innumerable issues to consider.

The patients often have a unique set of problems, questions, and concerns. They face a wide range of challenges encompassing both physical and emotional adjustments. Preoperative preparation and education are imperative as these patients will be learning a whole new set of behaviors related to caring for the ostomy, adapting to changes in body image, and experiencing other emotional issues that reach well beyond the patient and involving significant others and/or family members—challenges that can even impact the physicians and nursing staff caring for the patient.

This chapter focuses on preoperative preparation of the patient who will, or possibly will, undergo surgery requiring an ostomy, as well as postoperative follow-up in the ambulatory clinic setting. Discussion will include preoperative counseling, stoma site marking, postoperative clinic visits, ostomy management issues, stomal, and peristomal complications.

PREOPERATIVE MANAGEMENT

Once a diagnosis is made, the preoperative evaluation must focus on minimizing the patient's overall operative risk. Along with the orders for testing and medical exam, it is essential to explain the surgical procedure and expectations in as much detail as possible to the patient. It is important to explain this in terms that the patient will understand. It may require more than one explanation as the patient may not be able to process all of the information at this time since the period of time between learning of the need for surgery and the scheduled operation is one of the most difficult times for the patients. They may be dealing with a devastating diagnosis, a surgical procedure, and the idea of an ostomy. This is a very emotional time for patients and their family members as fears, questions, concerns, and uncertainties surface. Allowing ample time to discuss questions, fears, and concerns is often difficult in the office setting; however, it is a very important step toward success.

Education, while very important at this point, may be difficult as this is a time when the patient may find it hard to concentrate well enough to listen and remember much of the discussion. It may even be necessary to arrange for a second appointment for further discussion when the patient can better focus on ostomy-related information. Written information and resources provide an opportunity to review and reinforce what has been discussed.

Thorough preoperative preparation including teaching and knowledgeable counseling are key elements in preparing the patient for positive outcomes. Having access to a certified Wound Ostomy Continence Nurse (WOCN/Enterostomal Therapist) is a great advantage for the busy surgeon, and for the patient, as a WOCN has the education and training to evaluate the patient's readiness for learning, answer questions, counsel, and mark the proposed ostomy site. If a WOCN is not available, it will be the surgeon's responsibility to provide the required information and mark the stoma site.

PREOPERATIVE COUNSELING, STOMA SITE SELECTION, AND MARKING

Preoperative counseling and stoma site marking are critical components in preparing the patient for surgery and fostering positive outcomes. This preoperative visit provides an opportunity to instruct the patient and family members regarding the planned surgical procedure and expected results. It will also allow an opportunity to answer any questions the patient might have. The physician should initiate discussion by assessing the patient's knowledge of the diagnosis and surgical procedure as well as feelings concerning the surgery and family support system, and evaluate whether the person is receptive to information and how much information is desired. Some patients ask for as much information as possible, while other patients want very little. The physician should direct the discussion to accommodate individual needs, beliefs, cultural parameters, and language. In addition, the physician should consider physical disabilities or any limitations that could impact self-management such as vision or hearing problems, manual dexterity, skin sensitivities and allergies, emotional and mental status, psychosocial issues, language barriers, cultural and spiritual beliefs, and use of a prosthesis.

Ascertaining the patient's education level, type of employment, and normal physical activities aids individualizing information related to various aspects of living with an ostomy is also important. One should provide basic information about the stoma appearance, ostomy appliances, and stoma care. With the aid of pictures, diagrams, and pouching system components, the patient can better visualize procedures in an effort to increase understanding while simultaneously reducing fears. Written patient education materials are readily available from ostomy product manufacturers and from reliable internet sites (listed at the end of this chapter). Providing prepared materials eases the burden for the patient to remember all of the discussion and from having to search on their own for information. Patients may get anecdotal information from friends, neighbors, or unreliable internet sites with negative comments about poor outcomes regarding similar surgeries. This, in turn, increases fears and concerns. Patients who remain negative about surgery may not realize that they can live well without the body parts that need to be removed and may benefit from meeting or talking with someone who has successfully recovered from a similar surgery (1). Of note, the United Ostomy Association of America has a visitor program that can be accessed from their web site.

SITE MARKING

Preoperative stoma site selection is a critical component in preparing all patients scheduled for ostomy surgery regardless of whether the intended ostomy is temporary or permanent, and even if it is only a possibility that a stoma will be created. It is one of the most important factors in fostering optimal results and decreasing the possibility of ostomy-related complications. Eliminating this vital step can result in a stoma located in a position that makes it difficult, if not impossible, to allow normal activity and to manage without fear of leakage (2).

A difficult seal and leakage of effluent onto the skin can create further complications of denuded skin, pain, and increased physical and emotional stress on the patient, as well as increased time and money spent on supplies for ostomy care; poor placement can even lead to reoperation. Thus, preoperative stoma site marking can reduce many potential adverse outcomes.

Selecting and marking the best site for ostomy placement should be done by a qualified WOCN or the surgeon. In facilities that do not have a WOCN, the surgeon must thoroughly examine the patient's abdomen for folds, creases, scars, and other prostheses that can make pouch application and maintenance difficult.

Choosing the Site

The planned surgical procedure generally dictates the anatomic location by the type of stoma that will be created. Standard accepted practice supports siting an ileostomy or ascending colostomy on the right and a descending or sigmoid colostomy on the left. However, existing scars or certain irregular abdominal contours may prevent using the preferred sites. If there is a preexisting or potential urinary ostomy, it is generally sited on the right and the fecal ostomy on the left. If two sites are to be marked, one for fecal and the other for urinary diversion, the two sites are marked on different planes in case a belt is needed for one or the other.

There may be instances when the exact surgical procedure cannot be determined until after the abdomen is opened, thus creating the need to mark alternate sites. Optimal stoma site location parameters are within the rectus muscle to decrease chances of parastomal hernia or prolapse, on the apex of the infraumbilical mound, 3 to 4 inches from the planned incision, and within the patient's visual field. Placement of a stoma on or near scars, skin folds and/or deep creases, bony prominances, the umbilicus or waistline/beltline, costal margins, underside of a protuberant abdomen, pendulous breasts, or hanging/sagging abdominal pannus should be avoided. If a patient has any prostheses or supportive devices such as a brace, support belt, or uses a wheelchair, it is best to select the stoma site with the patient actually using the device.

With the above parameters in mind, the abdomen should be examined in the sitting, standing, and lying positions to identify the rectus muscle, belt line, and skin folds. The abdomen should be observed during position changes to detect any major creases, shifting skin folds or other factors that may interfere with pouch adherence. Drawing lines with a washable pen helps indicate any identified factors while searching for an area of the abdomen with at least 2 to 3 inches of even skin around any potential stoma site to allow for adequate adherence of the appliance seal (3). A faceplate (wafer) from an ostomy pouching system should be used as a guide to mark the site.

Once an optimal site has been determined, the patient should be able to see it. If pendulous breasts or a large abdomen obstruct visualizing the site, it may need to be altered; alternatively, a mirror may be necessary during pouch changes.

Special Considerations

A mucous fistula should be positioned 3 inches away from a functioning stoma or it will interfere with the appliance seal of the functioning stoma. If a patient is wheelchair bound, the site should be marked higher to increase visualization and allow for flow of effluent. In addition, pendulous breasts may chafe or cause difficulty in placing the pouching system, and obese patients may need to be marked in upper quadrants.

Except in emergency situations, it is unacceptable to determine stoma placement when the patient is supine on the operating table. No matter how perfect the site may appear when lying down, it can change dramatically when the patient is sitting or standing [Fig. 1(**A**)–(**C**)] (3).

Marking the Stoma Site

There are three generally accepted methods for marking the stoma site: tattoo, indelible marker, and laceration (Table 1) (4). Choosing the optimal method depends on the surgeon or patient preference as well as the amount of time between the marking session and the date of surgery.

Henna tattooing has been evaluated as an alternative to the permanent tattoo in marking stoma sites. A Henna tattoo may last longer than an indelible pen marker and also has the advantage that it is not permanent.

PLAN THE WELL-CONSTRUCTED STOMA

Although the intended stoma is only a part of the planned surgical procedure, it will need to be managed on a daily basis. The technique for constructing the stoma can make a considerable difference in whether the end result will be a well-functioning or problematic stoma. The amount of protrusion and location of the lumen play critical roles in preventing peristomal skin complications.

The ideal stoma has a centrally located lumen with some degree of protrusion and is created in the site that is most appropriate for successful management. Positioning the stomal lumen at skin level is a set-up for failure. A moderate length of 1 to 3 cm allows the effluent to flow into the ostomy pouch. A stoma that is less than 1 cm or flush with the skin can be very difficult to manage as there is not enough projection for flow of effluent directly into the pouching system. This is especially true during peristalsis when the stoma may retract, allowing leakage under the pouch faceplate, causing skin irritation and embarrassment. Conversely, a stoma that is very long can be psychologically disturbing to the patient as well as more difficult to disguise under clothing. It is also potentially more prone to injury from laceration, trauma, or from bending in the pouching system.

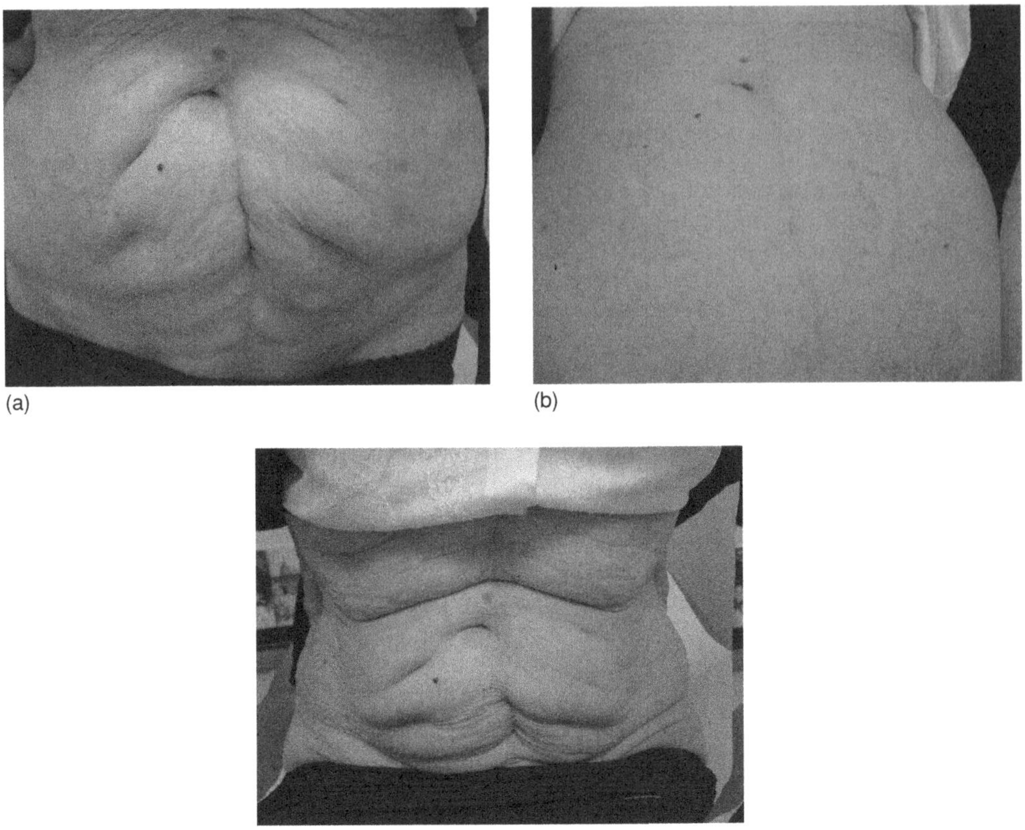

Figure 1 Stoma site marking: Patient in (**a**) standing, (**b**) lying, and (**c**) sitting positions, demonstrates importance of evaluating abdomen in different positions. Abdomen looks smooth lying down.

POSTOPERATIVE MANAGEMENT

Adjustment to living with an ostomy occurs gradually over time. Shortened hospital stays allow little time for the patient to learn complete self-management. Home health care is often ordered for continued teaching and assessment; however, not all patients take advantage of or have access to this type of service. Increased constraints on delivery of home care and varying insurance coverage can affect some aspects of care (5). All of these considerations lead to an increased need for evaluation in the outpatient ostomy clinic; ostomy patients should be seen in the clinic as early as two to four weeks after surgery, and for follow-up at 3, 6, and 12 months (6). If there are any complications, follow-up appointments should be set up, as needed. At each postoperative visit, the appliance should be removed, the stoma should be measured, and the stoma and surrounding skin should be inspected.

BASIC OSTOMY CARE

A number of different pouching systems are available for ostomy care (Table 2). Each system has a barrier that adheres to the skin with adhesive and is meant for a single use. There are a few adhesive systems that can be reused, those that employ a belt rather than adhesive; however, generally, adhesive-based systems are used. Most pouching systems are worn for three to seven days, depending on the type of effluent, the patient's skin type, and daily activities. In any event, the appliance should be kept in place for at least 24 hours to prevent skin trauma from frequent removal.

In the first six to eight weeks postoperatively, a cut-to-fit pouching system should be used as the size of the new stoma will gradually decrease. The wafer or skin barrier must be cut or

Table 1 Methods for Marking the Stoma Site

Method	Technique	Advantages	Disadvantages
Tattoo	*Methylene blue*—inject 0.01 mL of dye intradermally with a tuberculin syringe and 25-gauge needle. *India ink*—apply drop of India ink on the site. Puncture the skin through the drop of ink with a 25-gauge needle. Stretch the skin for better introduction of ink into the subcuticular tissue. Remove residual ink and apply a small dressing if needed.	A tattoo is permanent, easily recognized and cannot be erased during showers, presurgical abdominal preparation or operating room scrub.	Pain associated with needle puncture Permanent (if site is not used, the patient is left with lifelong permanent tattoo) Some patients object to needle puncture and/or permanent tattoo Certain cultural beliefs oppose tattoo marking More than one puncture may be necessary for clear visualization
Indelible marker	An X or circle is made with an indelible marking pen. Cover the mark with a transparent dressing to protect it from washing away.	Can remain visible 5–10 days (may send marker and dressing home with patient; instruct patient/family to darken if necessary).	It is necessary to scratch the mark on the skin with a needle or scalpel after the patient anesthetized so site still visible after abdominal preparation
Laceration	Scratch the skin surface with a sterile needle or lacerate the site superficially with a scalpel	Most often used in surgical setting just prior to surgical scrub to help identify the site as scrub may remove indelible ink marking.	This method is not recommended in the office setting as it is painful and because of risk of infection.

molded to the correct size and shape of the stoma. The most common skin complication after ostomy surgery is peristomal skin irritation from contact with effluent as the stoma size changes. Therefore, the patient should be shown how to adjust the appliance opening accordingly in order to protect the skin.

CHOOSING AN OSTOMY POUCHING SYSTEM

Ostomy pouching systems may be flat or convex and flexible or rigid, with varying degrees of convexity and flexibility. The goal in all cases is to provide a secure seal with predictable wear time to protect the skin from damaging effluent, protect the stoma from trauma, and prevent damage caused by products used for pouching. Determining the pouching system that is most appropriate for a given stoma depends on the degree of stoma protrusion, abdominal contour, size and shape of the stoma, the location of the stoma lumen (i.e., centered, to the side, skin level) and the type of effluent. Consideration should also be given to the patient's level

Table 2 Ostomy Appliances/Pouching Systems

One-Piece	Flat	Cut-to-fit
		Pre-cut
	Convex	Pre-cut
Two-Piece	Flat	Cut-to-fit
		Pre-cut
		Mold-to-fit
	Convex	Pre-cut
		Mold-to-fit

Notes: Most one and two-piece systems are available with a drainable or closed-end pouch. There are also specialty pouching systems for patients with severe reactions to adhesive systems or with unusual abdominal contour.

Table 3 General Guidelines for Choosing an Ostomy Pouching System

Characteristic	Challenge	Pouching system
Flat, firm abdomen	Convex systems sit too high on skin	Use a flat pouching system
Soft abdomen	Soft abdomen may shift with movement	Use a rigid faceplate or wafer to support soft abdomen around stoma. May also need to use belt or binder
Hard round abdomen	Pouching system needs to conform to shape	Use a flexible flat seal to conform to shape of abdomen. (The most flexible pouches are one piece)
Flushed, recessed, or retracted stoma	Effluent flows at skin level, erodes, and loosens pouch seal causing irritation to the skin	Use a convex faceplate to press down on skin to increase skin/adhesive contact and help increase degree of stoma protrusion to prevent undermining. Convexity comes in both rigid and flexible forms and with varying degrees of convexity from shallow to deep. Match the degree of convexity to the contour of the abdomen around the stoma
Deep creasing	Difficult to maintain adequate pouch seal	Need flexible pouching system and additional measures to increase adherence such as belt, double faced adhesives or contact cement
Stoma close to incision, scar, dip, or gully	Difficult to maintain adequate pouch seal	Use ostomy paste, barrier wafers, adhesive rings, and paste strips to fill in the defect to provide a flat area for sealing
Stoma fistula, peristomal fistula	Undermining of pouch adhesive seal Erosion of skin	Cut opening to allow fistula effluent to flow into pouch. Protect skin with barrier film, barrier wafer or paste strips. If fistula is a distance away from stoma, may need multiple pouches, smaller flanges or overlap adhesive portions of pouches

of physical activity, manual dexterity, visual acuity, mental awareness, and very importantly, patient preference.

Specific guidelines are used to determine the most appropriate system for different abdominal contours and degree of stomal protrusion (Table 3). Other factors to consider include matching the pouch to the contour of the patient's abdomen and that flexible pouching systems fold with the patient skin folds. In patients with a soft abdomen, creases can be matched or eliminated with a firm faceplate, by using convexity or a belted system. Patients with a very obese abdomen with large skin folds, creases, and a protuberant abdomen have a difficult time seeing the stoma. In these cases, a mirror or caregiver assistance may be needed. Finally, the use of adjunct products and creative measures increases pouch adherence (i.e., paste, cement, seals, belts) and fills in defects.

OUTPATIENT CARE

The initial outpatient visit should include removal of the appliance to assess the stoma appearance, function, and type of effluent, the adequacy of the pouching system (success or failure), and the peristomal skin. In addition, one should assess how well the patient is adjusting to having and caring for an ostomy. This is also the time to answer questions related to return to activities, sex and intimacy, travel, odor, and to discuss frequency of emptying as well as any night-time emptying that may be interrupting sleep.

POUCH REMOVAL AND APPLICATION TECHNIQUE

The patient should be taught the proper technique of caring for a stoma. This technique includes removing the old pouch by lifting a corner of the skin barrier wafer or tape edge, and avoiding trauma to the skin by pressing the skin away from the adhesive rather than pulling the pouch barrier away from the skin. A wet washcloth or gauze can be used to press the skin away. Adhesive remover may be used and is especially helpful for patients with sensitive skin or hair growth on the abdomen. The skin is then cleansed with warm water. The use of soaps are discouraged as deodorant soaps can be very drying to skin, while soaps with moisturizers may interfere with obtaining a secure seal. The stoma is measured to determine the exact size to cut the appliance opening. Measuring cards can be obtained from product manufacturers and are included in each box of pouches or wafers. If ostomy paste is used, it should be applied around the opening in order to come in contact with the skin only proximal to the stoma. The pouching system is then applied to dry skin and pressed to seal. The patient should be asked to apply light pressure with the palm of the hand to warm the appliance seal for increased adherence to the skin. It should be ascertained that the pouch tail is clamped or closed.

Pouch change frequency depends on the type of stoma, the location of the stoma, and the consistency of effluent. Most pouching systems are made to be worn for three to seven days. Liquid output may shorten wear time to an average of three to five days, while a sigmoid colostomy may average five to seven days. The patient with a colostomy that functions only once or twice per day may be able to use a disposable pouch that is removed daily after evacuation. The patient can be instructed to examine the barrier upon removal to determine length of wear time. The timing of pouch changes can be challenging. Choosing a time of day when the stoma is least likely to be functioning makes the change less frustrating. Generally, the stoma is less active before eating or drinking in the morning or at least two hours after a meal.

PROBLEMS IN STOMA MANAGEMENT

Problematic stomas require additional time and energy for care. Due to shorter wear time, the number of stomal supplies increases, thus increasing the cost. This makes it more difficult for the patient to provide self-care and may ultimately create further emotional stress. Management issues generally arise with any of the following: a poor stoma site, the stoma is flush with the skin, the stoma budded, but the lumen is at skin level to the bottom or to the sides, the stoma is lying in or near skin folds and creases, the stoma is located close to an open wound, is recessed, retracted, or a fistula or parastomal hernia develops. Changes in weight may also affect pouch wear time.

Stomal and peristomal complications in ostomy patients can be the result of surgical technique, disease processes, medical management, changes in body contour, or patient self-care practices. Due to improvements in surgical techniques and supplies for ostomy management, complications occur less frequently than in the past, and those who are caring for the patient with an ostomy must be knowledgeable regarding preventative measures, management options, and appropriate surveillance to ensure that further problems do not recur.

Complications can create painful skin problems, increase fear of leakage or odor, and restrict activities. Effective care must be directed toward recognizing and understanding complications, as well as initiating early interventions while teaching both the patient and caregivers. Periodically examining the patient helps identify and correct techniques that may create the risk for developing complications; however, this often occurs only when another condition or disease process that brings the patient into the hospital or clinical office.

Stomal Complications

Stoma Necrosis

Stoma necrosis is described as dark discoloration (purple, dark red, brown, or black) most often occurring in the immediate post-op period that can be caused by mesenteric tension, overzealous trimming of the mesentery from the bowel end, or by interruption of blood flow by trauma to the stoma (7). Damage to the stoma can vary and may be circumferential or scattered on the mucosa. If the necrosis extends to the fascial level, emergent surgical intervention is indicated. A stoma with necrosis that remains viable will exhibit sloughing of the dead tissue, resulting in a flush or slightly retracted stoma (Fig. 2). Interventions include follow-up in the outpatient setting for thorough ongoing assessment, avoiding trauma to the stoma, and allowing ample space between the pouch opening and the stoma to prevent constriction of the stoma.

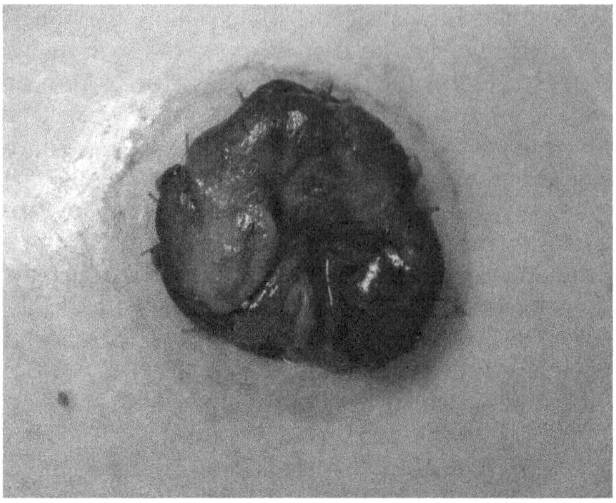

Figure 2 Stoma necrosis.

Mucocutaneous Separation

This occurs as a result of the breakdown of the suture line between the stoma mucosal tissue and the abdominal surface. Malnutrition, corticosteroids, tension at the suture line, and poor blood supply are among factors that predispose a patient to having this problem. Mucocutaneous separation may be partial or circumferential (Fig. 3). Interventions include cleansing the area thoroughly with each pouch change, filling in the separated area with skin barrier powder, paste or absorbent dressing such as calcium alginate or hydrofiber to absorb drainage, applying skin barrier paste circumferentially directly around the stoma, cutting the pouch barrier opening exactly to stoma size so it will cover and protect the separated area, and increasing the frequency of pouch changes to every two to three days to treat the affected area.

Parastomal Hernia

A parastomal hernia describes loops of the intestine protruding through the fascial defect around the stoma which can result as a bulge beside or around the stoma. A parastomal hernia can result from loss of muscle tone (as with obesity or aging), high intra-abdominal pressure (as with chronic cough, sneezing, heavy lifting), an excessively large fascial defect, placement of the stoma outside of the rectus muscle, or in the midline incision (Fig. 4). Interventions include the use of an appliance belt if the hernia is mild, the use of an ostomy/hernia support belt (elastic binder with an opening for the pouch), discontinue the use of irrigation to regulate stool (if patients is using irrigation for elimination), possibly modify the pouching system to accommodate changes in the abdominal contour, or surgical repair of the parastomal hernia may be necessary if there is any obstruction to elimination or ischemia.

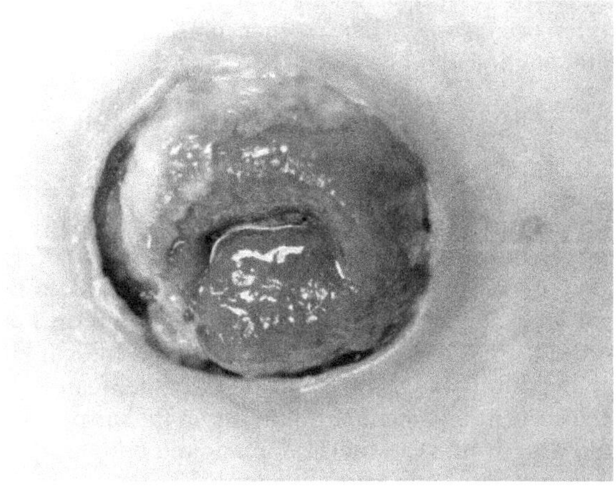

Figure 3 Mucocutaneous separation.

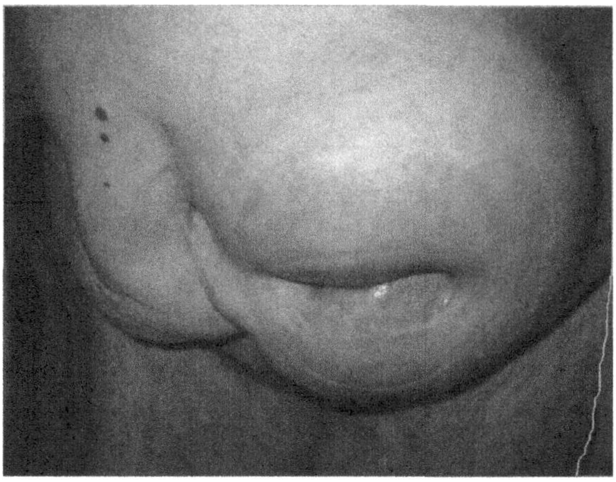

Figure 4 Parastomal hernia.

Stoma Prolapse

Prolapse of a stoma occurs because of telescoping of the intestine through the stoma. The prolapse can be partial (sliding) or complete (irreducible) and can be either short or very long. Stomal prolapse can result from an excessively large opening in the abdominal wall, inadequate fixation of the bowel to the abdominal wall, or high abdominal pressure (Fig. 5). Interventions include the use of larger pouching system to accommodate the increased length and diameter of the prolapsed stoma, the use of a flexible one-piece pouching system that can be cut to an adjusted size if the stoma size further increases by cutting slits in the barrier opening to allow for potential enlargement without constricting the stoma, avoiding a two-piece pouching system as flange can be rigid and less flexible for stoma expansion, instructing the patient in how to reduce the stoma size by using cold compress or table sugar if it becomes edematous, applying the pouching system with patient lying down to help reduce the stoma for pouch application, using an ostomy support binder with prolapse overbelt to help secure it in place, or surgical intervention if the stoma becomes ischemic, congested, too difficult to manage, or restricts the flow of stool.

Stoma Retraction

Stoma retraction is a reduction in the normal stomal protrusion to skin level or below skin level (Fig. 6). Interventions include adding an ostomy appliance belt to increase the adherence of the pouching system, refitting to a convex pouching system by choosing the system that best fits the contour of the peristomal area (i.e., shallow, deep, rounded, pointed), or surgical intervention, if necessary.

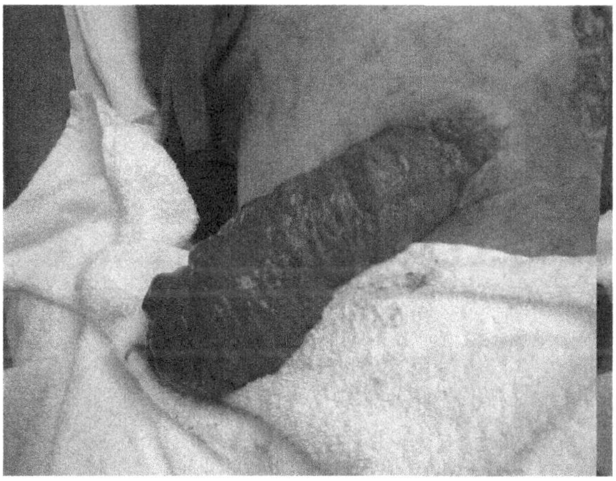

Figure 5 Stoma prolapse.

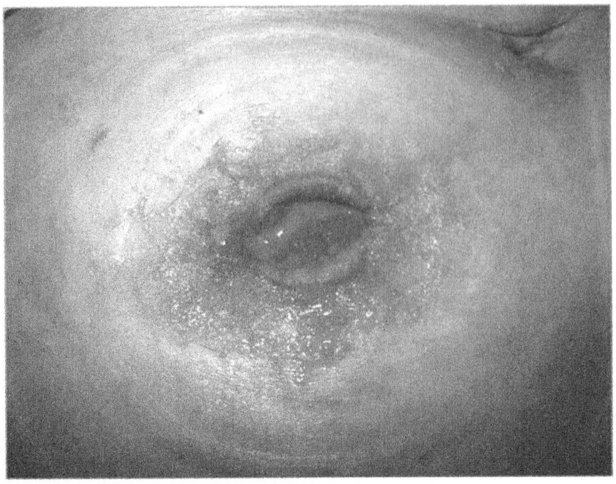

Figure 6 Stoma retraction.

Stoma Stenosis

Stenosis, or narrowing or contracting of the skin or fascia around the stoma, can cause impaired drainage of effluent from the stoma (Fig. 7). Interventions include the addition of a low-residue diet, stool softeners (if colostomy), and increased fluid intake, stomal dilatation, or surgical revision, if necessary.

Stoma Fistula

A stoma fistula is an abnormal opening either in peristomal skin or through stoma from intestinal lumen, most often associated with ileostomies. It can occur following peristomal abscess, from injury to the ileum from an appliance faceplate, suturing too deep into the ileum at the fascial level, or may be related to recurring Crohn's disease. A stomal fistula may make it difficult to maintain a pouch seal and may cause damage to the peristomal skin (Fig. 8). Interventions include adjusting the opening of appliance system to allow the fistula effluent to drain into pouch, protecting the skin with barrier film, barrier wafer or paste strips (if fistula is a distance away from stoma, it may need multiple pouches, smaller flanges, or overlap adhesive portions of pouches), or surgical resection or relocation.

Stoma Trauma

Injury to the mucosa that has the appearance of a cut or scaring on the outer edge of stoma anywhere from the base to the tip is considered stoma trauma (Fig. 9). Causes include cutting the flange opening too small, trapping the stoma mucosa when connecting the two-piece equipment, wearing tight clothing or a belt over the stoma, and nicking the stoma with a fingernail or equipment while cleaning during pouch changes. Interventions include identifying the causative factor and modifying the pouching system, instructing the patient to use careful technique during appliance changes, and scheduling a re-evaluation of the traumatized area.

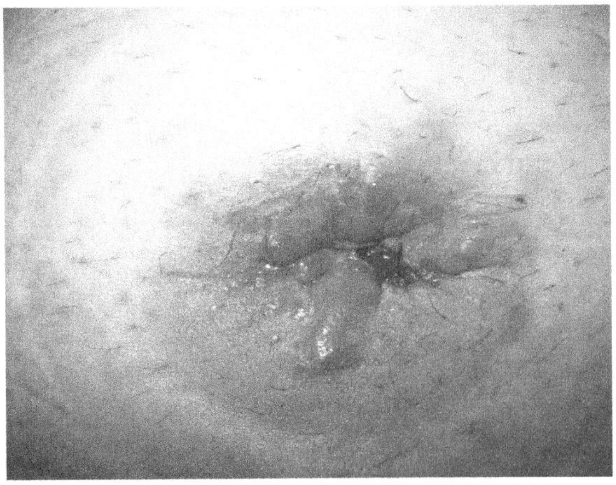

Figure 7 Stoma stenosis.

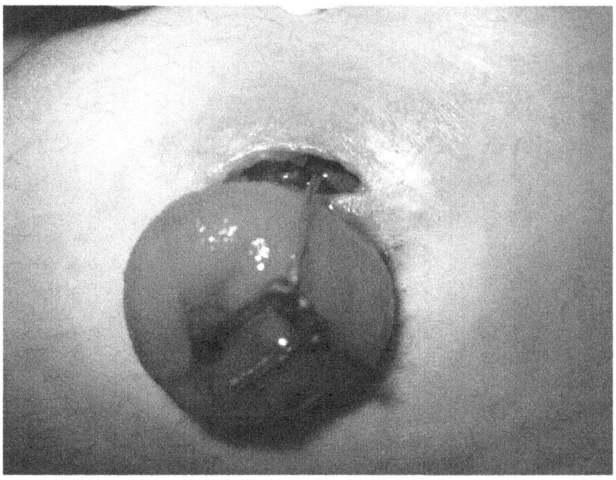

Figure 8 Stoma fistula.

PERISTOMAL COMPLICATIONS

Contact Dermatitis

Chemical Irritant Contact Dermatitis

Chemical irritant contact dermatitis causes erythema, skin erosion, or ulcers accompanied by itching, burning, or pain. Skin damage results from exposure to a chemical such as stool, urine, solvents, soaps, pastes, or sealants. This is one of the most common peristomal skin complications and is often due to poor fitting, loosening, or inadequate seal of the pouching system allowing seepage of effluent onto the skin. Prolonged or chronic contact with effluent may result in hyperplasia or thickening of the epithelium with a grayish white warty appearance (Fig. 10). Interventions include determining the cause by evaluating the affected skin and adhesive barrier of the removed pouching system that exhibits where the leakage occurs, questioning the patient about their usual wear time, amount and consistency of effluent, changes in weight, as well as pouch application and removal technique, checking for peristomal creases with changes in the position from standing to sitting, refitting to a proper pouching system for abdominal contour, maintaining skin care using skin barrier powder to absorb moisture from the eroded skin and seal with no-sting skin sealant, and eliminating exposure to the offending substance thereby allowing the skin to heal.

Allergic Contact Dermatitis

Allergic contact dermatitis is a sensitivity to a part of the appliance or any other product used for care of the ostomy. Allergic contact dermatitis may occur immediately or develop over a

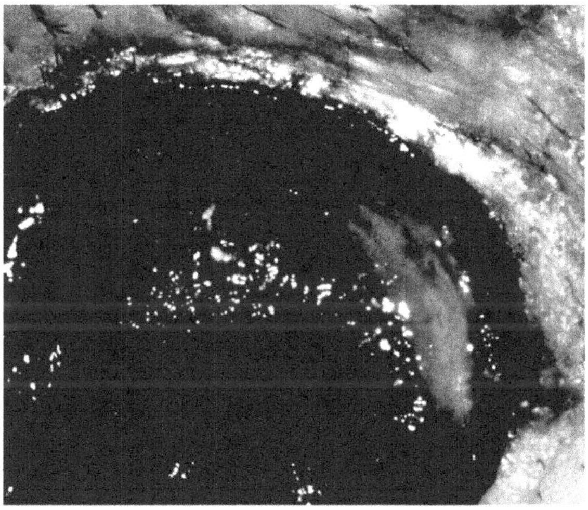

Figure 9 Stoma trauma.

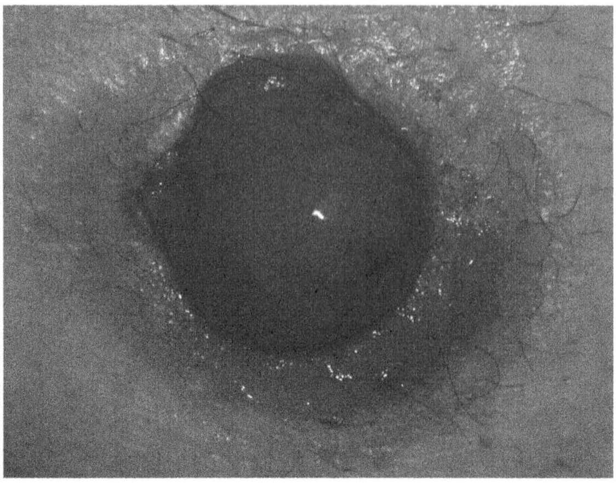

Figure 10 Chemical Irritant Contact Dermatitis.

period of time as a delayed response. It presents as erythema, edema, or erosion in the area where the product has come in contact with the skin. This may be accompanied by weeping or bleeding, itching, burning, or stinging (Fig. 11). Interventions include inspecting the skin and all components of the removed pouching system to determine any pattern that reflects contact with a certain product, patch testing in the clinic or by instructing the patient to apply small pieces of all products/materials that they have been using on the skin on the opposite side of the abdomen from the stoma, cover with hypoallergenic tape, and remove after 48 hours for assessment (using the abdomen provides an area with the same skin thickness, skin temperature, and exposure to friction as the area where the stoma is or will be), eliminating the offending agent or minimizing contact between the skin and the offending agent, treating the inflamed area with a steroid cream for a short period of time, switching to another formula or different brand if the current pouch system barrier is the offending product, using another brand, moldable seal rings, or eliminating paste altogether if skin paste is the offending product, or using a pouch cover if the problem results from the pouch plastic touching the skin.

Peristomal Candidiasis

Candidiasis is a common peristomal skin complication involving an overgrowth of the Candida organism that thrives in an occluded, warm, dark, and moist environment such as the peristomal area. It is characterized by solid areas of erythema or darker pigmentation with surrounding red satellite pustules with white tops. The skin may have a whitish superficial coating and frequent itching and/or burning and most common under the adhesive seal of the pouching system where the environment is moist. Predisposing factors include antibiotic therapy, corticosteroid therapy, diabetes, immunosuppression, and use of oral contraceptives. Damaged skin is more susceptible to Candida (Fig. 12). Interventions include topical application of an antifungal powder with each pouch change. The powder is rubbed into the skin and the excess powder

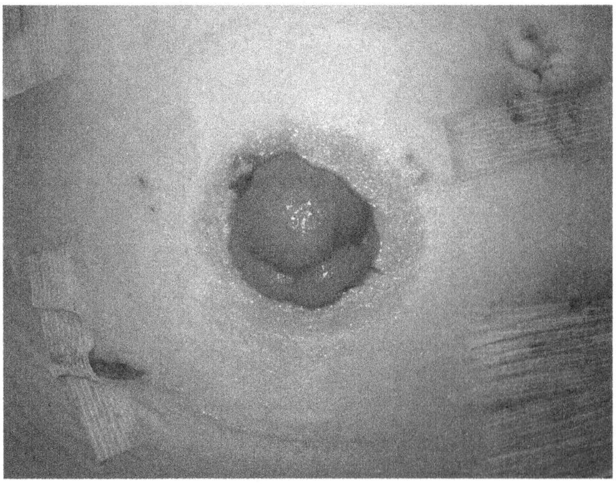

Figure 11 Allergic contact dermatitis.

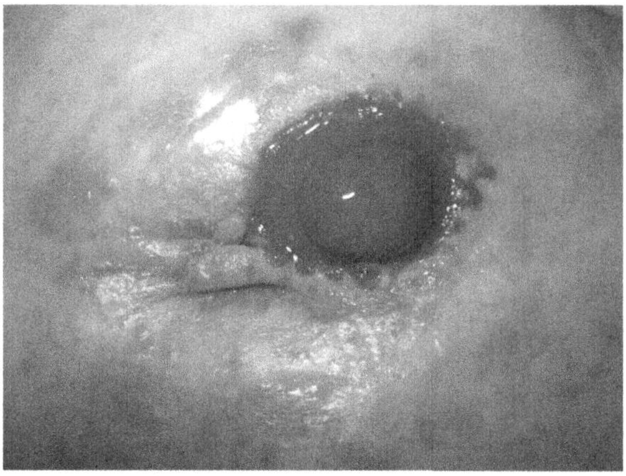

Figure 12 Peristomal candidiasis.

must be brushed away to allow the appliance to seal. The powder may need to be sealed with nonstinging skin barrier film. The patient should also be instructed of the possible need to change the pouching system more frequently in order to treat the affected area.

Folliculitis

Folliculitis is a bacterial infection or inflammation of hair follicles, often associated with repeated traumatic hair removal from traumatic pouch removal, poor shaving technique, or shaving too frequently. Other predisposing factors include diabetes, immunosupression, malnutrition, or use of corticosteroids. Isolated pustules, erythema, or darker pigmentation at the hair follicles are the primary identifying factors. The pustules may progress to papules and crust formation (Fig. 13). Interventions include observing the patient's technique for pouch removal and peristomal hair removal, instructing the patient to avoid shaving the affected area and trimming peristomal hair with scissors or an electric clipper, using adhesive removers to ease release of adhesives to avoid pulling out hairs, applying antibacterial powder and rubbing into the skin (may seal with skin barrier film), and the use of antibacterial soap may also be helpful.

Peristomal Trauma

Peristomal trauma is a result of skin loss or skin stripping from a traumatic pouch system removal (Fig. 14). Stripping the epidermis leaves skin surface moist and painful. Skin injury can also occur from pressure from use of convex faceplates, belts, and belt tabs. Interventions include eliminating the cause of the trauma, applying a skin barrier powder to open areas, and covering with a thin hydrocolloid, instructing the patient to push skin away rather than tear pouch off skin, limiting the amount of extra products used to increase adhesive effect, using an adhesive remover to help loosen seal during tape and barrier removal, avoiding scrubbing or

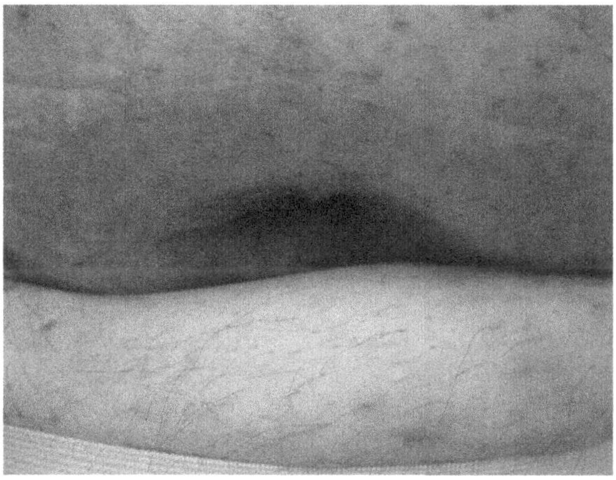

Figure 13 Folliculitis.

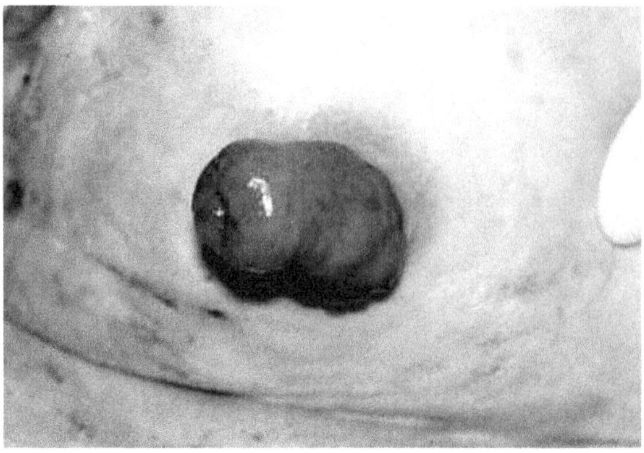

Figure 14 Peristomal Trauma.

picking residue of paste and adhesives from peristomal area, and, if there is pressure trauma, refitting the faceplate and/or belt.

Peristomal Psoriasis

Peristomal psoriasis appears as erythema with whitish patches of scaly plaques. Psoriasis generally occurs in sites of repeated minor trauma such as on the scalp, elbows, knees, and soles of the feet. It can also occur on the peristomal skin and is most often found in patients who have a history of psoriasis in other areas of the body (Fig. 15). Interventions include the use of topical steroid creams (rub into skin, allow to absorb, and then remove excess prior to pouch application) or topical immunomodulators such as picrolimus cream (i.e., Elidel); these should be applied to the affected area with each pouch change. Referral to dermatology may also be helpful.

Bacterial Infections

Bacterial infections are present as large patchy or solid areas of erythema with weepiness and/or crusting (Fig. 16). These often occur under tape areas where the plastic of the pouching system traps moisture on the skin and from inadequate drying of the skin after swimming or showering. Other predisposing factors include diabetes, immunosuppression, malnutrition, or use of corticosteroids. Isolated pustules, erythema, or darker pigmentation at the hair follicles are the primary identifying factors and the pustules may progress to papules and crust formation. Interventions include observing the patient's technique for pouch removal and peristomal hair removal, instructing the patient to avoid shaving the affected area and trimming peristomal hair with scissors or electric clipper, using adhesive removers to ease release of adhesives to avoid pulling out hairs, applying antibacterial powder and rubbing into the skin (may seal with skin barrier film), and using an antibacterial wash with each pouch change for persistent cases.

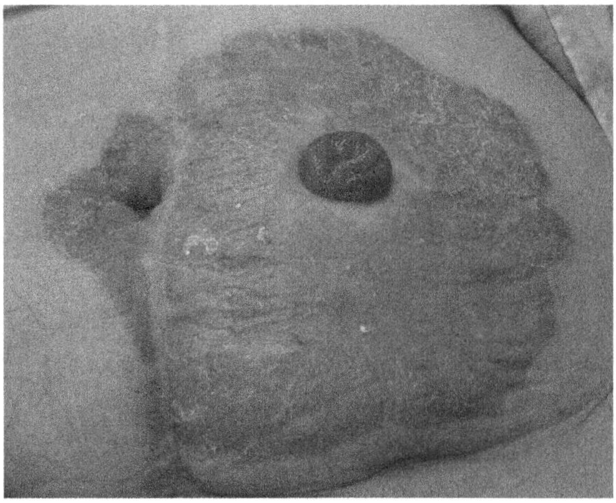

Figure 15 Peristomal psoriasis.

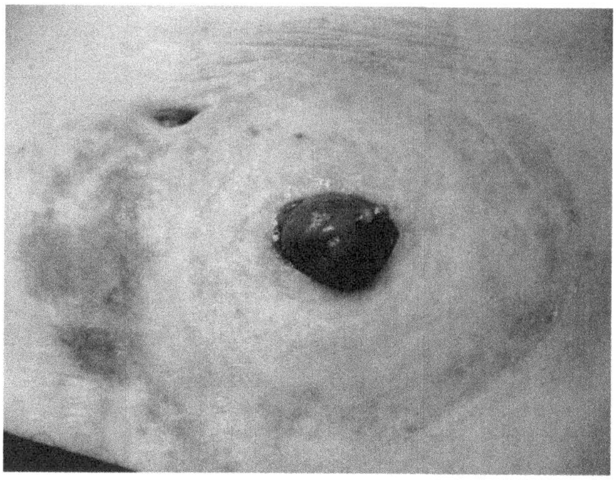

Figure 16 Bacterial Infections.

Mucosal Transplantation

Mucosal transplantation occurs when viable intestinal mucosa transplanted or seeded into the abdominal skin surface when the bowel is sutured to the epidermis, rather than the dermis, during stoma construction. It appears as small islands of mucosa in the immediate peristomal skin area. Mucosal transplants produce mucous and may interfere with the seal of the pouching system (Fig. 17). Interventions include applying absorptive hydrocolloid skin barrier powder or dressing to provide a dry surface for pouch adherence, or stoma revision for cases that are difficult to manage.

Peristomal Varices

Peristomal varices are bluish-purple discolorations of the peristomal skin related to dilated veins from portal hypertension. Bleeding at the stoma-skin junction can occur spontaneously either in the pouch or during pouch changes (Fig. 18). Interventions includes applying gentle skin care and careful pouch removal with an adhesive remover, refitting the stoma appliance opening to avoid rubbing on the stoma, avoiding tight clothing that could constrict or rub on the stoma precipitating a bleed, and using a flexible one-piece pouching system that will not apply direct firm pressure to the peristomal area. Interventions to stop peristomal bleeding include applying direct pressure, cauterization with silver nitrate, or application of gel foam or epinephrine soaked gauze. Suture ligation may be needed in severe cases.

Pseudoverrucous Lesions (Hyperplasia)

Pseudoverrucous lesions are wart-like lesions protruding above skin level in the proximal peristomal area (sometimes referred to as hyperplasia, or proud flesh) as a result of chronic exposure to moisture from an ill-fitting pouching system (Fig. 19). The size of the lesion depends on how long and how much skin is exposed to prolonged contact with effluent. The raised or

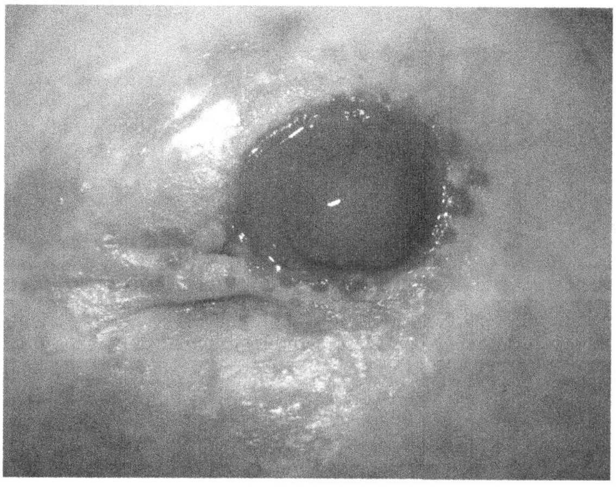

Figure 17 Mucosal transplantation.

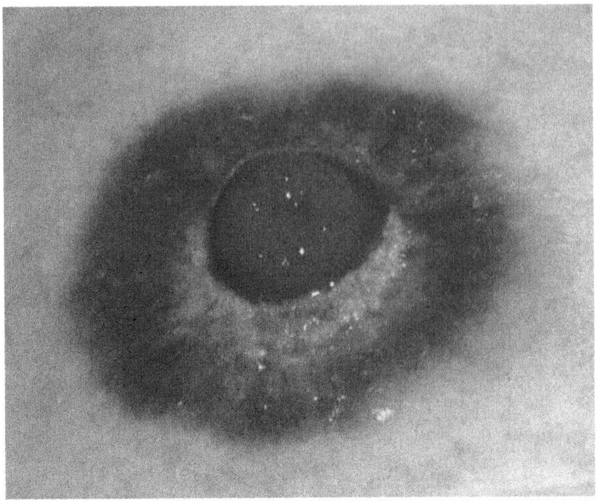

Figure 18 Peristomal varicies.

thickened epithelium has a grayish white warty appearance. The affected skin and the removed adhesive barrier of the pouching system should be assessed; in addition, assessment should be made for peristomal creases, and folds in sitting and/or standing positions. The patient should be questioned about their usual wear time, amount and consistency of effluent, changes in weight, as well as pouch application and removal technique. Interventions include refitting to an appropriate pouching system that mirrors the abdominal contour, cutting the pouch opening to the stoma size and shape (covering the lesions and eliminating exposure to effluent allows skin to heal), adding skin barrier paste around opening of pouch barrier (if the patient is not already using barrier paste), using hydrocolloid powder to absorb moisture from eroded skin, and the patient should be instructed to increase frequency of pouch changes.

Peristomal Pyoderma Gangrenosum

Peristomal pyoderma gangrenosum is a painful irregular ulcer with ragged reddish-purple borders. The lesion may begin as a small pustule and progress to a full thickness wound with a necrotic center; the base of the lesion is generally very painful. There may be single or multiple lesions that can enlarge by tunneling under the epidermis. This often occurs with underlying systemic diseases such as inflammatory bowel disease. On assessment, the appearance and clinical manifestations of the lesions are the most important for diagnosis (Fig. 20). Interventions include keeping the area clean and provide topical wound care to absorb drainage, using an absorptive skin barrier powder to absorb drainage, using creative pouching techniques to maintain pouch barrier seal, and using topical immunomodulators such as tacrolimus ointment (i.e., Protopic) or picrolimus cream (i.e., Elidel). These should be applied to the lesions and covered with nonadherent (telfa) and pouch over dressing. For an even more superior adherence, ointment can be mixed with a paste (i.e., Orabase). Intralesional steroid injections or topical

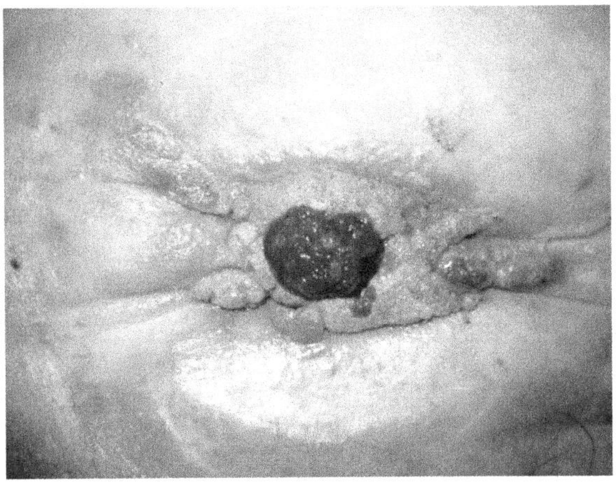

Figure 19 Pseudoverrucous Lesions (Hyperplasia).

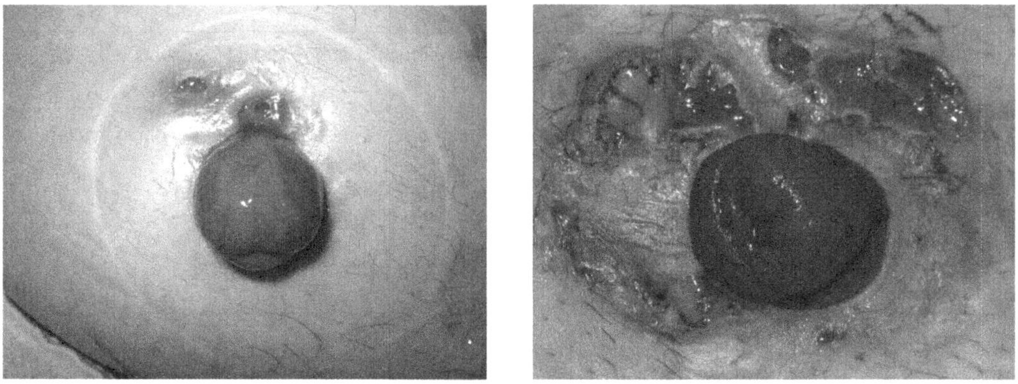

Figure 20 Peristomal pyoderma gangrenosum.

steroid cream may aid healing. Topical anesthetic may be needed during exam and/or care due to pain, and biopsies may be done to exclude other skin diseases. Management of underlying disease processes generally leads to improvement of the skin lesions.

Problem Solving

When removing a stoma pouch from a patient's abdomen, the stoma, abdomen, and pouch should all be assessed. Examining skin contours, the skin, and the angle at which the stoma empties is important. The adhesive surface of the pouch barrier that is removed should also be assessed. Skin problems often mirror what is seen on the removed pouch seal and identifies where the pouch seal was lost. These are the areas that may need to be built up with paste, paste strips, and/or barrier rings to fill in crevices and creases. Tables 4 and 5 outline problem management guidelines and pouch seal considerations.

Some tips to facilitate office visits include instructing patients to bring supplies to their office visits so the pouch can be removed to inspect the stoma and the peristomal skin. It is also helpful to keep a small variety of supplies on hand for those patients who forget to bring their own supplies. A custom cut one-piece pouch may be used in many different situations until the patient can apply their own at home. It is also important to instruct patients and caregivers on when to call the doctor and when to go to the emergency room.

DIETARY CONSIDERATIONS

Most patients having ostomy surgery express concerns regarding diet before and after surgery. There is no special diet for a person with an ostomy. In most cases there are few, if any, restrictions. However everyone is unique and can tolerate different foods. It must first be considered if the

Table 4 Problem Management Guidelines

Deep peristomal creasing
Match pouch to patient's skin contours
Flexible pouching system (folds with patient)
Measures to increase adherence (e.g., bonding cement, tacky skin barrier)
Soft abdomen-match or eliminate creases with firm faceplate, convexity, or belted system
Flushed, retracted, or budded stoma with opening at skin level will likely need a convex pouching system that will press on the skin around the stoma to help the stoma protrude more. This helps reduce risk of pouch seal undermining and leaking.
Creasing to one side—barrier strips, wedges to create even surface
Scars, gullies, defects
small defects—fill with barrier paste
large defects—use moldable barrier wedges, strips, rings
High output stoma—may need high output pouch that holds larger volume
When possible provide templates and written instructions

Table 5 Pouch Seal Considerations

Many skin problems are caused by keeping a pouch on too long. Pouch changes should be scheduled rather than waiting for leakage.
Changes in climate affect wear time
Changes in weight—if skin contour or protrusion of stoma changes, it may need a different pouching system to obtain a good seal
Pregnancy and parastomal hernia cause changes in abdominal contour
Patients with very, oily, or diaphoretic skin may need to change more often
Be sure skin is clean and dry when applying a new pouch
If using ostomy paste, apply around the opening rather than the outer edges of the barrier
Avoid belt or tight waistband directly over the stoma

patient's diet has been previously restricted because of any other disease processes such as diabetes, cardiac disease, allergies, or other medical problem; if so, those restrictions still apply regardless of ostomy surgery.

While the digestive system is recovering, the patient may notice decreased hunger and may feel full quickly. Frequent small meals or snacks may improve food intake in the first few weeks. For patients with small intestine ostomies, a low-residue diet, avoiding high-fiber foods such as raw vegetables, nuts, corn, or any foods with heavy skin or seeds, may be used in the first two weeks. It is important to instruct patients with any intestinal surgery to chew all foods well.

Regardless of what type of ostomy surgery the patient has undergone, in some way the intestine has been manipulated and resected. The patient needs to know what part of the bowel has been removed and how it affects absorption of nutrients, fluid, and electrolytes. It is also essential to note that one cannot slow or stop the bowel from working by not eating or drinking. Skipping meals leaves the bowel empty and causes gas.

Enteric coated and time release capsules that are designed to be absorbed along the full length of bowel may be incompletely absorbed in the person with an ileostomy because of decreased bowel length. Patients should be informed of this and, if necessary, a chewable or liquid that is readily absorbed may be prescribed.

FOOD BLOCKAGE

Food blockage can occur in patients following abdominal surgery, and occurs most often in patients with ileostomy. Eating high-fiber foods too quickly or in large amounts tends to form a mass that is difficult to pass through the intestine. Blockage is characterized by crampy abdominal pain, thin watery output, diminished flow of waste, increased stool odor, or abdominal swelling and/or vomiting.

ILEOSTOMY LAVAGE

Ileostomy lavage may be used to help dislodge the fibrous mass when a patient with an ileostomy develops a food blockage that does not respond to conservative measures such as peristomal massage or soaking in a warm bath. A small hole or slit can be made in the upper area of a drainable pouch, or an irrigation sleeve can be used to collect the fluid during the procedure. Specifically, a lubricated 14 or 16Fr catheter is inserted into the stoma to the point of the blockage and 30 to 50 mL of saline is gently instilled. The catheter is then removed; a flow should resume within a few minutes. The above steps should be repeated if necessary until the blockage is resolved.

COLOSTOMY IRRIGATION

Descending or sigmoid colostomies may be cleansed or flushed by a procedure known as irrigation. Similar to an enema, colostomy irrigation is the instillation of fluid into the colon via the stoma using a cone-tipped catheter. The irrigating fluid, usually warm water, distends the bowel causing the bowel to contract and empty. Colostomies may be irrigated as a washout procedure, before a test or surgery, to administer therapeutic solutions or to stimulate peristalsis.

Colostomy irrigation can also be used as a management option to regulate bowel elimination. It enables a patient to empty their colon at a convenient time and thereby increasing their independence and security. If the procedure works well, the person with a descending or sigmoid colostomy can count on regular evacuations and the need for a pouch is minimized. The patient who irrigates successfully may wear only a small stoma cap or gauze square over the stoma between irrigations; some patients wear a small pouch for ensured security.

Colostomy irrigation is not always appropriate or even desirable for every patient who has a sigmoid or descending colostomy. The patient's age, physical and mental ability to learn and perform the procedure, the disease process, and whether or not the ostomy is temporary or permanent are all factors that need to be considered. Irrigation is contraindicated with stomal prolapse due to an increased risk further prolapse, parastomal hernia because of an increased risk for bowel perforation and poor evacuation results, in children or young adults as routine irrigation may create bowel dependency, after pelvic or abdominal radiation, because of the extreme risk of bowel perforation. Irrigation should not be done until all bowel friability has resolved, normal bowel function is restored and the mucosa of the stoma is healthy. In addition, irrigation should be avoided in patients with extensive diverticulosis due to the risk of bowel perforation and in patients with limited manual dexterity, poor learning ability, poor bowel regularity before surgery, and extremely ill or terminally ill patients.

Once the patient's candidacy for irrigation has been determined, the patient should be counseled concerning his or her options. Advantages and disadvantages of using routine irrigation to regulate bowel elimination should be discussed. The chief advantage is that the patient regains control over fecal elimination. If irrigation is successful, the patient may choose not to wear a pouch and only use a small protective covering. Successful management of the colostomy with irrigation may assist in the psychosocial adjustment to the colostomy. Disadvantages include the time required for the procedure since not all patients can achieve complete control with irrigation. If elimination patterns change or become unpredictable, the patient may not be free of bowel movements between irrigations.

Regulation of the colostomy using irrigation is a personal matter, and the final decision of whether to use this method should be made by the patient with proper guidance from healthcare professionals. Only those patients who meet the established criteria for irrigation should proceed with using this method of bowel management. Table 6 outlines the irrigation procedure.

QUALITY OF LIFE ISSUES FOR OSTOMY PATIENTS

Quality of life can be described as the degree of satisfaction or contentment and the ability to cope with life. How an illness and its treatment affect quality of life is determined by how it is perceived by the patient (2). The reason for the surgery and whether the stoma is temporary or

Table 6 Irrigation Procedure

Gather equipment
Fill irrigation container with 1 L warm water. Run water through the tubing to remove any trapped air
Hang container at shoulder height with patient sitting on toilet or chair near toilet
Remove old pouch or covering from stoma
Attach irrigation sleeve over stoma
Lubricate cone irrigator and gently insert into stoma. Hold cone gently but firmly against stoma to prevent backflow of water
Open clamp and allow water to flow. If cramping occurs, shut off water flow, keeping cone in place until cramp subsides, then continue
After water has been instilled, gently withdraw cone and close top of irrigation sleeve
Allow 15–20 min for most of return, dry and clamp bottom of sleeve. Patient may proceed with other activities
Leave sleeve in place for approximately 20 min
When evacuation is complete, remove sleeve, clean peristomal skin and apply pouch or protective covering
Wash equipment

Table 7 Ostomy Organizations

American Cancer Society—www.cancer.org
American Dietetic Association—www.eatright.org
American Society of Colon and Rectal Surgeons—www.fascrs.org
Crohn's and Colitis Foundation of America—www.ccfa.org
National Cancer Institute—www.cancer.gov
United Ostomy Association of America—www.uoaa.org
Wound Ostomy and Continence Nurse Society—www.wocn.org

permanent can affect the rate of adjustment. Returning to presurgery quality of life requires a number of steps toward returning back to normal. Access to appropriate supplies and information will assist the patient in managing self-care and provide the equipment for increasing the patient's feeling of well-being.(8)

Quality of life is directly impacted by the amount of time that has lapsed since surgery, the patient's age, and emotional adaptability; however adjusting to an ostomy also significantly depends on meeting the desired goals for pouching the ostomy including obtaining a secure leak-proof pouch seal, attaining a predictable, sustainable wear time, being able to physically manage the ostomy, and choosing a pouching system that is discrete and compatible with the patient's lifestyle.

Ostomy surgery involves a major physical change to the body and the patient with a stoma faces a number of issues and concerns. Body image, security of the pouch seal, noise, diet, odor, confidence in self-care, sex and intimacy, night-time emptying, interruption of sleep, sleep positioning, and travel are among the main concerns. While the patient recovers physically, the emotional, psychological, and learning needs of the patient must be met. Returning to presurgery quality of life takes time, but most importantly requires availability of resources for learning self-care, having access to appropriate supplies, and follow-up care. The patient's adjustment to an ostomy also depends not only on information or misinformation and preconceived notions, but also on the response of family, friends, and personnel caring for the patient.

In helping patients cope with ostomy surgery, caregivers must also be able to cope. This means having adequate knowledge of the emotional needs of the patient, ostomy pouches and other supplies, community resources, and available educational material. There are many professional and voluntary organizations that provide materials and information on ostomy patient education such as health-care professionals within local communities, gastroenterologists, WOCNs, dieticians, pharmacists, social workers, trained lay visitors, and psychotherapists, among others. In addition, manufacturers and suppliers of ostomy equipment produce patient education materials. Table 7 lists organizations that provide a variety of useful information related to ostomy patient education and may have local chapters, support services, or representatives in the community.

Education and support are the components of care that will lay the foundation to guide the person with an ostomy toward an optimal level of adjustment. Health-care professionals should make it a practice to address quality of life issues and make referrals for resources that can support the patient in attaining adequate access to appropriate supplies, information, and assistance toward managing self-care, taking the steps toward getting back to normal, and returning to a productive and satisfying life.

REFERENCES

1. Carmel J, Goldberg M. Preoperative and postoperative management. In: Colwell JC, Goldberg J, Carmel M, Carmel J, eds. Fecal and Urinary Diversions: Management Principles. Philadelphia: Mosby, 2004:207–239.
2. Vasilevsky C, Gordon P. Gastrointestinal Cancers: Surgical Management. In: Colwell JC, Goldberg M, Carmel J, eds. Fecal and Urinary Diversions: Management Principles. Philadelphia: Mosby, 2004:126–135.
3. Lerner J, Eisenstat T, Spear J. Pitfalls of Stoma Placement. Departments of Surgery and Nursing, University of Maryland Hospital, Baltimore, Maryland.
4. Broadwell D, Jackson B. Principles of Ostomy Care. St. Louis: Mosby, 1982:329–339.

5. Colwell JC, Goldberg M, Carmel J. The state of the standard diversion. JWOCN 2001; 28(1): 6–17.
6. Harford FJ, Harford DS. Intestinal stomas. In: Beck DE, Welling DR, eds. Patient Care in Colorectal Surgery. New York: Little, Brown and Company, 1991:95–111.
7. Duchesne JC, Wang YZ, Weintraub SL, et al. Stoma complications: a multivariate analysis. Am Surg 2002; 68(11):961–986.
8. Grant M, Ferrell B, Dean G, et al. Revision and psychometric testing of the City of Hope Quality of Life-Ostomy questionnaire. Qual Life Res 2004; 13:1445–1457.

25 Perioperative Pain Management

Lawrence Frank
Division of Anesthesiology, Cleveland Clinic Florida, Weston, Florida, U.S.A.

INTRODUCTION

Ambulatory surgery and procedures now constitute the majority of surgeries performed in the United States (1). In fact, many of the procedures described in this text have been performed on an outpatient basis for decades. Pain control is, many times, the key to success in delivering the ambulatory outcome for these procedures. Delayed discharge and unplanned admissions are often related to the degree of pain control (2–4). Early and effective treatment for pain and nausea decreases the time spent in the postanesthesia care unit (PACU), while increasing patient satisfaction. Although the majority of patients remain free of moderate-to-severe pain, 5% to 33% of patients may suffer considerable postoperative pain (2,5). Pain is the most common cause of hospital admission, or a visit to the emergency room after discharge (6). Indeed, pain is the number one complaint patients have following ambulatory surgery (Fig. 1).

The Joint Commission on Accreditation of Healthcare Organization (JCAHO), which accredits hospitals in the United States, implemented pain measurement standards several years ago (7). Patient outcomes are no longer viewed in terms of major morbidity and mortality, but now also include endpoints such as patient satisfaction, quality of life, and quality of recovery. Thus, it is necessary for all physicians involved in the surgical procedure to be informed of current postoperative pain management modalities. This chapter will review and summarize state of the art pain management as it pertains to ambulatory colorectal surgery.

PAIN ASSESSMENT

Postoperative pain management actually begins preoperatively. There must be discussion between patient and caregiver as to their expectation for the relief of pain. It is not realistic for the patient to believe there will be no postoperative pain. Misconceptions must be clarified as early as possible to allay any anxieties. Documentation should be made of the patient's current pain level and locations before surgery. This provides a baseline for preexisting levels of pain and will serve as a reference point to monitor postoperative pain control effectiveness. Clinical assessment of postoperative pain includes its effect on function as well as comfort and should be described in sufficient detail to accomplish certain goals: (1) to ensure a correct diagnosis and to quantify postoperative pain, (2) to select the appropriate therapy, and (3) to evaluate response to therapy.

The most common reason for under-treatment of postoperative pain is the failure of clinicians to fully assess pain (8). Pain should be assessed and documented frequently in the immediate postoperative period, along with the other vital signs; this makes pain the fifth vital sign. The most reliable indicator is the patient's self-reporting of pain. Pain is a subjective experience and, as such, it should be the patient's perceptions that are noted, rather than the clinicians'. It should also be kept in mind that measures of pain intensity are meant to compare the intensity of pain in one patient at any given time with the intensity at another given time; it is not meant as a comparison between different patients.

Postoperative pain has several unique features. Unlike many other pain syndromes, acute surgical pain is predictable, and its intensity can be correlated with the operative site and the extent of the surgical procedure. This differs from other pain symptoms in that it is transient and usually improves after a short period of time. The pain may also be different during activity, deep breathing and coughing, and that should also be documented. During recovery from surgery, it must not be assumed that all pain is originating from the surgical wound; indeed,

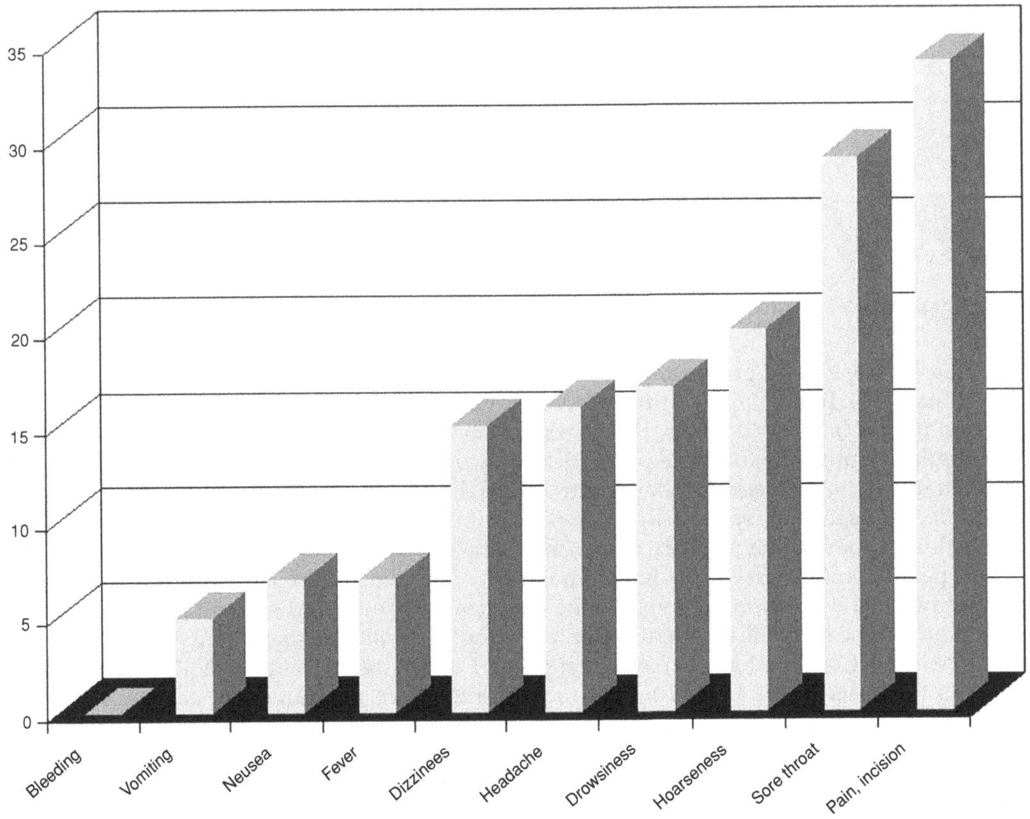

Figure 1 Overall percentage of patients with postoperative symptoms 24 hours after surgery. *Source*: From Ref. 75.

it may be other causes of pain. The clinician should always be open to alternative diagnoses and complications when patients exhibit uncontrolled or unexpected pain. This may indicate new complications (e.g., bleeding) or a comorbid condition (e.g., angina). A patient on chronic pain medication is a special case and will be discussed later. Finally, neuropathic pain may be developing. This can occur within days after the original injury and will also be addressed later in this chapter. Pain is a complex, multimodal/dimensional symptom, determined not only by the physical presence of tissue injury, and the resulting nociceptor injury, but also by prior experience, personal beliefs, motivations, and environment.

There is no true objective measurement of pain. It is essentially self-reporting. Theoretically, postoperative pain should be evaluated using multiple parameters such as location, intensity, quality, and emotional consequences. Multidimensional scales have been developed for that purpose, but they are far too complex for widespread and repetitive use in surgical patients. Thus, the uni-dimensional scale measurement is generally used.

The uni-dimensional scaling technique is the oldest form of a pain measurement tool. Basically, the patient is asked to describe their current pain experience from a list of adjectives that reflect graduations of pain intensity (9). The scale may contain between two and seven words. Generally, a four descriptor verbal reading scale (VRS) is commonly used: none, mild, moderate, or severe. Other descriptors could include discomfort, distressing, horrible, excruciating, etc.

More accurate, the numerical rating scales (NRSs) are the simplest and most commonly used scales. The numerical scale is most commonly presented horizontally, on a scale of 0 to 10, with 0 denoting no pain and 10 denoting the worst pain imaginable. The patient selects a number (verbal version) or marks the scale (written version), corresponding to the pain. This is a simplified version of the visual analog scale (VAS), which is a 1 to 100 linear scale, long employed by psychologists, and validated over a long period of time. It has been shown in several studies that the postoperative patient is generally cognitively impaired, and this leads

No Pain	0	1	2	3	4	5	6	7	8	9	10	Worst Pain Imaginable

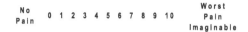

Figure 2 Numerical rating scale (NRS).

to an imprecision of plus or minus 20 in measurements in a postoperative setting (10). Thus, the simplified scale is justified (Fig. 2).

A newer innovation is a picture scale (Fig. 3). This tool consists of a series of four to six faces depicting different expressions ranging from a happy smiling face to a sad teary face. Patients reportedly prefer to use the face scale over the NRS or VAS scales because it is easier and may be particularly useful in the patient with a communication problem (e.g., hard of hearing, language fluency).

Thus, pain is assessed before the operation or intervention and again immediately after the operation; it is subsequently measured at regular intervals. Repeated pain assessment is a fundamental tool for improving the quality of acute pain management. It is important that the measurement be patient self-reported because health-care providers tend to underestimate the patient's pain. Since patients have the right to appropriate pain management, pain assessment is no longer optional.

PAIN MEDICATION

In this section, the pharmacodynamics and pharmacology of the various drugs available to the clinician will be addressed, and dosing schedules, routes of administration, side-effects, and metabolic pathways relevant to the clinician will be reviewed. Unfortunately, with the voluntary withdrawal of the very promising COX-2 inhibitors, we have a more limited, but well-known selection of agents.

Opioids

Opioid drugs are the most commonly used analgesics in clinical practice. Their pharmacological effects were well known to ancient civilizations and have been cited in the literature of many cultures. The word opium is derived from the Greek word juice because it was obtained from the juice of the poppy, *Papaver Somniferum*. Morphine was isolated from opium in 1803 by Serturner. The term opioid refers to substances, natural and synthetic, that have morphine-like properties. Their low cost, easy availability, and effectiveness have lent to their widespread use for pain mangement.

Opioids produce their effects by binding to specific membrane receptors. There are three families of opioid receptors (ORs): (1) the μ opioid receptor (MOR), (2) the κ opioid receptor (KOR), and (3) the δ opioid receptor (DOR). These receptors, in varying degrees, appear at all levels of the central nervous system, including the cortex, medulla, and spinal cord. They have even been found in peripheral tissues (11).

Most of the commonly used opioids are listed in Table 1. Their pharmacodynamics are listed in Table 2. In general, opioids are absorbed when given by all routes of administration, including transdermal, spinal, buccal, inhalational, parenteral, oral, and rectal, to name a few. The liver is the main site of metabolism for most opioids. Metabolism is very dependent on liver blood flow. Some of the metabolites have pharmacological activity.

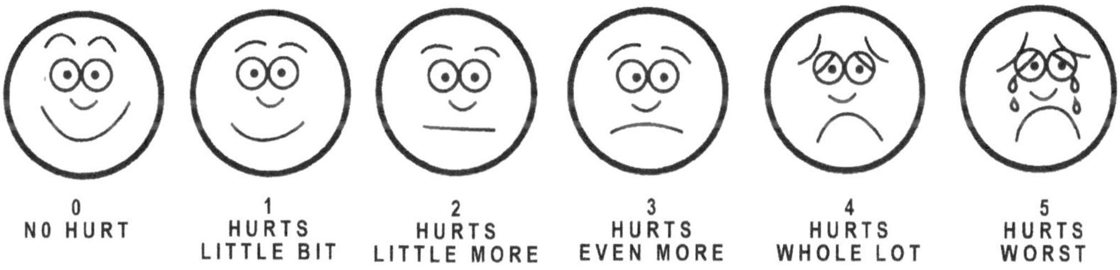
0
NO HURT
1
HURTS
LITTLE BIT
2
HURTS
LITTLE MORE
3
HURTS
EVEN MORE
4
HURTS
WHOLE LOT
5
HURTS
WORST

Figure 3 Faces pain scale.

Table 1 Commonly Used Opioids in the Perioperitive Period

Agonist	Morphine
	Hydromorphone (Dilaudid)
	Fentanyl
	Oxycodone
	Hydrocodone
	Propoxyphene (Darvon)
	Codeine
	Meperidine
Partial agonist	Buprenorphine
	Tramadol (?)
Agonist–antagonist	Butorphanol (Stadol)
	Pentazocine (Talwin)
	Nalbuphine (Nubain)
	Buprenorphine (Buprenex)
Pure antagonist	Naloxone (Narcan)
Combinations	Oxycodone/acetaminophen or ASA (Percodan)
	Hydrocodone/acetaminophen or ASA (Vicodin)
	Propoxyphene/acetaminophen or ASA (Darvocet)
	Codeine/acetaminophen or ASA (Tylenol #3)

Abbreviation: ASA, Acetylsalicyclic acid.

Morphine remains the gold standard in opioid analgesia for moderate-to-severe pain (12). It should be administered via the intravenous route. At the present time, meperidine (Demerol) is no longer recommended in postoperative pain, owing to significant adverse effects, especially the accumulation of neurotoxic metabolites (13). Hydromorphone (Dilaudid) is a semi-synthetic derivative of morphine. When administered intravenously, it has a more rapid onset (less than five minutes) and a shorter time to peak effect (less than 10 minutes) than morphine (14).

Tramadol (Ultram), a relatively new opioid, is said to be an atypical opioid because it acts centrally, but is relatively weak when compared to morphine, about 1/10 as effective (15). In the United States, tramadol is not a controlled substance, although it still requires a prescription. Because of its unusual agonist action, it was thought to be free of the usual side-effects of opioids. However, this has not been the case. It has all the usual side-effects, including postoperative nausea and vomiting (PONV), of the currently prescribed opioids.

Several opioids including morphine, hydrocodone, oxycodone, and tramadol are available as a controlled release (CR) oral preparations which significantly extend plasma half-life, thus giving patients a longer pain-free interval (16). These medications are usually given over an 8 or 12 hour redosing schedule and at a reduced amount (50–75%).

Significant benefits have been found by combining opioids (tramadol, codeine, oxycodone, hydrocodone) with acetaminophen and/or acetylsalicylic acid, the so-called compounded analgesics. The compounded opioids have been found to be two to three times as effective as they

Table 2 Opioid Pharmacodynamics

Opioid	Equipotent IV dose (mg)	Equipotent PO dose (mg)	Effective duration (hr)
Morphine	5	10–30	3–4
Hydromorphone	2	2–3	3–6
Fentanyl	0.075	N/A	0.5
Meperidine	50	150	2–3
Codeine	30	30–60	2–4
Oxycodone	5	5–10	4–6
Hydrocodone	5	5–10	4–6
Propoxyohene	N/A	65–100	3–4
Tramadol	N/A	100	4–6
Butorphanol	2	2	3–4
Buprenorphine	0.3	0.6	4–6

Abbreviation: N/A, not applicable.

would be alone. Their use, however, must be limited to a maximum daily dose of aspirin or acetaminophen (17).

Opioids can induce adverse side-effects. Thus, outside of its use for clinical analgesia, there is no other indication for administering opioids. Careful titration will reduce the incidence and severity of side-effects. The worst potential side-effect is respiratory depression, which is thought to occur less than 1% of the patients. Opioids decrease both respiratory rate and tidal volume, together called the minute ventilation (18). The main effect is to decrease the brain's responsiveness to carbon dioxide. Patients may even be awake, but apneic. Opioids also inhibit the respiratory response to hypoxia (19). Fortunately, respiratory depression can be reversed with naloxone (Narcan). Careful titration (50 μg boluses) will reverse respiratory depression, but allow continued pain control.

Another potential side-effect of opioids may induce a transitory pruritis, possibly related to histamine release. The precise mechanism is unknown, and may be related to a central itch center (20). Many pharmacological therapies such as antihistamines, 5-HT receptor antagonists, opioid antagonists, propofol, NSAIDS, and droperidol, have been studied with no clear choice.

Opioids cause urinary effects since they change the nature of ureter and bladder contractions. The response in humans is variable and unpredictable. Finally, opioids can also cause hemodynamic effects by inducing vasodilation of peripheral arterioles and veins. Hypotension may occur when the patient is moved from the supine position. In addition, there are some direct effects on the heart, particularly bradycardia, which may reduce cardiac work load and diastolic pressure (21).

Gastrointestinal (GI) effects and PONV will be covered later in this chapter in significant detail due to its particular relevance.

Cyclooxygenase Inhibitors for Analgesia (Nonopioid Analgesics)

The medications described in this section has traditionally been referred to as "nonopioid analgesics" or nonsteroidal anti-inflammatory drugs (NSAIDs). Recent research has shown that all their actions are through the inhibition of different cyclo-oxygenase (COX) enzymes, and are now subdivided into COX-1, COX-2, or COX-3. Comparing the analgesia produced by COX inhibition to opioids is difficult. Opioids have no ceiling effect. That is, the clinician can relieve virtually any pain with enough opioid, albeit with concomitant sedation or other unwanted side-effects. Conversely, the COX inhibitors do have a ceiling effect, especially in patients with severe pain, where increases in dose will not provide any patient benefit.

Nonselective COX Inhibitors

Aspirin is the prototype for all COX inhibitors. It is unique among the medications in its class since it covalently binds with COX enzymes, resulting in permanent inhibition. Since platelets do not make produce COX enzyme, aspirin essentially renders them useless. Aspirin also produces a myriad of GI effects. Soon after ingestion, heartburn, nausea, or vomiting may occur. After days to weeks, ulcers may form in the GI tract, leading to either bleeding, sometimes silent, but may also lead to vomiting blood or melanotic stools. As such, aspirin is not recommended for long-term use of pain management.

A recent study of aspirin for postoperative pain control suggested that a dose of 1000 mg is needed for a clinical effect, with a daily maximum dose of 2500 mg (22). This is approximately equal to acetaminophen on milligram for milligram comparison.

Ibuprofen, a reversible nonselectable COX inhibitor (Motrin, Advil, Nuprin) is the original modern NSAID. Its spectrum of GI toxicity is much lower than aspirin. Ibuprofen's effects on platelets are reversible once the drug has been discontinued. It has a relatively short duration of action (half-life = 2 hrs) and dosing must be repeated every four hours. Newer agents such as naproxen (Naprosyn, Anaprox, Aleve) or diflunisal (Dolobid) are essentially clinically identical to ibuprofen but have much longer effective half-lives, allowing a 12-hour dosing schedule (Table 3).

Ketorolac (Toradol) has had a significant impact on the treatment of postoperative pain. For the first time, clinicians have a parenterally administered drug that is an alternative to opioids. Ketorolac is the first drug in its class that could reliably substitute for morphine. Several studies have shown that 30 mg of ketorolac provides relief similar to 10 mg of morphine (23). To minimize side-effects, there is a recommended dosing schedule of not more than 30 mg IV or IM every six hours, for up to five days. Naturally, onset is faster and duration is shorter

Table 3 Nonopioid Analgesics

Generic name	Trade name	PO dose (mg)	Effective duration (hr)	Maximum 24 hr dose (mg)
Prescription				
Naproxen	Anaprox	250–500	8–12	1200
	Anaprox DS	500		
	Aleve			600
Diclofenac	Voltaren	100	24	100
	Arthotec	50, 75	8	300
Celecoxib	Celebrex	200	12	None
Ketorolac	Toradol	PO: 10	6	40
		IM/IV: 30–60		120
Fenoprofen	Nalfon	300–600	6	3200
Diflunisal	Dolobid	500–1000	8–12	1500
Nonprescription				
Ibuprofen	Advil, Motrin, Nuprin	200–400	4–6	1200
Acetominophen	Tylenol	325–1000	3–6	4000
Acetylsalicyclic acid (ASA)	Aspirin, Empirin, Ecotrin	325–1000		4000

Abbreviation: PO, per os.

with intravenous injection versus intramuscular administration. Ketorolac is also available in a PO formulation, but the maximum daily dose is limited to 40 mg. In general, the nonselective COX inhibitors should only be considered a postoperative intervention. They all have a risk of inhibiting platelet formation and may increase the risk of surgical bleeding. Their risk of use should always be weighed against potential benefits.

COX-3 Inhibitors

The mechanism of action of acetaminophen (Tylenol) is solely due to reversible COX-3 enzyme inhibition, and it exhibits analgesic and antipyretic qualities. However, it has no anti-inflammatory action, but, more importantly, has no action on platelet COX enzymes; platelets retain their function. It also has no known GI or renal side-effects. In fact, acetominophen may be used all throughout pregnancy since it does not cause premature closure of the ductus arteriosis in the fetus.

The only drawback with acetaminophen is that it may cause fatal hepatic necrosis; this is a dose-related adverse event. The fatal dose in adults is in excess of 10 g, the usual daily dose is 1000 mg every four hours with a maximum daily dose of 5 g. These doses are reduced in children and patients with compromised liver function.

Acetaminophen is available as a compounded drug and works quite synergistically to produce superior analgesia when combined with codeine (Tylenol with codeine), oxycodone (Percocet) (17), and hydrocodone (Hydrocet).

COX-2 Inhibitors

Unfortunately, the recently released and highly effective COX-2 inhibitors have been withdrawn from use. However, while in use, rofecoxib (Vioxx) and valdecoxib (Bextra) were very effective. The only COX-2 inhibitor still available is celecoxib (Celebrex), but is only approved for arthritic pain, not postoperative pain. It has a very slow absorption from the GI tract, and time to peak effect is several hours, making it unsuitable as an acute postoperative medication. However, one recent study reported good results when administered as a loading dose of 400 mg, two hours preoperatively, followed by 200 mg every 12 hours for up to 14 days (24). It should be stressed, however, that this is an off-label use of this medication.

New and Novel

Over the past several years, a new and novel use of gabapentin (Neurontin) has emerged for acute preoperative pain control. Gabapentin's use in neuropathic pain is well established (25). Its mechanism is through calcium channel blocking by binding reversibly to the subunit receptors, blocking the development of hyperalgesia locally and diminishing central sensitization. Recent studies have shown that it is effective in reducing acute postoperative pain as well as reducing the concomitant use of opioids. Not surprisingly, the opioid side-effects of PONV, respiratory depression, and pruritis are reduced (25). The only drawback is an increased risk of sedation. Whether this sedation prolongs "street readiness" is presently unknown.

The most optimal results are obtained with a very simple regimen: the patient takes a one time PO dose of 1200 mg gabapentin two hours prior to surgery. Divided doses or lower doses are not nearly as efficacious. The widespread use of gabapentin has yet to occur, but these types of drugs are clearly the wave of the future. Of note, postoperative pain is an off-label use of this medication.

STATE OF THE ART PAIN MANAGEMENT: MULTIMODAL ANALGESIA

All the previous sections of this chapter related to patient education, patient assessment, and pain reduction have led to the concept of pain management. Pain management is most effective using a multimodal approach (26,27). That is, applying agents and techniques that operate through different mechanisms. Multimodal therapy for pain control is part of a broader clinical approach, not unlike that seen in therapies developed for treatment of neoplasia, infection, and hypertension.

The benefits of multimodal analgesia in terms of drug sparing has been reviewed by a panel of experts convened to evaluate the literature. They concluded that using multimodal analgesia regimens not only improved patient management, but because of opioid sparing, also reduced the incidence of PONV (28).

Postoperative pain occurs as a result of diverse etiologies and mechanisms. Surgery is accompanied by anxiety, fasting, anesthetic agents, pain, and immobilization, each of which exerts incremental effects of discomfort. Surgical trauma produces a neurohumoral inflammatory response, resulting in the release of intracellular contents (proteases, bradykinins, prostaglandins) from both damaged and inflammatory cells. This heightens the sensitivity of the injured nerve fiber at the surgical site—the nociceptor. Pain is transmitted to the brain via different pathways through the spinal nerves and cord. Thus, there is a valid rationale for using different modalities to alleviate the perception of pain by modulating the mechanisms at the different sites.

A multimodal strategy for postoperative analgesia should begin prior to surgery. Patients should be educated in the importance and rationale for using different analgesics. Patients will also benefit from an explanation of how much and what type of pain can be expected after the procedure (29).

Preemptive analgesia refers to the concept of administering the medication or performing an intervention prior to surgical tissue injury. This effect has been demonstrated in animal models, but definitive randomized clinical trials in patients have not always shown this technique to be efficacious (30,31). As discussed previously, in recent studies, only gabapentin has shown preemptive analgesic effects. The theoretical basis for prevenative analgesia relates to hyperalgesia from acute tissue injury. Anti-inflammatory analgesics, local anesthetic infiltration, nerve blocks, or small doses of opioids prior to surgical incision modulate this hyperalgesic effect (32,33).

There are essentially two methods of delivering current multimodal therapy: fixed dose versus flexible dose combination. There are several FDA-approved fixed dose combination drugs which include an opioid and usually acetaminophen or occasionally aspirin (Table 4). Patients can also be prescribed opioids and nonopioid adjuncts; however, in this scenario, patients must adhere to a more complicated pain medicine schedule, which may not be realistic.

Each operation and each patient are unique situations and thus the clinician must tailor a suitable regimen of pain control. One thing is clear in many postoperative pain audits: monotherapy is generally unsatisfactory from the patient's perspective.

POSTOPERATIVE NAUSEA AND VOMITING

Adequate control of PONV is one of the major goals of ambulatory surgery. The overall incidence has remained constant over the past two decades in the 20% to 30% range (34,35). It is estimated that 0.2% of all patients may experience intractable PONV, leading to a delayed recovery or even unanticipated hospital admission (36). In most surveys, PONV is among the most unpleasant experiences of surgery and is associated with poor patient satisfaction (37). In addition, PONV

Table 4 Common Opioid/Analgesic Combinations and Controlled Opioids

Generic name	Trade name	Dose (mg)	Daily maximum tablets	Effective duration (hr)
Codeine/ acetaminophen	Tylenol #3, 4	30, 60/300	12	3–4
Codeine/ASA	Empirin #3, 4	30, 60/325	12	3–4
Oxycodone/ acetaminophen	Percocet	2.5–10/325–650	6–12	4–6
Oxycodone/ASA	Percodan	4.88/325	12	4–6
Hydrocodone/ acetaminophen	Vicodin	5/500	8	4–6
Hydrocodone/ ibuprofen	Vicoprofen	7.5/200	6	4–6
Propoxyphene/ acetaminophen	Darvocet	65,100/650	8	4–6
Controlled release opioids				
Oxycodone-CR	Oxycontin	10, 20, 40, 80	2	12
Morphine-CR	MS Contin	15, 30, 60	2	12
Tramadol-ER	Ultram ER	100	3	24

Abbreviation: ASA, acetylsalicyclic acid.

may also be rarely associated with serious complications such as wound dehiscence, aspiration, hematoma at the surgical site, dehydration, electrolyte imbalance, Mallory–Weiss tear, and esophageal rupture (37–39).

Anesthetics, especially opioids, delay gastric emptying and increase large and small bowel transit times. While the exact mechanisms are unknown, these agents affect the central vomiting reflex of the medulla, which is in close proximity to the visceral and somatic pathways responsible for vomiting (40,41). Vomiting is the actual physical phenomenon of the forceful expulsion of gastric contents from the mouth. Retching, while it looks similar, is defined as a labored, spasmodic, rhythmic contraction without expulsion of gastric contents.

Predicting in advance which patients may be at high risk for PONV allows the clinician to selective prophylaxis for those patients who will have the most benefit (42). Table 5 lists all identified risk factors for increased susceptibility to PONV, and Table 6 outlines a formula to calculate the risk factors (42). As can be seen, a number of strategies are available (Table 7).

Great strides have been made in the treatment of PONV with the introduction of 5-HT3 receptor antagonists. These agents act directly on the chemo-receptor trigger zone (CTZ) of the brain. Their lack of sedation and other side-effects when compared to the older agents make them an ideal choice for ambulatory surgery. Ondansetron (Zofran), the first agent of this group, is effective given at the end of surgery in a 4 to 8 mg dose (43,44). Another popular agent in the United States is granisetron (Kytril) and has been used in a dose of 0.1 to 3 mg (45,46). Most studies have shown PONV efficacy in a 1 mg dose, but one study has recently successfully described its use in a dose as low as 0.1 mg (47). It appears that there is a wide dose range for these very safe medications.

The use of steroids as an antiemetic is common, although its mechanism is unknown. Dexamethasone (Decadron) is the drug of choice because it is nonsedating, long-acting, and inexpensive. The recommended dose is 5 to 10 mg in adults. It appears to be most effective when administered prior to the start of the procedure (48).

Droperidol, a butyrophenone, has been used extensively in the prevention of PONV in low doses (0.625–1.25 mg), which does not cause sedation or prolongation of the PACU stay. Doperidol is best administered at the completion of surgery (49). In 2001, the FDA issued a

Table 5 Risk Factors for Postoperative Nausea and Vomiting

Anesthetic factors	Patient factors	Surgical factors
Volatile agents	Female	Lengthy procedure
Nitrous oxide	Previous PONV	Type of surgery[a]
Opioids	History of motion sickness	
Neostigmine (>2.5 mg)	Moderate-to-severe postoperative pain	
	High anxiety	
	Nonsmoker	

[a] Intra-abdominal; major gynecologic; breast; ENT; strabismus.
Abbreviation: PONV, postoperative nausea and vomiting.

Table 6 Simple Postoperative Nausea and Vomiting Risk Scoring

Risk factors	Risk of PONV
Female	10% if zero factors
Previous PONV	21% for one factor
Previous history of motion sickness	39% for two factors
Nonsmoker	61% for three factors
Postoperative use of opioids	79% for four factors

Abbreviation: PONV, postoperative nausea and vomiting.

warning related to an association of droperidol with a potentially fatal cardiac arrhythmia, with about 74 in 11 million chance. Many experts in the field have challenged the FDA on this issue, and droperidol continues to be an excellent rescue drug for PONV (50,51).

In the benzamide group, the most common antiemetic is metoclopramide (Reglan). It is considered to be a pro-kinetic agent because it increases GI motility, and lowers esophageal sphincter tone. It also acts centrally at the CTZ. All these effects can precisely counter opioid side-effects (52). However, recent studies have cast doubt on the low doses (10 mg) frequently employed in postoperative use to reduce the incidence of adverse side-effects. The recommended dose now is 20 mg (53).

There are several older medications available which are quite effective, but generally produce some sedation in clinical doses. Of these, the anticholinergic scopolamine is the most potent. It is available as a convenient transdermal preparation and should be applied the evening before, or four hours prior to the completion of surgery (54). The antihistamine diphenhydramine (Benadryl, 10–50 mg IV), and the priperazine, hydroxyzine (Vistaril, 25–50 mg, IM only) act at similar central sites and are quite effective, but their side-effects may prolong recovery room stay. Finally, phenothiazine, prochlorperazine (compazine, 5–10 mg PO), and promethazine (Phenergan, 25 mg, PO, IM, IV) can serve as rescue regimens, as long as the patient is informed of what to expect and accepts the plan to be discharged while still somewhat sedated (see Table 8 for summary) (55).

Strategies to Prevent PONV

The clinician should determine the risk of PONV for each patient. Patients who are high risk or undergoing procedures associated with a higher risk (Tables 5 and 6) for complications from vomiting such as facial plastic surgery should receive PONV prophylaxis. Combination

Table 7 Suggested Therapeutic Options for Postoperative Nausea and Vomiting

A. Pharmacologic
 a. Monotherapy
  i. Older antiemetics
   1. Phenothiazines: promethazine (phenergan), prochlorperazine (Compazine)
   2. Butyrophenones: droperadol (Inapsine)
   3. Benzamides: metaclopramide (Reglan)
   4. Anticholinergic: scopolamine (Scope)
   5. Antihistamine: diphenhydramine (Benadryl), cyclizine (Marzine), hydroxyzine (Vistaril)
  ii. New antiemetics
   1. Serotonin 5-hydroxytryptamine 3 (5-HT_3) receptor antagonists: ondansetron (Zofran), granisetron (Kytril)
  iii. Nontraditional antiemetics: dexamethasone (Decadron), propofol (Diprovan)
 b. Combination of two or more of the above agents
  i. 5-HT_3 receptor antagonist + droperidol
  ii. 5-HT_3 receptor antagonist + dexamethasone
  iii. Virtually any combination the clinician is comfortable with
B. Other measures with antiemetic effect
 a. Supplemental oxygen
 b. Adequate hytration
 c. Good pain relief
 d. Anxiolytic
C. Alternative techniques: acupuncture, acupressure or laser stimulation of the P6 point, hypnosis
D. Multimodal approach using the above options

Table 8 Agents for Postoperative Nausea and Vomiting with Initial Dose

Generic name	Trade name	Initial dose (mg)	Duration (hr)
Ondansetron	Zofran	4	4
Granisetron	Kytril	0.1	8
Dexamethasone	Decadron	5	24
Droperidol	Inapsine	0.625	2
Metoclopramide	Reglan	20	2
Scopolamine	Scop (transdermal)	0.4	72
Diphenhydramine	Benadryl	25	4
Hydroxyzine[a]	Vistaril	25	6
Prochlorperazine	Compazine	5	4
Promethazine	Phenergen	25	8
Propofol	Diprovan	10	0.2

[a]NOT for intravenous use—intramuscular or per os only. All others available, IV, IM, PO formulations available.

antiemetic therapy is superior to single-agent therapy for PONV prophylaxis (56). Unfortunately, for the patient with unresolved PONV, there is scant randomized clinical trial data that have identified a specific working therapy. Current clinical rational is to choose an agent of a different mechanism than what was previously used. (Agents are summarized in the above Table 8).

SPECIAL CONSIDERATIONS

There are two patient populations that merit extra detail: the elderly patient and the drug-dependent patient.

Since the population in the United States is aging, all caregivers are dealing with older patients. However, the older patient is rather heterogeneous. Many have aged well and seem to be chronologically and physically well preserved, while others may have a range of chronic conditions and can be taking several medications. In addition, older patients are frequently under-treated for pain for many unfounded reasons, including: some pain is a normal part of aging, older patients are not complaining of pain and are therefore not in pain, opioids are more dangerous in older patients, older patients use pain complaints as an attention-seeking device, and addiction results from opioid use.

Physiologically, as we age, the two organs of excretion—the liver and the kidney—have decreased function. Organ blood flow is decreased by about 10% per decade after the age of 60. Thus, the use of COX inhibitors should be especially adjusted. As with all patients, we must be cognizant of liver function impairment in elderly patients, and reduce opiate use accordingly. The rule of thumb in the older patient is to start low and frequently assess. There is some evidence that elderly patients respond better to verbal rather than visual scales of pain assessment. This is because approximately 80% of elderly patients have some visual impairment, 75% have some hearing impairment, and approximately 22% have significant impairments in both (57).

Drug-Dependent Patients

Many patients who present for ambulatory surgery are chronic users of habituating medications, especially opioids and benzodiazepines. The use of opioids dramatically increased after the 1997 consensus statement from the American Academy of Pain Medicine which concluded that using opioids for chronic "nonmalignant" pain was appropriate. We are now regularly encountering patients who are chronically taking morphine (MS Contin) or oxycodone (Oxycontin) and concurrently with diazepam (Valium) or lorazepam (Ativan). These patients seem to have a greater response to surgical pain. The opioid-dependent patient's tolerance may be responsible for the increased pain sensitivity and local hyperalgesia. Not realizing this, and unfamiliar with the large doses sometimes taken by these patients, clinicians frequently under-treat these patients, with resultant patient dissatisfaction (58,59).

The occasion of surgery should not be a time for withdrawal, whether intentionally or not. On the day of surgery, these patients should take their medication, including the sustained release formulation. These are generally on a 12-hour schedule and should keep the patients

Table 9 Important Predictors of Severe Postoperative Pain

Most important factor	Preoperative pain levels Younger age Type of surgery (abdominal and orthopedic surgery are 3 × more painful than laparoscopic)
Moderately important factor	Preoperative anxiety level Preoperative questioning level
Less important factor	Incision size (larger more painful than smaller) Female gender

Source: From Ref. 42

at baseline. If missed, equivalent doses should be given intraoperatively (Table 2). It is also important to remember that these patients will require more opioid analgesia postoperatively, and at more frequent intervals than the physician is accustomed to prescribing. At the present time, there are no prospective studies for the best preoperative management to follow for these patients, other than rational judgment.

CHRONIC POSTOPERATIVE PAIN

One of the reasons for ensuring patient comfort after surgery is the potential for developing a chronic pain syndrome. This has only started to be recognized over the last 10 to 15 years. This depends on many factors, but can occur from 4% to 50% of patients postoperatively (60,61). Precise mechanisms, prevention, and treatment of chronic postsurgical pain are under active study, both clinically and in animal studies in the laboratory. While much is still unknown, we can glean some useful data to guide us.

In the simplest model, we need only think of persistent postoperative pain as the causative agent in a neuropathic pain complex. It is thought that nerve injury from transection, or even stretching or constriction, can cause it. However, even soft tissue injury can change local nociceptors and produce a hyperalgesia. This can quickly lead to a central nervous system change in the usual conduction and pain perception. That is the bad news. The good news is that there are currently very good predictors of who may develop persistent postoperative surgical pain and what procedures may cause this phenomenon (Table 9) (62,63,64). There is also believed to be a strong polymorphic genetic component, as seen in both human trials and animal studies (64). Some of these factors, especially the level of the patient's pain both pre- and postoperatively, are under the physician's control and should be aggressively treated to help prevent this symptom complex.

NEW USEFUL MODALITIES AND ALTERNATIVE MODALITIES

Any postoperative pain modality should satisfy several obvious criteria. It must be safe, more effective than placebo, cost effective and be easily understood by the patient. One approach that easily meets these criteria is local anesthetic wound and incision infiltration. Besides providing pain relief through its primary property of anesthesia, it is now known that local anesthetics provide local anti-inflammatory action, which may be even more important. Although single infiltration techniques have been in use for a long time, more recently, incisional catheter techniques have been developed and FDA-approved for ambulatory use. The easiest, most cost effective, and safest device (Fig. 4) is probably the elastomeric pump. In this technique, a small plastic catheter is placed in the wound and then sutured closed. The pump delivers an infusion of long-acting local anesthetic into the wound. By use of a simple clamp, it then becomes a patient controlled analgesic (PCA) device. This provides nonopioid analgesia and all the resultant adverse effects of opioids are greatly reduced (65).

The application of local topical anesthetics has also proven efficacious. Although these are available in a variety of preparations, the most widely used is lidoderm 5%. Patients can be discharged while still comfortable after local wound infiltration with instructions to apply

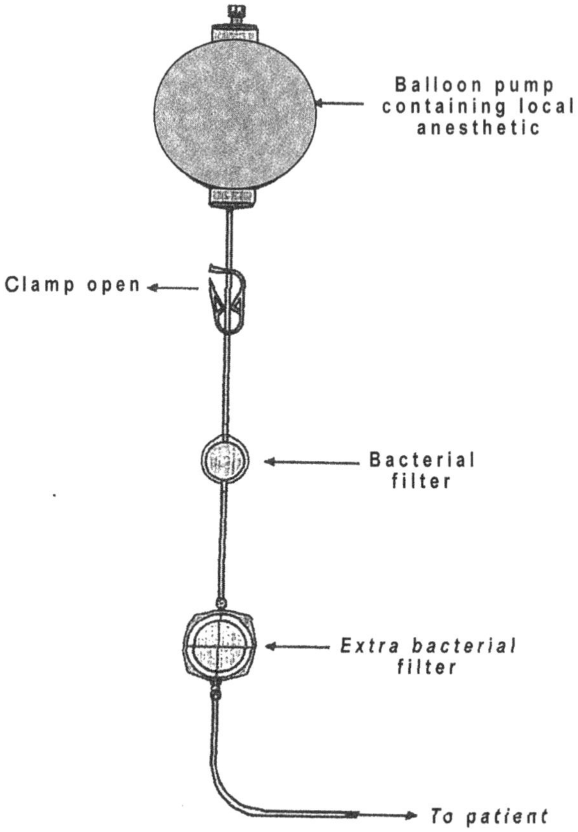

Figure 4 Elastomeric pump.

lidoderm as the anesthesia wears off. It is shown to be quite effective as a short-term solution after a variety of procedures.

Certainly the most novel device, recently FDA-approved for inpatient use and soon to be approved for outpatient use, is an iontophoretic transdermal system (ITS) (66,67). Iontophoresis is a technology by which a tiny electrical current is used to drive an ionized drug through the skin and into the capillary bed. Through clinical testing, ideal analgesia has been determined for mild to almost severe pain at 40 μg of fentanyl delivered every 10 minutes, on demand. The ITS is only slightly larger than the passive transdermal fentanyl patch, essentially a miniature PCA device. It is designed to give a maximum of 200 doses or last for 24 hours before becoming inactive. The main drawback is the potentially high cost, which is yet to be determined.

There are also some alternative medical modalities that have received some validity through traditional randomized clinical trials. Acupuncture is one such modality. It is a traditional Chinese medical practice that has been in use for three millennia. Manual, thermal, or electrical stimulation can be applied to the needles. There are several treatments that may be useful. Needle placement in the area of an incision with an application of electrical current can alleviate acute and chronic pain and provide analgesia (68). Auricular acupuncture, where the mechanism is less obvious, has been shown to provide pain relief in procedures other than those covered within this text (69). These needles are sometimes left in place as small tacks, which the patient can stimulate and obtain relief. There is also a device to provide electrical stimulation to auricular points which is very small and worn by the patient postoperatively to help provide pain relief (70).

In the very anxious, but appropriate patient, perioperative acupuncture has been found to reduce operative anxiety and reduce perioperative opioid use (71). Acupuncture is also commonly used for management of nausea after surgery or chemotherapy. Some studies have shown near equivalence between acupuncture point P6 and common antiemetic agents (72,73). Since

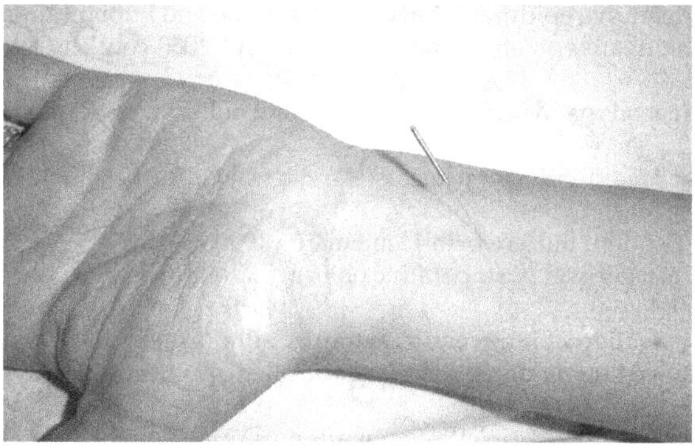

Figure 5 Acupuncture point P6: Defined by two of the patient's thumb widths (the Chinese CUN measurement) proximal to the most prominent wrist crease on the ventral aspect of the arm between the tendons of the flexor carpi radialis and the palmaris longus.

acupuncture is becoming increasingly known to patients, the clinician may want to consider making it an available option for pain management (Fig. 5).

Another modality or pain management is the various relaxation techniques. An extrapolation of this concept is adequate preoperative patient education. The so-called mind–body therapies are a rather heterogeneous group of techniques which include yoga, music therapy, positive-thought therapy, and guided imagery. There are studies showing perioperative pain score reduction using these nonpharmacological interventions and may be useful in specific situations (74). This was included in this section to remind caregivers that we are still a long way from mastering all possibilities for postoperative pain relief, and should keep all scientific philosophies open to the new and varied ideas.

REFERENCES

1. Joshi GP. Postoperative pain management. Am J Orthop 2004; 33:128–135.
2. Pregler J, Kapur P. The development of ambulatory anesthesia and future challenges. Anaesthesiol Clin North Am 2003; 21:207–228.
3. Rawal N, Hylander J, Nydahl PA, et al. Survey of postoperative analgesia following ambulatory surgery. Acta Anaesthesiol Scand 1997; 41:1017–1022.
4. Chung F, Ritchie E, Su J. Postoperative pain in ambulatory surgery. Anesth Analg 1997, 85, 808–816.
5. Mitchell M. Pain management in day-case sugery. Nurs Stand 2004; 18:33–38.
6. Coll AM, Ameen JR, Moseley LG. Reported pain after day surgery: a critical literature review. J Adv Nurs 2004; 46:53–65.
7. Joint Commission on Accreditation of Healthcare Organizations. Comprehensive Accreditation Manual for Behavioral Health Care (CAMBHC) Pain Assessment and Management Standards 2001–2002. Oakbrook Terrace, IL: JCAHO, 2002:1–14.
8. Max MB, Payne R, Edwards WT, et al. Principles of Analgesic Use in the Treatment of Acute Pain and Cancer Pain. 4th ed. Glenview, IL: American Pain Society, 1999.
9. Hobbs GJ, Hodgkinson V. Assessment, measurement, history and examination. In: Rowbotham Dj, Macintyre P, eds. Acute Pain. London: Arnold, 2003:93–111.
10. DeLoach LJ, Higgins MS, Caplan AB, et al. The visual analog scale in the immediate postoperative period: intrasubject variability and correlation with a numeric scale. Anesth Analg 1998; 86:102–106.
11. Stein C, Yassouridis A: Peripheral morphine analgesia. Pain 1997; 17:119–121.
12. McQuay HJ, Carroll D, Moore RA. Injected morphine in postoperative pain: a quantitative systematic review. J Pain Syptom Manage 1999; 17:164–174.
13. Latta KS, Ginsberg B, Barkin RL. Meperidine: a critical review. Am J Ther 2002; 9:53–68.
14. Coda BA, O'Sullivan B, Donaldson G, et al. Comparative efficacy of patient-controlled administration of morphine, hydropmorphone, or sufentanil for the treatment of oral mucositis pain following bone marrow transplantation. Pain 1997; 72:333–346.
15. Shipton EA. Tramadol- present and future. Anesth Intensive Care 2000; 28:363–374.
16. Hale ME, Fleischmann R, Salzman R, et al. Efficacy and safety of controlled-release versus immediate-release oxycodone: randomized double-blind evaluation in patients with chronic back pain. Clin J Pain 1999; 15:179–183.
17. Edwards JE, Moore RA, McQuay HJ. Single dose oxycodone and oxycodone plus paracetamol (acetaminophen) for acute postoperative pain. Cochrane Database Syst Rev 2000; 4: CD002763.

18. Rygnestad T, Borchgrevink PC, Eide E. Postoperative epidural infusion of morphine and bupivacaine is safe on surgical wards: organization of the treatment, effects and side effects of 2000 consecutive patients. Acta Anesthesiol Scand 1997; 41:868–876.
19. Babenco HD, Conard PF, Gross JB. The pharmacodynamic effect of a remifentanil bolus on ventilatory control. Anesthesiology 2000; 92:393–398.
20. Szarvas S, Harmon D, Murphy D. Neuraxial opioid-induced pruritus: A review. J Clin Anesth 2003; 15:234–239.
21. Estafanous F, ed. Opioids in Anaesthesia II. London: Butterworth-Heinemann, 1990:93–109.
22. Edwards JE, Oldman AD, Smith LA, et al. Oral aspirin in postoperative pain: a quantitative systematic review. Pain 1999; 81:289–297.
23. Ready LB, Brown CR, Stahigren LH, et al. Evaluation of intravenous ketorolac administered by bolus or infusion for treatment of postoperative pain: a double-blind, placebo-controlled, multicenter study. Anesthesiology 1994; 80:1277–1286.
24. Reuben SS, Ekman EF, Charron D. Evaluating the analgesic efficacy of administering celecoxib as a component of multimodal analgesia for outpatient anterior cruciate ligament reconstruction surgery. Anesth Analg 2007; 105(1):222–227.
25. Kok-Yuen Ho, Tong JG, Ashraf SH. Gabapentin and postoperative pain- a systematic review of randomized controlled trials. Pain 2006; 126:91–101.
26. Joshi GP, White PF. Management of acute and postoperative pain. Curr Opin Anaesthesiol 2001; 14(4):417–421.
27. Chilvers CR, Nguyen MH, Robertson IK. Changing from epidural to multimodal analgesia for colorectal laparotomy: an audit. Anaesth Intensive Care 2007; 5(2):230–238.
28. Gan TJ. Consensus guidelines for managing postoperative nausea and vomiting. Anesth Analg 2004; 97:62–71.
29. Acute Pain Management Guideline Panel. Acute Pain Management: Operative or Medical Procedures and Trauma. Clinical Practice Guideline, Rockville, MD: Agency for Health Care Policy and Research, Public Health Service, U S. Department of Health and Human services, 1992.
30. Woolf CJ, Chong MS. Preemptive analgesia—treating postoperative pain by preventing the establishment of central sensitization. Anesth Analg 1993; 77:362–379.
31. Dahl JB, Kehlet H: The value of pre-emptive analgesia in the treatment of postoperative pain. Br J Anaesth 1993; 70(4):434–439.
32. Ejlersen E, Anderson HB, Eliasen K, et al. A comparison between preincisional and postincisional lidocaine infiltration and postoperative pain. Anesth Analg 1992; 74:495–498.
33. Dahl JB, Hjorsto NC, Stage JG, et al. Effects of combines perioperative epidural bupivacaine and morphine, ibuprofen, and incisional bupivacaine on postoperative pain, pulmonary, and endocrine function after minilaparotomy cholecystectomy. Reg Anesth 1994; 19:199–205.
34. Bonica J, Crepps W, Monk B, et al. Post-anesthetic nausea, retching and vomiting. Anesthesiology 1958; 19:532–540.
35. Cohen MM, Duncan PG, DeBoer DP,et al. The postoperative interview: assessing risk factors for nausea and vomiting. Anesth Analg 1994; 78:7–16.
36. Gold BS, Kitz DS, Lecky JH, et al. Unanticipated admission to the hospital following ambulatory surgery. J Am Med Assoc 1989; 262:3008–3010.
37. Myles PS, Williams DL, Hendrata M, et al. Patient satisfaction after anaesthesia and surgery: results of a prospective survey of 10,811 patients. Br J Anaesth 2000; 84:6–10.
38. Watcha MF, White PF. Postoperative nausea and vomiting: its etiology, treatment, and prevention. Anesthesiology 1992; 77:162–184.
39. Wilder-Smith OH, Martin NC, Morabia A. Postoperative nausea and vomiting: a comparative survey of the attitudes, perceptions, and practice of Swiss anesthesiologists and surgeons. Anesth Analg 1997; 84:826–831.
40. Wang SC, Borrison HL. A new concept in the organization of the central emetic mechanisms: recent studies on the site of action of apomorphine, copper sulfate and cardiac glycosides. Gastroenterology 1952; 22:1–12.
41. Andrews PLR. Vagal afferent innervation of the gastrointestinal tract. In: Cevero F, Morrison JFB, eds. Progress in brain research, vol 67. London: Elsevier, 1986:65–86.
42. Apfel CC, Laara E, Kiovuranta M, et al. A simplified risk score for predicting postoperative nausea and vomiting: conclusions from cross-validations between two centers. Anesthesiology 1999; 91:693–700.
43. Tramer MR, Reynolds DJ, Moore RA, et al. Efficacy, dose-response, and safety of ondansetron in prevention of postoperative nausea and vomiting: a quantitative systematic review of randomized placebo-controlled studies. Anesthesiology 1997; 87:1277–1289.
44. Tang J, Wang B, White PF, et al. The effect of timing of ondansetron administration on its efficacy, cost effectiveness, and cost-benefit as a prophylactic antiemetic in the ambulatory setting. Anesth Analg 1998; 86:274–282.

45. Wilson AJ, Diemunsch P, Lindeque BG, et al. Single-dose I. V. granisetron in the prevention of postoperative nausea and vomiting. Br J Anaesth 1996; 76:515–518.
46. Mikawa K, Takao Y, Nishina K, et al. Optimal dose of ganisetron for prophylaxis against postoperative emesis after gynecological sugery. Anesth Analg 1997; 85:652–656.
47. Taylor AM, Rosen M, Diemunsch PA,et al. A double-blind, parallel-group, placebo-controlled, dose-ranging multicenter study of intravenous granisetron in the treatment of postoperative nausea and vomiting in patients undergoing surgery with general anesthesia. J Clin Anesth 1997; 9:658–663.
48. Henzi I, Walder B, Tramer MR. Dexamethasone for the prevention of postoperative nausea and vomiting: a quantitative systematic review. Anesth Analg 2000; 91:1404–1407.
49. Henzi I, Sonderegger J, Tramer MR. Efficacy, dose-responce, and adverse effects of droperidol for prevention of postoperative nausea and vomiting. Can J Anaesth 2000; 47:537–551.
50. Habib AS, Gan TJ. Food and Drug Administration black box warning on the perioperative use of droperidol: a review of cases. Anesth Analg 2003; 96:1377–1379.
51. Gan TJ, White PF, Scuderi PE, et al. FDA "black box" warning regarding the use of droperidol for postoperative nausea and vomiting: is it justified? Anesthesiology 2002; 97:287.
52. Harrington RA, Hamilton CW, Brogden RN, et al. Metoclopramide: an updated review of its pharmocolological properties and clinical use. Drugs 1983; 25:451–494.
53. Quaynow H, Raeder JC. Incidence and severity of postoperative nausea and vomiting are similar after metoclopramide 20 mg and ondansetron 8 mg given by the end of laparoscopic cholecystectomies. Acta Anaesthesiol Scand 2002; 46:109–113.
54. Kranke P, Morin AM, Roewer N, et al. The efficacy and safety of transdermal scopolamine for the prevention of postoperative nausea and vomiting: a quantitative systematic review. Anesth Analg 2002; 95:133–143.
55. Khalil S, Philbrook L, Rabb M, et al. Ondansetron/promethazine combination or promethazine alone reduces nausea and vomiting after middle ear surgery. J Clin Anesth 1999; 11:596–600.
56. Habib AS, Gan TJ. Combination therapy for postoperative nausea and vomiting – a more effective prophylaxis? Ambu Surg 2001; 9:59–71.
57. Prowse M. Postoperative pain in older people: a review of the literature. J Clin Nursing 2007; 16:84–97.
58. Brill S, Ginosar Y, Davidson EM. Perioperative management of chronic pain patients with opioid dependency. Curr Opin Anesth 2006; 19:325–331.
59. Rozen D, DeGaetano NP. Perioperative management of opioid-tolerant chronic pain patients. J Opioid Manag 2006; 2(6):353–363.
60. Wilder-Smith OHG, Arendt-Nielsen L. Postoperative hyperalgesia: its clinical importance and relevance. Anesthesiology 2006; 104:601–607.
61. Lavand'Homme P. Perioperative pain. Curr Opin Anesthesiol 2006; 19:556–561.
62. Kalkman CJ, Visser K, Moen J, et al. Preoperative prediction of severe postoperative pain. Pain 2003; 105:415–423.
63. Kehlet H, Jensen TS, Woolf C. Persistent postsurgical pain: risk factors and prevention. Lancet 2006; 367:1618–1625.
64. Seltzer Z, Wu T, Max MB, et al. Mapping a gene for neuropathic pain-related behaviour following peripheral neurectomy in the mouse. Pain 2001; 93:101–106.
65. Zohar E, Fredman B, Phillipov A, et al. The analgesic efficacy of patient-controlled bupivacaine wound instillation after total abdominal hysterectomy with bilateral salpingo-oophorectomy. Anesth Analg 2001; 93:482–487.
66. Mayes S, Ferrone M. Fentanyl HCl patient-controlled Iontophoretic transdermal system for the management of acute postoperative pain. Annals Pharm 2006; 4:2178–2186.
67. Power I. Fentanyl HCl iontophoretic transdermal system (ITS): clinical application of iontophoretic technology in the management of acute postoperative pain. Br J Anaesth 2007; 98(1):4–11.
68. Lin YC. Perioperative usage of acupuncture. Pediatr Anesth 2006; 16:231–235.
69. Buckley N. Auricular acupuncture for analgesia after arthroscopy. CMAJ 2007; 176(2):193–194.
70. Sator-Katzenschlager SM, Michalek-Sauberer A. P-Stim auricular electroacupuncture stimulation device for pain relief. Expert Rev Med Devices 2007; 4(1):23–32.
71. Kotani N, Hashimoto H, Sato Y, et al. Preoperative intradermal acupuncture reduces postoperative pain, nausea and vomiting, analgesic requirement, and sympathoadrenal responses. Anesthesiology 2001; 95:349–356.
72. Gan TJ, Parillo S, Fortney JT, et al. Comparison of electroacupuncture and ondansetron for the prevention of postoperative nausea and vomiting. Anesthesiology 2001; 95:A22.
73. Coloma M, White PF, Ogunnaike BO, et al. Comparison of acustimulation and ondansetron for the treatment of established postoperative nausea and vomiting. Anesthesiology 2002; 97:1387–1392.
74. Tusek DL, Church JM, Strong SA, et al. Guided imagery: a significant advance in the care of patients undergoing elective colorectal surgery. Dis Colon Rectum 1997; 40:172–178.
75. Chung F. Recovery pattern and home-readiness after ambulatory surgery. Anesth Analg 1995; 80:896–902.

26 Perioperative Counseling

Norma Daniel
Department of Colorectal Surgery, Cleveland Clinic Florida, Weston, Florida, U.S.A.

Arlene Segura
Surgical Services, Cleveland Clinic Florida, Weston, Florida, U.S.A.

INTRODUCTION

The introduction of managed care has resulted in the redesigning of the health-care delivery system with the focus of delivering quality care by cost-effective means. This shifting paradigm now relocates surgical procedures from inpatient to outpatient settings, permitting the patient to arrive at the hospital on the day of surgery and be discharged that same day to continue self-management at home. Consequently, ambulatory surgery has placed the responsibility on patients for their presurgical and postsurgical care. Therefore, patient education is vital in making informed decisions as a significant part of their care has been transferred from the monitored in-patient setting to the patient's home. This can impact the surgical experience. Perioperative counseling should focus on equipping patients with the tools necessary to assist them in successful recovery throughout the perioperative process.

The Joint Commission on Accreditation of Health Care Organization stresses that it is essential for nurses in ambulatory settings to become involved in the delivery of perioperative teaching programs (1). The perioperative care must be patient oriented. It is the responsibility of the perioperative nurse to assess, plan, implement, and evaluate the care given to patients undergoing ambulatory colorectal surgery, and to work toward producing observable and measurable outcomes. Interventions must be implemented preoperatively to prevent complications, as ambulatory colorectal surgery encompasses a wide range of diseases and disorders which are discussed in detail in other chapters within this textbook. The most common procedures performed are those affecting the anus and rectum. There should be teaching literature available in the physician's office, as the more informed the patient and family, the more positive the surgical experience.

PREPARING THE PATIENT

Patient preparation for ambulatory colorectal surgery goes beyond the provision of information; it should include influencing emotions and attitudes in order to alter behavior (2). The manner of preparation will have a profound impact on the postoperative recovery and on the smooth functioning of the surgical unit. Patient care should be individualized, as no surgical experience is considered minor. Any functional disturbance in the body can influence emotions and attitudes, and alter behaviors and continuity of care. As a result, meeting the physiological and psychological needs of the patient is vital in ensuring a favorable outcome of the surgical experience (2). Therefore, in preparing the patient for ambulatory colorectal surgery, the overall goal of the nurse is to be a skilled communicator, knowledgeable, sensitive, a keen listener, and avid teacher.

Meeting with the patient and the family at least one week prior to the date of surgery is important, as it establishes a rapport with both the patient and family. It is during that phase that all related data are collected and reviewed, and the patient is given instructions and emotional support as the stress level is much lower at that time than on the day of surgery. When sitting face to face with the perioperative nurse, the patient is much more relaxed and cooperative in assisting to create an individualized plan of care. Potential problem areas can be identified, and plans for intervention to ensure successful resolution can be initiated. This session may be the most memorable part of the surgical experience (3).

Preoperative Investigation

The cornerstone of an effective evaluation is a detailed history and physical. This is a valuable tool in assessing any premorbid conditions that may have a negative impact on the patient's perioperative experience and recovery. The patient should be medically cleared, including documenting any knowledge of the patient's living conditions, special needs, social issues, or family status that may affect the ambulatory surgical experience. Furthermore, many patients may have difficulty obtaining preoperative test results as they must go to the provider contracted by their insurance carrier, and these are usually performed at separate sites. For older adults, this sometimes results in confusion and difficulty in collecting information and their declining to attend the preoperative interview. This leads to the need for a telephone interview, which is an inefficient method of assessment for identifying needs and related problems. Many older adults may appear to be cognitive and functionally competent during telephone interview, and the interviewer may not be aware of any deficits which may require special attention during surgery (4).

Recent laboratory values, radiological reports, and electrocardiograms are essential in obtaining the patient's baseline medical status, while identifying and correcting any potential problems to decrease the incidence of perioperative morbidity and mortality. This practice will reduce the number of cancellations on the day of surgery, minimize potential complications by correcting preoperative abnormalities, and improve efficacy of the surgical process. All preoperative testing should be reviewed at least one week prior to surgery to allow for ample time to correct abnormal values, arrange for referrals, and provide for anticipated postoperative needs.

Using the anesthesia guidelines of each institution will assist in obtaining the required preoperative tests along with the surgeon's orders. In reviewing the patient's history, particular attention should be given to any history of mitral valve disorders, cardiac pacemakers, serious systemic disease or recent joint replacements, indwelling implants or stents, any currently prescribed steroid use, or blood dyscrasia. Should any of these premorbid conditions be present, appropriate clearances and recommendations should be obtained from the specialist involved in that area of service. Guidelines are followed for preoperative intravenous antibiotics for patients with mitral valve disorders and prosthetic implants and subacute bacterial endocarditis prophylaxis is given, if warranted.

At the time of the preoperative interview, the patient's chart should contain a complete history and physical with recommendations, and documentation of the clearance status of the patient for the proposed surgery. Copies of laboratory reports, radiological and anorectal physiology studies, stress tests, echocardiogram, and implant identification cards should also be attached to the medical record.

Anesthesia protocols usually advise that on the morning of surgery, patients should take their antihypertensive, antianginal, antiarrhythmic, antiparkinson, and antiepileptic medications with a small sip of water. All nonsteroidal anti-inflammatory medications should be withheld 7 to 10 days prior to surgery, to prevent alteration in platelet and coagulation function. Coumadin should be withheld at least five days prior to the procedure (3). The need for shorter term angicoagulation should be determined prior to discontinuation of Coumadin. Patients on insulin are usually instructed to withhold their insulin or to administer half of their normal dose, as recommended by their internist. Inquires should be made regarding herbal medications as they could directly affect body function. Vitamin E taken in large doses of 400 IU per day can have an antiplatelet effect resulting in slow wound healing. Over the counter medications, such as herbal medications and vitamins, including garlic and fish oils, should be reviewed as they can cause bleeding, thus patients should be advised to stop these preparations 7 to 10 days prior to surgery (3).

Preoperative Counseling

A preoperative visit is perhaps the most important tool for establishing a trusting relationship between the patient and nurse, which is very effective in reducing anxiety. The goal of this visit is to improve perioperative outcomes. Research has shown that patient education is an important component of the perioperative process, as it positively impacts on postoperative recovery and results in better coping ability, improved compliance, decreased anxiety and pain, and a more rapid return to recovery (3). A study of 100 patients who received preoperative teaching revealed a decrease in pain and depression, an earlier return to activities of daily living, an increase in patient compliance, and a heightened sense of patient satisfaction (5).

During the preoperative visit, the nurse assesses the patient's ability to process information, perception of the illness, and the ability to learn. The patient's readiness to learn can then be evaluated.

Thus, the amount of information given depends on the patient's readiness to receive or not receive. Forcing information on a patient who is not receptive only causes increased anxiety, which could result in an increased pulse, blood pressure, and respiratory rate. Sometimes moderate-to-high levels of anxiety interferes with the ability to process information resulting in confusion and the inability to cope. It is important to understand that behavioral tendencies are different in each patient. Preoperative counseling, therefore, prepares the patient mentally and emotionally for the intended procedure, in order to eliminate stress and anxiety. Otherwise, concerns can generate extreme physiological stress in patients who are already filled with preconceived notions about the implications of the procedure. This could eventually lead the patient to cancel the proposed surgery.

The preoperative nurse needs to ascertain that the patient understands the surgeon's explanation of the proposed surgery, and there is no lack of specific information. The patient needs to know the risks, benefits, alternatives, and possible complications, after which the consent is secured. The role of the perioperative nurse is to enhance, reinforce, clarify, and interpret this information for the patient (2). Preoperative counseling provides the patient with information and explanation of the intended surgical procedure, and the expected patient outcomes. Explanation of the pertinent nursing activities is given throughout the preoperative, intraoperative, and postoperative phase of the surgical experience, and it is during that period that reassurance is given to allay the patient's fears and anxieties.

During the preoperative interview, patients are screened in order to identify problems or special needs they may require prior to surgery. For example elderly patients may have difficulty arranging transportation. Most patients view the upcoming surgery with uncertainty, ignorance, and a vast majority express fear. It is vital that the preoperative information be geared to alleviate some of these anticipated emotions and expected patient behaviors, to ensure a well-informed and confident patient.

Preoperative teaching equips the patient with coping skills which help regain control of his or her life processes. Instructions, verbal and written, are given regarding the bowel preparation to be self administered on the day prior to surgery. The patient is advised to have nothing to eat or drink after midnight on the day prior to the surgical procedure. Prescription for oral antibiotics, if indicated, is given and any mechanical preparation, if indicated, is taken on the day prior to the surgery. The bowel preparation of most ambulatory colorectal surgery patients is usually two cleansing enemas or, depending on the magnitude of the procedure, an oral administration with polyethylene–glycol electrolyte solution (HalfLytely® or Golytely®; Braintree Labs Inc, Braintree, Maryland, U.S.A.) or Fleet® Phospho Soda (Fleet®, Lynchburg, Virginia, U.S.A.) oral laxative preparation. It is the patient's right to know what the total perioperative experience involves, thus an explanation of the sequence of events on the day of the surgery should be outlined. Written and verbal instructions are given to the patient regarding time of arrival, location of the hospital, admitting/registration office, family waiting room, number of family members allowed in the ambulatory care unit (ACU), the duration of surgery and the appropriate length of time in the operating room, and post anesthesia care unit (PACU) before being discharged (3). At this juncture, the opportunity is given for questions and answers regarding nursing care. The patient is advised to make arrangement for a designated caregiver to be available for transport on discharge.

The ACU: Patient Expectations

The patient is made aware of the preoperative protocol in the ACU and is reminded that this will involve assessment by the preoperative nurse and anesthesiologist, a further chart review of tests, surgical consents, and the need for intravenous access. A preoperative visit by the surgical team helps generate patient confidence and reassurance. Family members and friends are allowed to remain with the patient until escorted to the operating room.

Because the patient under general anesthesia is always susceptible to nerve injury which may result from pressure, obstruction, and stretching because of faulty positioning (6), the operating room team depends heavily on the information in the patient's medical record. Any pertinent information documented during the preoperative interview which would impact patient positioning is a major consideration during the intraoperative phase.

INTRAOPERATIVE CONSIDERATIONS

During the preoperative counseling, the nurse should be aware that, on entering the operating room, the patient may exhibit great stress and anxiety when leaving the familiar faces of family and friends and suddenly being surrounded by unfamiliar masked individuals, bright overhead lights, a large assortment of instruments, and high-tech equipment. Verbal reassurance should be given regarding the efficiency and competence of the surgical team, and information about the progress of the surgery relayed to designated family members or caregivers who will be in the family waiting room.

A large majority of patients are placed either in the prone jacknife position or the modified lithotomy positions which may place tremendous strain on certain areas of the body. As anesthetic agents and muscle relaxants depress the pain receptors, the patient loses the ability to compensate (6). Therefore, any disease process that will impact patient positioning should be documented and brought to the attention of the surgical team. Any such documentation will alert the surgical team to ensure safety in patient positioning and to vigilantly monitor for any exaggerated or abnormal movements of the patient's body.

The patient is given a brief explanation of what to expect before succumbing to general anesthesia, with the reassuring knowledge of awakening in the PACU with a nurse in vigilant attendance. At the completion of surgery, the surgeon will be available to give a report and reassurance of a successful procedure to the family members or designated caregivers.

DISCHARGE PLANNING

Discharge planning should begin in the physician's office at the time of preoperative patient counseling, and should be integrated in all aspects of patient care. Because some anesthesia medication causes amnesia, postoperative home going instructions should be discussed with the patient and family members. The Joint Commission on Accreditation of Healthcare Organization recommends that patients be discharged when a specified set of discharge criteria is met. This includes mobility, wound management, drain, setons, packing, voiding, diet, and information regarding what to expect postdischarge. Studies show that in 1996, one third of the population undergoing ambulatory surgical procedures were about 65 years of age or older, and these patients were prone to multiple chronic problems or limitations which hindered their ability to manage activities of daily living. In addition, approximately 80% of older adults have significant comorbidities, and would need postoperative assistance; therefore adequate preoperative assessment should be geared to meeting the special needs of these patients (4).

Another important aspect of discharge is pain management, and the patient must be reassured that pain will be controlled with oral analgesics (7). Previous experiences can affect a patient's perception; therefore, reassurance should be given that pain will be controlled before discharge, and a 24 hour number will be given to call if a problem should arise (7). Pain medications and any other pertinent drugs which are usually prescribed postoperatively can be called in to a pharmacy, and family members or caregivers should be available to have prescriptions filled prior to or immediately after surgery.

Patients scheduled for ambulatory colorectal surgery often do not appreciate the need for an escort, as their conception of the procedure is minimal surgery. These patients must be told that, although they are being discharged on the same day, depending on the nature of the surgery, they may experience an extended recovery time, and must plan ahead for care at home.

Returning to work is another important aspect in the recovery process and depends on the nature of the surgery; therefore discussion regarding postoperative restrictions should allow patients to plan ahead for work and duties at home.

A telephone call to the patient is initiated within 24 to 48 hours postoperatively for feedback on patient status and to identify problems to be addressed and resolved; in addition, many older patients live alone and may have difficulty managing the illness and medication changes. Home-going instructions should be reviewed with the patient and caregivers with instructions to contact the physician's office at a designated time to ensure adequate postoperative evaluation.

FUTURE CONSIDERATIONS OF AMBULATORY SURGERY

With the constant advancement of technology, continued refinement of instrumentation and public acceptance, greater numbers of colorectal procedures will be performed in ambulatory care settings. Because of the wide variety of disorders associated with this specialty, the new approaches, and changing patterns of the delivery of health care, it is wise to anticipate future trends in order to effectively deliver quality care. The transition of surgical care from in-hospital to out-patient will continue to accelerate; therefore, preoperative counseling of patients undergoing colorectal surgery in ambulatory settings will continue to play a major role.

REFERENCES

1. Eddy ME, Coslow BI. Preparation for ambulatory surgery: a patient education program. J Post Anesthes Nurs 1991; 6:5–12.
2. Fortner PA. Preoperative patient preparation: psychological and educational aspects. Semin Perioper Nurs 1998; 7:3–9.
3. Dunn D. Preoperative assessment criteria and patient teaching for ambulatory surgery patients. J Perianesthes Nurs 1998; 13:274–291.
4. Tappen RM. Preoperative assessment and discharge planning for older adults undergoing ambulatory surgery. AORN J 2001; 73:467, 469–470.
5. Brumfield VG, Kee CC, Johnson JY. Perioperative patient teaching in ambulatory surgery settings. AORN J 1996; 64(6):941–952.
6. Stoelting, RK, Miller RD. Basics of Anesthesia Positioning. 2nd ed. New York: Churchill Livingstone, 1998:201–208.
7. Doyle Christine E. Preoperative strategies for managing postoperative pain at home after day surgery. J Perianesthes Nurs 1999; 14(6):373–379.

Index

Abdominal sacrocolpopexy, 175–176
Abdominoperineal resections (APRs), 18, 277–278
Abscess drainage, 193, 197
Acceptable ambulatory procedures, 2
Acellular dermalmatrix (ADM), 275, 276
Acetaminophen, 310
Acetominophen, 310
Acetylsalicyclic acid (ASA), 308, 312
Acquired immunodeficiency syndrome (AIDS), 245
Acticon Neosphincter®, 137
Acupuncture, 183–184, 316–317
Acute anal fissures, 103
Acute eczematous dermatitis, 241
Acute Physiology and Chronic Health Evaluation (APACHE), 3
Acyclovir triphosphate, 246
Adjunctive biofeedback treatment methods, 73
Advancement flap, 106
Advil, 309, 310
Aerobes, 217
Alcock's canal. *See* Pudendal canal
Allergic contact dermatitis, 241, 293–294
Allis or Kocher clamps, 177
Alosetron, 124
Altemeier's procedure (perineal rectosigmoidectomy), 155
Alvenor®, 81
Ambulatory care unit (ACU), patient expectations, 323–324
Ambulatory colorectal surgery, 1
  anesthesia protocols, 322
  discharge planning, 324–325
  intraoperative considerations, 324
  perioperative counseling
    preparing the patient, 321–324
  perioperative pain management
    chronic, 315
    modalities, 315–317
    multimodal analgesia, 311
    nausea and vomiting, 311–313
    pain assessment, 305–307
    pain medication, 307–311
    special considerations, 314–315
Ambulatory surgery, 1
  future prospects, 325
American Society of Anesthesiologists Classification (ASA), 2
Amitiza (lubiprostone), 127, 147
Amitriptyline, 125
Ampicillin, 253
Anaerobes, 217
Anal adenocarcinoma, 242
Anal canal, anatomical characteristics of
  anal verge, 12
  anus or anal orifice, 12
  external muscle layer, 188
  inner muscle layer, 188
  linings, 12
  muscle groups
    conjoined longitudinal muscle (CLM), 13
    external anal sphincter, 13–14
    internal anal sphincter, 13
    levator ani, 14–15
Anal canal sensation, 117
Anal cancer, 104
Anal carcinoma, 227
Anal continence plugs, for FI, 130
Anal dilation, 106
Anal fissures
  alternative pathologies, 104
  clinical history, 103
  in Crohn's disease patients, 225–227
  definition, 103
  diagnosis, 103–104
  medical therapy, 104–105
  physiology, 103
  surgical procedure
    advancement flap, 106
    anal dilation, 106
    lateral internal anal sphincterotomy (LIS), 105–106
  treatment, 104
Anal fistula, 187, 191, 195, 197
Anal fistula plugs, 211–212
Anal glands, 187
Anal herpes, 246
Anal incontinence, 93, 109–111, 114, 123
  characterization of, 111
Anal intraepithelial neoplasia (AIN), 247
  association with anal SCC, 260
  and Bowen's disease, 259
  clinical approach, 261–263
  pathologists' interpretation of, 261
Anal malignancy, 104
Anal manometry, 116–117, 143, 148, 208
Anal pap smear technique, 263
Anal pruritis, 241, 242
Anal SCC, 260
Anal sphincter electromyography (EMG)
  background and basic concepts, 27
  clinical application and indications, 30
  findings and interpretation, 29

Anal sphincter electromyography (EMG) (*cont.*)
instrumentation and technique
concentric needle, 28
monopolar wire electrode, 28–29
single-fiber EMG electrode, 28
surface plugs, 28
Anal sphincters, 46
Anal stenosis, 226
Anal stretch method, 93
Anal submucosa, 88
Anal ulcers, 245, 103, 104
in Crohn's disease patients, 226, 232
Anal vasodilatation, 104
Anal verge, 188
Anal warts, 248
Anesthesia, complication of, 4
Anesthetics, local, 80
Anismus, 55, 143, 147
Anorectal abscess
anatomy and pathophysiology, 188–190
complications
incontinence, 198
necrotizing infection, 198
recurrence, 197–198
epidemiology, 191
etiology, 190
histology and pathophysiology, 187–188
microbiology and antibiotics, 191
predisposing conditions and causes of, 190
special considerations, 198–199
symptoms and clinical evaluation, 191–193
treatment
catheter drainage, 196–197
for fistula, 197
incision and drainage, 193–196
postoperative care, 197
primary closure, 196
Anorectal angle (ARA), 33–34
Anorectal coordination maneuver, 69–70
Anorectal lesions, 25
Anorectal manometry (ARM), 55, 229
basic concepts, 21
clinical application, 27
measurements for
Cough Reflex Test, 25
high pressure zone (HPZ), 24
rectal capacity, 24–25
rectal compliance, 25
Rectoanal Inhibitory Reflex (RAIR), 24
resting pressure, 23
sensory threshold, 24
squeeze pressure, 24
pitfalls, 26–27
systems used to perform
fluid or air-filled balloon systems, 21–22
microtransducers, 22–23
sleeve catheters, 23
water-perfused catheters, 23
water-perfused systems, 22
technique for evaluation
continuous pull-through method, 26
cough reflex, 26
measuring pressure during attempted defecation, 26
monitoring of wave patterns, 25
stationary pull-through method, 26
Anorectal pain
differential diagnosis for, 193
evaluation, 181–182
levator ani syndrome, 182
management, 183–184
in patients with pelvic floor prolapse, 181
proctalgia fugax, 182
pudendal neuropathy, 182
Anorectal physiological testing, 198
Anorectal STDs, 245
Anorectal strictures, 226, 232
Anorectal surgery, 1
Anorectal ultrasound (AUS), 45
in abscesses, 51
equipment, 45
fistulae
ANO, 52
in extrarectal masses, 52
rectovaginal, 52
imaging
accuracy in predicting sphincter defects, 50–51
accuracy in predicting the tumor stage, 48–49
for rectal mass, 47
for rectal tumor, 46–47
for sphincter defects, 50
procedure, 45–46
Anorexia, 141
Anoscopy, 143, 192, 206, 245
Anterior colporrhaphy, 175
Anterior levatorplasty, 136
Anterior sphincteroplasty, 136–137
Anterior vaginal wall prolapse, repair, 174, 175
Antibiotics, 272
Antibody testing, 254
Anticholinergics, 167
Antidiuretic hormone (ADH), 173
Antihistamines, 242, 309
Antimetabolites, 230–231
Antiplatelet therapy, 2
Antipruritics, 80
Aquacel-AG, 269
Arcus tendineous fascia pelvis (ATFP), 175
Ardium®, 81
Arthrotec®, 127
Artificial bowel sphincter, 137
Arvenum 500®, 81
Aspergillosis, 231
Aspirin, 5, 254, 309–310
Astringents, 80
Atopic dermatitis, 242
Atrophicus, 240
Atropine, 124
Autologous tissues, 172
Azathioprine, 230
Azithromycin, 252, 253, 254, 255

Bacillus spp., 191
Bacterial infections, ostomy, 296–297
Bacterial lesions, 251

Bacteroides, 198
Bacteroides spp., 191
Baden–Walker half-way system, 163
Balloon expulsion, for constipation, 73
Balloon expulsion test, 144
Barium enema, 144, 229
Barium suspension, 33
Basic metabolic panel (BMP), 4
Benadryl, 313, 314
Beta-hemolytic infection, 241
Bichloroacetic acid, 248
Bicycling, 182
Bile acid binders, 136
Bile acid malabsorption, 122
Biofeedback therapy, 136, 147, 152, 169, 183
  adjunctive
    balloon expulsion for constipation, 73
    coordination training for FI, 73
    sensory discrimination training technique, 73
  for colon and rectal practice
    behavioral component, 65
    behavioral strategies, 65–67
    PMR component, 67–71
    technical component, 62–64
    therapeutic component, 65
  for constipation, 60–61
  data acquisition, 63
  defined, 61–62
  efficacy of, 56–60
  failure, 147
  fecal incontinence, 61
  feedback display, 63
  management of FI, 129
  manometric, 147
  monitoring abdominal muscle activity, 64
  monitoring pelvic muscle activity, 64
  sessions, 71–73
  studies, 57–59
Bioplastique™, 131
Bipolar scissors hemorrhoidectomy, 92
Bladder paresis, 18
Bladder retraining, 169
Bladder sensation, normal, 168
Botulinum toxin injections, 104, 105, 183
Botulinum toxin type A injection, 148
Bovine glutaraldehyde cross linked collages (GAX), 172
Bowen's disease, 241, 242, 259
Bulimia, 141
Buprenorphine, 308
Burgio's urge suppression strategies, 67
Butorphanol, 308

Calcium-channel blockers, 105
Calibration, 38
Campylobacter infections, 255
Cancer screening criteria, 261
Candidiasis, 241, 294
Capasaicin, 243
Capiven®, 81
Carbon-coated zirconium beads, 172
Cardiac evaluation, prior to surgery, 5
Catheter drainage, 196–197
CCF-FI Grading Scale, 110
CD4+ T-lymphocyte, 245, 249, 263
Cefotaxime, 253
Ceftazidine, 253
Ceftriaxone, 253, 254
Celecoxib, 310
Celiac sprue, 122
Cellulitis, 255
Cephalad, 15
Cerebrovascular accidents, 111
Cervical cancer, 259–260
Cervical intraepithelial neoplasia (CIN), 259
C fiber sensory affert neurons, 243
Chagas' disease (trypanosomiasis), 141
Chancres, 254
Chancroid infections, 253–254
Chemical irritant contact dermatitis, 293
Chemotherapy, 223
Chlamydia infections, 251–252
Chloramphenicol, 253
Chocolate agar plates, 253
Choice of the procedure, 1
Cholecystectomy, 122
Cholestyramine, 124
Chronic anal fissures, 103
Cilansetron, 125
Cinedefecography, 55, 144–145, 150–152, 153–155
Ciprofloxacin, 230, 255
Cipromyacin, 253
Circular anal dilator (CAD), 93
Clean granulating wound, 271
Cleveland Clinic Florida Fecal Incontinence (CCF-FI) scale, 110, 136
Clinical enigma, 182
Clonidine, 124
Closed Ferguson technique, 88–89
Closure of the skin, after draining abscess, 196
CMV-related perianal ulceration, 249
Coccydioidomycosis, 231
Coccygodynia, 181
Codeine, 308, 310
Cognitive behavioral therapy (CBT), 130
Cognitively training breathing patterns, 71
Cognitively training hand temperature, 71
CO_2 laser hemorrhoidectomy, 92
Colchicine, 147
Colestipol, 125
Collagen plug, 213–214
Collection bags, 38
Colonic inertia, 37, 55, 143, 158
Colonic transit, 36–37
Colonoscopy, 248
Colon surgery, 272
Colorectal surgery, 1
Colostomy, 235–236
Colostomy irrigation, 300–301
Colpexin ball or sphere, 174
Compounded analgesics, 308
Computerized tomography (CT), 181, 183, 192, 207, 227, 229
Concomitant fissurectomy, 105
Condyloma, 247
Condyloma accuminata, 247

Congestive heart failure, 2
Connective tissue disorders, 111
Constipation, 122
  anal manometry, 143
  balloon expulsion for, 73
  balloon expulsion test, 144
  biofeedback therapy for, 60–61
  breath hydrogen concentration test, 146
  chronic, 126
  cinedefecography, 144–145
  colonic transit study, 146
  defined, 126
  definitions and criteria, 142
  dosing guidelines, 126–127
  dynamic magnetic resonance imaging (MRI) defecography, 145
  electromyography, 145
  epidemiology and economical impact, 141–142
  failure of conservative treatment
    biofeedback therapy, 147
    laxatives, 146
    pharmacotherapy, 147
  following hemorrhoidectomy, 97
  functional, 143
  functional analysis of, 144
  IBS-related, 143
  initial approach for treatment of, 143
  initial colorectal evaluation
    diagnosis of functional constipation, 144
    differential diagnosis, 142–143
    physical examination, 143
  management of specific forms of
    cul-de-sac hernias, 152
    paradoxical puborectalis contraction, 148–149
    rectal intussusception, 153
    rectal prolapse, 155
    rectocele, 149–150
    slow transit, 158
    solitary rectal ulcer, 155–158
  perineal examination, 143
  pudendal nerve terminal motor latency (PNTML), 145–146
  results of surgical treatment, 158
  scintigraphic defecography, 146
  slow transit, 143
  structural etiology of, 143
Continence, 55–56
Continuous Positive Airway Pressure (CPAP) device, 4
Contraindications, to ambulatory surgery, 2
Cooper's ligament, 170
Coordination training, for fecal incontinence, 73
COX inhibitors, 309–310, 314
COX-2 inhibitors, 307, 310
COX-3 inhibitors, 310
Crohn's disease, 6, 104, 190, 197
  clinical presentation, 225
  diagnosis, 227–229
  examination under anesthesia (EUA), 227
  history and physical examination, 227
  medical management, 232–233
  nonfistulous conditions, 232–233
  physical findings
    anal fissures, 225–226
    anal stenosis and anorectal stricture, 226
    anal ulcers, 226
    carcinoma, 227
    perianal abscesses and fistulas, 226
    rectovaginal fistulas, 226–227
    skin tags, 225
    symptomatic fecal incontinence, 227
  surgical management, 230–232
  treatment of fistulas
    endorectal advancement flap (EAF), 233–234
    fibrin glue, 235
    fistula plug, 235
    gracilis muscle transposition, 235
    ileostomy and colostomy (temporary diversion), 235–236
    limited fistulotomy, 233
  wounds related to, 271
Crohn's fistulae, 209
Cryotherapy, 83–84, 93, 248
Cryptoglandular disease, 203, 212, 217
Cryptoglandular fistula management algorithm, 214
Cryptoglandular theory, 187
Cul-de-sac hernias, 152
Cutting seton, 208
Cyclooxygenase inhibitors for analgesia, 309
Cyclosporine A, 231
Cystocele, 163
Cystometry, 168–169
Cystoscopy, 170
Cytomegalovirus, 248–249

Daflon®, 81
Dakin's solution, 273
Decadron. *See* Dexamethasone
Deep postanal space abscesses, 6
Defecation disorders, functional, 55
Defecography (evacuation proctography), 115–116
  background and basic concepts, 32
  clinical applications, 36
  findings and interpretations
    anorectal angle (ARA), 33–34
    measurements, 33
    perineal descent (PD), 34
    puborectalis length (PRL), 34
  instrumentation
    commode, 32
    contrast media, 33
  structural and anatomic findings, 34–36
  technique, 33
Defibrillator, 2
Definitive therapy, 217
Dehisced wound, 274–276
Delorme's operation (mucosectomy), 155
Delorme's procedure, 158
Denonvilliers'fascia, 18, 19
Dermal inclusion cysts, 217
Desmopressin, 173
Detralex®, 81
Detrusor contractions, 166, 169, 170, 172
Detrusor overactivity, 166, 167
Detrusor pressure, 168

Dexamethasone, 312, 314
Diabetes, 111, 167, 241
Diabetic-associated diarrhea, 122
Diabetic wounds, 268
Diagnostic colonoscopy, 143
Diaphragmatic breathing, 71
Diarrhea, 231
  etiologies of, 122
Diazepam, 314
Diclofenac, 127, 310
Dietary modification, 67
Diflunisal, 310
Digital maneuvers, 157
Digital rectal examination, 182, 245
Diltiazem, 105
Diltiazem ointment, 104–105
Diphenhydramine, 313, 314
Diphenoxylate, 124, 136
Direct fluorescent antibody (DFA) testing, 252
Disseminated infection, 253
Distal peripheral sensory neuropathy, 230
Diuretics, 167
DNA-chain termination, 246
Donovanosis, 254–255
Douglas pouch, 152
Doxycycline, 252, 255
Draining seton, 209
Droperidol, 309, 312–313, 314
Dull ache, 56
Durasphere™, 131
Dyskinetic puborectalis, 147
Dyssnergia, 71
Dyssynergic defecation, 143, 147
Dysynergia, 136

Edema, 221, 294
Elatec®, 81
Elective hemorrhoidectomy, 2
Elective inguinal hernia repair, 1
Elective surgical treatment, 232
Electrical stimulation, 170
  for FI management, 130
Electrocardiogram (ECG), 4
Electrocautery, 10, 89
Electrogalvanic stimulation (EGS) therapy, 183
Electromyography-based biofeedback, 183
Electromyography (EMG), 51, 55, 109, 117
EMLA cream, 248
Enck's critical review, on biofeedback, 55, 61
Endoanal MRI, 116
Endoanal ultrasound (EAUS), 109, 115, 182, 193
Endorectal advancement flap (EAF), 209–210, 233–234
Endoscopy, 229
Enema, 45, 127
Enema®, 219
Enteric pathogens infections, 255
Enterobius Vermicularis, 240
Enteroceles, 36, 144, 152, 177–178
Enterocystocele, 177
Epinephrine, 90
E7 protein, 248
Erythematous swelling, 191
Erythromycin, 252, 255
Escherichia coli, 191
Estrogen deficiency, 166
Estrogen therapy, 172–173
Evaluation under anesthesia (EUA), 192
External anal sphincter (EAS), 50
Extrarectal masses, 52
Extrasphincteric abscess, 204–205

Famcilovir, 246
Fascial dehiscence, 274
Fasciocutaneous flap, 221
Fast twitch muscle fibers, 70
Fecal contamination, 239
Fecal diversion, 232, 235
Fecal Incontincence Severity Score, 122
Fecal incontinence (FI), 55–56, 135
  ambulatory procedures for, 131–132
  biofeedback therapy, 129–130
  biofeedback therapy for, 61
  causes, 110
  cognitive behavioral therapy (CBT), 130
  and constipation, 126–128
  diagnostic testing, 114–115
  and diarrhea, 123–126
  differential diagnosis of, 122
  and disordered defecation with incomplete evaluation, 129
  functional, 121–123
  history, 109–111
  imaging
    defecography, 115–116
    endoanal ultrasound, 115
    MRI, 116
  medical treatment, 135–136
    anal continence plugs, 130
    electrical stimulation, 130
    improvement of hygiene in fecal seepage, 130
  neuromuscular functions
    anal manometry, 116–117
    electromyography, 117
    pudendal nerve terminal motor latency (PNTML), 117–118
    rectal and anal sensory testing, 117
  physical examination, 114
  surgical management
    anterior sphincteroplasty, 136–137
    artificial bowel sphincter, 137–138
    assessment, 135
    sacral nerve stimulation (SNS), 138–139
    stimulated graciloplasty, 139
  symptomatic, 227
Fecal Incontinence Quality of Life Scale (FIQL), 111, 113–114
Fecal Incontinence Severity Index, 112
Fecal seepage, 129
Fenoprofen, 310
Fentanyl, 308, 316
Ferguson technique, 96
Fiber supplementation, 124, 128
Fibrin glue, 211, 235
Fibrosis, 182
Fissures, 104, 240

Fistula-in-ano, 187
  classification, 203–205
  differential diagnosis, 204
  etiology, 203
  evaluation
    anal manometry, 208
    physical examination, 206
    radiological examinations, 207
    symptoms, 206
  incidence, 203–204
  treatment
    advancement flaps, 209–211
    fibrin glue, 211
    fistula plug, 211–212
    fistulotomy, 208
    setons, 208–209
Fistula plugs, 211–212
Fistulas, 226–227, 240
Fistulography, 207
  conventional, 229
Fistulotomy, 203, 208
Fistulous tracts, with AUS, 52
Flebotropin®, 81
Fleet®, 219
Fleet™, 143
Fleet® Phospho Soda, 323
Flexion of the hips and pelvis, 66
Fluid or air-filled balloon systems, 21–22
5-Fluorouracil, 262
Foley catheter, 136, 171
Folliculitis, 241, 295
Foreign body, in surgical wound, 276
Fournier's disease, 198
Fournier's gangrene, 105, 198
French soft latex mushroom catheter, 196–197
Functional anorectal pain, 56
Functional constipation, 55
Functional gastrointestinal disorders
  fecal incontinence (FI), 55–56
  functional anorectal pain, 56
  pelvic floor dyssynergia, 55
Functional incontinence, 166

Gabapentin, 310–311
Gastric emptying, 146
Gastrocolic reflex, 66
Gastrograffin, 229
Gastrointestinal Health Diary, 123
Gastrointestinal motility disorder, 37
Gastrointestinal Quality of Life Index, 111
Gelfoam, 97
Genital ulceration, with *H. ducreyi*, 253
Genital warts, role of HPV in, 247
Germinal center hyperactivity, 47
Giemsa staining, 246
Glossitis, 230
Gluteal cleft, 218
Gluteal pain, 196
Gluteus maximus myocutaneous flap, 223
Glycerin suppositories, 128
Glyceryl trinitrate cream, 104
Goldman cardiac risk index, 2
Golytely®, 323
Goodsall's rule, 206
Gracilis muscle transposition, 235
Graciloplasty, 137
Granisetron, 312, 314
Granulation tissue, 267
Granuloma inguinale (donovanosis), 254–255

H. ducreyi infection, 253
Habit training, 66
HalfLytely®, 323
Hand warming, 71
Hanley procedure, 195
Harmonic Scalpel, 92
Hematological disorders, 198–199
Hematuria, 167, 172
Hemorrhoidal bundle, 89
Hemorrhoidal disease
  classification, 80
  clinical symptoms, 79
  comparison studies, 84–85
  cryotherapy, 83–84
  etiology, 79
  evaluation, 79–80
  grading, 80
  infrared coagulation, 84
  injection sclerotherapy, 83
  medical treatment
    diet counselling, 80
    micronized purified flavonoid fractions (MPFFs), 81
    topicals, 80–81
    Warmsoaks and sitz baths, 80
  physical examination of, 79–80
  predisposing factors, 79
  rubber band ligation, 81–84
  surgical treatment
    anal stretch, 93
    closed Ferguson technique, 88–89
    complications, 97–98
    conventional hemorrhoidectomy, 87
    cryotherapy, 93
    laser hemorrhoidectomy, 92
    Ligasure™ hemorrhoidectomy, 92
    modified Whitehead hemorrhoidectomy, 91–92
    open milligan morgan technique, 89
    stapled hemorrhoidopexy, 93–96
    submucosal Park's hemorrhoidectomy, 90–91
  thrombosed external, 84
    management of, 97
Hemorrhoidal pedicle, 89
Hemorrhoidal plexus, 15, 90
Hemorrhoidectomy, 84, 232
  conventional, 87
  procedure, 87
Hemorrhoids, 240, 241
Hemostasis, 89
Hemostat, 217
Henkle James SR anoscope, 143
Henna tattooing, 285
Herpes simplex virus (HSV), 246
Hidradenitis suppurativa, 198, 217
Highly active antiretroviral therapy (HAART), 245

High pressure zone (HPZ), 24
Hirschsprung's disease, 142, 143
Histamine, 239
Histoplasmosis, 231
History of patient, significance in surgery, 1–2
Hormonal deficiency, in menopausal women, 240
Hormone therapy, 172–173
HPV-16, 248
5-HT receptor antagonists, 309
Human immunodeficiency virus (HIV), 104, 245
Human papillomavirus (HPV), 246–248
Hydrocodone, 308, 310
Hydrocortisone cream, 242
Hydrofiber plus silver, 269
Hydrogen peroxide, 52
  injection, 193
Hydromorphone (Dilaudid), 308
Hydroxyzine, 313, 314
Hypertonia, 72
Hypertrophic cardiomyopathy, 191
Hypoalbuminemia, 268
Hypochondriacs, 182
Hypogastric nerves, 17–18
Hypogastric plexus, 17–18
Hypoproteinemia, 268
Hypothyroidism, 142

Ibuprofen, 254, 309, 310
Iceberg syndrome, 158
Ileocolitis, 248
Ileorectal anastomosis, 158
Ileostomy, 235–236
Ileostomy lavage, 300
Imiquimod, 248, 262
Immune suppression, 255
Immunosuppressive disorders, 6
Infected wound, 272
Inferior hemorrhoidal artery. *See* Inferior rectal artery (IRA)
Inferior rectal artery (IRA), 16
Inflammatory bowel disease (IBD), 122
Inflammatory nodes, 47
Inflammatory phase, in wound healing process, 267
Inflammatory plaques, 241
Infliximab, 231
Infrared coagulation, 84
In-hospital drainage, 193
Initial Italian Sacral Neurostimulation Group Experience, 138
Injection sclerotherapy, 83–84
Innervation, autonomic
  anal canal, 19
  rectum, 17–19
  sensory, 19
In situ carcinoma, 259
Integral Theory, 171
Internal anal sphincter (IAS), 50, 103, 187
Internal pudendal artery, 16
Internal sphincterotomy, 89
Intersphincteric abscess, 195, 204–205
Intersphincteric space, 15, 136, 188
Intra-abdominal colorectal surgery, 1
Intraepithelial squamous neoplasia, 259
Intravenous fluid requirements, 1
Intussusception, 35
Iontophoretic transdermal system (ITS), 316
Ipsilateral ileopectineal line, 170
Iron persulphate, 83
Irritable bowel syndrome (IBS), 122, 143
Ischioanal space, 188
Ischiococcygeal line (ICL), 152
Ischiorectal abscess, 51, 192, 194, 197
Ischiorectal fossa, 15
Ischiorectal space, 15
Island Flap Anoplasty, 211, 212
Itch–scratch–itch behavior, 239

Jacobson's progressive muscle relaxation strategy, 71–72
Jarish–Herxheimer reaction, 254
Jeep's disease, 217
Joint Commission on Accreditation of Healthcare Organization (JCAHO), 305

Kanamycin, 253
Karydakis flap technique, 222–223
Kegel exercises, 68, 69, 72, 174
Keratolytics, 80
Ketorolac, 309–310
Ketorolac tromethamine (Toradol), 97
Klebsiella spp., 191

Laceration, 287
Lactose or fructose intolerance, 122
Laparoscopic wound, 279
Laser epilation, 218
Laser hemorrhoidectomy, 92
Lateral internal anal sphincterotomy (LIS), 105–106
Latissimus dorsi-serratus flap, 277
Laxatives, 146
Leak point pressures, 169
Leukocytosis, 192
Levator ani symptoms, 56
Levator ani syndrome, 182
Levator spasms, 182
Lichen sclerosis, 240
Lichen sclerosus, 240, 242
Lidocaine, 90, 243
  injection, 248
Ligasure™ hemorrhoidectomy, 92
Limberg flap repair, 221
Limited fistulotomy, 233
Liquid nitrogen, 83–84
Lithotomy position, 210
Loperamide, 124, 136
Lorazepam, 314
Lubiprostone, 147
Lymphatic drainage, 17
Lymph nodes, 49
Lymphoscintigraphy, 17

Macroplastique, 172
Magnetic resonance imaging (MRI), 116, 207, 227
Malignant hyperthermia, 4
Manchester Health Questionnaire, 111

Manometric biofeedback, 147
Manometric testing, 182
Marcaine, 219
Marshall—Marchetti–Krantz procedure, 170
Marsupialization, 219
Maturational phase, in wound healing process, 267
McCall culdeplasty, 178
Medical colostomy, 210
Medullary canal remnants, 217
MEN IIb syndrome, 142
Meperidine (Demerol), 308
Metabolites, 307–308
Metallic taste, 230
Methacrylate-coated capsules, 146
Methylene blue injection, 243
Meticulous hemostasis, 269
Metoclopramide, 313, 314
Metronidazole, 230
MHA-TP, 254
Microscopic colitis, 121, 122
Microtransducers, 22–23
Milligan–Morgan system, related the fistula tracks, 203
Mind–body therapies, 317
Misoprostol, 127, 147
Mitral valve prolapse, 191
Mixed Incontinence, 166
Morphine, 308, 314
Motrin, 309
6-MP, 230
MRI, 45, 51, 116, 126, 129, 145, 188, 195, 207, 207, 212
Mucocutaneous separation, 290
Mucosal transplantation, 297
Mucosal ulcerative colitis, 104
Mucosal ulcers, 254
Multifactorial concomitant PFM dysfunction, 72
Multiple sclerosis, 110, 111, 142
Musculocutaneous latissimus dorsi flap, 277
Mushroom-tip catheter, 234
Myocardial infarction, 2

Naloxone (Narcan), 309
Naproxen, 309
Natal clefts, 217
Nausea, 230, 305, 311–314
Necrotic tissue, 273
Necrotic wound, 273–274
Necrotizing infection, 198
Neisseria gonorrhea infections, 252–253
Neodymium:yttrium–aluminum garnet (Nd:YAG), 92
Neurostimulation, 138
Neurosyphilis, 254
Neutrophil counts, 198
Nifedipine, 105
Nitroglycerin preparations, 104
Nodules of Gerota, 17
Nonabsorbable sugars, 126, 128
Noncodeine analgesics, 197
Non-fermenters, 38
Nonrelaxing puborectalis syndrome, 34–35
NSAID, 309
Nuprin, 309
Nurse, preoperative, 323

Obesity, 3, 166
Obstructive defecation, 143, 147
Obstructive sleep apnea (OSA), 3–4
Obturator internus muscle contracts, 69
Ondansetron, 314
Open Milligan morgan technique, 89
δ opioid receptor (DOR), 307
κ opioid receptor (KOR), 307
μ opioid receptor (MOR), 307
Opioids, 307–309
Organ-specific risk-assessment indexes, 2
Ostomy management, in ambulatory setting
  basic care, 286–287
  colostomy irrigation, 300–301
  constructing the stoma, 285–286
  dietary considerations, 299–300
  food blockage, 300
  ileostomy lavage, 300
  issues with
    mucocutaneous separation, 290
    parastomal hernia, 290
    stoma fistula, 292
    stoma necrosis, 289
    stoma prolapse, 291
    stoma retraction, 291
    stoma stenosis, 292
    stoma trauma, 292, 293
  outpatient care, 288
  peristomal complications
    allergic contact dermatitis, 293–294
    bacterial infections, 296
    chemical irritant contact dermatitis, 293
    folliculitis, 295
    mucosal transplantation, 297
    peristomal candidiasis, 294–295
    peristomal psoriasis, 296
    peristomal pyoderma gangrenosum, 298
    peristomal trauma, 295
    peristomal varices, 297
    pseudoverrucous lesions, 297–298
  postoperative management, 286
  pouching systems, 288
  pouch removal and application technique, 288–289
    tips, 299
  preoperative management, 283
    counseling, 284
    stoma site marking, 284–285
  quality of life issues, 301–302
Ostomy pouching systems, 287–288
Outlet obstruction, 143
Overflow incontinence, 166
Overstaging, 48
Oxidation reaction, 52
Oxycodone, 308, 314

Paget's disease, 240, 242
Palpation, 206, 245
Pan-enteric inertia, 146
Papanicolaou smear, 255
Papulosquamous disorders, 242

Paradoxical puborectalis contraction (PPC), 148–149
Paradoxical puborectalis syndrome, 36
Paranal spaces, 15–16
Pararectal spaces, 15–16
Parastomal hernia, 285
Parasympathetic fibers, 163
Paravaginal defect repair, 175
Paresthesias, 230
Parkinson's disease, 111, 142
Park's classification system, 203
Park's cryptoglandular theory, 226
Park's hemorrhoidectomy, 90–91
Partial thromboplastin time (PTT), 4
Pathological lymph nodes, 47
Patient controlled analgesic (PCA) device, 315
Patient evaluation, for ambulatory surgery, 1–3
- choice of the procedure, 1
- physical examination, of patient, 2
- preoperative work-up, 4–6
- special considerations, 3–4

Patient preparation, for ambulatory colorectal surgery
- establishing rapport with patient and family, 321
- patient expectations of ACU, 323–324
- preoperative counseling, 322–323
- preoperative investigation, 322

PDS-2 sutures, 269
Pelvic CT, 229
Pelvic floor dysfunction
- neuromuscular mechanisms of continence, 163
- pelvic organ prolapse (POP)
  - evaluation tools, 163–164
  - treatment, 173–177
- urinary incontinence
  - demographics, 164–166
  - diagnosis and evaluation, 166–169
  - risk factors, 166
  - treatment, 169–173
  - types, 166

Pelvic floor dyssynergia (PFD), 55, 60, 143, 147
Pelvic floor exercises, 174
Pelvic floor functions, 163
Pelvic floor muscles (PFMs), 56
- activities, 168
- Burgio's urge suppression strategies, 67
- patient education and behavior modification of anatomy, 65–66
- sEMG evaluation, 64, 65

Pelvic floor muscle training (PFMT), 169
Pelvic floor-oscopy, 145
Pelvic floor physiotherapy, 169
Pelvic laxity, 36
Pelvic MRI, 229
Pelvic muscle exercise training principles, 68
Pelvic nerves, 18
Pelvic pain, 71
Pelvic plexus, 17–18
Pelvic relaxation, 36
Pelvic rotator cuff (PRC), 69
Penicillinase-producing gonorrhea species, 253
Peptostreptococcus spp., 191
Perianal abscesses, 189, 191, 226
Perianal cellulites, 241
Perianal Crohn's disease. *See* Crohn's disease
Perianal space, 15
Perineal descent (PD), 34
Perineal pressure, 150
Perineal sepsis, surgery for, 231–232
Perineal wound, 277–279
Peristomal candidiasis, 294–295
Peristomal psoriasis, 296
Peristomal pyoderma gangrenosum, 298
Peristomal trauma, 295
Peristomal varices, 297
Pessaries, for POP, 174
Petroleum-based gauze, 275
Pezzer catheter, 210
Pfannensteil, 170
PFM denervation, 65
Phenergan, 313
Phenol (5%) in vegetable oil, 83
Phenothiazine, 313
Photodynamic therapy, 262, 263
Physiological and Operative Severity Score for enUmeration of Mortality (POSSUM), 3
Physiological quieting, 71
Pilonidal abscess, 217–218
Pilonidal cyst, 217
Pilonidal disease
- acute presentation, 217–218
- chronic presentation
  - gluteus maximus myocutaneous flap, 223
  - Karydakis flap technique for, 222–223
  - limberg flap repair, 221
  - pilonidal sinus, 218–219
  - primary excision and closure by granulation, 219–221
  - sinus excision, 219
- epidemiology, 217
- follow-up visits and surveillance, 224
- malignant degeneration of pilonidal sinus, 223–224

Pilonidal sinus, malignant degeneration of, 223–224
Pinworm infection, 240
Pneumonia, 231, 255
Podophyllin, 247
Podophyllotoxin, 247
Polyethylene–glycol electrolyte solution, 323
Polypropylene tape, 171
Post anesthesia care unit (PACU), 305, 323
Posterior colporrhaphy, 177
Posterior vaginal wall prolapse, 177
Postligation bleeding, 82
Postoperative nausea and vomiting (PONV), 311–314
- prevention strategies, 313–314

Postoperative pain management, 1
Preemptive analgesia, 311
Preganglionic fibers, 17
Pregnancy testing, 5
Preoperative complete blood count (CBC), 4
Preoperative patient assessment and optimization, 1
Preoperative work-up, for surgery, 4–6

Presacral fascia, 11
Presacral veins, 11
Pressure-regulating balloon, 137
Probiotics, 125
Prochlorperazine, 313, 314
Proctalga fugax
  symptoms, 56
Proctalgia fugax, 182
Proctectomy, 232
Proctitis, 251, 254
Proctocolectomy, 232
Proctological disorders, 240
Proctoscope, 45–46
Proctoscopy, 245
Proctosigmoidoscopy, 197
Prognostic Nutritional Index, 3
Prolapse, stages of, 163–164
Prolapsed rectal mucosa, 240
Prolapse grading system, 163
Proliferative phase, in wound healing process, 267–268
Prolonged ileus, 1
Promethazine, 313
Propofol, 309, 314
Propoxyohene, 308
Prostaglandin E, 127
Protectants, 80
Prothrombin time (PT), 4
Providone–iodine solution, 88
Proximate Hemorrhoidal Circular Stapler, 93
Pruritus ani
  etiologic factors, 241
  evaluation of, 241–242
  physical examination, 241
  primary (idiopathic), 239
  secondary, 239–241
  treatment, 242–243
Pseudomembranous colitis, 248
Pseudoverrucous lesions, 297–298
Psoriasis, 240, 241
Psychotropic medications, 167
Pubococcygeal line (PCL), 145
Puborectalis, 50, 114
Puborectalis length (PRL), 34
Puborectalis muscle, 198
Puborectalis syndrome, 147
  nonrelaxing, 35
Pudendal canal, 15
Pudendal nerve afferents, 170
Pudendal nerve entrapment, 182
Pudendal nerve terminal latency (PDTL), 137
Pudendal nerve terminal motor latency (PNTML), 30–32, 109, 115, 117–118
  background and basic concepts, 30
  clinical application, 32
  instrumentation
    electromyographic equipment, 30–31
    St Mark's electrode, 30–31
  technique, 31
  testing, 109
Pudendal neuropathy, 182
Pulmonary disease, 167

Quinine, 83
Quinolones, 253

Radiation therapy, 223
Radiologic studies, for ambulatory surgery, 5
Radiologic tests, 1
Radionucleotide white cell scanning, 192
Radio-opaque markers, 146
Rectal and anal sensory testing, 117
Rectal emptying, 115–116
Rectal intussusception, 153, 154–155
Rectal (or hemorrhoidal) arteries, 16–17
Rectal prolapse, 155, 157
Rectal ulcer syndrome, 158
Recto-anal inhibitory reflex (RAIR), 24, 117
Rectoanal intussusception, 35, 36
Rectoceles, 35, 55
Rectopexy, 152
Rectovaginal fistulae, 52, 153, 226–227, 233
Rectum, anatomical characteristics of
  anterior, 8
  characteristics, 7
  facial attachments, 9–11
  fascia propria of, 9
  folds, 7
  lateral curves, 7
  lower third of the rectum, 7
  mesorectum, 8, 9
  middle, 7
  posterior, 8
  upper third of the, 7
  valves, 7
Reglan. *See* Metoclopramide
Relaxation and quieting, of muscle activity, 70
Relax exercises, 70
Retropubic colposuspension, 170
Retropubic sling procedures, 170–172
Retrorectal space, 16
Risk-assessment system, 1
Rome II criteria of functional gastrointestinal disorders, 142
Rome II criteria for PFD, 129
Rome II diagnostic system, 55
  criteria for diagnosis of constipation, 56
  criteria for pelvic floor dyssynergia, 56
Rotational flaps, 218
RPR test, 254
Rubber band ligation, 81–82

Sacral nerve stimulation (SNS), 138–139
Sacral neuromodulation, 138
Sacrococcygeal pain, 181
Sacrospinous ligament fixation, 176–177
Sacrotuberous ligament, 188
Salicylazosulfapyridine, 146
Saline laxatives, 127, 128
Saline-moistened gauze, 272
Scabies infestation, 241
Scissors hemorrhoidectomy, 92
Scopolamine, 313
Seborrhea, 240
Seborrheic dermatitis, 242
Secca procedure, 131–132

SEMG activity, from the pelvic musculature, 62
SEMG Instrumentation, 62
SEMG PRM treatment goals, 67
Sensory discrimination training technique, for FI, 73
Seroma formation, 221
Serotonin reuptake inhibitors, 147
Setons, 208–209, 232
Sexual complications, after rectal surgery, 19
Sexual dysfunction, after proctectomy, 18
Sexually transmitted diseases (STDs)
  bacterial
    Chancroid, 253
    Chlamydia, 251–252
    enteric pathogens (shigella, campylobacter), 255
    granuloma inguinale (donovanosis), 254–255
    Neisseria gonorrhea, 252–253
    syphilis, 253–254
  viral
    cytomegalovirus, 248–249
    herpes simplex virus (HSV), 246
    human papillomavirus (HPV), 246–248
Shigella infections, 255
Short bowel syndrome, 122
Sigmoid loop, 36
Sigmoidoceles, 36, 55, 144, 152, 154
Sigmoidoscopy, 255
Signal detection, in biofeedback therapy, 62
Signal processing, in biofeedback therapy, 62–63
Silk, 208
Sitz baths, 84, 197, 199, 209, 218, 104
Sitzmark™, 37, 146
Skin grafting, 218
Sleeve catheters, 23
Slow transit constipation, 143
Small-bowel bacterial overgrowth, 122
Small bowel transit, 37–39
Sodium morrhuate, 83
Sodium tetradecyl sulfate, 83
Solitary rectal ulcers, 144, 155–158
Sphincter deficiency, 168, 169
Squamous cell carcinoma (SCC), 240, 259
SRS Orion PC/12, 71
Staphylococci spp., 191
Stapled hemorrhoidopexy, 93, 96–97
Stapled transanal rectal resection (STARR) procedure, 153
Stapling devices, 1
Static defecography, 145
Static transperineal ultrasound, 228–229
Steroids, 80
Stimulated graciloplasty, 139
St Mark's electrode, 30, 31
Stoma creation, 272
Stoma fistula, 292
Stoma prolapse, 291
Stoma retraction, 291
Stoma stenosis, 292
Stoma trauma, 292
Stool bulk forming agents, 197
Stress urinary incontinence, 166, 168, 170
Submucous space, 15
Suboptimal delineation, of the rectal wall, 49
Subtotal colectomy, 152, 158
Sulfamethoxazole, 255
Sulfapyridine, 146
Sulphonomides, 253
Superficial postanal space, 16
Suppositories, 127
Supralevator abscess, 51, 196
Supralevator spaces, 16, 188
Suprasphincteric abscess, 204–205
Surgery, for stress urinary incontinence, 8
Surgical planning, 1
Syphilis infections, 253–254
Systemic hormone therapy, 173
Systemic infections, 111

Tacrolimus, 230
Teflon-coated silver wire monopolar electrode, 28
Tension-free vaginal tape (TVT), 171
Tetracycline, 253
Thayer–Martin agar plates, 253
Three-column ligation, 82
Three-dimensional ultrasound (3-DUS), 45
Thrombosis, 84
TIME principle, 269
Tincture of Opium, 125
Tramadol, 308
Transanal digital massage, 183
Transanal endoscopic ultrasound (EUS), 228
Transitional zone, of anal, 187
Transit studies
  colonic, 36–37
  small bowel, 37–39
Transobturator slings, 171–172
Transsphincteric abscess, 204–205
Transsphincteric fistula, 197, 208
Transvaginal repair, 152
Treponema, 254
Trichloroacetic acid, 248
Trimethoprim, 255
Tuberculosis, 231

Ulcerative colitis, 248
Ulcers, 246
Ultram. *See* Tramadol
Uni-dimensional scaling technique, 306
Unmyelinated C-fibers, 239
Urea hydrochloride, 83
Urethral pressure profile, 169
Urge suppression strategies, 67
Urinary incontinence
  among Caucasian women, 166
  bimanual examination, 167
  defined, 164
  demographics, 164–166
  diagnosis and evaluation, 166–169
  laboratory examination, 168
  neurological examination, 167
  pelvic examination, 167
  physical examination, 167–168
  rectal examination, 167
  risk factors, 166
  speculum examination, 167

Urinary incontinence (*cont.*)
  surgical procedure, 170–172
  treatment, 169–173
  types, 166, 170
Urinary tract infections, 167
Urodynamics, 168
Uroflowmetry, 168
Urogenital atrophy, 166, 174
Uterosacral ligament suspension, 176, 177
UT1 tumors, 47–48
UT2 tumors, 47–48
UT3 tumors, 47
UT4 tumors, 47

VAC system, 221
Vacuum Assisted Wound Closure system (VAC), 270, 275, 277
Vagina, identifying points in the, 163
Vaginal bulging, 150
Vaginal vault prolapse repair, 175
Vaizey scale, 110–111
Valacyclovir, 246
Valsalva leak point pressure (VLPP) measurements, 169
Valsalva maneuver, 64, 72, 79, 114
Valsava maneuver, 69
Variton®, 81
Vasoconstrictors, 80
VDRL test, 254
Venitol®, 81
Verbal reading scale (VRS), 306
Versafoam, 277
Vestigial sex glands, 217
Vicryl mesh, 275
Videoendoscopic elastic band ligation (VE-EBL), 82
Viral DNA, 246
Vircryl suture, 269
Visceral hypersensitivity, 127
Viscero–fascial layer, 9
Vistaril, 313
Visual analog scale (VAS), 306
Vitamin E, 322
Voiding dysfunction, 71
Volitional contraction, 169
V-shaped cruciate incision, 90

Water-perfused catheters, 23
Western diet, 126
Wet anus, 91
Whitehead deformity, 91
Whitehead hemorrhoidectomy, modified, 91–92
Whitney's "cryptitis" theory, 187
Wound assessment, 270–271
Wound dressings, 269–270
  types and properties of, 270
Wound healing process, 267–268
  factors impeding, 268–269
  principles, 269
Wound Ostomy Continence Nurse (WOCN/Enterostomal Therapist), 283
Wound with enterocutaneous fistula, 276–277

Zero-vicryl sutures, 177
Zoloft®, 127
Z-plasty, 218

Printed in the United States
by Baker & Taylor Publisher Services